W9-CCY-694

Thrombolytic Therapy

edited by Gerald C. Timmis, M.D.

FUTURA

**Futura Publishing
Company, Inc.**
Armonk, NY
1999

Published by
Futura Publishing Company
135 Bedford Road
Armonk, NY 10504

ISBN#: 087993-426-3

Every effort has been made to ensure that the information in this book is as up to date and accurate as possible at the time of publication. However, due to the constant developments in medicine neither the author, nor the editors, nor the publisher can accept any legal or any other responsibility for any errors or omissions that may occur.

All rights reserved.

No part of this book may be translated or reproduced in any form without written permission from the publisher.

Printed in the United States of America on acid-free paper.

Table of Contents

Preface

Acute myocardial infarction may be considered to be the quintessential "20th Century Disease." At the beginning of this century, while the connection between coronary occlusion and myocardial infarction was being established by physiologists in the animal laboratory, clinicians considered coronary occlusion to be uniformly and immediately fatal. In the second decade, the connections between coronary thrombosis and the clinical and pathologic findings of myocardial infarction were made and it became clear that survival was possible. Early treatment was limited to strict bed rest to allow the injured myocardium to heal. However, acute mortality remained high, exceeding one-third in patients who lived long enough to be admitted to the hospital. Indeed, by mid-century acute myocardial infarction was recognized as the most common cause of death in developed nations.

There have been two major breakthroughs in the treatment of acute myocardial infarction in this century. The first, in the early 1960s, was the development of the coronary care unit, in which the high mortality in hospitalized patients from primary arrhythmias was virtually eliminated. The second—thrombolytic reperfusion of occluded coronary arteries—came along approximately two decades later, and in appropriately selected patients has caused a further substantial reduction in mortality.

This excellent monograph captures well the dramatic developments of coronary thrombolysis. This mode of therapy represents a triumph of cardiology, hematology, and evidence-based medicine. This fascinating story is 'must reading" for cardiologists and clinical trialists alike.

As the century comes to a close, the incidence of acute myocardial infarction, though still high, appears finally to be declining. The mortality in patients with this condition who reach the hospital has been radically reduced. A major lesson learned from thrombolytic therapy is the importance of achieving full myocardial reperfusion as rapidly as possible, irrespective of the method of opening the occluded artery. The application of this important principle is certain to continue to improve the outcome in patients with myocardial infarction during the 21st century.

Eugene Braunwald, M.D.
Distinguished Hersey Professor of Medicine
Faculty Dean and Vice-President for
Academic Programs at Brigham & Women's
Hospital and Massachusetts General
Hospital
Boston, MA

Foreword

by Gerald C. Timmis, M.D.

It has been a daunting but not unwelcome task to chronicle the saga of thrombolytic therapy, and to organize the chronology of those key contributions made by the innovative and courageous investigators as this important therapy has evolved. Without fear of being indicted for hyperbole, I believe most would conclude that myocardial reperfusion in acute myocardial infarction by thrombolytic agents ranks among the more majestic medical achievements of this century. In recounting this therapeutic journey I have attempted to avoid the controversies with which this odyssey has abounded as we have pursued the ideal therapeutic agents and strategies. On the other hand, before our readers have concluded their study of this material we will have addressed the issue of mechanical reperfusion for acute coronary syndromes, especially in the context of its having been compared with thrombolytic therapy.

Without attesting to the accuracy of the exact fiducial point defining the ensuing sequence of events pertaining to the development of thrombolytic therapy (Chapter 1), I must acknowledge the seminal contributions of A.P. Fletcher, our beloved Sol Sherry and his colleague Alkjaersig, who in the late 1950s began their exploration of the thrombolytic state in man.[1,2] Shortly thereafter, Polivoda, our friend Ralph Schröder, and his colleague Heckner, explored this therapy in Germany.[3] As is so frequently the case in medicine, their collective efforts garnered little clinical attention for more than a decade when the intracoronary instillation of fibrinolytic agents was then explored.[4] Peter Rentrop was particularly instrumental in capturing our fancy and focusing our interest on this new therapeutic departure.[5]

In the later 1960s and early 1970s several multicenter trials were performed by the European Working Party exploring various "initial doses" of intravenous streptokinase followed by maintenance infusions ranging from 24 to 72 hours. Compared to a control group in whom only the infusion of heparin was employed following an initial loading dose, a survival advantage was variously shown, especially after the first 24 hours of infarction (perhaps the earliest identification of the early hazards phenomenon as has been further discussed by the ISIS trialists).[6,7] The subsequent historical highlights of the European Cooperative Study Group, an outgrowth of the European Working Party, are tabulated in Chapter 2. The 1980s ushered in the use of intravenous streptokinase administered by short-term infusion for acute myocardial infarction.[8,9] However, the first relatively large prospective investigation of an intravenous lytic agent, the ISAM study,[10] failed to anneal thrombolytic therapy as the successful solution for myocardial reperfusion that it has ultimately become (Chapter 3).

Although much of the seminal work with lytic therapy was done in Europe, interest was being focused on this same therapeutic adventure in America by a number of agencies, including the Western Washington Trialists, who also explored the efficacy of both intracoronary and intravenous streptokinase.[11,12] The MITI investigators, an outgrowth of the Western Washington group (Chapter 4), were among the early explorers of prehospital initiation of thrombolytic therapy.[13]

In the meantime, the ISIS investigators (Chapter 5) in their second international trial further explored intravenous streptokinase in a randomized double-blind protocol. In multifactorial fashion, they also investigated the acute and sustained administration of oral aspirin in the early hours of myocardial infarction employing four randomization arms of more than 4,000 patients each (placebo infusion and tablets, aspirin alone, streptokinase alone, and combination therapy). This landmark study demonstrated the now famous huge survival advantage of both streptokinase and aspirin compared with patients receiving neither agent and further surprisingly showed that the therapeutic achievements in terms of survival with aspirin rivaled that of streptokinase.[14] This same investigational consortium subsequently compared streptokinase to tissue plasminogen activator (tPA) and anistreplase with and without heparin against background therapy with aspirin, showing comparable effects on survival of all three agents (ISIS-3).[15]

The Italian contingent, which was originally a part of the ISIS consortium, similarly examined the efficacy of intravenous streptokinase compared with no thrombolytic treatment in almost 12,000 patients (GISSI; Chapter 6). They also observed a significant survival advantage in the recipients of thrombolytic therapy, and as was the case in the ISIS-2 trial this was particularly true of those treated in the earliest hours after the onset of myocardial infarction.[16] As was the case with the ISIS-3 trial when they subsequently compared streptokinase to recombinant tissue plasminogen activator, they demonstrated no significant differences in total events including death, clinical heart failure, global and regional ventricular impairment, or electrocardiographic changes.[17]

Although the inaugural revelations of the first large mortality trial of thrombolytic therapy were inauspicious, Rolf Schröder, its senior investigator, discusses the chronology of a series of subsequent studies of thrombolytic agents designed to establish myocardial reperfusion. The trials that he addresses in Chapter 7 firmly establish lytic reperfusion as the mainstay of modern therapy for myocardial infarction.

Back in North America further spectacular exploration of thrombolytic therapy was achieved by the TIMI study group,[18] beginning in the decade of the 1980s with a comparison of streptokinase and tPA (favoring the latter) and subsequently with a strategy of early versus delayed angioplasty in a multifactorial model with either early or delayed beta blocker therapy, all layered upon thrombolytic therapy (TIMI 2).[19,20] In brief, there was no advantage shown when aggressive mechanical intervention was employed in conjunction with tPA. The same was true at one year of beta blocker therapy. An encyclopedic series of TIMI trials followed as tabulated in Chapter 8.

An equally ambitious investigation of the relative advantages of thrombolytic and mechanical reperfusion was spearheaded by the TAMI trialists in temporal tandem with the TIMI group.[21] As was the case with TIMI 2 they observed that immediate angioplasty conferred no additional benefit following successful thrombolysis. A variety of TAMI trials followed as tabulated in Chapter 9 comparing combination lytic agents (tissue plasminogen activator and urokinase), thrombolysis with immediate versus delayed heparin, and tPA with adjunctive prostacyclin as well as a number of other adjuncts.

There were other early important players such as the U.S./Canadian TEAM investigators who focused on a relatively new thrombolytic agent, the longer acting anistreplase, comparing it with other agents such as streptokinase and tPA (Chapter 10). Briefly, this agent was shown to be somewhat more effective than intravenous streptokinase achieving patency rates similar to those of intracoronary streptokinase. On the other hand, both regional and global ventricular function and therefore infarct size appeared to be more favorably affected by tPA although patency with this agent was no greater than with anistreplase at 24 hours.[22-24]

Even back in the era of intracoronary streptokinase the question of the need for and efficacy of intravenous heparin adjunctive to a thrombolytic agent was raised.[25] Based on the anticoagulant effect of fibrinogen degradation products it was suggested that, at least with streptokinase, heparin be delayed for 12 hours.[26] More recently, others have raised a question as to whether heparin contributes to the efficacy of thrombolytic therapy.[27,28] Nevertheless, the first GUSTO trial was designed in part to emphasize the importance of intravenous heparin because of the earlier revelations of the HART trial comparing heparin with low-dose oral aspirin as adjunctive to tPA for acute myocardial infarction.[29] This study showed that patency rates from 7 to 24 hours after beginning tPA infusion were measurably greater with heparin than with aspirin alone.

The first GUSTO trial (Chapter 11) was primarily designed to test the hypothesis that rapid and durable infarct artery patency correlates with survival. It further explored different approaches to the use of heparin with thrombolytic agents by randomizing patients to one of four arms including streptokinase with subcutaneous heparin, streptokinase with intravenous heparin (the standard U.S. approach) front-loaded tPA with intravenous heparin, and the combination of streptokinase and tPA with intravenous heparin.[30] This was a hugely important study involving over 41,000 people showing that 30-day survival was best preserved by the strategy employing accelerated tPA with adjunctive intravenous heparin. A very important component of this trial was the angiographic substudy of more than 2,400 people showing that complete restoration of myocardial reperfusion (TIMI grade 3 flow) was associated with a lower mortality rate than was the case with TIMI grade 0, 1 flow and even better than TIMI grade 2 flow.[31] Subsequent GUSTO trials are enumerated in Table 1 of Chapter 11. Not mentioned in this table is the SPEED trial (GUSTO IV pilot), in which a reduced dose of reteplase plus abciximab has been explored in acute myocardial infarction in patients presenting with chest pain of less than 6 hours duration. This trial suggested that abciximab with 10 units of rPA administered as a bolus dose achieved higher TIMI grade 3 patency rates at 90 minutes (52%) than that measured in a meta-analysis of twelve trials of tPA at the same interval (45%).[32]

Although, as stated above, the early implementation of prehospital thrombolysis from North America was chronicled by the MITI trialists, this activity already was well underway abroad.[33,34] One of the earliest ventures into "immediate" or prehospital administration of streptokinase occurred in Israel in the mid 1980s, as discussed in Chapter 12. One of the earliest, and certainly at the time the largest, prospective randomized trial exploring this strategy was reported by the European Myocardial Infarction Project Group who used anistreplase because of its ease of administration.[35] While less than a resoundingly positive experience, this study clearly supported the earliest possible administration of thrombolytic therapy in acute myocardial infarction if not establishing the superiority of prehospital therapy. At about the same time the GREAT trialists demonstrated that in the UK anistreplase could be administered safely and effectively by general practitioners using domiciliary anistreplase before hospitalization.[36]

Not only was the effect of thrombolysis on survival one of the key revelations as this therapeutic strategy matured, but interest additionally focused on the impact of reperfusion on myocardial function (Chapter 13).[37,38] Several studies suggested that the gain in ventricular function is a result of early recapture of infarct-related coronary artery patency whether by thrombolysis, angioplasty, or both.[39,40] Moreover, while some synergy may exist in this regard between angioplasty and thrombolytic agents, the important point is that whether achieved by either or both, the establishment of unrestricted reperfusion (TIMI grade 3 flow) at the earliest possible juncture is the key.[40]

A variety of new thrombolytic agents have been developed through molecular explorations and remodeling (Chapter 14). Reteplase, TNK-tPA and lanoteplase have been developed from mutations of wild-type tPA. Staphylokinase and dsPA, a species of plasminogen activator extracted from the saliva of the vampire bat (desmodus rotundus) are examples of thrombolytic agents deriving from processes other than genetic or molecular manipulations of wild-type tPA. Most of the former, that is, derivatives of wild-type tPA including reteplase, lanoteplase and TNK-tPA have been explored in phase II and phase III clinical trials. Because of various new properties such as a longer biologic half-life, resistance to plasminogen activator inhibitor and fibrin specificity, these agents can be given in one or two bolus doses. Excellent patency rates have been observed for reteplase in the RAPID trials,[41,42] the INJECT trial,[43] and GUSTO III[44] (Chapter 15). The same has been shown to be true with various rate adjusted doses of lanoteplase in the InTIME trials.[45] The derivative most similar to native tPA (wild-type) is TNK-tPA which has been explored clinically in the TIMI 10A dose-ranging trial and in ASSENT 1 patency and safety trials, respectively.[46,47] Chapter 15 also discusses the transition of achieving myocardial reperfusion from enzymatic to mechanical strategies and adjunctive therapies therein.

The foregoing brings us to one of the final chapters of this presentation (Chapter 16) which deals at length with the therapeutic efficacy (superiority?) of primary angioplasty in acute myocardial infarction. This question was first addressed in the mid 1980s at two institutions, Beaumont Hospital and the University of Michigan.[48] This small study compared angioplasty to the intracoronary instillation of streptokinase and found that while early coronary reperfusion rates were similar, angioplasty was better at preserving ventricular function as measured globally and regionally approximately 7 days thereafter. The first PAMI trial began in 1991 and when reported in 1993 showed that in those institutions armed with highly sophisticated interventional cardiologists and catheter laboratory facilities, immediate primary angioplasty for acute myocardial infarction yielded a better survival, improved ventricular function and fewer recurrent ischemic events than the thrombolytic alternative (tPA).[49] Similar observations have been made comparing angioplasty to other thrombolytic agents (streptokinase).[50] In the second PAMI trial it was shown that superior survival rates could be achieved whether performed in high-risk or low-risk myocardial infarction.[51,52] Currently the efficacy of primary stenting for acute myocardial infarction is being explored in the Stent-PAMI trial[53] and in the CADILLAC trial which are further discussed in Chapter 16 of this monograph.

To conclude, the introductory remarks in this foreword should not be construed as an exhaustive summary of the benchmarks heralding the evolution of thrombolytic therapy. I have not touched on a number of important contributions and trials such as APSIM,[54] ASSET,[55] GAUS,[56] PRIMI,[57] TAPS,[58] and STAR[59] to name but a few. Some of these derelictions are addressed in the final chapter (Chapter 17) which attempts to touch upon and summarize some of the more recent adventures that have found a permanent place in the mosaic of this unfolding story.

REFERENCES

1. Fletcher AP, Sherry S, Alkjaersig N. The maintenance of a sustained thrombolytic state in man. I. Induction and effects. J Clin Invest 1959;38: 1096B1110.

2. Fletcher AP, Sherry S, Alkjaersig N, et al. The maintenance of a sustained thrombolytic state in man. II. Clinical observations on patients with myocardial infarction and other thromboembolic disorders. J Clin Invest 1959;38: 1111B1119.

3. Polivoda H, Schröder R, Heckner S. Erste Erfahrungen mit der fibrinolytischen therapie des akuten herzinfarkts. Dtsch Med Wschr 1963;88:218B224.

4. Chazov EL, Mateeva LS, Mazev AV, et al. Intracoronary administration of fibrinolysin in acute myocardial infarction. Ter Arkh 1976;48:8B19.

5. Rentrop KP, Blanke H, Karsch KR, et al. Acute myocardial infarction: Intracoronary application of nitroglycerin and streptokinase. Clin Cardiol 1979;2: 354B363.

6. Amery A, Roeber G, Vermeulen HJ, et al. Single-blind randomised multicentre trial of comparing heparin and streptokinase in recent myocardial infarction. Acta Med Scand 1969;505:1B35.

7. European Working Party. Streptokinase in recent myocardial infarction: A controlled multicentre trial. Br Med J 1971;3:325B331.

8. Neuhaus KL, Köstering H, Tebbe U, et al. Intravenous kurzzeit-streptokinase-therapie beim frischen myokard-infarkt. Z Kardiol 1981;70:791B796.

9. Schröder R, Biamino G, von Leitner ER, et al. Intravenous short-term infusion of streptokinase in acute myocardial infarction. Circulation 1983;67: 536B548.

10. The ISAM Study Group. A prospective trial of intravenous streptokinase in acute myocardial infarction (I.S.A.M.). N Engl J Med 1986;314:1465B1471.

11. Kennedy JW, Ritchie JL, Davis KB, et al. Western Washington Randomized Trial of Intracoronary Streptokinase in Acute Myocardial Infarction. N Engl J Med 1983;309:1477B 1482.

12. Kennedy JW, Martin GV, Davis KB, et al. The Western Washington Intravenous Streptokinase in Acute Myocardial Infarction Randomized Trial. Circulation 1988;77:258B 352.

13. Weaver WD, Eisenberg MS, Martin JS, et al. Myocardial Infarction Triage and Intervention Project, Phase I: Patient characteristics and feasibility of pre-hospital initiation of thrombolytic therapy. J Am Coll Cardiol 1990;15: 925B931.

14. ISIS-2 (Second International Study of Infarct Survival) Collaborative Group. Randomised trial of intravenous streptokinase, oral aspirin, both, or neither among 17187 cases of suspected acute myocardial infarction: ISIS-2. Lancet 1988;2:349B360.

15. ISIS-3 (Third International Study of Infarct Survival) Collaborative Group. ISIS-3: A randomized comparison of streptokinase vs tissue plasminogen activator vs antistreplase and of aspirin plus heparin vs aspirin alone among 41299 cases of suspected acute myocardial infarction. Lancet 1992;339: 753B770.

16. Gruppo Italiano per lo Studio della Streptochinasi nell-Infarto Miocardico (GISSI). Effectiveness of intravenous thrombolytic treatment in acute myocardial infarction. Lancet 1986;ii: 397B402

17. GISSI-2 Gruppo Italiano per lo Studio della Streptokinasi nell-Infarto Miocarico. A factorial randomised trial of alteplase versus streptokinase and heparin versus no heparin among 12490 patients with acute myocardial infarction. Lancet 1990;;336:65B71.

18. TIMI Study Group. The Thrombolysis in Myocardial Infarction (TIMI) Trial: Phase I findings. N Engl J Med 1985; 312:932B936.

19. TIMI Research Group. Immediate vs delayed catheterization and angioplasty following thrombolytic therapy for acute myocardial infarction. TIMI II A results. JAMA 1988;260: 2849B2858.

20. TIMI Study Group. Comparison of invasive and conservative strategies after treatment with intravenous tissue plasminogen activator in acute myocardial infarction. Results of the Thrombolysis in Myocardial Infarction (TIMI) Phase II Trial. N Engl J Med 1989;320: 618B627.

21. Topol EJ, Califf RM, George BS, et al. A randomized trial of immediate versus delayed elective angioplasty after intravenous tissue plasminogen activator in acute myocardial infarction. N Engl J Med 1987;317:581B588.

22. Anderson JL, Rothbard RL, Hackworthy RA, et al., for the APSAC Multicenter Investigators. Multicenter reperfusion trial of intravenous anisoylated plasminogen streptokinase activator complex (APSAC) in acute myocardial infarction: Controlled comparison with intracoronary streptokinase. J Am Coll Cardiol 1988;11:1153B1163.

23. Anderson JL, Sorensen SG, Moreno FL, et al., and the TEAM-2 Investigators. Multicenter patency trial of intravenous anistreplase compared with streptokinase in acute myocardial infarction. Circulation 1991;83:126B140.

24. Anderson JL, Becker LC, Sorensen SG, et al., for the TEAM-3 Investigators. Anistreplase versus alteplase in acute myocardial infarction: Comparative effects on left ventricular function, morbidity, and 1 day patency. J Am Coll Cardiol 1992;20:753B766.

25. Timmis GC, Gangadharan V, Ramos RG, et al. Hemorrhage and the products of fibrinogen digestion after intracoronary administration of streptokinase. Circulation 1984;69:1146B 1152.

26. Timmis GC, Mammen EF, Ramos RG, et al. Hemorrhage vs rethrombosis after thrombolysis for acute myocardial infarction. Arch Intern Med 1986;146:667B672.

27. Ridker PM, Hebert PR, Fuster V, et al. Are both aspirin and heparin justified as adjuncts to thrombolytic therapy for acute myocardial infarction? Lancet 1993;341:1574B 1577.

28. Anderson JL, Karagounis LA. Does intravenous heparin or time-to-treatment/reperfusion explain differences between GUSTO and ISIS-3 results? Am J Cardiol 1994;74:1057B1060.

29. Hsia J, Hamilton WP, Kleiman N, et al. A comparison between heparin and low-dose aspirin as adjunctive therapy with tissue plasminogen activator for acute myocardial infarction. N Engl J Med 1990;323:1433B1437.

30. The GUSTO Investigators. An international randomized trial comparing four thrombolytic strategies for acute myocardial infarction. N Engl J Med 1993;329:673B682.

31. The GUSTO Angiographic Investigators. The effects of tissue plasminogen activator, streptokinase, or both on coronary-artery patency, ventricular function, and survival after acute myocardial infarction. N Engl J Med 1993;329:1615B1622.

32. Ohman EM. GUSTO IV pilot presented at Myocardial Reperfusion XI: Concepts and Controversies, Atlanta, Georgia, March 28, 1998.

33. Gotsman MS, Weiss AT. Immediate reperfusion in acute myocardial infarction. Bibltheca Cardiol 1986;40:30B51.

34. Gostsman MS, Weiss AT, Mosseri M, et al. Prehospital and very early hospital management of acute myocardial infarction by high-dose rapid infusion of streptokinase. In: Sleight P, ed. Streptokinase for Acute Myocardial Infarction: Results and Implications of the Major Clinical Studies. Kent England: MCS Consultants, 1989, pp 25B38.

35. The European Myocardial Infarction Project Group. Prehospital thrombolytic therapy in patients with suspected acute myocardial infarction. N Engl J Med 1993;320:383B389.

36. GREAT Group. Feasibility, safety and efficacy of domiciliary thrombolysis by general practitioners: Grampian Region Early Anistreplase Trial. Br Med J 1992;305:548B553.

37. Timmis GC, Westveer DC, Hauser AM, et al. The influence of infarction site and size on the ventricular response to coronary thrombolysis. Arch Intern Med 1985;145:2188B2193.

38. White HD, Norris RM, Brown MA, et al. Effect of intravenous streptokinase on left ventricular function and early survival after acute myocardial infarction. N Engl J Med 1987;317:850B855.

39. Guerci AD, Gerstenblith G, Brinker JA, et al. A randomized trial of intravenous tissue plasminogen activator for acute myocardial infarction with subsequent randomization to elective coronary angioplasty.

40. Ross AM. The plasminogen activator-angioplasty compablity trial (PACT) presented at Thrombolysis and Interventional Therapy in Acute Myocardial Infarction; the 13th International Workshop, Orlando, Florida, November 8, 1997.

41. Smalling RW, Bode C, Kalbfleisch J, et al. and the RAPID investigators. More rapid, complete and stable coronary thrombolysis with bolus administration

of reteplase compared with alteplase infusion in acute myocardial infarction. Circulation 1995;91:2725B2732.

42. Smalling RW, Bode C, Kalbfleisch J, et al. and the RAPID investigators. Improvement of global and regional LV-function by the bolus administration of recombinant plasminogen activator (r-PA) in acute myocardial infarction: A comparison with standard dose alteplase. (Abstract) Circulation 1994; 90(Suppl I):IB562.

43. International Joint Efficacy Comparison of Thrombolytics. Randomised, double-blind comparison of reteplase double bolus administration with streptokinase in acute myocardial infarction (INJECT): Trial to investigate equivalence. Lancet 1995;346:320B336.

44. GUSTO 3. A comparison of reteplase with alteplase for acute myocardial infarction. N Engl J Med 1997;337:1118B1123.

45. Liao WC, Beierle FA, Stoufer BC, et al. Single bolus regimen of lanoteplase (nPA) in acute myocardial infarction: Pharmakokinetic evaluation from inTIME 1 study. Circulation 1997; 96(Suppl I):IB260.

46. Cannon CP, McCabe CH, Gibson CM, et al. TNK-tissue plasminogen activator in acute myocardial infarction. Results on the Thrombolysis in Myocardial Infarction (TIMI) 10A dose ranging trial. Circulation 1997;21:95:351B356.

47. Preliminary data of ASSENT I were presented at the 70th Scientific Session of the American Heart Association, November 1997.

48. O'Neill W, Timmis GC, Bourdillon PD, et al. A prospective randomized clinical trial of intracoronary streptokinase versus coronary angioplasty for acute myocardial infarction. N Engl J Med 1986; 314:812B818.

49. Zijlstra F, Jan de Boer M, Hoorntje JCA, et al. A comparison of immediate coronary angioplasty with intravenous streptokinase in acute myocardial infarction. N Engl J Med 1993;328:680B684.

50. Grines CL, Browne KF, Marco J, et al. A comparison of immediate angioplasty with thrombolytic therapy for acute myocardial infarction. N Engl J Med 1993; 328:673B679.

51. Stone GW, Marsalese D, Brodie BR, et al. A prospective, randomized evaluation of prophylactic intraaortic balloon counterpulsation in high risk patients with acute myocardial infarction treated with primary angioplasty. J Am Coll Cardiol 1997;29:1459B1467.

52. Grines C, Marsalese D, Brodie B, et al., for the PAMI-II Investigators. Safety and cost effectiveness of early discharge after primary angioplasty in low risk patients with acute myocardial infarction. J Am Coll Cardiol 1998;31:967B972.

53. Grines CL, Morice MC, Mattos L, et al. A prospective multicenter trial using the JJIS heparin-coated stent for primary reperfusion of acute myocardial infarction. J Am Coll Cardiol 1997; 29(Suppl A):389A.

54. Bassand J-P, Machecourt J, Cassagnes J, et al. for the APSIM Study Investigators. Multicentrer trial of intravenous anisoylated plasminogen streptokinase activator complex (APSAC) in acute myocardial infarction: Effects on infarct size and left ventricular function. J Am Coll Cardiol 1989;13:988B997.

55. Wilcox RG, Lippe GV, Olsson DB, et al. Trial of tissue plasminogen activator for mortality reduction for acute myocardial infarction. Anglo-Scandinavian study of early thrombolytic therapy (ASSET). Lancet 1988;ii:525B530.

56. Neuhaus KL, Tebbe U, Gottwick M, et al. Intravenous recombinant tissue-plasminogen activator and urokinase in acute myocardial infarction: Results of the German Activator Urokinase Study (GAUS). J Am Coll Cardiol 1988;12:581B587.

57. PRIMI Trial Study Group. Randomized double-blind trial of recombinant prourokinase against streptokinase in acute myocardial infarction. Lancet 1989;i:863B868.

58. Neuhaus KL, von Essen R, Tebbe U, et al. Improved thrombolysis in acute myocardial infarction with front-loaded administration of alteplase: Results of the rt-PA-APSAC Patency Study (TAPS). J Am Coll Cardiol 1992;19:885B891.

59. Vanderschueren S, Barrios L, Kerdsinchai P, et al. For the STAR Trial Group. A randomized trial of recombinant staphylokinase versus alteplase for coronary artery patency in acute myocardial infarction. Circulation 1995;92:2044B2049.

Contributors

Jeffrey L. Anderson, MD
Merck & Company, Inc.
West Point, PA

Elliott M. Antman, MD
Cardiovascular Division
Department of Medicine
Brigham & Women's Hospital and
　Harvard Medical School
Boston, MA

Gregory W. Barsness, MD
Mayo Clinic
Rochester, MN

Eugene Braunwald, MD
Distinguished Hersey Professor of
　Medicine
Faculty Dean and Vice-President for
　Academic Programs at Brigham &
　Women's Hospital and Massachusetts
　General Hospital
Boston, MA

Robert M. Califf, MD
Professor of Medicine
Department of Medicine, Division of
　Cardiology, Director, Cardiac Care Unit,
　Duke University Medical Center
Durham, NC

Christopher P. Cannon, MD
Cardiovascular Division
Department of Medicine
Brigham & Women's Hospital and
　Harvard Medical School
Boston, MA

Nathan R. Every, MD
University of Washington
Seattle, WA

John K. French, MB, PhD
Cardiology Department
Green Lane Hospital
Auckland, New Zealand

Claudio Fresco, MD
Istituto "Mario Negri"
Milano, Italy

Barry S. George, MD
Associate Professor of Medicine
Ohio State University
Department of Cardiology
Riverside Methodist Hospital
Columbus, OH

Mervyn S. Gotsman, MD
David and Rose Orzen Professor of
　Cardiology
Director, Cardiology Department
Hadassah University Hospital
Jerusalem, Israel

Christopher B. Granger, MD
Assistant Professor of Medicine
Department of Medicine, Division of
    Cardiology, Co-Director, Cardiac Care
    Unit, Duke University Medical Center
Durham, NC

Cindy L. Grines, MD
Director, Cardiac Catheterization
    Laboratory
William Beaumont Hospital
Royal Oak, MI

Alfred P. Hallstrom, PhD
University of Washington
Seattle, WA

George P. Hanna, MD
Department of Internal Medicine
Division of Cardiology
The University of Texas Medical School
    and The Hermann Heart Center
Hermann Hospital
Houston, TX

Charles H. Hennekens, MD
Harvard Medical School
Chief, Division of Preventive
    Medicine
Brigham & Women's Hospital
Boston, MA

Thomas A. Hyde, MB, BS, BSc
Cardiology Department
Green Land Hospital
Auckland, New Zealand

J. Ward Kennedy, MD
Director, Division of Cardiology
Robert A. Bruce Professor of Medicine
University of Washington School of
    Medicine, University of Washington
    Medical Center, University of
    Washington
Seattle, WA

Dean J. Kereiakes, MD
Medical Director, The Carl & Edyth
    Lindner Center for Clinical Cardiology
    Research, Professor of Medicine, The
    University of Cincinnati College of
    Medicine, Interventional Cardiologist
Ohio Heart Health Center
Cincinnati, OH

Chaim Lotan, MD
Department of Cardiology
Hadassah University Hospital
Jerusalem, Israel

Aldo P. Maggioni, MD
Instituto "Mario Negri"
Milano, Italy

Jenny S. Martin, RN
Research Coordinator, MITI Coordinating
    Center, Division of Cardiology
University of Washington
Seattle, WA

Charles Maynard, MD
University of Washington School of
    Medicine, Department of Medicine and
    the University of Washington School of
    Public Health and Community Medicine
Seattle, WA

Carolyn H. McCabe, BS
Cardiovascular Division
Department of Medicine
Brigham & Women's Hospital and
    Harvard Medical School
Boston, MA

Morris Mosseri, MD
Department of Cardiology
Hadassah Univeristy Hospital
Jerusalem, Israel

Karl-Ludwig Neuhaus, MD
Städt Kliniken Kassel
Kassel, Germany

William W. O'Neill, MD
Director, Division of Cardiology
William Beaumont Hospital
Royal Oak, MI

E. Magnus Ohman, MD
Assistant Professor of Medicine,
  Department of Medicine, Division of
  Cardiology, Coordinator, Clinical Trials,
  Interventional Cardiology, Duke
  University Medical Center
Durham, NC

K. Peter Rentrop, MD
New York Medical College
St. Vincent's Hospital
New York, NY

Allan M. Ross, MD
Professor and Associate Chairman
Department of Medicine
Director, Cardiovascular Research Institute
George Washington University Medical
  Center
Washington, DC

Yoseph Rozenman, MD
Department of Cardiology
Hadassah University Hospital
Jerusalem, Israel

Rolf Schröder, MD
Department of Cardiology
Klinikum Steglitz
Free University
Berlin, Germany

Richard W. Smalling, MD, PhD
Professor and Co-Director Division of
  Cardiology, The University of Texas
Houston Health Science Center
Houston, TX

Gregg W. Stone, MD
Director, Cardiovascular Research and
  Education
Cardiovascular Research Foundation
Washington Hospital Center
Washington, DC

Ulrich Tebbe, MD
Städt Kliniken Kassel
Kassel, Germany

Gerald C. Timmis, MD
Clinical Professor of Health Sciences
  (Medical Physics)
Oakland University
Director of Research
Division of Cardiology
William Beaumont Hospital
Royal Oak, MI

Steven B.H. Timmis, MD
Division of Cardiology
William Beaumont Hospital
Royal Oak, MI

Gianni Tognoni, MD
Head, Lab of Clinical Pharmacology
Instituto "Mario Negri"
Milano, Italy

Eric J. Topol, MD
Chairman & Professor, Department of
  Cardiology; Director, Joseph J. Jacobs
  Center for Thrombosis and Vascular
  Biology, The Cleveland Clinic
  Foundation
Cleveland, OH

Sanjeev Trehan, MD
Division of Cardiology
University of Utah Health Science Center
Salt Lake City, UT

Pabio M. Turazza, MD
Instituto "Mario Negri"
Milano, Italy

Marc Verstraete, MD, PhD
Professor of Medicine
Center for Molecular and Vascular Biology
Katholieke Universiteit Leuven
Leuven, Belgium

Rainer von Essen, MD
Städt, Kliniken Kassel
Kassel, Germany

W. Douglas Weaver, MD
Division Head, Cardiovascular Medicine
Co-Director, Heart & Vascular Institute
Henry Ford Hospital
Detroit, MI

A. Teddy Weiss, MD
Aaron and Nettie Zuckerman Professor of
    Cardiology
Department of Cardiology
Hadassah University Hospital
Jerusalem, Israel

Harvey D. White, MB, DSc
Director, Coronary Care and
    Cardiovascular Research
Green Lane Hospital
Auckland, New Zealand

Doron Zahger, MD
Department of Cardiology
Hadassah University Hospital
Jerusalem, Israel

Chapter 1

Development and Pathophysiological Basis of Thrombolytic Therapy in Acute Myocardial Infarction: Part I. 1912–1977 The Controversy Over the Pathogenetic Role of Thrombus in Acute Myocardial Infarction

K. Peter Rentrop, M.D.

From St. Vincent's Hospital and Medical Center and Columbia-Presbyterian Medical Center, New York, New York

Although acute myocardial infarction (MI) was among the indications of Fletcher's 1959 safety study of thrombolytic therapy, this indication was not pursued in subsequent U.S. trials. The 1977 FDA approval of thrombolytic therapy did not include acute MI. The view that coronary thrombus, due to rupture of the underlying plaque and frequently associated with dissecting hemorrhage from the lumen into the plaque causes MI, had lost its dominance. Branwood had concluded that coronary thrombosis was not the cause but the consequence of MI, occurring in a minority of patients. Paterson had ascribed plaque hemorrhage to rupture of capillaries within the plaque. Autopsy studies in the mid-1960s provided fresh evidence that coronary thrombi were common in acute MI and that intimal fissuring caused both intraluminal thrombosis and plaque hemorrhage. Despite this, Robert's view that plaque fissures were artifacts resulting from sectioning arteries, and that coronary thrombosis resulted from a prolonged low output state associated with large infarcts, prevailed. Meanwhile, European investigators continued to explore thrombolysis in acute MI, although they believed that the lysis time for a coronary thrombus exceeded the time limit of myocardial tolerance of anoxia. They hoped to improve collateral flow and microcirculation by lysing microthrombi in capillaries and venules within and around the infarct zone. The reduction in blood viscosity associated with fibrinolytic therapy was expected to further improve collateral flow and to decrease myocardial oxygen demand by reducing afterload. The discussion about the pathogenesis of acute MI was limited by the inherent selection bias of autopsy studies and a paucity of in vivo angiographic data. (J Interven Cardiol 1998;11:255–263)

It was in February of 1977, when K.M., a 52-year-old man with an acute anterior wall myocardial infarction (MI) complicated by cardiogenic shock, was transferred to my service at the University of Goettingen, Germany. I was then head of the research team investigating surgical revascularization in patients with cardiogenic shock. Coronary angioplasty did not yet exist. Emergency coronary angiography revealed a total proximal occlusion of K.M.'s left anterior descending artery. His hemodynamics deteriorated progressively. As I accompanied him to the operating suite, he thanked me for my efforts. We both knew he was dying.

After the unsuccessful operation, I felt compelled to review his angiogram. The medical therapy at that time, consisting of bed rest, opiates, and management of arrhythmias, appeared woefully inadequate for patients in his condition, a mere exercise in palliation. The logistics of surgical revascularization were usually too complex and time consuming. With the coronary catheter, I had been within 2 cm of the arterial occlusion that was killing K.M. before my eyes and had been unable to help him. It seemed to me that I should have been able to extend my reach through that catheter just a little bit further.

I. The Introduction of Thrombolytic Therapy: Rationale and Early Experience

The clinical syndrome known today as acute MI was first clearly described and defined by J.D. Herrick in 1912.[1] In this landmark article, he also postulated the causative link between the clinical syndrome, localized myocardial necrosis, and coronary thrombosis, which came to be universally accepted. The terms "coronary thrombosis" and "myocardial infarction" were used synonymously until approximately 1940 when it became apparent that not each case of anemic myocardial necrosis manifests itself clinically, that not all infarctions are caused by coronary thrombosis, and that not all coronary thrombi cause infarction.

Blumgart and associates, whose necropsy studies provided many important insights into the human collateral circulation, demonstrated occlusive coronary thrombi that were not associated with infarctions in hearts with well-developed collateral channels.[2] They also found MIs in patients who, during their lifetime, had not experienced any of the clinical symptoms generally associated with evolving ischemic myocardial necrosis, i.e., patients who had suffered a "silent infarction."

Following isolated reports of cases in which both the clinical syndrome and autopsy findings of acute MI without coronary thrombi were present,[3,4] Friedberg and Horn published the first systematic study of infarction not caused by thrombosis in 1939.[5]

In 1,000 consecutive autopsies, these authors found that 31% of their cases of acute MI were not associated with recent coronary thrombosis. Atherosclerotic narrowing of the coronary arteries was combined with myocardial hypertrophy and abnormal circulatory dynamics due to associated diseases such as pulmonary embolism, aortic stenosis, or perioperative hypotension in most of their cases. The authors suggested that this combination of factors could reduce coronary blood flow sufficiently to cause myocardial necrosis. In some cases severe "coronary insufficiency" appeared to be "solely due to progressive coronary narrowing of extreme degree."

Infarcts without thrombosis consisted typically of small disseminated foci restricted to the subendocardial region, although in some cases large confluent areas of muscle necrosis were observed. The authors emphasized that the "clinical features and electrocardiographic alterations attributed to acute coronary thrombosis are actually due to the resulting myocardial damage" and that "it would appear more accurate to employ the clinical diagnosis myocardial infarction than coronary thrombosis."

The differences between infarctions that are associated with an occlusive coronary thrombus and those that are not were further clarified in 1951 by Miller and associates in a study of 143 consecutive necropsy cases of acute MI.[6] Acute thrombotic coronary occlusion was present in 94 of the 143 (66%) cases; the remaining 49 cases showed only atherosclerotic narrowing in the relevant coronary arteries. The severity and extent of coronary sclerosis were comparable in the two groups, but those cases without acute coronary occlusion showed markedly more myocardial hypertrophy than those with occlusion, possibly contributing to the development of "acute coronary insufficiency."

Among the 49 cases without total coronary occlusion, necrosis was limited to the subendocardial half of the myocardium in 82% (40/49). In contrast to Friedberg's and Horn's study, the subendocardial infarctions were generally confluent. In the group with total thrombotic occlusion, the necrosis involved not only the subendocardial layer of the myocardium, but also extended well into the subepicardial layer in 89% (84/94) of cases. The authors introduced the term "transmural infarction" to describe this finding and contrasted it with "subendocardial infarction." The mass of infarcted myocardium was larger in the hearts with total thrombotic occlusions; pericarditis and myocardial rupture occurred almost exclusively in this group.

These concepts were generally accepted by clinicians when Sherry and associates revolutionized the treatment of acute thromboembolic vascular diseases by dissolution of the causative thrombus or embolus using streptokinase. In the 1950s these investigators first induced "intense and prolonged thrombolytic states" in human volunteers by administering an intravenous infusion of streptokinase.[7] Subsequently, the investigators assessed the safety and therapeutic value of this treatment in several clinical syndromes felt to be thromboembolic in nature, including acute MI, pulmonary embolism, thrombophlebitis, and peripheral artery oc-

clusion.[8] In their patients with acute MI, the investigators hoped to achieve a "reduction of the final area of muscle infarction" by "rapid dissolution of a coronary thrombus."

In the first phase of their study, infarct patients were entered into a double-blind, randomized trial of intravenous streptokinase versus placebo. However, after enrolling 23 patients, the investigators abandoned this trial design because they felt it impeded data collection, and intravenous streptokinase was administered to an additional ten infarct patients in a nonrandomized fashion. Sherry and associates concluded that high levels of plasma thrombolytic activity are harmless to infarcted myocardium. Proof of clinical benefit was not possible due to the small study size, but it is noteworthy that the investigators found an earlier serum glutamic-oxaloacetic transaminase (SGOT) peak in streptokinase-treated patients than in controls. Today these findings would be considered indirect evidence of early reperfusion. However, such a conclusion was beyond the knowledge of enzyme kinetics at that time, and it was not drawn by the authors. Sherry and associates abandoned their research of thrombolysis in acute MI after publication of their study in 1959. They thereafter focused their efforts on the other thromboemobolic syndromes, leading ultimately to the 1977 Food and Drug Administration approval of thrombolytic therapy for the treatment of pulmonary embolism, deep vein thrombosis, peripheral artery thrombosis, thrombosed dialysis fistulae, and thrombosed intravenous catheters. Approval of thrombolytic therapy for acute MI was not sought.

II. The Rationale for Thrombolytic Therapy in Acute Myocardial Infarction Is Challenged; Are Coronary Thrombi Secondary Phenomena?

A provocative hypothesis proposed in 1956 by Branwood and Montgomery, which reversed the cause-and-effect relationship between coronary thrombosis and MI had become increasingly accepted.[9] These investigators reported that among 61 cases of MI, coronary thrombosis was found in only 13 (21%). By histologic criteria, many of the occlusive thrombi were younger than the related infarcts. The authors concluded that occlusive coronary thrombosis is not the cause of, but rather a terminal event occurring in, a minority of patients after an MI has developed. A low incidence of coronary thrombi in acute MI was soon confirmed in several necropsy studies.[10–12] Furthermore, investigators reported an increase in the incidence of coronary artery thrombosis with a longer time interval between the onset of infarction and death.[10,13] Radioactive fibrinogen, injected in a patient while in the coronary care unit (CCU) after onset of infarction, could be demonstrated in all portions of the coronary thrombus of those patients who subsequently died, indicating that the thrombus had developed only after onset of infarction.[14]

The revolutionary hypothesis derived from these studies was completed by W. Roberts, who in his own necropsy studies noted that fatal acute MI was regularly associated with severe, diffuse coronary artery disease (CAD), whereas arterial thrombosis was present in only 8% of patients who had died within 6 hours of infarction and approximately 50% of those who died later.[12] "The degree of luminal narrowing of coronary arteries by old atherosclerotic plaques" was found to be "identical in patients with fatal acute myocardial infarction who have coronary thrombi and in those without coronary thrombi."[15] Roberts concluded that "even totally occluding thrombi, when found in arteries more than 90% occluded by old atherosclerotic plaques, may have little functional significance." If "nothing new appears" in the coronary arteries "at the time of acute myocardial infarction in most patients stricken,"[15] what would be the cause of myocardial necrosis?

Roberts suggested that in the presence of severe and diffuse CAD "even minor disturbances in coronary artery perfusion could shift the balance from adequate to inadequate flow producing ischemia and necrosis in the myocardium."[15] He noted that the majority of infarctions begin during decreased activity, such as sleep or rest, which may be associated with slowed blood flow.

A mechanism for secondary thrombosis was suggested by Walston et al.'s finding that low output syndromes were present prior to death in 90% (17/19) of patients with coronary thrombi but in only 39% (7/18) of those without coronary thrombi at autopsy.[16] Building on these observations, Roberts explained the formation of thrombi after onset of infarction by a combination of prolonged and profound decrease in coronary flow in those patients in whom extensive myocardial necrosis had decreased cardiac output and aggregation of platelets at points of luminal narrowing where high velocity gradients can activate platelets.[15]

These concepts dominated the thinking of U.S. clinicians until the early 1980s (and that of the U.S. trained author until 1977) and are responsible for the lack of interest in thrombolytic therapy among cardiologists in the land of its inception. Instead, large resources were committed to studies that attempted to limit infarct size by reducing myocardial oxygen demand. These studies yielded disappointing results.[17]

III. The European View: Collateral Flow, Microcirculation, and Afterload Reduction

Entirely different concepts guided European clinicians who conducted several randomized mortality trials of prolonged intravenous streptokinase, and later urokinase, infusion in acute MI during the 1960s and 1970s. Although these trials were too small to determine the benefits and risks of this therapy unequivocally, many European clinicians adopted the treatment of acute MI with intravenous infusion of thrombolytic agents. The concept of evaluating new therapies with randomized trials of appropriate size was not yet fully developed.

This author became familiar with the pathophysiological concepts of the European investigators as an intern at the University of Giessen, Germany, in 1968 (prior to his clinical training in the United States) where H.G. Lasch headed an influential group of researchers. These investigators had not abandoned the hypothesis that MI is caused by coronary thrombosis, but they did not believe that myocardium could be salvaged by dissolving the causative coronary thrombus. Prolonged intravenous thrombolytic therapy had been found to recanalize peripheral artery thrombi at a rate of 7 cm/24 hours.[18] In animal models, dissolution of coronary artery thrombi was found to occur 3–7 hours after initiation of thrombolytic therapy.[19,20] It was felt that this dissolution time exceeded the time limit of myocardial tolerance of anoxia.[19] However, these studies also described microthrombi in the capillaries and venules of the infarcted tissue and its marginal zones, which were not present in animals treated with thrombolytic agents. It appeared that these microthrombi could be dissolved more rapidly by fibrinolytic therapy than the large thrombus in the subtending coronary artery, and it was hypothesized that myocardium could be salvaged by restoring the microcirculation and improving collateral flow.[19,20] Other investigators noted that blood viscosity was reduced in patients treated with intravenous streptokinase, primarily due to the breakdown of fibrinogen, a large protein. Neuhoff et al. suggested that the reduction in blood viscosity would further improve collateral flow.[21] An additional benefit of decreased blood viscosity was seen in the concomitant reduction in afterload. The resultant decrease in myocardial oxygen demand was expected to enhance preservation of myocardium.

A prolonged intravenous infusion of streptokinase was used to achieve and main-

tain these benefits. Typically, an initial rapid infusion of 250,000 U of streptokinase, which was administered to overcome antistreptokinase titers from preceding streptococcal infections, was followed by a 12- to 24-hour infusion of 100,000 U/hour to maintain a prolonged thrombolytic state.

In 1979 Verstraete and his colleagues of the European Cooperative Study Group published the results of the last trial in which a prolonged infusion of intravenous streptokinase versus placebo was assessed in the *New England Journal of Medicine*.[22] Among their 512 medium-risk patients, they found a significantly lower 6-month mortality rate in the streptokinase group (15.6%) than in the control group (30.6%). They attributed this important mortality benefit to an improvement in cardiac microcirculation and a reduction in total peripheral resistance. Dissolution of the causative thrombus was not discussed as a possible mechanism.

In spite of its strongly positive result, this trial failed to change the skeptical attitude of U.S. clinicians toward thrombolytic therapy in acute MI. In an editorial accompanying the publication, it was pointed out that other similar trials had had negative results, that the mechanisms of benefit remained speculative, and that afterload could be reduced in safer and more easily controlled ways than by use of thrombolytic agents.[23]

IV. Changes in the Vessel Wall at the Site of Coronary Thrombosis

Thus Herrick's concept had become irrelevant, for different reasons, to clinicians on both sides of the Atlantic. However, among pathologists, the pathogenetic role and etiology of coronary thrombosis in acute MI continued to be discussed vigorously. While some investigators attributed coronary artery thrombosis to systemic factors such as slow blood flow[15,16] or hypercoagulability,[24,25] others stressed local factors, among which plaque rupture[26–29] and subintimal hematoma[30,31] were the most important ones.

Benson was the first investigator to observe breaks in the vascular intima at the site of coronary artery thrombosis, which were sometimes associated with "dissecting hemorrhage from the lumen into the plaque"; he suggested that these changes in the vessel wall may be the cause of thrombus formation.[26] Koch and Kong noted that coronary thrombosis almost always covers a ruptured, ulcerated plaque into which bleeding has occurred, where the contents of the atheroma were in direct contact with the thrombus.[27] These observations were extended by Leary,[28] Saphir et al.,[29] and others, leading to the hypothesis that coronary thrombosis is caused by disruption of the intima and the attendant exposure of blood to the highly thrombogenic contents of the underlying atherosclerotic plaque.

This view was challenged by Paterson, who proposed the hypothesis that *thrombi are caused by subendothelial hemorrhages*.[30,31] This hypothesis came to be widely accepted. These hemorrhages were seen as a consequence of vascularization of the intima resulting from intimal thickening. The normal intima and the inner portion of the media are avascular and receive their nutrients by diffusion directly from the arterial lumen, whereas the outer portions of the vessel wall are perfused by vasa vasorum. However, as first shown by Winternitz,[32] diffusion from the arterial lumen can extend only to a certain limit, which was determined to be 0.35 mm for coronary arteries.[33,34] Once atherosclerotic thickening of the intima exceeds this limit, vascularization of the intima occurs. Paterson suggested that vascularization of the intima originates not only from the vasa vasorum but also directly from the vessel lumen. Thus, thin-walled capillaries, which are poorly supported by tissue within the plaque (which is frequently necrotic), are exposed to arterial pressure. Rupture of these vessels and hemorrhage into the plaque were regarded as an inevitable and frequent consequence. Paterson proposed three mechanisms to explain the formation of intraluminal thrombi above subendothelial plaque hemorrhages:

1. Activation of the coagulation process by diffusion of procoagulant ("thromboplastic") factors from a superficial hematoma into the vessel lumen.
2. Necrosis of the intima above a superficial hematoma.
3. Retrograde extension of an intraplaque thrombus through connecting capillaries into the lumen.

Paterson's view lost its dominance in the mid-1960s due to three publications that deepened the understanding of plaque rupture.[35–37] In an autopsy series of 30 acute MI cases and 28 cases of sudden death, D. Sinapius[35] at the University of Goettingen, Germany, sectioned the coronary arteries transversely at 2- to 3-mm intervals and found intracoronary thrombus in 93% (28/30) of the infarct cases and 57% (16/28) of the sudden death cases. He estimated the age of the different parts of the thrombus by histologic criteria. The oldest part of the thrombus was assumed to identify the site of its origin. At this site "luminal narrowing" of the vessel was calculated. Calculation of luminal narrowing was based on planimetric measurements, identical with those now used in the interventional laboratory to calculate "plaque burden" with intracoronary ultrasound. A "luminal narrowing," or in today's terminology "plaque burden," of at least 75% was found at the site of origin of all 24 thrombi in the MI group and in 9 of the 12 cases with thrombus in the sudden death group.

In agreement with Paterson and others, Sinapius found subendothelial hemorrhages within the plaque at the site of coronary thrombosis in all but two of his cases. Furthermore, Sinapius confirmed Paterson's observation of sinusoidal channels extending from the lumen into the superficial layers of the plaque. But his conclusions about the relationships between these phenomena were radically different from those of Paterson. Sinapius did not consider the sinusoids to be true capillaries since they did not drain into venules and were not connected with the capillary networks subtended by the vasa vasorum. He concluded that these sinusoids were remnants of the process of thrombus organization and that they did not contribute to the nutrition of the intima. Furthermore, he never observed major plaque hemorrhage close to these sinusoids.

Instead, Sinapius noted that he could regularly trace the plaque hematoma to a site of intimal disruption. Intimal tears were found within the thrombosed segment of the artery in 21 of the 24 cases in the acute MI group and in 11 of the 12 cases of the sudden death group. All intimal tears were associated with dissecting hemorrhages close to the vessel lumen (Fig. 1). The depth of these intimal tears varied between 0.1 and 2 mm.

Some were large, complete tears of the fibrous cap above an atheroma, exposing a plaque ulcer to blood as described by Koch and Kong[27]; others were small, confined to superficial layers of connective tissue. The intimal tears were located at the site of the oldest portion of the thrombus in 16 of 24 cases. In five cases, an intimal tear was found outside of the oldest part of the thrombus but still within the thrombosed segment of the artery; organization at the base of the thrombus was advanced to a point that healing of the plaque rupture at this site was likely to have occurred. In only three cases from the acute MI group and in one case from the sudden death group did the intima appear intact throughout the entire extension of the thrombus. Based on these findings, Sinapius concluded that *intimal disruption is the overriding mechanism, causing both the dissecting plaque hematoma and the coronary thrombus.*

Since intimal tears were primarily lo-

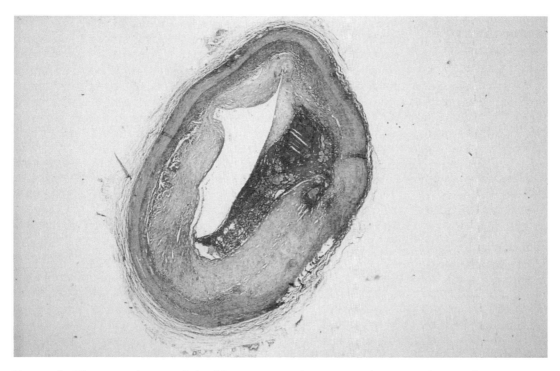

Figure 1. Plaque with tear of the fibrous cap and extensive dissecting hemorrhage into the atheroma (Courtesy D. Sinapius).

cated in the thin capsule above fatty deposits and at the margins of atheromatous plaques, Sinapius postulated that they were caused by mechanical factors, such as increased wall stress on a thin fibrous cap, pressure gradients between the arterial lumen and the fatty deposits within the plaque, or shear forces at the margins of plaques. This view has recently been expanded.[38–40]

One month after Sinapius' publication, Chapman reported that for each one of the 19 occlusive coronary thrombi examined at autopsy, "a point of attachment could be demonstrated between the thrombus and the exposed atheromatous debris."[36] In 1966 Constantinides reported that "all of the 17 recent coronary thrombi studied at autopsy were attached to cracks in the atheromatous wall" and that "16 of 17 thrombi were accompanied by hemorrhages in the surrounding plaques, all of which could be traced to plaque fissures."[37] Constantinides also found minor hemorrhages, which resulted from the rupture of intraplaque capillaries, not connected to the lumen in addition to the major hemorhages associated with plaque fissure.

While these publications succeeded in refuting Paterson's hypothesis that coronary thrombosis results from plaque hemorrhage, they failed to settle the argument about the cause and effect relationship between coronary thrombus and MI. It was pointed out that plaque fissures could represent an artifact, resulting from preparation and sectioning of the artery.[12]

V. The Temporal and Spacial Relationships Between Coronary Thrombi, Myocardial Infarction, and Preinfarction Angina

In a 1972 study of 206 necropsy cases of MI, Sinapius analyzed the temporal and spacial relationships between coronary thrombi and myocardial infarcts.[41] Occluding coronary thrombus was found in 96.5% (164/170) of transmural infarcts and in 55.6% (20/36) of smaller infarcts. Sinapius

noted that all thrombi were located in the artery subtending the infarcted myocardium. He, and later Chapman,[42] argued that this constant spacial relationship refutes the hypothesis that intracoronary thrombus is caused secondarily by systemic factors that result from MI, such as shock, slow blood flow, or activation of the coagulation system. As a result of these mechanisms, a random distribution of thrombi in the three coronary arteries would be expected.

Furthermore, Sinapius noted that in 90% of his cases, the thrombus was located in the proximal segment of the subtending artery. The infarcted myocardium was always separated from the thrombus by a segment of artery that was free of thrombus. Sinapius stated that this finding is incompatible with the hypothesis that the infarcted myocardium causes secondary thrombosis by a direct effect on the subtending artery.

Studying serial transverse sections of occlusive thrombi, Sinapius noticed a multilayered structure in many thrombi, which indicated protracted and episodic growth according to histologic criteria. The oldest portion of the thrombi either antedated the on-set of infarct symptoms or coincided with them. In no case had thrombus formation begun after onset of infarction, a result that expanded an earlier study by Sinapius[43] but contradicted the studies of Branwood and Montgomery[9] and Ehrlich and Shinohara.[11]

Finally, in contrast to Spain and Bradess,[10] Popper and Feiks,[13] and Roberts and Buja,[12] Sinapius noted that in his series, the frequency of coronary thrombi did not increase with survival time. Sinapius concluded that the constant spacial and temporal relationships between thrombi and infarcted myocardium support the hypothesis that nearly all transmural infarcts are caused by occlusive thrombi and not the reverse.

From the multilayered structure of thrombi, Sinapius concluded that the majority of plaque ruptures do not immediately cause an occlusive thrombus but are sealed off by a nonocclusive, parietal thrombus. Sinapius suggested that prein-farction angina could have its anatomical basis in plaque rupture, the attendant dis-secting hematoma, and parietal thrombus formation. These phenomena would cause an abrupt decrease in vessel lumen.[42,43] Such lesions can stabilize although they tend to recur. Transmural infarction results only from subsequent total occlusion of the vessel, the likelihood of which increases as the residual lumen decreases.

VI. The 1973 National Heart, Lung and Blood Institute (NHLBI) Workshop

Thus by 1972, two seemingly incom-patible hypotheses about the role of coro-nary thrombosis in the pathophysiology of acute MI had been fully developed, and each view was represented by renowned investigators. In 1973 the NHLBI organized an important international workshop that brought together leading proponents of the two hypotheses: W. Roberts and L.R. Erhardt represented the view that thrombo-sis is a secondary event, while D. Sinapius, I. Chapman, and C.J. Schwartz postulated that thrombus is an important causative factor in the pathogenesis of acute MI.[42]

Agreement was reached that in cases of multifocal subendocardial infarction, the frequency of thrombotic occlusion is low. The investigators agreed further that multi-focal subendocardial infarcts occurring in the presence of advanced coronary sclerosis without thrombotic occlusion can be caused by severe ischemia resulting from either a sudden increase in myocardial oxy-gen demand or a decrease in myocardial perfusion from an extrinsic cause.

It was also agreed that coronary thrombi are much more prevalent among cases of transmural infarction than among cases of subendocardial necrosis. It became evident that the observed differences in the frequency of coronary thrombosis between the different series were in part due to different inclusion criteria, which had resulted in varying pro-portions of subendocardial infarcts. The workshop focused on transmural infarcts.

It was pointed out that the estimation of infarct and thrombus age by histologic criteria is difficult, precluding firm conclu-sions. The estimation of the age of the thrombus by means of administering ra-dioactive 125 iodine-tagged fibrinogen was found to be questionable as well, since plasma containing radioactive fibrinogen could perfuse a preexisting thrombus. While all participants of the workshop con-firmed the consistent spacial relationships between thrombi and infarcts as outlined above, it was emphasized that this finding alone does not exclude the possibility of a secondary origin of thrombus. "If the thrombus is primary, its location at any given point in the artery must be ex-plained." Plaque rupture at the site of thrombosis provides an explanation. The investigators concluded cautiously that "most evidence continues to affirm the ba-sic concept that myocardial infarction can result from acute ischemia produced by thrombotic occlusion of a coronary artery."

However, several important issues re-mained unresolved. The frequency of thrombosis in acute transmural infarction varied from 54%–96.5% in the different se-ries presented at the workshop. No satisfac-tory explanation for this discrepancy could be found. While all investigators found a significant plaque burden at the site of thrombi, unanimity did not exist concern-ing changes within the plaque; thus, Roberts found associated plaque hemor-rhage in only 27% of his cases. Accordingly, the participants of the workshop also con-cluded that the "idea that coronary throm-bosis is a secondary event following infarc-tion is provocative and deserves serious consideration."

VII. Coronary Artery Bypass Surgery, Intraortic Balloon Counterpulsation, and Initial Experience with Coronary Angiography in Acute Myocardial Infarction

There was agreement in the 1970s that MI results from an acute imbalance between oxygen supply and demand. Researchers agreed that in transmural infarcts, oxygen supply is limited by an obstructive process in the corresponding coronary artery, although the etiologic role of thrombus continued to be debated.

The only method to normalize myocardial blood supply known at the time was coronary artery bypass surgery, introduced by Favaloro and associates at the Cleveland Clinic in 1967 for the treatment of angina pectoris. Favaloro soon extended coronary artery bypass surgery to the treatment of evolving MI in a small pilot study, which indicated that this therapy was feasible and safe.[44] This author witnessed first-hand this pioneering development during his training at the Cleveland Clinic, 1970–1973.

Encouraged by reports from the Cleveland Clinic, Berg and associates in Spokane, Washington, initiated the first major study of coronary artery bypass grafting (CABG) for the treatment of acute MI in 1971.[45] The investigators achieved restoration of coronary flow by saphenous vein grafting within the first 6–8 hours of infarction. They reported a hospital mortality of 4.6% in their first 65 patients, which compared favorably to the 15% mortality in a medically treated matched control group from the same institution.

The low mortality rate of the surgically treated patients did not appear to reflect a selection bias since 27% (17/65) of the patients presented in cardiogenic shock; the 15% mortality in the medical group was consistent with general experience at the time.

CABG for the treatment of acute MI complicated by cardiogenic shock was further explored by several groups. It was learned that bypass surgery was feasible in shock patients if hemodynamics could first be stabilized by intra-aortic balloon counterpulsation. The Massachusetts General team reported a 47% survival rate in patients revascularized surgically within 24 hours of shock onset.[46] This result was encouraging compared to historical controls.

Coronary angiography was performed prior to surgical revascularization without apparent increase in mortality or morbidity in hemodynamically stable patients. In shock patients, coronary angiography was found to be safe following stabilization with intraaortic balloon counterpulsation.

Drs. Hutter and associates[46] from the Massachusetts General Hospital reported that surgical revascularization improved myocardial function only if coronary angiography demonstrated "some vascularity" of the infarct area, either through collateral channels or via antegrade flow. Coronary angiography prior to emergency surgery provided the first in vivo data on the frequency of total coronary artery occlusion in patients with acute MI. Berg et al.[45] reported that the incidence of total occlusion of the infarct-related artery was 77% (50/65) in their study group. The high incidence of total occlusions within the first hours of infarction reported in their study was at odds with the autopsy findings of Roberts et al., who reported a low incidence of total occlusion in the early hours of MI[12] and in remarkable agreement with the findings of Sinapius and other pathologists who believed that infarcts are caused by occlusive thrombi.[35–37]

The Spokane surgeons were able to remove thrombus and/or atheromatous material from the infarct artery in 16 cases by Fogerty catheter extraction, the first direct in vivo evidence of intracoronary thrombus. However, neither the authors nor other investigators drew conclusions regarding the pathogenesis of infarction at that time.

Surgical revascularization in acute MI was carried out by only a few groups, and randomized trials of this technique were never conducted. Cost and logistics made this treatment inaccessible to the majority of patients. The lack of a broad interest in acute surgical revascularization was reflected in the 1977 "Report of the Ad Hoc Committee On The Indications For Coronary Angiography," which specified that coronary angiography was contraindicated during acute MI. Angiography prior to acute surgical revascularization was not considered.[47]

References

1. Herrick JB. Clinical features of sudden obstruction of the coronary arteries. JAMA 1912;59:2015-2020.
2. Blumgart HL, Schlesinger MJ, Davis D. Studies on the relation of the clinical manifestations of angina pectoris, coronary thrombosis, and myocardial infarction to the pathologic findings. Am Heart J 1940;19:1-91.
3. Libman E. The importance of blood examinations in the recognition of thrombosis of the coronary arteries and its sequelae. Am Heart J 1925;1:121-123.
4. Buechner F. Die Rolle des Herzmuskels bei der Angina pectoris. Beitr z path Anat u z allg Path 1932;89:644-667.
5. Friedberg CK, Horn H. Acute myocardial infarction not due to coronary artery occlusion. JAMA 1939;112:1675-1679.
6. Miller RD, Burchell HB, Edwards JE. Myocardial infarction withand without acute coronary occlusion. Arch Intern Med 1951;88:597-604.
7. Fletcher AP, Sherry S, Alkjaersig N. The maintenance of a sustained thrombolytic state in man I. Induction and effects. J Clin Invest 1959;38:1096-1110.
8. Fletcher AP, Sherry S, Alkjaersig N, et al. The maintenance of a sustained thrombolytic state in man II. Clinical observations on patients with myocardial infarction and other thromboembolic disorders. J Clin Invest 1959;38:1111-1119.
9. Branwood AW, Montgomery GL. Observations on the morbid anatomy of coronary artery disease. Scot Med J 1956;1:367-375.
10. Spain DM, Bradess VA. The relationship of coronary thrombosis to coronary atherosclerosis and ischemic heart disease. Am J Med Sci 1960;240:701-710.
11. Ehrlich JC, Shinohara Y. Low incidence of coronary thrombosis in myocardial infarction. Arch Pathol 1964;78:432-445.
12. Roberts WC, Buja LM. The frequency and significance of coronary arterial thrombi and other observations in fatal acute myocardial infarction. Am J Med 1972;52:425-443.
13. Popper L, Feiks FK Herzinfarkt und Koronarthrombose. Wien Klin Wochenschr 1961;73:421.
14. Erhardt LR, Lundman T, Mellstedt H. Incorporation of 125I-labelled fibrinogen into coronary arterial thrombi in acute myocardial infarction in man. Lancet 1973;1:387-390.
15. Roberts WC. The pathology of acute myocardial infarction. Hosp Pract 1971;12:89-104.
16. Walston A, Hackel DB, Estes EH. Acute coronary occlusion and the "power failure" syndrome. Am Heart J 1970;79:613-619.
17. Rude RE, Muller JE, Braunwald E. Efforts to limit the size of infarctions. Ann Intern Med 1981;95:736-761.
18. Lasch HG. Die Therapie des Herzinfarkts. Therapiewoche 1970;3:107-114.
19. Ruegsegger P, Nydik I, Abarquez R, et al. Effect of fibrinolytic (plasmin) therapy on the physiopathology of myocardial infarction. Am J Cardiol 1960;6:519-524.
20. Nydik I, Ruegsegger P, Bouvier C, et al. Salvage of heart muscle by fibrinolytic therapy after experimental coronary occlusion. Am Heart J 1961;61:93-100.
21. Neuhof H, Hey D, Glaser E, et al. Hemodynamic reactions induced by streptokinase therapy in patients with acute myocardial infarction. Eur J Intensive Care Med 1975;1:27-30.
22. European Cooperative Study Group. Streptokinase in acute myocardial infarction. N Engl J Med 1979;301:797-802.
23. Sullivan JM. Streptokinase and myocardial infarction. N Engl J Med 1979;301:836-837.
24. Cooperberg AA, Teitelbaum JI. The concentration of antihemophilic globulin (AHG) in patients with coronary artery disease. Ann Intern Med 1961;54:899-907.
25. Dintenfass L. Some rheologic factors in pathogenesis of thrombosis. Lancet 1965;2:370.
26. Benson RL. The present status of coronary arterial disease. Arch Pathol Lab Med 1926;2:876-916.
27. Koch W, Kong LC. Ueber die Formen des Coronarverschlusses, die Aenderungen im Coronarkreislauf und die Beziehungen zur Angina Pectoris. Beitr z Path Anat u z allg Path 1932;90:21-34.

28. Leary T. Experimental atherosclerosis in the rabbit compared with human (coronary) atherosclerosis. Arch Pathol 1934;17:453-492.

29. Saphir O, Priest WS, Hamburger WW, et al. Coronary arteriosclerosis, coronary thrombosis, and the resulting myocardial changes. An evaluation of their respective clinical pictures including the electrocardiographic records, based on the anatomical findings. Am Heart J 1935;10:567-595.

30. Paterson JC. Vascularization and hemorrhage of the intimaof arteriosclerotic coronary arteries. Arch Pathol 1936; 22:313-324.

31. Paterson JC. Capillary rupture with intimal hemorrhage as a causative factor in coronary thrombus. Arch Pathol 1938;25:4744-4787.

32. Winternitz MC, Thomas RM, LeCompte PM. The Biology of Atherosclerosis. Springfield, IL: Charles C. Thomas, 1938.

33. Geiringer E. Intimal vascularization and atherosclerosis. J Path Bact 1951; 63:201-211.

34. Geiringer F. The mural coronary. Am Heart J 1957;41:359-368.

35. Sinapius D. Ueber Wandveraenderungen bei Coronarthrombose. Klin Wochenschr 1965;16:875-880.

36. Chapman I. Morphogenesis of occluding coronary artery thrombosis. Arch Pathol 1965;80:256-261.

37. Constantinides P. Plaque fissures in human coronary thrombosis. J Atheroscler Res 1966;6:1-17.

38. Falk E. Plaque rupture with severe preexisting stenosis precipitating coronary thrombosis: Characteristics of coronary atherosclerotic plaques underlying fatal occlusive thrombi. Br Heart J 1983; 50:127-134.

39. Richardson PD, Davies MJ, Born GVR. Influence of plaque configuration and stress distribution on fissuring of coronary atherosclerotic plaques. Lancet 1989;2:941-944.

40. Cheng GC, Loree HM, Kamm RD, et al. Distribution of circumferential stress in ruptured and stable atherosclerotic lesions: A structural analysis with histopathological correlation. Circulation 1993;87:1179-1187.

41. Sinapius D. Beziehungen zwischen Koronarthrombosen und Myokardinfarkten. Dtsch Med Wochenschr 1972; 12:443-448.

42. Chandler AB, Chapman I, Erhardt LR, et al. Coronary thrombosis in myocardial infarction. Am J Cardiol 1974; 34:823-833.

43. Sinapius D, Haeufigkeit und Morphologie der Coronarthrombose und ihre Beziehungen zur antithrombotischen und fibrinolytischen Behandlung. Klin Wochenschr 1965;43:37-43.

44. Favaloro RG, Effler DB, Cheanvechai C, et al. Acute coronary insufficiency (impending myocardial infarction and myocardial infarction): Surgical treatment by saphenous vein graft technique. Am J Cardiol 1971;28:598-605.

45. Berg R, Everhart FJ, Duvoisin G, et al. Operation for acute coronary occlusion. Am Surg 1976;42:517-521.

46. Hutter AM, Gold HK, Leinbach RC, et al. Various uses of intraaortic balloon pump in acute myocardial infarction: The first 24 hours in myocardial infarction. Witzstrock, New York-Baden-Baden-Koeln, 1977.

47. Bristow JD, Burchell HB, Campbell RW, et al. Report of the Ad Hoc committee on the indications for coarteriography. Circulation 1977;55:969A-974A.

Development and Pathophysiological Basis of Thrombolytic Therapy in Acute Myocardial Infarction: Part II. 1977-1980 The Pathogenetic Role of Thrombus Is Established by the Goettingen Pilot Studies of Mechanical Interventions and Intracoronary Thrombolysis in Acute Myocardial Infarction

K. Peter Rentrop, M.D.

From St. Vincent's Hospital and Medical Center and Columbia-Presbyterian Medical Center, New York, New York

Between 1977 and 1980, our group performed immediate coronary angiography in 158 patients admitted with acute myocardial infarction (MI) at the University of Goettinger, Germany. From June 1978 to May 1979, our pioneering study of mechanical transcatheter recanalization of acute total coronary artery occlusions using guidewires and tapered catheters was performed. Restoration of antegrade flow in 7 of 13 patients was associated with an improvement in left ventricular function not seen in historical controls. From June 1979 to December 1980, the pathogenetic role of thrombus and spasm in acute coronary syndromes was explored in our pioneering study of intracoronary streptokinase infusion. Following injection of nitroglycerin, streptokinase was selectively infused at a rate of 2000 U/minute for 50-95 minutes. Only four of the initial 22 infarct patients showed improvement of antegrade flow following intracoronary nitroglycerin alone. Reopening of the completely obstructed vessel or increase in lumen diameter at the site of subtotal occlusion occurred in 22 of 29 infarct patients within 15-90 minutes of streptokinase infusion but in none of the five patients with unstable angina. Chest pain was alleviated and left ventricular function was improved significantly after successful lysis. The first presentation of both our mechanical and pharmacological interventions in acute MI to a large international audience at the annual American Heart Association meeting in 1979 convinced clinicians of the etiologic role of fibrin-rich coronary thrombus in acute MI. The demonstration of rapid restoration of antegrade flow initiated a worldwide renaissance in the application of thrombolytic therapy and paved the way for primary angioplasty in acute MI. (J Interven Cardiol 1998;11:265-285)

From January 1977 to December 1980, this author, as head of the group investigating new therapies in acute MI at the University of Goettingen, Germany, conducted a series of protocols that involved immediate cardiac catheterization and coronary angiography in 158 patients admitted with the diagnosis of acute MI. The following sections will describe in historical sequence the evolution of these protocols and the insights we derived from each series. Drs. H. Blanke, K.R. Karsch, and H. Kaiser formed the core of the team.

I. Preliminary Studies (January 1977 to June 1978): Coronary Angiography in Cardiogenic Shock and Evolving Myocardial Infarction

In the initial protocol, it was attempted to assess the efficacy of intra-aortic balloon counterpulsation and coronary artery bypass surgery for the treatment of cardiogenic shock. The protocol was initiated by Dr. H. Kreuzer, Chairman of the Department of Cardiology at the University of Goettingen.[48] This author formally structured the cardiac catheterization team to provide care at the CCU level. Dedicated personnel monitored and managed hemodynamics, electrical stability, and chest pain.[49] The total amount of dye was limited to 1 mL/kg body weight in order to minimize volume loading and negative inotropic effects.[49] Nonionic dyes, which we evaluated in separate studies,[50] were soon used in this protocol.

Between January and October 1977, nine patients were enrolled. Intra-aortic balloon counterpulsation, which was initiated prior to angiography in eight patients, resulted in at least transient stabilization of hemodynamics in all cases. During angiography, hemodynamics did not worsen except for the one patient in whom intra-aortic balloon counterpulsation was not used. In spite of the initial stabilization achieved in eight patients, only two were discharged from the hospital.[48]

In keeping with larger studies,[46] this author concluded that cardiac catheterization can be performed safely, even in very ill patients with acute MI, as long as they are appropriately supported.[48] However, intra-aortic balloon counterpulsation and surgical revascularization were ultimately futile in patients with completed infarction. If there was any hope to stabilize patients in cardiogenic shock long-term, it was by revascularizing viable ischemic myocardium. Although it had not been proven in humans as yet, the importance of time in the evolution of infarction had been increasingly appreciated by groups performing surgical infarct revascularization.[46,48]

Therefore, this author curtailed the original study. In a new protocol, the efficacy of surgical revascularization for treating *early* cardiogenic shock was to be tested. The study was extended to patients with evolving infarction who were *not* in cardiogenic shock in order to assess the efficacy of intra-aortic balloon counterpulsation in limiting infarct size.[49] Patients who presented within 6 hours of onset of ischemic chest pain lasting more than 30 minutes were enrolled. Patients presenting 6-12 hours after symptom onset were enrolled only if they had on-going symptoms of ischemia. In order to minimize delays before intervention, the "objective" admission criteria of infarct studies performed at that time were abandoned, and confirmation of the diagnosis of infarction by changes in the ECG or enzyme release was not awaited. These parameters were used retrospectively only to confirm the admission diagnosis. We maintained these enrollment criteria in all our subsequent studies.

There were two additional in-hospital deaths among our initial group of 35 patients. No death occurred during angiography or appeared to be related to it. The only complication possibly related to acute angiography was ventricular fibrillation, which occurred in five patients and which was easily controlled. We concluded that coronary angiography is ethically justifiable in a research project.

Total occlusion of the infarct-related artery was found in 74% (26/35) of the patients,[49] confirming the in vivo results of Berg et al.'s study[45] and the postmortem findings of Sinapius.[41] In the remaining patients, lesions of ≥ 90% severity with at least partial antegrade filling of the infarct artery were found. The incidence of total occlusion among patients who were hemodynamically stable was comparable to that among patients in cardiogenic shock. This observation was not consistent with the postmortem studies of Walston et al. and at odds with their conclusion that thrombotic coronary artery occlusion results from a decrease in coronary flow in patients with low cardiac output.[16]

Necropsy studies were performed in all nonsurviving patients by Dr. D. Sinapius, Head of the Division of Angiopathology at the University of Goettingen. Sinapius consistently demonstrated to this author a coronary thrombus at the site at which in vivo angiography had identified an acute total occlusion. These thrombi were not just superimposed upon a severe coronary lesion as one would expect if they had been formed as a result of slow flow[15,16]; rather, they were all firmly attached to a ruptured plaque. A ruptured plaque complicated by a dissecting subintimal hemorrhage (Fig. 2B) was also found by Sinapius in all cases in which in vivo angiography had shown a subtotally occluded infarct lesion (Fig. 2A). These demonstrations made the publications of

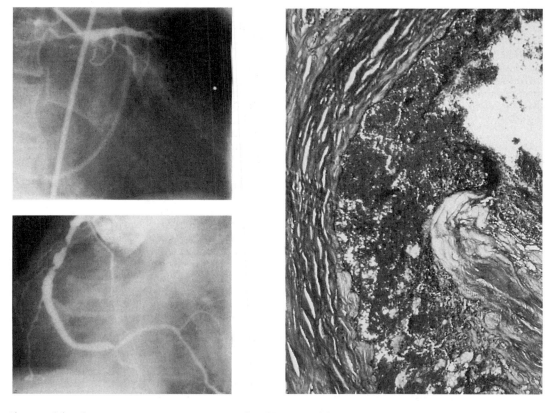

Figure 2A. Acute coronary angiogram of a 61-year-old man with an inferior wall infarct in cardiogenic shock. Chronic total occlusions of the left anterior descending and left circumflex branches (upper panel); severe lesions in the right coronary artery (lower panel). **Figure 2B.** Cross-section of the right coronary artery at the level of the first subtotal lesion showing plaque rupture and extensive subintimal hemorrhage.

Sinapius strikingly concrete to this author, and they exerted a profound impact on his further work.

II. The First Goettingen Pilot Study (June 1978 to June 1979): Acute Transluminal Coronary Artery Recanalization

The exploration of intra-aortic balloon counterpulsation and surgical revascularization in acute MI came to an abrupt end at the University of Goettingen in June 1978 when this author recanalized, in an unplanned emergency procedure, an acute total coronary occlusion.[51] This author is indebted for support of the subsequent phases of his work to Dr. H. Bretschneider, Chairman of the Department of Physiology, and Chairman of the "Sonderforschungsbereich," i.e., the Federal Research Fund (Score Grant) at the University of Goettingen.

Recanalization of an Iatrogenic Coronary Artery Occlusion with a Guidewire.

On June 13, 1978, a 45-year-old truck driver who had been admitted to the University Hospital in Goettingen with unstable angina pectoris underwent coronary angiography. At 12:15 p.m., immediately after contrast injections into the right coronary artery, which had demonstrated a subtotal occlusion (Fig. 3A), the patient complained of severe, persistent chest pain, and new inferior ST elevations were noted. This author was called, and repeat visualization of the right coronary artery revealed total occlusion at the site of the previous subtotal lesion (Fig. 3B).

Administration of large doses of nitroglycerin and opiates did not reverse the patient's clinical condition or restore antegrade flow. This author attributed the occlusion to a catheter-induced thrombus and pondered surgical revascularization and its inevitable loss of time. Perhaps this patient could be helped more effectively by restoring antegrade flow immediately using the catheter as a tool? After approximately 45 minutes of futile medical therapy, this author decided to attempt recanalization of the occluded right coronary artery using a modification of the "simple and effective technique," which had been developed by Dotter and Judkins in 1964 "for directly overcoming arteriosclerotic narrowing and occlusion in the arteries of the leg."[52] He gently advanced a 0.038-inch guidewire through the Sones catheter into the right coronary artery and across the occlusion without encountering significant resistance. Upon pullback of the wire, the patient reported instant cessation of chest pain, and the ECG reverted to baseline. Contrast injection demonstrated restoration of brisk antegrade flow at 1:00 p.m. (Fig. 3C). The episode of total right coronary artery occlusion had lasted 45 minutes.

The observations during this case were not compatible with W. Roberts' theory of the pathogenesis of acute MI according to which "even totally occluding thrombi when found in arteries more than 90% occluded by old atherosclerotic plaque may have little functional significance."[15] Both the abrupt progression from subtotal to total occlusion due to a catheter-induced thrombus and the recanalization of this artery by a simple guidewire maneuver had had profound clinical consequences.

Of more immediate concern to us, though, was the question of how to further treat our patient. How long would the channel, created by the wire, stay open? We were not aware of any publication at the time describing such a maneuver that we could have used as guidance. This author considered further dilatation of the lesion by recrossing it with the wire and advancing a small catheter over the wire (a modified Dotter technique), but ultimately decided against this because the patient was stable and the risks of transcatheter interventions in acute MI were unknown. Instead, he referred the patient for urgent surgical revas-

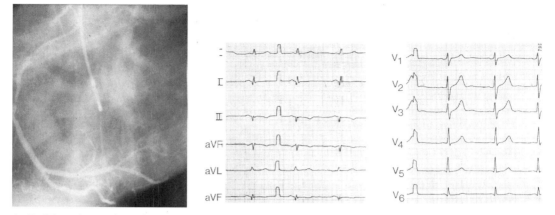

A. Lefthand panel: right coronary artery (RCA) in LAO projection, first injection. Righthand panel: ECG before angiography

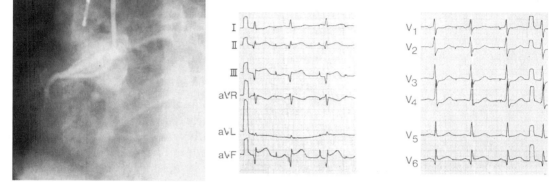

B. Right coronary artery and ECG after beginning of chest pain. (ECG calibration not optional due to emergency conditions.)

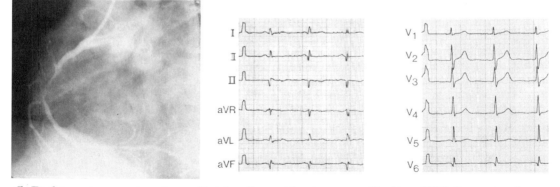

C. Right coronary artery immediately after guidewire recanalization; ECG 8 minutes later

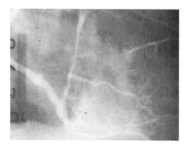

Figure 3. The first transluminal coronary artery recanalization in acute myocardial infarction. Use of a guidewire in an iatrogenic inferior wall infarct

D. Right coronary artery and vein graft 8 days after coronary artery bypass surgery

17

cularization. Heparin was administered during the 3-hour waiting period prior to surgery. The patient remained asymptomatic.

Follow-up angiography 9 days after surgery revealed patency of the saphenous vein graft to the right coronary artery *and of the recanalized right coronary artery* (Fig. 3D). Left ventriculography, as well as enzymatic, electrocardiographic, and thallium scintigraphic criteria indicated that this patient had not sustained any significant loss of myocardium during the 45-minute period of total coronary occlusion. This author concluded that revascularization of the infarct artery as an extension of the cardiac catheterization procedure had significantly shortened the period of ischemia and potentially salvaged myocardium when compared with the traditional revascularization option of emergent coronary artery bypass surgery. Therefore, this author decided to assess mechanical transcatheter interventions systematically in patients with acute evolving infarction and total occlusion of the infarct artery at acute angiography.[53] This departure from the standard medical therapy of the time, which consisted of bed rest, analgesics, and treatment of arrhythmias, was radical and criticized by some. However, the cardiac catheterization team, whom this author had trained during his studies of intra-aortic balloon counterpulsation and CABG for patients in cardiogenic shock and evolving infarction, was expertly prepared to perform these interventions without jeopardizing patient safety.

Acute Transluminal Coronary Artery Recanalization.

The only catheter-based technique for the treatment of CAD known at that time was percutaneous transluminal coronary balloon angioplasty, which had been introduced by Dr. A. Gruentzig et al. in 1977 to treat patients with stable angina pectoris.[54] It had not been used in acute MI.

The prototype balloon catheters manufactured at the time, which were made available in the spring of 1979 by Dr. A. Gruentzig to this author, had a short, stiff wire mounted at the tip of the balloon, which was not steerable. The devices were much more prone to cause vessel injury than were later, over-the-wire balloons. The risk was increased in patients with acute MI because there was no angiographic road map for advancing the balloon beyond the site of total occlusion. This author decided to defer the use of balloons in patients with acute MI and instead, modified Dotter's technique for recanalization of peripheral artery occlusions, using guidewires and nonballoon catheters, which were advanced over the wire. After testing various wires and catheters in animals, two techniques were used in the first series of patients:

1. The floppy tip of a 0.032-inch or a 0.038-inch guidewire was advanced beyond the total occlusion with careful attention to any indirect signs of impending dissection, such as wire buckling or the tactile sense of resistance. After pullback of the wire, changes in flow were assessed by repeat angiography (Fig. 4).

2. An end-hole recanalization catheter with a long taper from 1.7 mm at the shaft to 0.7 mm at the tip was combined with a 0.018-inch guidewire to recanalize and dilate the occlusion. The system was advanced through a preshaped guiding catheter with an internal diameter of 1.9 mm. Dye injections through the end-hole of the recanalization catheter were used to confirm correct intraluminal position of the system after the total occlusion appeared to have been crossed. Subsequently, the catheter was advanced far into the occluded vessel in order to dilate ("Dotter") the occlusion (Fig. 5). Following pullback of the recanalization catheter, the result of the intervention was documented by angiography.

Recanalization of a totally occluded infarct artery was attempted in 16 patients. In 1979

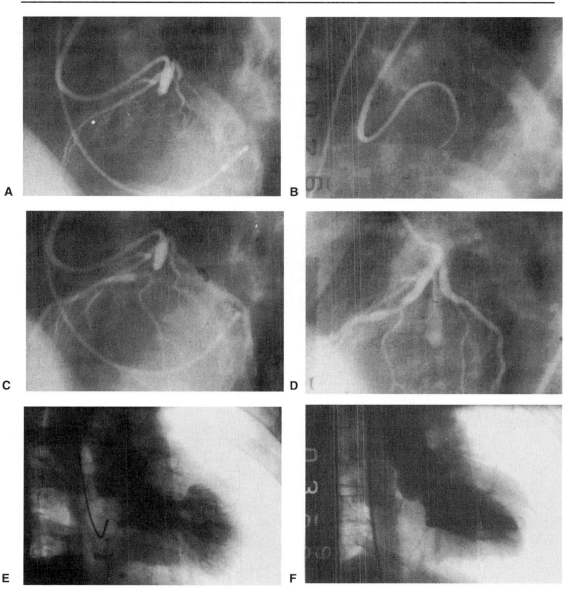

Figure 4. The first transluminal recanalization with a guidewire in a spontaneously occurring infarct. A. Subselective contrast injection into the totally occluded left anterior descending artery (LAD) through a Shirey catheter (LAO) cranial view). B. Special 0.038-inch guidewire advanced beyond the total occlusion. C. LAD immediately after withdrawal of the guidewire. Antegrade flow apparent. D. LAD 5 months later: spontaneous improvement of lumen. E. Left ventriculogram, RAO projection, end systole, before LAD recanalization. F. Left ventriculogram 5 months later.

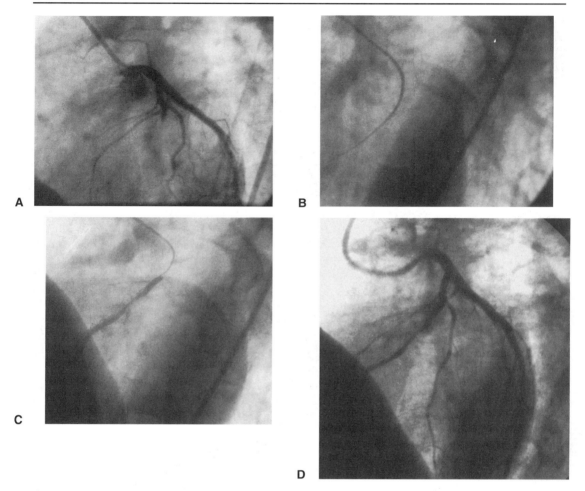

Figure 5. Transluminal recanalization in acute myocardial infarction with a modified "Dotter" technique. A. Preintervention angiogram LAO view: total occlusion of the left anterior descending artery (LAD). B. Recanalization catheter, which tapers from a 1.7-mm shaft to a 0.7-mm tip, has been advanced over a 0.018-inch guidewire across the occlusion. C. Selective dye injection into the recanalized LAD through the recanalization catheter, which has been pulled back into the proximal vessel.
D. Predischarge angiography of the left coronary artery

we published the results obtained in the first 13 patients, in whom the intervention was performed within 7.8 ± 8.3 hours of the onset of infarct symptoms.[53] There were no in-hospital deaths. One patient experienced an episode of asystole, and two patients had ventricular fibrillation during angiography; all were easily controlled. Dangerous reperfusion arrhythmias, as observed by Sommers and Jennings in animal experiments,[55] did not occur; in fact, there were no complications attributable to the recanalization attempts.

Injection of dye through the recanalization catheter enabled, for the first time, direct in vivo visualization of the coronary artery segment beyond the site of total occlusion. In two patients, mobile filling defects were observed, which extended distally from the total occlusion (Fig. 6). These mobile filling defects were interpreted as distal apposition thrombus, extending from the primary thrombus, which appeared firmly attached to the vessel wall. The most distal portion of the thrombus was separated from the region of the infarct by an

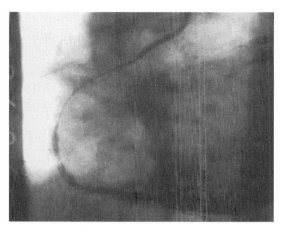

Figure 6. First in vivo visualization of a distal apposition thrombus in acute myocardial infarction. The tip of the recanalization catheter has been advanced just distal to the total occlusion of the right coronary artery. Injection of contrast media into the distal vessel revealed a mobile filling defect, attached to the site of total occlusion.

uninvolved segment of artery, an observation that confirmed previous necropsy reports[41,42] and that supported the notion that thrombotic coronary artery occlusion does not result from a direct effect of the infarcting myocardium upon the subtending coronary artery.

Restoration of antegrade flow after pullback of the recanalization device was observed in 7 of 13 patients. These patients were subsequently treated with heparin followed by long-term warfarin therapy. Repeat angiography in the chronic stage of infarction, which was performed in 6 of the patients who had experienced initial successful recanalization, revealed no reocclusion and further enlargement of the lumen in 4 of the 6 patients (Fig. 4).

Serial ventriculographic studies in the patients who had successful transcatheter revascularization revealed significant improvement in local wall motion and an increase in ejection fraction from $45\% \pm 6.5\%$ prior to intervention to $54.6\% \pm 11.6\%$ at chronic angiography (Fig. 7). It could not be determined whether this improvement of left ventricular function was attributable to the mechanical interventions, since the natural history of total coronary artery occlusion and left ventricular function in patients with acute MI was unknown at the time.

Spontaneous Coronary Artery Recanalization Following Acute Myocardial Infarction Demonstrated by Serial Angiography (Fall 1978 to June 1979).

We used serial angiography to study the spontaneous evolution of total coronary occlusion and left ventricular function in nine patients with acute MI. In these patients recanalization had not been attempted because acute angiography had been performed prior to the introduction of recanalization techniques or they had unfavorable anatomy for a recanalization attempt.[53]

Restoration of antegrade flow had not occurred during acute angiography in any of the nine patents when contrast injections were repeated in different planes. However, angiography in the chronic stage of infarction documented brisk antegrade flow in 4 of the 9 infarct vessels with residual lesions between 80% and 95% (Figs. 8 and 9).

However, serial ventriculographic studies in these nine patients demonstrated

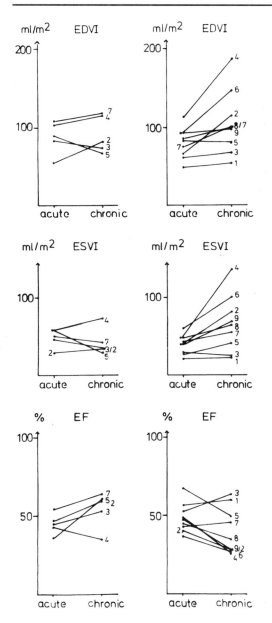

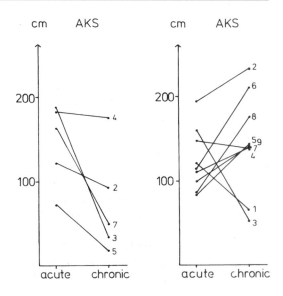

Figure 7. Changes of left ventricular function determined by biplane cineventriculography in the acute and chronic stages of infarction. Left panel: after transluminal coronary artery re-canalization; Right panel: in a comparison group. A. End diastolic volume index (EDVI). B. End systolic volume index (ESVI). C. Left ventricular ejection fraction (EF). D. Length of the akinetic segment (AKS).

results that were significantly different from those observed in the mechanical recanalization group. Local wall motion had deteriorated significantly and ejection fraction had decreased from 48.9% ± 9% to 40.9% ± 14.5% (Fig. 7).

The finding of spontaneous recanalization in nearly half of the totally occluded infarct vessels was new and had important pathophysiological implications. We con-

cluded that the mechanical interventions that we had introduced had accelerated a process that would occur spontaneously in many cases. Furthermore, we hypothesized that the acceleration of recanalization could preserve left ventricular function by salvaging jeopardized myocardium.[53]

Both spontaneous recanalization of total occlusions and spontaneous improvement of lumen following mechanical re-

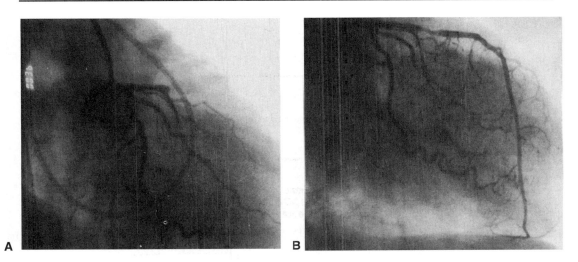

Figure 8. Spontaneous coronary artery recanalization demonstrated by serial coronary angiography in a patient with acute anterior wall infarction. A. Left coronary artery, 10 hours after onset of infarct symptoms: total occlusion of the left anterior descending artery. B. Three months later: 80% lesion in the left anterior descending artery.

canalization were compatible with the hypothesis that acute infarction is caused by coronary thrombosis. Necropsy studies had shown that retraction of coronary artery thrombi from the intact portion of the intimal surface and dissolution of thrombus by activation of the endogenous thrombolytic system can occur within 2-14 weeks after MI.[56,57]

Does Coronary Spasm Play a Central Role in the Pathogenesis of Acute Myocardial Infarction?

In 1977 Oliva and Breckinridge reported that intracoronary injection of nitroglycerin within 10.5 hours after onset of acute MI restored antegrade flow in 40% (6/15) of their study patients. They concluded that spasm exits in at least 40% of patients within 10.5 hours from the onset of infarct symptoms.[58]

The possible role of spasm in the pathogenesis of acute MI was further explored by Maseri et al. in 1978, in a study of eight patients who were assessed during attacks of preinfarction angina pectoris with transient ST-T changes and who subsequently developed MI.[59] Hemodynamic monitoring indicated that the episodes of preinfarction angina were caused by transient decreases in coronary flow and not by increases in myocardial oxygen demand, leading to the concept of *dynamic* coronary stenosis. Coronary angiography during anginal attacks revealed a total or subtotal coronary occlusion with absent or poor distal filling and restoration of prompt distal filling after administration of sublingual nitroglycerin in all patients. Maseri et al. concluded that the dynamic stenosis was due to a focal vasospasm, superimposed, in most cases, on an atherosclerotic lesion. Thallium scintigraphy during anginal attacks showed a transient massive transmural deficit of tracer uptake in the ventricular wall corresponding to the transient ST-T changes. All subsequent infarcts occurred in the area that showed electrocardiographic changes during the anginal attack. Postmortem examination in one patient and coronary angiography after infarction in two patients revealed complete, thrombotic occlusion of the branch that had had reversible occlusion during the anginal attack. The authors concluded that occlusive vasospasm and the attendant stagnation of blood flow may be responsible for thrombosis and MI.

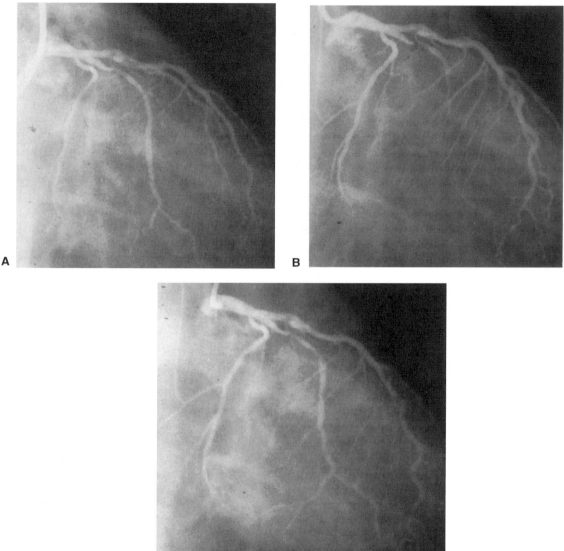

Figure 9. Serial angiography in a patient with lateral wall infarction. A. Left coronary artery during episode of unstable angina 2 weeks prior to infarction. The intermediate branch is severely narrowed but fills promptly and completely. B. During acute myocardial infarction, the intermediate branch is subtotally occluded and fills with delay and incompletely. C. Four weeks after acute myocardial infarction: prompt and complete antegrade filling of the lateral branch.

Our observation of spontaneous recanalization of infarct vessels could be explained by spontaneous release of coronary spasm as well as by endogenous thrombolysis. Thus, the hypothesis of the central role of plaque rupture and coronary thrombosis in the pathogenesis of acute MI was challenged again. Our angiographic observations and mechanical interventions had provided important, but still rather indirect, data concerning the pathogenesis of acute MI. Perhaps more direct evidence could be obtained from pharmacological interventions aimed at selectively reversing the different mechanisms that might be responsible for acute coronary artery occlusion.

III. The Second Goettingen Pilot Study (June 1979 to December 1980): Intracoronary Thrombolytic Therapy

On June 22, 1979, this author initiated a clinical study designed to determine the pathogenetic roles of thrombus and spasm in acute MI.[60] The approach tested in this study had evolved during a 9-month period of intense discussions among members of our group and was greatly influenced by the studies of Dr. D. Sinapius, with whom this author was privileged to work at the time.

The Composition and Length of Occlusive Coronary Thrombi.

The generally held conviction of the 1960s and 1970s that thrombolytic therapy was not a useful method to restore antegrade flow in occluded coronary arteries was based on small and inconclusive studies of the composition and length of coronary thrombi. Hampton reported that occlusive arterial thrombi are composed primarily of platelets, and he concluded that the paucity of fibrin may make them a poor target for thrombolytic therapy.[61] Lasch suggested that coronary thrombi are too long to allow the rapid restoration of antegrade flow required to salvage my-

ocardium.[18] The first large autopsy study using appropriate methodology to assess the composition and length of occlusive coronary thrombi was published in 1972 by Sinapius.[62] In 91 cases of acute MI, Sinapius differentiated three groups of thrombi. There were 41 *coagulation thrombi,* which contained primarily erythrocytes and only very small amounts of platelets. Usually, there was a well-developed network of fibrin in such thrombi. There were 14 *platelet thrombi.* which contained primarily platelets and only small amounts of fibrin. *Mixed thrombi,* a combination of coagulation and platelet thrombi, were found in 36 cases. The majority of mixed thrombi contained large quantities of fibrin. Adding the coagulation thrombi and the mixed thrombi with large amounts of fibrin, Sinapius concluded that approximately 80% of occlusive coronary thrombi would be appropriately targeted by thrombolytic therapy; 20% would be expected to be resistant to such an intervention.

The average length of an occlusive coronary thrombus was found to be 20.2 mm. Thrombi in the LAD were shorter (16.6 mm) than were those in the RCA (24.3 mm). In fact, 76% of the LAD thrombi were 12 mm or less. Extrapolating from data published regarding the duration of femoral artery recanalization by intravenous thrombolytic therapy, Sinapius estimated that the shorter coronary thrombi could be dissolved in 1-2 hours with an intravenous streptokinase infusion.

Sinapius' study failed to influence the thinking of clinicians until the end of 1978, when this author designed a study that would use coronary angiography to assess the speed and frequency of coronary artery recanalization achieved with standard intravenous streptokinase therapy. However, prior to its initiation, this protocol was to undergo an important change based on further analysis of the biochemical composition of coronary thrombi and the mechanisms of thrombolysis. Dr. H. Koestering, the hematologist on our team, contributed importantly to this analysis.

Exolysis and Endolysis.

The plasminemia caused by intravenous thrombolytic therapy results in breakdown of fibrin at sites exposed to the systemic circulation, i.e., the proximal and possibly the distal surface of the thrombus if collateral flow is present. This progressive dissolution of thrombus from the outside has been termed exolysis.

Thrombi contain a large amount of plasminogen, which is bound to the fibrin strands. In the 1970s several techniques were developed to activate the fibrin-bound plasminogen within the thrombus, a process called endolysis. These techniques were used to dissolve large chronic thrombi in peripheral arteries, which were difficult to dissolve with the standard intravenous application, requiring an infusion of a total of 2.5 million U of streptokinase daily for up to 5 days.

Mueller-Fassbender and Hess[63] in Munich, Germany, recanalized chronic peripheral artery thrombi with the transcutaneous catheter method developed by Dotter prior to intravenous thrombolysis in order to facilitate diffusion of streptokinase directly into the thrombus. They were able to recanalize 10 of 15 segmental occlusions of the femoral artery, which were 4-8 months old.[63]

Koestering et al. used a selective infusion technique to recanalize thrombosed Scribner shunts. They injected streptokinase, 20,000 U, every 5 minutes into the thrombosed artery and recanalized the vessels within 30-40 minutes.[64]

Coronary artery recanalization was attempted with a semiselective infusion technique in patients with acute MI as early as 1960 by Boucek and Murphy.[65] They positioned a catheter within the coronary sinus, close to the origin of the coronary artery that was presumed to be occluded. The selection of the coronary sinus was determined by electrocardiographic infarct location. They then infused 75,000 U of thrombolysin, a mixture of streptokinase and plasminogen, over 1 hour. In 6 of the 8 study patients, SGOT peaks occurred earlier and were lower than in conventionally treated patients, a finding that the authors interpreted as indirect evidence of rapid thrombolysis and salvage of myocardium by reperfusion. Contrast injections documenting coronary artery occlusion and recanalization were not performed.

In 1970 Moschos et al. assessed a selective coronary infusion technique in dogs.[66] They induced coronary artery thrombi and subsequently administered urokinase or thrombolysin, at a rate of 2,000 U/kg per hour, directly into the occluded vessel. Selective coronary angiography revealed that all seven acute coronary thrombi treated with this regimen were recanalized within 30-60 minutes, whereas intravenous infusion of 4,000 U/kg per hour for 4 hours in six animals failed to lyse the thrombi. Kordenat et al. also used an intracoronary infusion technique and achieved lysis of experimentally induced coronary thrombi in dogs within 15 minutes.[67] It appeared likely that the high concentration of thrombolytic agents achieved with intracoronary infusion resulted in diffusion of the drug into the thrombus, initiating endolysis.

Based on these studies, we hypothesized that an intracoronary, rather than an intravenous, infusion of streptokinase would be required to assess the full potential of thrombolytic therapy for the dissolution of occlusive coronary thrombi. Furthermore, use of a coronary catheter for selective drug delivery would allow angiographic documentation of the result as an integral part of the therapeutic intervention, whereas with intravenous application, diagnostic angiography would be an additional invasive procedure.

The total amount of fibrinolytic agent required to dissolve an arterial thrombus appeared to be much smaller using endolytic techniqes rather than the standard intravenous infusion. Verstraete[68] and Lopacius et al.[69] found only a minor decrease in fibrinogen levels following the intermittent application of streptokinase to a total dose of 250,000 U over 30 minutes.

Their finding suggested to us that the likelihood of catastrophic bleeding complications could be reduced by endolytic techniques.

Intracoronary Streptokinase Infusion in Evolving Myocardial Infarction: Protocol and Initial Results.

In the spring of 1979, we redesigned our protocol, abandoning intravenous infusion of streptokinase and adopting selective infusion techniques. Following coronary angiography, a nitroglycerin bolus, 0.15-0.45 mg would be injected into the infarct-related artery as per Oliva's and Breckinridge's protocol.[58] Subsequently, streptokinase would be selectively injected into the infarct artery at a rate of 2,000 U/min for 50-95 minutes. The infarct-related artery would be visualized after the nitroglycerin bolus and approximately every 15 minutes during the streptokinase infusion; if recanalization occurred, the infusion was to be continued until brisk antegrade filling (TIMI III in today's terminology) had been achieved. The most important adjunctive medications were heparin 10,000 U IV followed by long-term anticoagulation with warfarin. Since our observations in the first few patients had far-reaching impact on the further development of thromboytic therapy in acute MI,[60] they will be described again in some detail on the following sections.

The first study patient presented on June 22, 1979, with an acute anterior wall infarct. Coronary angiography revealed a subtotal lesion in the proximal segment of the left anterior descending artery. The lesion was concentric; there was no filling defect. Both intracoronary nitroglycerin and intracoronary streptokinase failed to change the angiographic appearance of the lesion or the clinical condition of the patient. He was ultimately stabilized with bypass surgery.

The second study patient presented on July 1, 1979, and also had an acute anterior

wall MI (Fig. 10A). His left anterior descending artery was totally occluded in the middle segment (Fig. 10B). Intracoronary administration of nitroglycerin failed to establish flow. Following perforation of the occlusion with a guidewire (Fig. 10C), incomplete antegrade filling of the artery was achieved (Fig. 10D). An intracoronary streptokinase infusion, 2,000 U/hour, was immediately initiated. The patient became asymptomatic within 5 minutes. The anterior ST-elevations decreased rapidly. Repeat dye injection after 50 minutes of streptokinase infusion revealed brisk, complete antegrade filling of the left anterior descending artery (Fig. 10E). In today's language, the guidewire recanalization had changed antegrade flow from "TIMI 0" to "TIMI I"; the streptokinase infusion had further improved flow to "TIMI III." The peak CPK value was 1,050 U/L.

Due to electrical instability, bypass surgery was performed the following day. Intraoperative inspection revealed no signs of infarction. A transmural myocardial biopsy was obtained from the anteroapical segment. Microscopic examination revealed acute, disseminated necrosis of individual myocytes in the subendocardial layer but no confluence of necrotic foci (Fig. 11). There was no evidence of myocardial hemorrhage. This pattern of necrosis was different from that typically associated with total occlusion of a coronary artery. We concluded from the clinical response and the histologic evidence that revascularization of the infarct-related artery within less than 4 hours of symptom onset had aborted an evolving infarct before it came to involve the full thickness of the myocardial wall.

The third study patient presented on July 13, 1979, with an acute inferior wall infarct. His dominant right coronary artery was completely occluded before the bifurcation. Intracoronary nitroglycerin, 0.15 mg, promptly resulted in the establishment of complete antegrade filling and a decrease in inferior ST-segment elevations. However, these benefits were only transient. It was the subsequent intracoronary

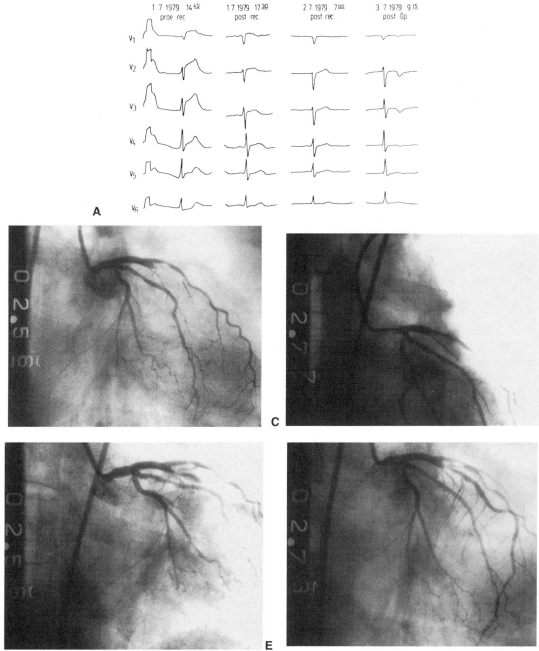

Figure 10. First coronary artery recanalization by combined mechanical and selective thrombolytic intervention (Patient A.B.). A. Electrocardiogram, chest leads of patient A.B. before recanalization of the left anterior descending artery (LAD) (pre-rec.), after recanalization of the LAD (post-rec.), and after coronary artery bypass surgery (post-op).B. Left coronary artery 2 hours and 20 minutes after onset of infarct symptoms; total occlusion of the left anterior descending artery. C. Guidewire is advanced across the total occlusion of the LAD 3 hours and 20 minutes after symptom onset. D. Incomplete antegrade filling of the LAD immediately after the guidewire has been pulled back. E. Prompt complete antegrade filling of the LAD after intracoronary infusion of 120,000 U of streptokinase over 50 minutes (4 hours, 10 minutes, after symptom onset).

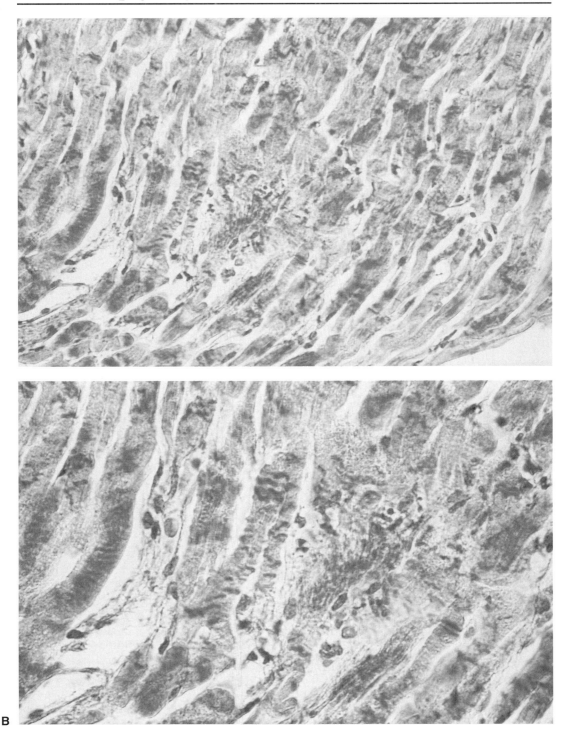

Figure 11. Intraoperative transmural myocardial biopsy obtained approximately 20 hours after recanalization of the left anterior descending artery from the anteroapical region (stain: Lie, modification of Tausch). Patient A.B. (see Fig. 10). A. Subendocardial layer showing mostly intact myocytes, and acute, focal necrosis of individual myocytes as well as beginning leucocyte exsudation. Magnification × 350. B. Subendocardial layer focusing on an area of myocyte necrosis. Magnification × 560.

infusion of streptokinase that resulted in progressive and sustained recanalization of the right coronary artery and sustained clinical improvement.

On August 6, 1979, when the fourth study patient presented also with an inferior infarction, we experienced the treacherousness of charting unknown territory. The left circumflex artery had a filling defect, which subtotally occluded it; antegrade flow was delayed and incomplete. Following intracoronary administration of nitroglycerin, 0.3 mg, antegrade flow became brisk, and the patient's pain resolved, although the filling defect did not change. Approximately 15 minutes after initiation of the streptokinase infusion, the patient became abruptly hypotensive and developed a complete left bundle branch block. Coronary angiography revealed a new filling defect, which completely occluded the proximal portion of the initially patent left anterior descending artery. The filling defect in the left circumflex artery had become smaller. With forceful repeat injection of dye, the filling defect in the left anterior descending artery disintegrated and embolized distally, prompt antegrade flow was restored, and the patient stabilized clinically. This author hypothesized that the transient occlusion of the left anterior descending artery had been caused by embolization of a platelet thrombus from the tip of the coronary catheter. In all future cases, aspirin, 1 g, was administered intravenously prior to acute interventions to prevent similar platelet thrombus formation.

The fifth patient presented on August 30, 1979, with an acute anterior wall infarct and total occlusion of the left anterior descending artery (Fig. 12). An acute bend in the proximal vessel precluded mechanical intervention with the instruments available at the time. Intracoronary administration of nitroglycerin, 0.3 mg, did not restore flow. However, 15 minutes after initiation of the intracoronary streptokinase infusion, multifocal PVCs were noted and angiography revealed complete, brisk antegrade filling of the left anterior descending artery. This was the first case in which rapid coronary artery recanalization was achieved solely with fibrinolytic therapy.

We concluded that thrombotic material, containing a significant amount of fibrin, was present at the site of acute obstruction in all three patients with total occlusion and in 1 of the 2 patients (patient 4) with subtotal occlusion in whom a filling defect was dissolved.

The effect of intracoronary nitroglycerin on the occlusions was much less impressive than that of selective thrombolysis. Intracoronary nitroglycerin failed to affect the degree of obstruction or distal filling in 3 of the 5 patients. The improved distal filling seen after intracoronary nitroglycerin in two patients could be regarded as evidence of spasm; however, it could also have resulted from an increase in caliber of the large conductance vessels.

After completion of thrombolytic therapy, residual lesions ranging between 60% and 90% severity persisted. This finding was in agreement with postmortem observations demonstrating that thrombotic coronary occlusion usually occurs at a site of significant atherosclerotic narrowing.

Roberts' hypothesis that coronary thrombosis in arteries severely narrowed by old plaque has little functional significance and is a secondary event after myocardial necrosis[12,15] had been seriously challenged by our previous observations of improvement in symptoms and left ventricular function following mechanical coronary artery recanalization. The new finding of rapid alleviation of chest pain and decrease of ST-elevations associated with restoration of antegrade flow by fibrinolytic therapy provided stronger evidence that occlusive coronary thrombosis can cause profound myocardial ischemia and infarction even if there is a severe preexisting stenosis.

Our findings and conclusions were published in October 1979 in *Clinical Cardiology*.[60] During the summer and fall of

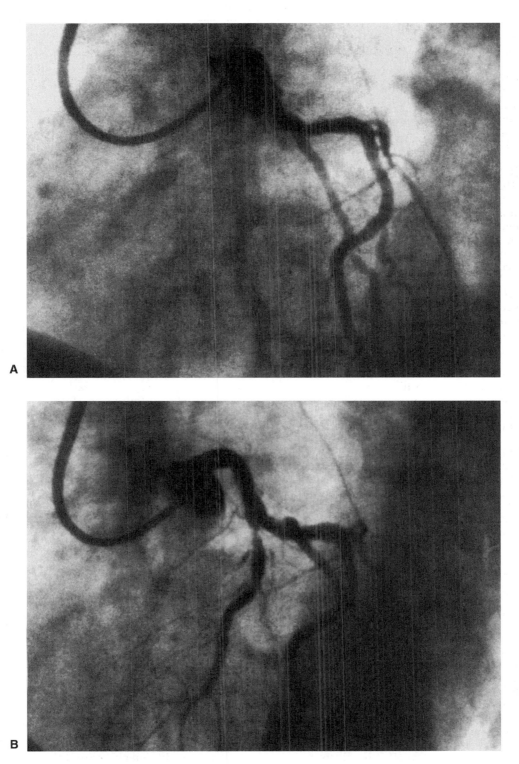

Figure 12. First recanalization of a coronary artery in acute myocardial infarction by intra-coronary streptokinase infusion alone. A. Left coronary artery, LAO cranial view before intervention. Total occlusion of the left anterior descending artery.

B. 15 minutes after beginning of intracoronary streptokinase infusion, 2000 U/min. Complete, prompt antegrade filling of the left anterior descending artery. Lucency at the site of previous total occlusion indicates residual thrombus.

1979, this author shared his observations with several investigators in Europe and the United States who were interested in duplicating his studies.

Demonstration of Coronary Artery Recanalization in Acute Myocardial Infarction at the American Heart Association (AHA) Meeting in Anaheim 1979.

The first presentation of our observations to a large international audience occurred the following month at the annual meeting of the AHA in Anaheim, California in 1979.[70] The printed abstract described the techniques and results of our mechanical revascularizations with guidewires and catheters but not our intracoronary thrombolytic interventions. Acceptance of this abstract had not come as a surprise since 1 year before, at the previous AHA meeting, Andreas Gruentzig had opened the minds of cardiologists to mechanical intravascular interventions with his presentation of the first percutaneous transluminal coronary angioplasty procedures in patients with stable angina pectoris.

The evening before his speech in Anaheim, this author decided to expand his presentation beyond the contents of the published abstract and to show angiograms of coronary artery recanalization with intracoronary streptokinase infusion as well. He felt that these angiograms provided crucial new evidence for the etiologic role of thrombus in acute MI. He was also concerned that his abstract reporting the first patients treated with intracoronary streptokinase, which had been submitted for the subsequent spring meeting of the American College of Cardiology in 1980, would not be accepted. Since coronary thrombus was still considered a consequence and not the cause of acute MI, there was not much interest in its lysis. The presentation in Anaheim turned out to be a watershed event. The angiograms of acute coronary artery recanalization convinced many clinicians and investigators of the etiologic role

of coronary thrombus. Much interest was expressed in learning the details of these techniques. Interventional cardiology, which had been restricted up to that point to angioplasty in stable angina pectoris, was now expanded to include the treatment of acute MI. Upon his return from Anaheim, this author found that the abstract reporting on intracoronary nitroglycerin and streptokinase application had indeed been rejected.

Expanding the Use of Intracoronary Streptokinase to Include Patients with Unstable Angina Pectoris.

During the subsequent 6-month period, we expanded our study at the University of Goettingen to 29 patients with acute MI. In addition, we enrolled five patients with unstable angina pectoris.[71] All five patients with unstable angina presented with subtotal coronary lesions. They failed to respond by clinical and angiographic criteria to both intracoronary spasmolytic and thrombolytic therapy.

Among the 29 patients with acute MI, total occlusions of the infarct vessel were found in 21 and subtotal lesions in 8. Total occlusion was successfully recanalized in 17 patients (81%). In 12 of these 17 patients, interventions preceding fibrinolytic therapy failed, and recanalization occurred within 15-90 minutes of intracoronary streptokinase infusion. All five patients in whom initially total occlusions were recanalized with intracoronary application of nitroglycerin (n = 3) or a guidewire maneuver (n = 2) demonstrated further improvement of lumen during the intracoronary streptokinase infusion.

Among the eight infarct patients with subtotal lesions of the infarct-related vessel, five exhibited improvement of lumen or flow. Four of these five patients responded to intracoronary streptokinase alone, and one showed some improvement of flow after intracoronary nitroglycerin and further improvement of lumen after the streptokinase infusion.

Left ventricular function improved immediately after restoration of antegrade flow among the infarct patients. LVEDP decreased from 20.4 ± 8.4 mmHg before the intervention to 15.7 ± 7.3 mmHg after the intervention (P < 0.005). Ejection fraction increased from 50.5% ± 12% to 54.6% ± 9% (P < 0.05). Repeat angiography in the chronic stage of MI revealed a further increase in ejection fraction to 56.6% ± 12%.

During aortocoronary bypass surgery, which was performed in six patients after the intervention, active contraction of the reperfused myocardium was noted; macroscopically, there was no evidence of transmural infarction. Myocardial biopsy obtained in two patients revealed only small foci of subendocardial necrosis (Fig 13).

These findings led to three conclusions and one hypothesis:

1. We concluded that lysis of acute coronary artery thrombi in humans by application of a thrombolytic agent does not require hours as was then generally believed[18] but could be achieved rapidly.
2. We concluded that the etiologic role of fibrin-rich coronary artery thrombi in the pathogenesis of acute MI was no longer questionable. Such thrombi cause the majority of infarcts. The role of fibrin containing thrombus remained uncertain in those patients who failed to respond to intracoronary thrombolysis. Failure of thrombolytic therapy was noted in only 19% (4/21) of infarct patients with total occlusions, but in 38% (3/8) of those with subtotal occlusions and in all five patients with unstable angina pectoris. A possible explanation for the failure of thrombolytic therapy in infarct patients with total occlusion was offered by Sinapius' autopsy finding that 20% of occlusive coronary thrombi consist exclusively or predominantly of platelets and contain very little fibrin.
3. We concluded that while the role of spasm in the pathogenesis of acute MI needed further investigation, spasmolysis was far less efficacious than thrombolyis in achieving sustained coronary artery recanalization in acute MI.

We hypothesized that rapid restoration of antegrade coronary flow by thrombolytic therapy in the early hours of MI can halt the progression of myo-cardial necrosis, resulting in salvage of jeopar-dized myocardium and preservation of myocardial function.

The results and conclusions derived from our expanded patient series were presented at the annual meeting of the AHA in 1980[72] and published as a full paper in *Circulation* in 1981.[71]

The Pathogenetic Role of Thrombus in Acute Myocardial Infarction Is Substantiated by Other Groups (1980).

The 1980 AHA meeting was also the first major international forum at which other investigators to whom this author had shown his angiograms in 1979 presented their results, including Drs. W. Ganz, H.K. Gold, and D. Mathey.[73-75] It was demonstrated that rapid coronary artery recanalization could be reproducibly achieved by the techniques developed by this author. The pathogenetic role of thrombus in acute MI was now generally accepted.

In October 1980, De Wood et al. from Spokane published a retrospective study of angiography in acute MI in the *New England Journal of Medicine*,[76] in which the authors expanded their previous reports of retrieval of thrombus from the infarct artery during emergency coronary artery bypass surgery.[45,77] Whereas their initial reports of intraoperative thrombus retrieval in 1974 and 1976 had not been widely noted, this finding was now embraced as further substantiation of the pathogenetic role of thrombus.[76]

De Wood et al. confirmed both their and our earlier findings of a high incidence

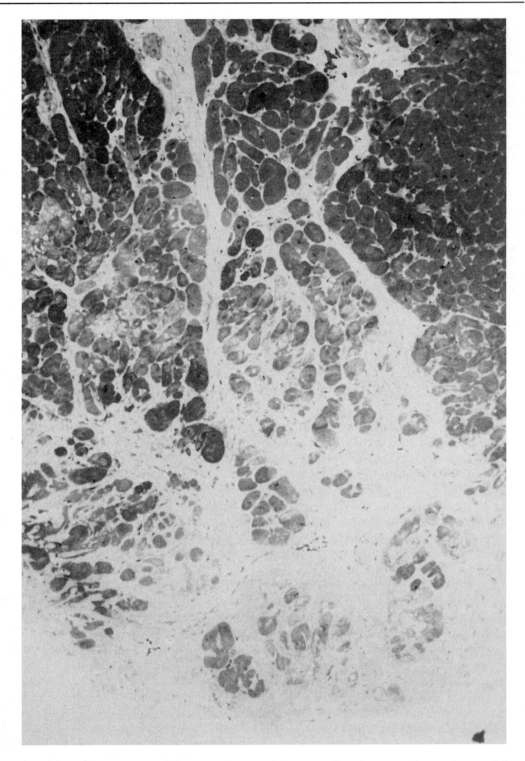

Figure 13. Myocardial biopsy from the center of the reperfused myocardium obtained during elective coronary artery bypass surgery several weeks after intracoronary streptokinase infusion. There is a subendocardial scar of < 1-mm thickness; otherwise, normal myocardium. (Stain: Toludin-blue; magnification × 140).

of total coronary occlusion in the early hours of infarction.[45,49,76] A new finding of De Wood et al.'s study was the significant decrease in the prevalence of total coronary occlusion from 87% (110/126) among patients evaluated within 4 hours of symptom onset to 65% (37/57) among those studied after 12-24 hours. De Wood et al. concluded that "coronary spasm or thrombus formation with subsequent recanalization or both may be important in the evolution of infarction." Quoting Oliva's and our studies, they suggested that intracoronary application of nitroglycerin or streptokinase "may help to define the contribution of spasm or thrombosis or both during the early hours of acute infarction."

We had documented spontaneous recanalization of totally occluded infarct arteries directly by serial angiograms in the same patients in an earlier study.[53] But we felt that the time frame of spontaneous recanalization might be different from that suggested by De Wood et al.'s study. The decrease in the frequency of total coronary occlusion during the initial 24 hours of infarction observed in De Wood et al.'s retrospective study could indicate a selection bias rather than spontaneous recanalization of total occlusion. We concluded that in future trials, the incidence of total occlusion in acute MI would need to be assessed prospectively by serial angiography in the same patients.[78]

References

48. Blanke H, Rentrop P, Karsch KR, et al. Invasive Diagnostik und Therapie im kardiogenen Schock. In: Bruckner JB, ed. Berlin-Heidelberg-New York: Springer-Verlag, 1980, pp. 373-378.

49. Rentrop KP, Blanke H, Karsch KR, et al. Koronarmorphologie und linksventrikulaere Pumpfunktion im akuten Infarktstadium und ihre Aenderungen im chronischem Stadium. Z Kardiol 1979;68:335-350.

50. Zipfel J, Baller D, Blanke H, et al. Reduktion kardialer Nebenwirkungen von Roentgenkontrastmitteln in der Angiokardiographie durch Zusatz von Kalzium und Verwendung eines nichtionischen Kontrastmittels. Klin Wochenschr 1980;58:1339-1346.

51. Rentrop P, DeVivie ER, Karsch KR, et al. Acute coronary occlusion with impending infarction as an angiographic complication relieved by a guide-wire recanalization. Clin Cardiol 1978;1:101-106.

52. Dotter CT, Judkins MP. Transluminal treatment of arteriosclerotic obstruction. Description of a technique and a preliminary report of its application. Circulation 1964;30:654-670.

53. Rentrop KP, Blanke H, Karsch KR. Initial experience with transluminal recanalization of the recently occluded infarct-related coronary artery in acute myocardial infarction-Comparison with conventionally treated patients. Clin Cardiol 1979;2:92-105.

54. Gruentzig AR, Myler RK, Hanna AS, et al. Perioperative dilatation of coronary artery stenosis: Percutaneous coronary transluminal angioplasty. (abstract) Circulation 1977;84:55-56.

55. Sommers HM, Jennings RB. The influence of procaine amide and oxygen on the onset of ventricular fibrillation following temporary occlusion of the left circumflex coronary artery. (Abstract) Fed Proc 1964;23:444.

56. Fulton WFM. The coronary arteries. Vol. III. Springfield, IL: Charles C. Thomas, 1965.

57. Chandler AP, Chapman J, Erhardt LE. "Salvage" with assisted circulation in acute myocardial infarction and shock. Am J Cardiol 1974;34:373-380.

58. Oliva PB, Breckinridge JC. Arteriographic evidence of coronary arterial spasm in acute myocardial infarction. Circulation 1977;56:366-374.

59. Maseri A, L'Abbate A, Baroldi G, et al. Coronary vasospasm as a possible cause of myocardial infarction. N Engl J Med 1978;299:1271-1277.

60. Rentrop KP, Blanke H, Koestering H, et al. Acute myocardial infarction: Intracoronary application of nitroglycerin and streptokinase in combination with transluminal recanalization. Clin Cardiol 1979;2:354-363.

61. Hampton JR. The potential of thrombolysis in the treatment of thrombotic coronary occlusion. Am Heart Assoc 1969, Monograph 27;231.

62. Sinapius D. Zur Morphologie Verschliessender Koronarthromben. Dtsch Med Wochenschr 1972;97:544-551.

63. Mueller-Fassbender H, Hess H. Spaetlyse-Behandlung chronischer arterieller Verschluesse: Ein neuer Weg zur Verbesserung der Ergebnisse. Muench Med Wochenschr 1975;117:1461.

64. Koestering H, Guerrero MA, Marschelke I, et al. Shuntthrombosen und ihre enzymatische Bereinigung. In: Marx R, Thjies HA, eds. Niere, Blutgerinnung und Haemostase. Stuttgart-New York: FK Schattauer, 1978, p. 311.

65. Boucek RJ, Murphy WP Jr. Segmental perfusion of the coronary arteries with fibrinolysin in man following a myocardial infarction. Am J Cardiol 1960;6:525-533.

66. Moschos CB, Burke WM, Lehan PH, et al. Thrombolytic agents and lysis of coronary artery thrombosis. Cardiovasc Res 1970;4:228-234.

67. Kordenat RK, Kezdi P, Powley D. Experimental intracoronary thrombosis and selective in situ lysis by catheter technique. Am J Cardiol 1972;30:640-645.

68. Verstraete M. Intermittent administration of streptokinase. Akt Probl Angiol 1978;37:95-103.

69. Lopacius S, Ziemski JM, Latallo ZS. Changes in blood clotting and fibrinolytic system during intermittent streptokinase therapy. Akt Prob Angiol 1978;37:87-94.

70. Rentrop P, Blanke H, Koestering H. Limitation of myocardial injury by transluminal recanalization of the infarct vessel in acute myocardial infarction. (abstract) Circulation 1979;60(Suppl. II) II-162.

71. Rentrop P, Blanke H, Kaiser H, et al. Selective intracoronary thrombolysis in acute myocardial infarction and unstable angina pectoris. Circulation 1981;63:307-317.

72. Rentrop P, Blanke H, Koestering H, et al. Intracoronary streptokinase infusion in 44 patients with acute ischemic syndromes. (abstract) Circulation 1980;62(Suppl. III):III-161.

73. Ganz W, Buchbinder N, Marcus H, et al. Intracoronary thrombolysis in evolving myocardial infarction in man. (abstract) Circulation 1980;62(Suppl. III):III-162.

74. Gold HK, Leinbach RC. Coronary flow restoration in myocardial infarction by intracoronary streptokinase. (abstract) Circulation 1980;62(Suppl. III):III-161.

75. Mathey D, Kuck KH, Tilsner V, et al. Non-surgical coronary artery recanalization in acute myocardial infarction. (abstract) Circulation 1980;62(Suppl. III):III-160.

76. De Wood MA, Spores J, Notske R, et al. Prevalence of total coronary occlusion during the early hours of transmural myocardial infarction. N Engl J Med 1980;303:897-902.

77. Duvoisin GE, Everhart FJ, Rudy LW, et al. Coronary embolectomy in 15 cases of acute myocardial infarction. (abstract) Circulation 1974;50(Suppl. III):III-12.

78. Feit F, Rentrop P. Thrombolysis in the treatment of acute myocardial infarction. In: Harrison's Principles of Internal Medicine. Update VI. New York, New York: McGraw-Hill, 1985, pp. 147-162.

Development and Pathophysiological Basis of Thrombolytic Therapy in Acute Myocardial Infarction: Part III. 1981-1985 Registries of Intracoronary Thrombolytic Therapy and Experimental Reperfusion Studies

K. Peter Rentrop, M.D.

From St. Vincent's Hospital and Medical Center and Columbia-Presbyterian Medical Center, New York, New York

The angiographic results of intracoronary thrombolysis were correlated with various outcome parameters in three registries. The West German Registry (n = 232) showed that mortality and improvement of left ventricular function were related to recanalization and prevention of reocclusion. This registry became the core database for the Food and Drug Administration (FDA) approval of thrombolytic agents for myocardial infarction in 1982. The European Registry (n = 414) analyzed changes in left ventricular ejection fraction further. A continuous model suggested that the functional benefit of reperfusion decreases rapidly and in a nonlinear fashion with delays in treatment during the first 3 hours. Reperfusion after > 6 hours was still associated with a significant benefit, which appeared to be related to collateral flow to the infarct zone. Myocardial salvage in experimental reperfusion studies and the reperfusion injury controversy are reviewed. In experimental studies performed by our group, it was found that thrombolytic agents did not exacerbate myocardial hemorrhage or increase infarct size. The Goettingen Registry (n = 152) demonstrated that reperfusion resulted in a steeper slope of the regression line between infarct size determined by ventriculography and cumulative serial creatine kinase release. Furthermore, reperfusion was associated with transient loss of R waves and transient development of Q waves. The implications of these findings regarding the reperfusion injury controversy and assessment of infarct size are discussed. Other analyses of the Goettingen data found that flow patterns to the infarct zone at preintervention angiography correlated with the duration of angina pectoris, incidence of antianginal therapy, and baseline ejection fraction. Assessment of the reliability of the admission ECG showed that half of the patients with infarction due to occlusion of the circumflex artery lacked diagnostic changes. The Goettingen Registery followed the first group of 70 patients ever treated with intracoronary thrombolytic therapy for 3 years. Mortality was low by the standards of the time. Reperfusion was associated with sustained improvement of left ventricular function and often dramatic clinical stabilization not seen before. (J Interven Cardiol 1998;11: 399-414)

I. The West German Multicenter Registry for Intracoronary Thrombolysis: Recanalization Rates and the Reocclusion Problem (1981)

Before organizing a prospective angiographic study, it appeared useful to pool the data available on intracoronary thrombolysis to assess recanalization rates, complications, and functional results. This author organized the first multicenter registry with four West German investigators (the West German Multicenter Registry), who pooled data obtained from 232 patients enrolled between June 1979 and March 1981.

Acute Recanalization Rates.

The angiographic registry data were published by W. Rutsch et al.[79] Preintervention angiography revealed complete occlusion of the infarct vessel in 80.5% (187/232) of the patients and a subtotal obstruction in the remaining 19.5% (45/232). The recanalization rate of total occlusions was 81% (151/187). In approximately 10% of these occlusions, the intracoronary streptokinase infusion followed perforation of the thrombus with a guidewire.

Recanalization occurred after 35.5 ± 8.4 minutes of thrombolytic therapy, requiring a mean dose of 71,000 U of streptokinase. Time to recanalization was related to duration of infarct symptoms. Recanalization occurred within 23 minutes among patients treated within 2 hours, within 31 minutes among those treated in 2-4 hours, and within 43 minutes among those treated after > 4 hours.

In an effort to achieve complete resolution of thrombus, the streptokinase infusion was routinely continued after initial documentation of reflow until antegrade filling was brisk and complete (TIMI III in today's terminology), and no further luminal improvement occurred. After completion of the streptokinase infusion, luminal

diameter remained reduced by at least 75% in three quarters of the patients. The severity of residual stenosis was related to patient age; in patients younger than 40 years, it was 62%; in those older than 40 years, it was > 80%.

Restoration of antegrade flow was associated with arrhythmias in one quarter of the cases. In contrast to experimental studies, in which abrupt release of a coronary ligation caused fatal arrhythmias,[55] the reperfusion arrhythmias associated with intracoronary streptokinase infusion were mostly self-limited and never fatal.

In-Hospital Mortality and Reinfarction.

W. Merx and colleagues of the University of Aachen reported on the in-hospital complications associated with intracoronary streptokinase infusion in the first 204 patients enrolled in the Registry, focusing on mortality, reinfarction, reocclusion, bleeding, and the timing of these complications.[80]

Hospital mortality was 10.3% (21/204). It was inversely related to the establishment of antegrade flow and directly related to the occurrence of reinfarction. Patients in whom recanalization was not achieved had a significantly higher hospital mortality (24% or 9/37) than those in whom a total occlusion was recanalized (7% or 9/179), and those with antegrade flow at baseline angiography (8% or 3/38). Five of the nine deaths in the reperfused group occurred in patients who experienced reinfarction and developed cardiogenic shock; two were sudden deaths, and two were noncardiac deaths.

Reinfarction occurred in 15% (32/204) of the total patient population. It tended to be more prevalent among patients in whom a total occlusion was recanalized: 19% (24/129) as compared to 8% (3/37) which had not been among those with total occlusions which had not been recanalized and 10% (4/38) among those who presented with antegrade flow at baseline angiography. The incidence of both death and reinfarction was dramatically higher in the coronary care unit (CCU) (8% or 16/204 and 13% or 27/204, respectively) than during the subsequent hospital stay (2.5% or 5/204 for each event).

The Reocclusion Problem.

Repeat angiography prior to hospital discharge in 79 patients in whom a total occlusion had been recanalized and who did not undergo early coronary artery bypass surgery revealed reocclusion of the initially recanalized vessel in 24% (19/79) of the cases. There was a significant correlation between reocclusion and reinfarction (Table 1). Among the 19 patients in whom reocclusion was documented, 14 had suffered reinfarction; only 5 patients had silent reocclusion. Among the 15 patients who experienced reinfarction after initial successful recanalization, reocclusion with complete loss of antegrade flow was found in 8 cases, whereas in 6 patients initially brisk antegrade filling (TIMI III) had become incomplete or delayed (TIMI I or II); only 1 patient showed normal flow in the infarct vessel.

Merx et al.'s study provided the first in-depth analysis of reocclusion of the infarct lesion and its clinical consequences after thrombolytic therapy.[80] Previous studies of intravenous thrombolysis in acute myocardial infarction (MI) had not identified this problem since restoration of antegrade flow had not been a primary goal.

The West German Registry investigators ascribed reocclusion after thrombolytic therapy to the persistence of a high grade lesion, which was unstable and tended to rethrombose. The decrease in the incidence of reocclusion after the first days was believed to be due to healing of the unstable plaque.

Hemorrhagic Complications.

The Registry participants explored several strategies to prevent reocclusion. All Registry participants treated their patients with high doses of heparin during the intervention and their CCU stay. The hematologist of our group initially voiced concern about using fulldose heparin during and shortly after thrombolytic therapy. In studies of intravenous streptokinase, breakdown of fibrinogen had been documented, and it was known that fibrinogen-split products inhibit platelet function. It was feared that adding heparin would cause an unacceptable increase in bleeding complications, although streptokinase doses infused selectively into the coronary artery were much lower than those administered intravenously.

The combination of streptokinase with heparin and aspirin was found to result in hemorrhage requiring transfusion in 7.4% (15/204) of the Registry patients. Bleeding usually occurred at the femoral puncture site and was significantly correlated with a decrease of fibrinogen level to < 100 mg/dL.

Table 1.

The Relation Between Reinfarction and Reocclusion in The West German Intracoronary Streptokinase Registry

		Reinfarction		
		Yes	No	All
Reocclusion	Yes	14	5	19
	No	1	59	60
	All	15	64	79

However, West German Registry patients in whom heparin was transiently discontinued or decreased due to bleeding complications exhibited a trend toward higher reinfarction rates. The investigators concluded that in order to prevent reocclusion, full dose intravenous heparinization for the first days after successful intracoronary thrombolytic therapy was essential, and the risk of bleeding from the groin puncture site must be accepted. Our group reduced the risk of bleeding by immediate surgical repair of the punctured femoral artery.

Hemorrhagic stroke occurred in only one patient (0.5%) who died of cardiogenic shock. The combination of full dose heparin with relatively low dose, selectively administered streptokinase did not increase hemorrhagic stroke. Later, it was the intravenous regimens utilizing large doses of thrombolytic agents, particularly clot-selective ones combined with heparin, which were found to increase the incidence of hemorrhagic stroke.

Coronary Artery Bypass Surgery and Angioplasty After Intracoronary Thrombolysis.

Since reinfarction occurred in some West German Registry patients in spite of aggressive anticoagulation, the investigators concluded that further interventions might be necessary to stabilize patients. D.G. Mathey and colleagues of the University of Hamburg reported on the results of coronary artery bypass grafting (CABG) performed in 48 Registry patients after successful recanalization.[81] The indications for surgery were either recurrent angina (n = 13) or a severe residual stenosis with a large amount of viable myocardium at risk (n = 35). The operation was performed on the day of thrombolytic therapy in 8 patients, within the subsequent 10 days in 26 patients, and > 10 days after the intervention in 14 patients. There were no deaths or other perioperative complications in any of the groups, and the authors concluded that CABG is both feasible and safe early after intracoronary thrombolytic therapy.

During the first 3-9 weeks after bypass surgery, there were 2 deaths, 2 nonfatal reinfarctions, and 2 of the 48 patients developed mild angina pectoris. The authors noted that CABG appeared to achieve better short-term and long-term stability after intracoronary thrombolytic infusion than medical therapy with its attendant in-hospital reinfarction rate of approximately 20%.

Treatment of the residual lesion by percutaneous balloon angioplasty was pioneered by J. Meyer and W. Merx et al. at the University of Aachen in a pilot study of 21 patients outside of the Registry.[82] Angioplasty was performed immediately after thrombolytic intervention in 19 of the study patients. There were no complications associated with angioplasty. During the follow-up period two patients suffered reinfarctions. The authors concluded that balloon angioplasty immediately after recanalization with intracoronary streptokinase was feasible and held promise as a method to reduce the incidence of reocclusion and reinfarction.

Two Pioneering Case Reports Are Discovered.

While collecting the Registry data, this author learned of two pioneering case reports that had anticipated some aspects of his work. They had been published in journals not commonly available to cardiologists outside of their country of origin.

A 1972 Brazilian publication, by Galiano et al., written in Portuguese, described mechanical recanalization of acute right coronary artery occlusions in two patients with cardiogenic shock.[83] Coronary artery recanalization was achieved by advancing an 8Fr Sones catheter in one case and a 7Fr Rodriguez Alvez catheter in the other, through the right coronary artery occlusion. This resulted in immediate clinical stabilization in both patients. The authors observed distal embolization of thrombus. Apparently, the authors did not pursue this approach any further.

A 1976 publication in a Soviet journal, by Chazov et al., written in Russian, reported on the use of intracoronary thrombolysis in two patients.[84] In one of the patients, recanalization had been documented. Soviet emissaries distributed a German translation of Chazov et al.'s article at several West German Universities (but not in Goettingen) after our initial publications had attracted world-wide attention. At the time, the first Western investigators were introduced to the concepts of mechanical recanalization and intracoronary thrombolytic therapy by this author and saw his recanalization films, Chazov et al.'s pilot study was not known to any of the leading investigators in the West. It was only after the appearance of these emissaries some 4 years after its publication that Chazov et al.'s work received the attention it deserved. However, by then, the time for small pilot studies had passed. It is perhaps a casualty of the Cold War era that a potentially far-reaching Russian pilot study did not influence other groups and remains merely a historical paper.[84]

Food and Drug Administration Approval for Thrombolytic Therapy.

In 1982, the U.S. Food and Drug Administration (FDA) implemented guidelines for "the use of thrombolytic agents for dissolving blood clots present during evolving myocardial infarction" based on the "pioneering investigations" of this author.[85] The FDA emphasized that it considered acceleration of coronary artery recanalization as the only proven benefit of thrombolytic therapy in acute MI. Salvage of myocardial tissue and reduction in mortality still remained to be proven in randomized trials.

Thus, more than 20 years after the first, prematurely curtailed clinical trial,[8] thrombolytic therapy for acute MI completed its tortuous journey and was finally available to patients in the country of its origin.

U.S. clinicians immediately embraced the concept that early reperfusion is beneficial, but were, with few exceptions,[86] not interested in investigating late reperfusion for the remainder of the decade. The 1987 edition of *Harrison's Principles of Internal Medicine* states: "If reperfusion is to be effective in salvaging jeopardized myocardium it must be carried out immediately after the onset of the clinical event; certainly within four hours, and preferably within two hours."[87]

Accordingly, thrombolytic therapy was generally not offered to patients presenting more than 4-6 hours after symptom onset. Furthermore, patients with antegrade flow at baseline angiography were not considered suitable for thrombolytic therapy.

Initial Studies of Changes in Ejection Fraction after Early and Late Reperfusion.

The West German Registry provided the opportunity to analyze changes in left ventricular function from preintervention to the chronic stage of infarction in patients with total occlusion at baseline angiography as a function of time to treatment.[88] We had included patients with persistent ischemic pain up to 12 hours after onset of infarction in our pilot studies. There was a significant increase in ejection fraction from $51\% \pm 12\%$ to $65\% \pm 6\%$ ($P < 0.025$) among those nine patients in whom permanent recanalization was achieved within 4 hours of symptom onset. This author found it noteworthy that among those 13 patients in whom permanent recanalization occurred > 6 hours after pain onset, ejection fraction also increased significantly, albeit less dramatically, from $52\% \pm 13\%$ to $56\% \pm 16\%$ ($P < 0.025$). In contrast, ejection fraction did not change among those nine patients who had experienced reocclusion of the infarct artery prior to chronic stage angiography. This analysis was obviously limited by its small sample size, and functional changes among patients with subtotal occlusion at baseline angiography were not assessed.

II. The European Registry for Intracoronary Streptokinase (1983)

This author expanded the West German Registry under the auspices of the European Society of Cardiology to include a total of 15 European and U.S. centers, which contributed data from 414 patients treated with intracoronary streptokinase.[89] Dr. K.R. Karsch organized the data. Analysis of the data was supported by the Department of Biostatistics of the Mount Sinai School of Medicine, New York, New York where this author and his team moved in 1981.

The European Registry focused on changes in left ventricular function. Left ventricular ejection fraction appeared to be a particularly useful endpoint since it correlates not only with infarct size, which cannot be measured directly in humans, but also with long-term survival. Detection of treatment effects with much smaller sample sizes than those required to determine mortality differences was possible.

Changes in Ejection Fraction as a Function of Angiographic Subset and Time to Reperfusion.

Changes in ejection fraction from preintervention to hospital discharge were assessed in three angiographic subgroups: (1) patients in whom a complete obstruction was recanalized and still patent at predischarge angiography; (2) patients in whom a complete obstruction of the infarct vessel was not recanalized; and (3) patients with initially incomplete obstruction. These groups were further subdivided according to the presence or absence of collateral flow to the infarct area prior to intervention. Finally, the time interval between onset of infarction and intervention was considered.

In 125 hospital survivors, ejection fraction had been determined by cineventricu-lography before the intervention and before hospital discharge and collateral status had been assessed prior to the intervention. Among those patients with initially complete obstruction of the infarct related coronary artery who experienced sustained recanalization (n = 89), ejection fraction increased significantly by 2.4% ± 1.3% (P < 0.05), whereas among those in whom complete obstructions were not recanalized or in whom reocclusion occurred (n = 17), a nonsignificant decrease in ejection fraction of 2.5% ± 9.3% was observed. In the group with incomplete obstruction at baseline angiography, ejection fraction increased significantly by 7.6% ± 14.1% (P = 0.03). Analysis of variance showed that the differences in ejection fraction changes between the recanalized, nonrecanalized, and incomplete obstruction groups were significant. Furthermore, in patients with collaterals at preintervention angiography, ejection fraction increased significantly (4.6% ± 10.6%; P < 0.01), whereas in those without collaterals there was no significant change (1.5 ± 12.2%).

It was concluded "that permanent coronary artery obstruction is usually associated with persistent loss of function, whereas improvement of function may occur in patients in whom recanalization occurs either spontaneously or due to an intervention."[89]

We hypothesized that the amount of functional benefit was related to both the time elapsed between coronary occlusion and reperfusion and the amount of myocardium at risk. Using the Registry data, we developed a continuous model relating change in ejection fraction to both duration of infarct symptoms before hospital admission and initial ejection fraction in patients in whom a complete coronary artery occlusion was permanently recanalized (Fig. 14). The largest increase in ejection fraction occurred when the initial ejection fraction was < 40% and treatment was initiated within the first hour of symptom onset. The fall-off of benefit was rapid and nonlinear in the first 3 hours. If treatment was delayed by >

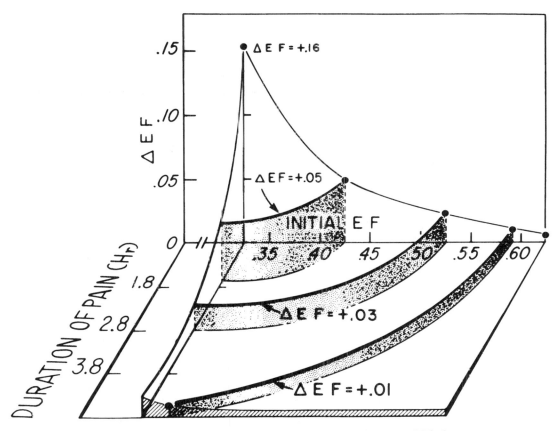

Figure 14. A conceptual model relating changes of ejection fraction (EF) from preintervention to chronic angiography to duration of infarct symptoms (hours) and preintervention ejection fraction (initial EF).

3 hours, the increase in ejection fraction became small although it remained positive even beyond 6 hours.

Among our patients presenting > 6 hours after onset of pain, collaterals to the infarct region were almost twice as frequent (54%; 13/24) as among patients presenting earlier (29%; 29/101). The patients treated > 6 hours after onset of chest pain were a select group since intracoronary streptokinase therapy was offered to them only if they had persistent chest pain, a criterion not considered essential for patients presenting earlier. We hypothesized that collateral blood flow to the infarct area slows the progression of myocardial necrosis and thereby prolongs the patient's ischemic pain and extends the time window

available for salvage of left ventricular myocardium by reperfusion.[89]

III. Reperfusion in the Experimental Animal

Myocardial Salvage.

We compared the time dependence of functional recovery after coronary artery recanalization in humans, as suggested by this model, with the progression of myocardial necrosis after temporary coronary artery ligation in the experimental animal. Reimer et al.[90] demonstrated in 1977, that after > 20 minutes, coronary ligation results in myocardial necrosis beginning in the subendocardial layer, which progresses over time toward the outer layers. After 4 hours of coronary ligation, MI is transmural and complete. Reperfusion within 4 hours salvages myocardium. The extent of salvage decreases with the duration of occlusion.[90]

These findings were confirmed by Schaper et al. in 1978 using a different methodology.[91] However, Schaper et al. did not confirm Jenning's observation that necrosis progressed in a linear fashion over time. In Schaper et al.'s model, 60% of the area at risk was already necrotic after 90 minutes of coronary occlusion; 75% of the area at risk was necrotic after 4 hours of occlusion, the same extent of necrosis as found after permanent occlusion. The rapid nonlinear progression of necrosis in Schaper et al.'s model was reminiscent of the rapid, irreversible loss of function observed within the first 3 hours in our ejection fraction model (Fig. 14).

In neither of these experimental models was the modifying influence of collateral flow upon infarct size considered. In another experimental study, Schaper showed that the proportion of myocardium at risk, which ultimately becomes necrotic after coronary occlusion, is inversely related to collateral blood flow per unit weight of ischemic myocardium.[92] Schaper identified four determinants of collateral flow:

1. Following occlusion of a coronary artery in the "in situ" beating heart collateral flow is inversely related to the size of the area at risk. Collateral flow is only 5 mL/min per 100 g following occlusion of a major coronary artery but 22 mL/min per 100 g after occlusion of a side branch. Schaper explained the relatively greater collateral flow after occlusion of small vessels by geometric factors. The density of collateral vessels in the dog heart is 10/cm^2. The number of collateral vessels entering into a cylinder of ischemic myocardial tissue increases in direct proportion to the radius of the ischemic area, whereas the mass of ischemic tissue increases to the square of the radius.

2. Following occlusion of a large coronary artery, collateral flow is inversely related to extravascular resistance, i.e., extravascular compression of the underperfused myocardium. In the isolated, empty, beating, blood-perfused heart, collateral flow was 25 mL/min per 100 g after occlusion of a major artery as compared to 5 mL/min per 100 g in the "in situ" beating heart. In other words, maximum unloading resulted in a five fold increase in collateral flow over that measured in the "in situ" beating heart.

3. There is a linear relationship between perfusion pressure and collateral flow.

4. Genetic factors that determine the number, size, and location of collateral vessels are directly related to collateral flow.

The collateral flow of 5 mL/min per 100 g observed after "in situ" occlusion of a major coronary artery provides only 1 mL oxygen/min per 100 g, which is insufficient to maintain tissue integrity and membrane function. Reduction of oxygen demand of the entire heart does not alleviate this critical limitation in oxygen supply. Myocardial salvage can be achieved only by those interventions that increase perfusion of ischemic myocardium.

In these experimental models, coronary occlusion was caused by abrupt ligation of a normal coronary artery. The models failed to take into account the period of progressive atherosclerotic narrowing, which often precedes total thrombotic occlusion in human coronary arteries. Khouri et al.[93] studied the effects of a slowly progressive coronary stenosis in a different animal model. They demonstrated growth of the collateral network, which limited or prevented myocardial necrosis following total occlusion of even a large coronary artery.

The Reperfusion Injury Controversy.

Striking changes following myocardial reperfusion in experimental studies sparked the reperfusion injury controversy. First, in the early 1970s, it was noted that reperfusion or reoxygenation of ischemic or hypoxic myocardium resulted in supercontraction of sarcomeres and prominent contracture bands, rapid cell swelling, severe damage of the sarcolemma, rupture of mitochrondria, and calcium overload of myocytes.[94-97] Hearse et al. concluded that these cellular changes indicated oxygen dependent exacerbation of tissue damage.[98,99] They suggested that the "reoxygenation phenomenon," as they termed it, was caused by oxygen-induced transmembrane calcium fluxes. Recent research has postulated a pathogenetic role of oxygen-free radicals,[100,101] proinflammatory cytokines,[102,103] and apoptosis.[104] Other investigators, however, have argued that these cellular changes affect only irreversibly injured myocytes.[105]

Second, Bresnahan et al.[106] described extensive myocardial hemorrhage after reperfusion in dogs, which was associated with a greater-than-predicted infarct size as assessed by serial creatine kinase values. They concluded that hemorrhage had caused infarct extension.[106] However, other investigators considered it unlikely that hemorrhage increased infarct size since they found that hemorrhage was restricted to zones with ischemic damage of the vasculature, and that the transmural extent of vascular injury was less than that of myocyte necrosis.[105,107,108]

Some autopsy studies suggested that myocardial hemorrhage was more extensive when reperfusion was achieved with thrombolytic therapy. Thus, Waller et al. reported hemorrhage extending beyond the zone of myocyte necrosis in patients reperfused with intracoronary streptokinase but not in those reperfused with primary angioplasty.[109] Mathey et al. found in necropsy studies extensive myocardial hemorrhage, which appeared to interfere with infarct healing after reperfusion with intracoronary streptokinase.[110] In our own patients, intraoperative inspection and transmural biopsies had not revealed any evidence of myocardial hemorrhage (Figs. 11 and 13 in Part II of this article).

We developed a dog model to assess infarct size, myocardial flow, and myocardial hemorrhage following reperfusion with intracoronary streptokinase.[111] Dr. K.R. Karsch was the principal investigator of this study, which was performed at the Max Planck Institute in Bad Nauheim, Germany, under its director, Dr. W. Schaper. A fixed stenosis severe enough to reduce reactive hyperemia to 50% of control was created in the left anterior descending or circumflex artery. This corresponds to a 75% to 80% stenosis over a length of 5 mm. The vessel was then totally occluded with a ligation distal to the stenosis. Thrombin was injected into the stenosed segment, and a second ligation proximal to the stenosis was made. Thus, a thrombotic occlusion was created at the site of a severe fixed stenosis. At 1, 2, 4, and 6 hours after occlusion, the ligations were released and streptokinase was infused selectively into the thrombosed coronary arteries for 1 hour. Reperfusion occurred in all 20 study dogs.

Infarct size increased with the duration of coronary occlusion to a similar degree as in dogs in which reperfusion was achieved by release of a mechanical obstruction without concomitant administration of thrombolytic agents. Hemorrhage was seen only in the 6-hour occlusion group, and it was limited to the central zone of necrosis in the subendocardial layer. These findings, too, were indistinguishable from those obtained in reperfusion studies in which a thrombolytic agent was not used.

Finally, the "no reflow" phenomenon, i.e., the absence of tissue perfusion following release of arterial occlusion, which was first observed in the brain,[112] was found to accompany myocardial reperfusion after coronary artery ligation lasting 60-90 minutes or more.[113-115] Bresnahan et al. suggested that the increase in interstitial pressure resulting from myocardial hemorrhage might worsen residual perfusion by compressing collateral vessels, veins, and lymphatics.[106] In our animal model, epicardial flow increased immediately after reperfusion to normal levels and did not change during the subsequent 2-hour observation period. Endocardial flow normalized slowly but began to decrease approximately 15 minutes after reperfusion. The delayed decrease in endocardial flow was statistically significant only in the group in which coronary occlusion had been maintained for 6 hours.[111] Kloner et al. found that the zone of "no reflow" corresponded to the zone of destruction of the microvasculature, was located internal to the zone of hemorrhage, and was smaller than the zone of myocyte necrosis.[113]

IV. The Goettingen Registry (1983-1985)

After analysis of the European Registry findings had been completed, the data of our four Goettingen pilot series were pooled within a Registry of 158 patients who had undergone acute coronary angiography between January 1977 and December 1980. The resultant Goettingen Registry contained more detailed clinical data than either the West German Registry or the Registry of the European Society of Cardiology. Articles published between 1983 and 1985, with the support of the Department of Biostatistics of the Mount Sinai School Medicine, investigated issues related to the controversy surrounding reperfusion injury and addressed patient selection criteria and trial design for reperfusion studies. Dr. H. Blanke was primarily responsible for organizing the Registry and analyzing its data.

Do Changes in the Serum Creatine Kinase Activity Curves after Reperfusion Indicate a Reperfusion Injury?

Bresnahan et al.'s conclusion that a greater-than-predicted creatine kinase release observed in reperfused dogs with myocardial hemorrhage indicated infarct ex-

tension[106] led to controversy about whether Shell and Sobel's model for calculating infarct size from serial measurements of serum creatine kinase activity[116,117] was applicable after reperfusion. Shell and Sobel's model was based on animal studies in which infarction was caused by permanent coronary occlusion.[117,118] In these studies, myocardial creatine kinase depletion had been found to be quantitively related to myocardial infarct size determined by both gross pathology and histology.[118] Furthermore, a linear relationship had been established between myocardial creatine kinase depletion and the amount of creatine kinase appearing in blood over 24 hours.[116]

Following reperfusion during evolving infarction, a change in the serum creatine kinase blood curve had been observed in both animal and human studies, consisting of a rapid rise to an early peak. This was attributed to rapid wash out of the enzyme.[119-122] There was controversy over whether reperfusion increases the total amount of creatine kinase recovered in blood per unit infarcted myocardium, which, if true, would invalidate the standard model of calculating infarct size from enzyme release. Experimental studies by Bresnahan et al.[106] and Jarmakani et al.[119] indicated that this was not the case. Vatner et al., on the other hand, found an increase in the amount of creatine kinase appearing in blood per gram of infarcted myocardium following reperfusion. This resulted in a different linear relationship between calculated and measured infarct size than that found among nonreperfused animals.[120] Human studies addressing this issue were not available.

Therefore, we assessed the kinetics of creatine kinase release in 27 patients of our Goettingen Registry who had successful recanalization of a total coronary artery occlusion after receiving intracoronary streptokinase therapy and in a conventionally treated comparison group of 24 patients with total coronary occlusion who had undergone acute coronary angiography before the advent of reperfusion techniques.[123] We investigated the relations between creatine kinase release and angiographic parameters of infarct size determined in the chronic phase of MI in both groups.

The time elapsed between onset of infarct symptoms and peak creatine kinase levels was significantly shorter for patients reperfused with coronary streptokinase (13.5 ± 5.3 hours vs 22.9 ± 7.4 hours, P = 0.0001). Both cumulative creatine kinase release and peak creatine kinase were found to correlate significantly with the length of the noncontracting segment, determined in the chronic stage of infarction, among conventionally treated patients and among reperfused patients. The relationships were linear in both groups (Fig. 15). However, the slopes of the regression lines were significantly steeper in the streptokinase group than in the comparison group, i.e., 199 versus 85 (P = 0.004), for cumulative creatine kinase release (Fig. 15). Inverse relationships were found between ejection fraction in the chronic stage and both cumulative creatine kinase release and peak creatine kinase in the two groups. Again, the slopes of the regression lines were significantly steeper in the streptokinase group.

We concluded that early reperfusion by intracoronary streptokinase in humans

alters the shape of the serial creatine kinase blood curve in a manner similar to that demonstrated by Vatner et al. in the experimental animal.[120] The steeper slope of the regression line between angiographically determined infarct size and cumulative creatine kinase release in reperfused patients indicated that more creatine kinase appears in serum per unit of infarcted myocardium. The difference in enzyme release between reperfused and nonreperfused patients increases with infarct size.

This latter finding was not consistent with the assumption in Shell's model of a constant serum entry ratio of creatine kinase in nonreperfused infarcts. Other investigators had questioned the validity of this assumption. More creatine kinase was found to enter the serum in dogs with patchy infarcts than in those with homogeneous infarcts of comparable size, presumably due to better residual perfusion and wash out of enzymes.[124] Less creatine kinase release was demonstrated from the center of large confluent infarcts, where regional flow was severely reduced.[125] This finding suggested that the size of large infarcts is underestimated by Shell and Sobel's formula, at least in the dog model.[125]

Reperfusion should improve blood flow to the central ischemic zone of large

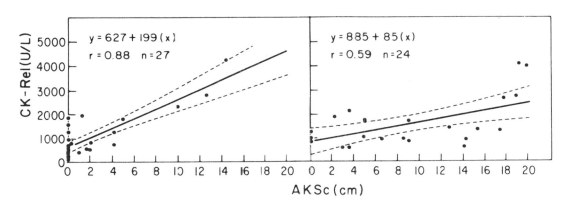

Figure 15. Correlation between cumulative creating kinase release (CK-Rel) and the length of the akinetic segment in the chronic stage of infarction (AKSc). Streptokinase group (left); comparison group (right). Dotted lines represent the 95% confidence intervals.

infarcts and increase enzyme wash out unless there is a "no reflow" phenomenon. Our finding that the difference in enzyme release between reperfused and conventionally treated patients increased with infarct size was not compatible with a "no reflow" phenomenon in large infarcts. Furthermore, it indicated that in conventionally treated patients, the serum entry ratio of creatine kinase is not a constant but is inversely related to infarct size. Our findings demonstrated that in humans, as in the dog model,[125] large, nonreperfused infarcts are underestimated by enzymatic assessment. Within the context of reperfusion, this means that cumulative and peak creatine kinase values determined after successful thrombolytic therapy indicate smaller infarcts than comparable creatine kinase values among conventionally treated patients. The reperfusion injury controversy was not resolved by our findings since enzyme wash-out would occur both in the presence and absence of such an injury. However, Bresnahan's argument that a greater-than-expected enzyme release following reperfusion is proof of a reperfusion injury was refuted.

Do Electrocardiographic Changes after Streptokinase-Induced Coronary Artery Revascularization Indicate Reperfusion Injury?

A rapid decrease of ST segment elevations following coronary artery recanalization had been described in experimental[67,126-129] and clinical studies beginning with ours.[51,60,71,121] While some investigators interpreted this finding as evidence of resolution of ischemia,[121] others suggested that it might indicate acceleration of myocardial necrosis.[129] Rapid appearance of Q waves and loss of R waves after reperfusion were interpreted by some as further evidence of reperfusion injury.[129]

The early clinical studies evaluating the electrocardiographic changes following intracoronary streptokinase infusion were inconclusive since they lacked control groups. Therefore, we assessed electrocardiographic changes in 37 patients from our Goettingen Registry with total occlusion of the left anterior descending artery at acute angiography. In 15 patients, the occlusion had been recanalized with intracoronary streptokinase infusion; the comparison group of 22 patients had undergone acute angiography prior to the advent of interventional techniques.[130] Electrocardiographic and ventriculographic parameters of infarct size were correlated.

We restricted the study to patients with occlusion of the left anterior descending artery since we had found that the sensitivity of the ECG for acute MI is greatest with occlusion of this vessel.[131] Furthermore, a close correlation between the sums of ST elevation, Q wave areas, and R wave areas assessed in both the six anterolateral leads and the 35-lead precordial map had been found.[132]

In each patient, six 12-lead ECGs were obtained: (1) immediately before angiography, i.e., approximately 5 hours after onset of infarct symptoms; (2) 3 hours after angiography; (3 ,4, 5) approximately 12, 24, and 48 hours after angiography; and (6) in the chronic stage of infarction.

The sum of ST elevations in leads V_1-V_6 was comparable in the two groups prior to angiography. Immediately after angiography, the sum of ST elevations had decreased significantly by 60% in the recanalized group, but only by 13% (n.s.) in the comparison group (Fig. 16).

The sum of R wave height (Fig. 17) and the number of pathological Q waves in the precordial leads (Fig. 18) were comparable in the two groups prior to angiography. In the streptokinase group, the sum of R waves decreased, and the number of Q waves increased throughout the initial 12 hours following reperfusion, a finding indistinguishable from that seen in the nonreperfused comparison group during the same period of time. Divergence between the groups became evident after 24 hours.

Among comparison patients, a plateau had been reached by 12 hours; the sum of R

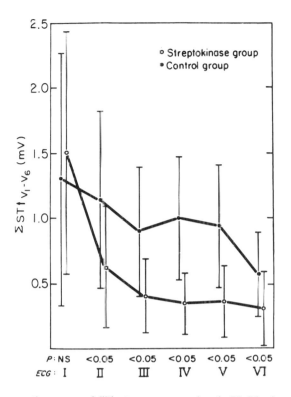

Figure 16. Changes in the sum of ST elevations in leads V_1-V_6 during the study period in patients in whom total occlusion of the left anterior descending artery was recanalized with intracoronary streptokinase and a comparison group not receiving the drug. (I) Before angiography, about 5 hours after infarct onset; (II) 3 hours after angiography; (III), (IV), and (V) 12, 24, and 48 hours after angiography; and (VI) chronic infarct stage.

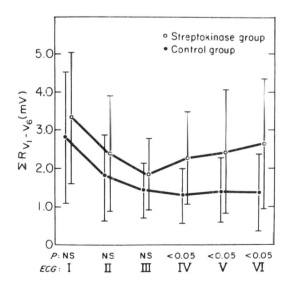

Figure 17. Changes in the sum of R wave height in V_1-V_6. Patient groups and times as in Figure 16

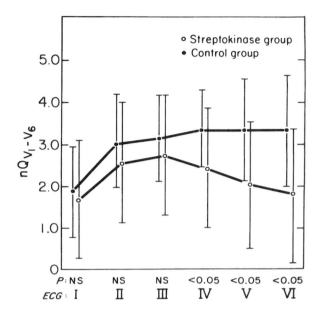

Figure 18. Changes in the number of pathological Q waves in V_1-V_6. Patient groups and times as in Figure 16.

waves and the number of Q waves did not change further with entry into the chronic stage of infarction. In the chronic stage, the sum of R waves was significantly smaller and the number of Q waves significantly larger than before angiography. No differences were noted between patients with persistent occlusion and those with spontaneous recanalization.

Among patients reperfused by intracoronary streptokinase, a significant increase in the sum of R waves (Figs. 10a and 17) and a significant decrease in the number of Q waves occurred between 12 hours after angiography and the third week after infarction (Fig. 18). Three weeks after infarction, the sum of R waves and the number of Q waves were not significantly different from the values obtained prior to angiography. In the follow-up period, the group reperfused with streptokinase displayed a significantly greater sum of R waves and significantly smaller number of Q waves than did the comparison group.

These electrocardiographic changes were paralleled by changes in left ventricular function. In the group reperfused with streptokinase, there was a significant increase in ejection fraction between the initial and the follow-up stage; the length of the akinetic segment decreased significantly. Neither ejection fraction nor the length of the akinetic segment changed in the comparison group.

Significant correlations were noted at follow-up between each of the electrocardiographic parameters of infarction (sum of R waves, number of Q waves) and each of the parameters of left ventricular function (ejection fraction, length of the akinetic segment), a finding confirming earlier studies.[133-135]

Transient Q waves and a short-term decline in the sum of R and S wave heights had been described in animal models when reperfusion was induced within 1 hour.[67,128,136] Clinicians had observed transient Q waves in conditions characterized by a brief episode of severe ischemia, e.g., Prinzmetal's angina, during bypass surgery, coronary angiography, and exercise stress testing.[137-141]

Disappearance of Q waves and reappearance of R waves in established MI had been described as rare occurrences in the prethrombolytic literature.[142-150] Q waves usually disappeared only weeks to years after MI; in a study of 775 patients, this phenomenon was observed in 6.7% by the end of the second year.[150] The mechanisms are unknown.

Our finding that Q waves disappear and R waves reappear frequently after reperfusion with intracoronary streptokinase was new. The time frame of these electrocardiographic changes was different from that reported in conventionally treated patients. In our streptokinase-treated patients, the signs of myocardial necrosis started to disappear within 24 hours after reperfusion. The mechanisms are unknown, although it is noteworthy that in a canine model, Theroux et al.[151] observed deterioration in left ventricular function immediately after reperfusion followed by an improvement after 24 hours. They ascribed the transient impairment in function to local edema, inflammatory reaction, and hemorrhage,[151] mechanisms that might also be responsible for the transient appearance of Q waves and loss of R waves in reperfused patients.

The finding of a significant correlation between the electrocardiographic parameters of infarct size and left ventricular function in the chronic stage suggests that the number of pathological Q waves and sum of R waves can be used to assess infarct size in reperfused patients. However, the timing of these electrocardiographic measurements is important; among conventionally treated patients, these parameters reflect infarct size as early as 18 hours after symptom onset, whereas among reperfused patients, infarct size would be overestimated if determined at this time.

The finding of a smaller infarct size in the streptokinase group as determined by electrocardiographic and ventriculographic parameters in the chronic stage of infarction indicates that ischemic myocardium was salvaged by reperfusion. If a reperfusion injury occurred, which is not excluded by our findings, it did not affect all of the myocardium at risk.

Salvage of myocardium by reperfusion does not imply that reperfusion-induced myocardial hemorrhage is innocuous. As discussed earlier, myocardial hemorrhage occurs frequently if reperfusion is achieved > 6 hours after onset of MI. It has been suggested that myocardial hemorrhage is responsible for the "early hazard" of late thrombolytic therapy[152] by predisposing patients to an increased risk of myocardial rupture.[153-155] Furthermore, the transient depression of local function associated with hemorrhage, which is evident in animal models,[15] could cause hemodynamic decompensation in patients with severely compromised left ventricular function.

Correlations Between Baseline Angiographic Patterns and the Duration of Angina Pectoris, Antianginal Therapy, and Baseline Left Ventricular Function.

The availability of residual flow to the infarct zone had been found to determine the effectiveness of various interventions to limit infarct size, such as coronary artery bypass surgery,[46] intraaortic balloon counterpulsation,[156] beta receptor blockade,[157] and intracoronary streptokinase infusion.[88] The two patterns of residual flow, i.e., antegrade residual flow through an incomplete obstruction or retrograde through collateral channels, were considered to be equivalent by some authors.[158]

We grouped the patients of the Goettingen Registry with enzymatically confirmed infarction and complete baseline data (n = 130) into three angiographic subsets based on the preintervention angiogram: (1) those with antegrade flow through an incomplete obstruction (28%, n = 36); (2) those with retrograde flow through collateral channels (43%, n = 56); and (3) those with an avascular infarct (29%, n = 38). We investigated whether the groups differed in distribution of baseline variables,[159] i.e., cardiac history, extent of CAD, and acute left ventricular function.

We found that the groups did not differ in the incidence of previous infarction, Killip classification, or distribution of infarct vessels.

Patients with avascular infarction differed significantly from the other groups with respect to three baseline variables: (1) the incidence of single vessel disease (79%) was significantly greater than in the groups with collateralized total occlusion (57%) or subtotal obstruction (64%); (2) the time interval from the initial onset of angina pectoris to infarction was significantly shorter (0.7 ± 3.1 months) than among patients with a collateralized total occlusion (14.2 ± 21.4 months) or those with subtotal obstruction (6.5 ± 16.1 months); and (3) antianginal drugs were used significantly less frequently (16%) than in the groups with collateralized total occlusions (54%) or subtotal occlusions (56%).

As is known, new onset angina pectoris indicates that a coronary artery lesion has reached the degree at which it critically interferes with myocardial blood supply. Our finding that the history of angina pectoris was shorter in patients with avascular infarction than among those with collateral flow suggested that the time interval from the development of a critical stenosis to thrombotic occlusion was also shorter in this angiographic subset. This conclusion was further supported by Fulton's autopsy studies.[160] In a canine model, Khouri et al. found that a critical coronary artery lesion stimulates the enlargement of collateral channels, a process that requires time.[93] Thus, our findings further suggested that among patients with avascular infarctions, the time interval from development of a critical stenosis to thrombotic occlusion was shorter than the time required for the growth of angiographically detectable collaterals. The lack of antianginal therapy prior to infarction in 84% of patients with avascular infarction suggested that many of these patients were asymptomatic prior to

the index event and experienced thrombotic occlusion of a lesion that was not previously critical.

Patients with antegrade flow through a subtotal occlusion differed from the other angiographic subsets by having significantly better left ventricular function at baseline. Their ejection fraction was 55% ± 13% versus 48% ± 13% for the group with collateral flow and 50% ± 10% for those with avascular infarcts. Since the incidence of previous infarction and the distribution of infarct vessels was nearly identical among the three groups, this finding suggested that antegrade flow through subtotal lesions was greater than retrograde flow through collateral channels at the time of angiography.

Thus, the three angiographic subsets differed from one another in important baseline variables. We decided to factor these angiographic subsets into the design of our reperfusion trials as covariates.

Reliability of the Admission Electrocardiogram in Diagnosing Acute Myocardial Infarction and Identifying the Infarct Artery.

In research and clinical practice, reperfusion therapies were offered only to patients presenting with both prolonged ischemic chest pain and electrocardiographic changes suggestive of acute ischemia or infarction. However, Rude et al. showed in 1983 that 21% of 3,697 patients in the Milis Study, who had confirmed acute MI, lacked the "classic" electrocardiographic abnormalities, i.e., abnormal Q waves and ST segment elevations, in their serial ECGs.[161] Sullivan, Ward, and colleagues concluded from their postmortem studies that infarction of the lateral wall of the heart caused by disease of the left circumflex artery rarely presents with classic electrocardiographic changes.[162,163] In vivo studies had correlated acute electrocardiographic changes with the findings of coronary angiograms performed after infarct healing.[164-168] We had shown that, at this time, the infarct-related lesion has frequently undergone important changes, such as spontaneous recanalization or progression to total occlusion.[53,80]

The Goettingen Registry afforded us the opportunity to correlate changes on the admission ECG with coronary angiographic findings obtained within several hours of infarct onset.[131] The primary goal of this study was to assess the reliability of the admission ECG in diagnosing acute MI and determining the infarct related artery. Acute angiography was performed if a patient had chest pain lasting > 30 minutes, which was considered indicative of myocardial ischemia by a cardiologist. Patients were not excluded if infarct signs on the admission ECG were not evident.

The diagnosis of acute MI was confirmed by enzymatic criteria in 152 of the 158 Goettingen Registry patients. The 146 patients in whom the infarct related artery could be determined based on angiographic criteria comprised the study group. Coronary angiography was performed 6.3 ± 6 hours after the onset of pain. Standard 12-lead ECGs were recorded during the hour preceding cardiac catheterization.

"Classic" electrocardiographic signs of anterior or inferior infarction were defined as abnormal Q waves or ST segment elevations of at least 0.1 mV in two adjacent leads. True posterior infarction was diagnosed if, in lead V_1, R was > S or if R was > 5 mm in the presence of an upright T wave.

Classic electrocardiographic changes were found in 81% (118/146) of the study patients, remarkably similar to the incidence reported by Rude et al.[161] The incidence of classic patterns of infarction was 94% (77/82) for patients with occlusion of the left anterior descending artery, 77% (30/39) for those with occlusion of the right coronary artery, and 44% (11/25) for those with occlusion of the left circumflex artery.

The most common electrocardiographic abnormality for all three infarct related arteries in patients with classic patterns was ST segment elevation. This abnormality occurred most commonly in

lead V_2 in patients with left anterior descending artery involvement (83% or 68/82), in lead III in those with right coronary artery involvement (59% or 23/39), and in lead V_6 in those with left circumflex artery involvement (36% or 9/25). There was no difference in the incidence of ST segment elevations and abnormal Q waves between patients with total and subtotal occlusions of the infarct artery.

In the group of 28 patients without a "classic" infarct pattern on the admission ECG, MI was caused by occlusion of the left circumflex artery in 14 patients, the right coronary artery in 9 patients, and the left anterior descending artery in 5 patients. The most common abnormalities among patients with left circumflex artery involvement were ST segment depressions in the lateral precordial leads and T wave abnormalities. In two patients with circumflex disease, the admission ECG was normal.

In conclusion, in 18% of patients (28/152) with a myocardial infarct by pain and enzymatic criteria, the admission ECG lacked classic infarct abnormalities. Exclusion from thrombolytic therapy of patients with typical infarct symptoms on the basis of the admission ECG will deprive approximately half of the patients with MI caused by occlusion of the left circumflex artery of their chance to benefit from reperfusion. Finally, the admission ECG does not distinguish between patients with subtotal occlusion and those with total occlusion regardless of the identity of the infarct related artery.

The First Group of Patients Treated with Intracoronary Thrombolytic Therapy: Short-Term and Long-Term Follow-Up.

Following our radical departure from the accepted standard of care for patients with acute MI in 1978, concerns were expressed regarding the safety of cardiac catheterization in acute MI[169] and short- and long-term adverse effects of intracoronary thrombolytic therapy. Additionally, the issue of a learning curve had to be considered in this historical patient group. In 1983 we completed follow-up of the 158 patients who had undergone immediate coronary catheterization at the University of Goettingen between January 1977 and December 1980.[170] We compared the outcome in those 70 patients with enzymatically confirmed acute MI who had been treated with intracoronary streptokinase with that of 66 patients who had had emergency coronary angiography performed prior to the introduction of intracoronary intervention techniques. Excluded from this study were those six patients who did not fulfill enzymatic criteria of acute MI and those 16 patients who had participated in our study of mechanical recanalization with catheter-based techniques; the uneventful hospital course and improvement in left ventricular function seen in these patients have been described earlier.

Baseline clinical and angiographic variables, including Killip class, were comparable in the study group and the comparison group. Reperfusion was achieved in 85% of the streptokinase-treated patients. Arterial entry sites were repaired surgically in those patients in whom reperfusion was achieved. We used coronary artery bypass surgery aggressively if there was clinical or angiographic evidence of significant myocardium at risk. Surgery was performed in 37% (26/70) of patients treated with intracoronary streptokinase and in 27% (18/66) of the patients in the comparison group. Hospital mortality was 11% in the streptokinase group and 18% in the comparison group. During the follow-up period of 35 ± 5 months (range: 24-45 months) for the streptokinase-treated group and 48 ± 9 months (range: 28-82 months) for the comparison group, the annual mortality rate was approximately 3% in both groups, similar to the ranges reported by other investigators at that time for patients with comparable left ventricular function and coronary anatomy.[171]

Left ventricular ejection fraction increased in the streptokinase-treated group from $50\% \pm 4\%$ prior to intervention to $58\% \pm 12\%$ (P = 0.005) at hospital discharge. Patients in the comparison group experienced a decrease in left ventricular ejection fraction from $51\% \pm 10\%$ at acute angiography to $47\% \pm 12\%$ (P= 0.049) at hospital discharge. This difference between the groups persisted during long-term follow-up.

In contrast to other investigators,[79,80,169] we did not observe any major complications that were attributable to acute cardiac cathetherization. Acute, major bleeding occurred in only one streptokinase-treated patient. Nonfatal reinfarction occurred in five patients in the streptokinase-treated group and in seven patients in the comparison group.

Autopsy carried out by Dr. D. Sinapius in all patients who died during the hospital phase (except for one patient in the comparison group) revealed a single myocardial rupture in a patient in the comparison group. The lack of myocardial rupture among streptokinase-treated patients was reassuring in view of concerns that thrombolytic therapy might increase the incidence of this complication.[153-155] We speculated that we had prevented myocardial rupture by excluding patients in whom myocardial necrosis appeared complete at the time of initial evaluation.

We concluded that there was no evidence of any major adverse effects associated with the initial efforts at achieving coronary artery recanalization in acute MI. Adverse learning curve effects were not apparent. In fact, we felt that our patients had benefited from participating in our pioneering studies of mechanical recanalization and intracoronary thrombolytic therapy since their hospital mortality was low by the standards of the time, they experienced improvement of left ventricular function, and they frequently demonstrated dramatic clinical improvement following reperfusion. The need for randomized studies to further assess these therapies and adjunctive interventions was obvious.

References

79. Rutsch W, Schartl M, Mathey D, et al. Percutaneous transluminal coronary recanalization: Procedure, results, and acute complications. Am Heart J 1981;102:1178-1181.

80. Merx W, Doerr R, Rentrop KP, et al. Evaluation of the effectiveness of intracoronary streptokinase infusion in acute myocardial infarction: Post-procedure management and hospital course in 204 patients. Am Heart J 1981;102:1187-1191.

81. Mathey DG, Rodewald G, Rentrop KP, et al. Intracoronary streptokinase thrombolytic recanalization and subsequent surgical bypass of remaining atherosclerotic stenosis in acute myocardial infarction: Complementary combined approach effecting reduced infarct size, preventing reinfarction, and improving left ventricular function. Am Heart J 1981;102 1181-1187.

82. Meyer J, Merx W, Schmitz H, et al. Percutaneous transluminal coronary angioplasty immediately after intracoronary streptolysis of transmural myocardial infarction. Circulation 1982;66:905-913.

83. Galiano N, Macruz R, Arie S, et al. Enfarte agudo do miocardio e choque-tratamento por recanalizacoa arterial atraves do caterismo cardiaco. Arq Bras Cardiol 1972;25:197-204.

84. Chazov EI, Mateeva LS, Mazaev AV. Intracoronary administration of fibrinolysin in acute myocardial infarction. Ter Arkh 1976;48:8-19.

85. Letter on file.

86. Kennedy JW, Ritchie JL, Davis KB, et al. Western Washington Randomized Trial of intracoronary streptokinase in acute myocardial infarction. N Engl J Med 1983; 309:1477- 1482.

87. Pasternak R, Braunwald E, Alpert JS. Acute myocardial infarction. In: Harrison's Principles of Internal Medicine. New York, New York: McGraw-Hill, 1987, pp. 982-993.

88. Rentrop P, Blanke H, Karsch KR, et al. Changes in left ventricular function after intracoronary streptokinase infusion in clinically evolving myocardial infarction. Am Heart J 1981; 102:1188-1193.

89. Rentrop KP, Smith H, Painter L, et al. Changes in left ventricular ejection fraction after intracoronary thrombolytic therapy. Circulation 1983; 68(Suppl. I):I-55-I-60.

90. Reimer KA, Lowe JE, Rasmussen MM, et al. The wave front phenomenon of ischemic cell death. I. Myocardial infarct size vs duration of coronary occlusion in dogs. Circulation 1977; 56:786-792.

91. Schaper W, Frenzel H, Hort W, et al. Experimental coronary artery occlusion II. Spatial and temporal evolution of infarcts in the dog heart. Basic Res Cardiol 1979;74:233-239.

92. Schaper W. Experimental coronary artery occlusion. III. The determinants of collateral blood flow in acute coronary occlusion. Basic Res Cardiol 1978;73:584-594.

93. Khouri EM, Gregg DE, McGranahan GM Jr. Regression and reappearance of coronary collaterals. Am J Physiol 1971; 220:655-661.

94. Jennings RB, Sommers H, Smyth GA, et al Myocardial necrosis induced by temporary occlusion of a coronary artery in the dog. Arch Pathol 1960; 70:68-78.

95. Shen AC, Jennings RB. Kinetics of calcium accumulation in acute myocardial ischemic injury. Am Pathol 1972; 67:441-452.

96. Kloner RA, Ganote CE, Whalen D, et al. Effect of a transient period of ischemia on myocardial cells. II. Fine structure during the first few minutes of reflow. Am J Pathol 1974;74:399-413.

97. Whalen DA, Hamilton DG, Gante CE, et al. Effect of a transient period of ischemia on myocardial cells. I. Effects on cell volume regulation. Am J Pathol 1974;74:381-397.

98. Hearse DJ, Humphrey SM, Nayler WG, et al. Ultrastructural damage associated with reoxygenation of the anoxic myocardium. J Mol Cell Cardiol 1975;7:315-324.

99. Hearse DJ. Reperfusion of the ischaemic myocardium. J Mol Cell Cardiol 1977;9:605-616.

100. Ambrosio G, Flaherty JT, Duilio C, et al. Oxygen radicals generated at reflow induce peroxidation of membrane lipids in reperfused hearts. J Clin Invest 1991; 87:2056-2066.

101. Bolli R, Zughaib M, Li XY, et al. Recurrent ischemia in the canine heart causes recurrent bursts of free

radical production that have a cumulative effect on contractile function: A pathophysiological basis for chronic myocardial 'stunning.' J Clin Invest 1995;96:1066-1084.

102. Kukielka GL, Smith CW, Manning AM, et al. Induction of interleukin-6 synthesis in the myocardium: Potential role in postreperfusion inflammatory injury. Circulation 1995; 92: 1866-1875.

103. Krown KA, Page MT, Nguyen C, et al. Tumor necrosis factor alpha-induced apoptosis in cardiac myocytes: Involvement of the sphingolipid signaling cascade in cardiac cell death. J Clin Invest 1996;98:2854-2865.

104. Fliss H, Gattinger D. Apoptosis in ischemic and reperfused rat myocardium. Clin Res 1996;79:949-956.

105. Jennings RB, Reimer KA. Factors involved in salvaging ischemic myocardium: Effect of reperfusion of arterial blood. Circulation 1983;68(Suppl. I):I-25-I-36.

106. Bresnahan GF, Roberts R, Shell WE, et al. Deleterious effects due to hemorrhage after myocardial reperfusion. Am J Cardiol 1974;33:82-86.

107. Fishbein MC, Y-Rit J, Lando U, et al. The relationship of vascular injury and myocardial hemorrhage to necrosis after reperfusion. Circulation 1980; 62:1274-1279.

108. Kloner RA, Rude RE, Carlson N, et al. Ultrastructural evidence of microvascular damage and myocardial cell injury after coronary artery occlusion: Which comes first? Circulation 1980; 62:945-952.

109. Waller BE, Rothbaum DA, Pinkerton CA, et al. Status of the myocardium and infarct-related coronary artery in 19 necropsy patients with acute recanalization using pharmacologic (streptokinase, r-tissue plasminogen activator), mechanical (percutaneous transluminal coronary angioplasty) or combined types of reperfusion therapy. JACC 1987;9: 785-801.

110. Mathey DG, Schofer J, Kuck KH, et al. Transmural, haemorrhagic myocardial infarction after intracoronary streptokinase. Clinical, angiographic, and necropsy findings. Br Heart J 1982; 48:546-541.

111. Karsch KR, Hofmann M, Rentrop KP, et al. Thrombolysis in acute experimental myocardial infarction. JACC 1983; 1:427-435.

112. Ames A III, Wright RL, Kowoods M, et al. Cerebral ischemia II. The no-reflow phenomenon. Am J Pathol 1968; 52: 437-447.

113. Kloner RA, Ganote CE, Jennings RB. The "no-reflow" phenomenon following temporary coronary occlusion in the dog. J Clin Invest 1975;54:1496-1508.

114. Camilleri JP, Joseph D, Fabiani JN, et al. Microcirculatory changes following early reperfusion in experimental myocardial infarction. Virchows Arch [Anat Pathol Anat Histol] 1976; 369:315-333.

115. Gavin JB, Seelye RN, Nevalainen TJ, et al. The effect of ischemia on the function and fine structure of the microvasculature of myocardium. Pathology 1978;10:103-111.

116. Shell WE, Kjekshus JK, Sobel BE. Quantitative assessment of the extent of myocardial infarction in the conscious dog by means of analysis of serial changes in serum creatine phosphokinase activity. J Clin Invest 1971; 50:2614-2625.

117. Sobel BE, Bresnahan GF, Shell WE, et al. Estimation of infarct size in man and its relation to prognosis. Circulation 1972;46:640-648.

118. Kjekshus JK, Sobel BE. Depressed myocardial creatine phosphokinase activity following experimental myocardial infarction in rabbit. Circ Res 1970;27:403-414.

119. Jarmakani JM, Limbird L, Graham TC, et al. Effect of reperfusion on myocardial infarct, and the accuracy of estimating infarct size from serum creatine phosphokinase in the dog. Cardiovasc Res 1976;10:245-253.

120. Vatner SF, Baig H, Manders WT, et al. Effects of coronary artery reperfusion on myocardial infarct size calculated from creatine kinase. J Clin Invest 1978;61:1048-1056.

121. Ganz W, Ninomiya K, Hashida J, et al. Intracoronary thrombolysis in acute myocardial infarction: Experimental background and clinical experience. Am Heart J 1981;102: 1145-1149.

122. Anderson JL, Marshall HW, Bray BE, et al. A randomized trial of intracoronary streptokinase in the treatment of acute myocardial infarction. N Engl J Med 1983;308:1312-1318.

123. Blanke H, von Hardenberg D, Cohen M, et al. Patterns of creatine kinase release during acute myocardial infarction after nonsurgical reperfusion: Comparison with conventional treat-

ment and correlation with infarct size. JACC 1984; 3:675-680.

124. Cairns JA, Missirlis E, Fallen EL. Myocardial infarction size from serial CPK: Variability of CPK serum entry ratio with size and model of infarction. Circulation 1978;58:1143- 1153.

125. Swain JL, Cobb FR, McHale PA, et al. Nonlinear relationship between creatine kinase estimates and histologic extent of infarction in conscious dogs: Effects of regional myocardial blood flow. Circulation 1980;62:1239-1247.

126. Maroko PR, Libby P, Ginks WR, et al. Coronary artery reperfusion 1. Early effects on local myocardial function and the extent of myocardial necrosis. J Clin Invest 1972;51: 2710-2716.

127. Muller JE, Maroko PR, Braunwald E. Evaluation of precordial electrocardiographic mapping as a means of assessing changes in myocardial ischemic injury. Circulation 1975; 52:16-27.

128. Smith GT, Soeter JR, Haston HH, et al. Coronary reperfusion in primates. Serial electrocardiographic and histologic assessment. J Clin Invest 1974; 54:1420-1427.

129. Capone RJ, Most AS. Myocardial hemorrhage after coronary reperfusion in pigs. Am J Cardiol 1978;41:259-266.

130. Blanke H, Scherff F, Karsch KR, et al. Electrocardiographic changes after streptokinase-induced recanalization in patients with acute left anterior descending artery obstruction. Circulation 1983;68:406-412.

131. Blanke H, Cohen M, Schlueter GU, et al. Electrocardiographic and coronary arteriographic correlations during acute myocardial infarction. Am J Cardiol 1984;54:249-255.

132. Zmyslinski RW, Akiyama T, Biddle TL, et al. Natural course of the S-T segment and QRS complex in patients with acute anterior myocardial infarction. Am J Cardiol 1970;43:29-34.

133. Awan NA, Miller RR, Janzen VZ, et al. Noninvasive assessment of cardiac function and ventricular dyssynergy by precordial Q wave mapping in anterior myocardial infarction. Circulation 1977;55:833-838.

134. Askenazi J, Parisi AF, Cohn PF, et al. Value of the QRS complex in assessing left ventricular ejection fraction. Am J Cardiol 1978;41:494-499.

135. Palmeri ST, Harrison DG, Cobb FR, et al. A QRS scoring system for assessing left ventricular function after myocar-

dial infarction. N Engl J Med 1982; 306:4-9.

136. Gross H, Rubin IL, Laufer L, et al. Transient abnormal Q waves in the dog without myocardial infarction. Am J Cardiol 1964;14:669-674.

137. Roesler H, Dressler W. Transient electrocardiographic changes identical with those of acute myocardial infarction accompanying attacks of angina pectoris. Am Heart J 1954; 47:520-526.

138. Haiat R, Chiche P. Transient abnormal Q waves in the course of ischemic heart disease. Chest 1974;65:140-144.

139. Meller J, Conde CA, Donoso E, et al. Transient Q waves in Prinzmetal's angina. Am J Cardiol 1975;35:691-695.

140. Klein HO, Gross H, Rubin IL. Transient electrocardiographic changes simulating myocardial infarction during open-heart surgery. Am Heart J 1970;79:463-470.

141. Bateman T, Gray R, Maddahi J, et al. Transient appearance of Q waves in coronary diseases during exercise electrocardiography: Considerations of mechanisms and clinical importance. Am Heart J 1982;104:182-184.

142. Gittler R, Schack JA, Vesell H. The electrocardiogram one year after acute myocardial infarction. Am Heart J 1956; 51:246.

143. Pappas MP. Disappearance of pathological Q waves after myocardial infarction. Br Heart J 1958;20:123.

144. Kaplan BM, Berkson DM. Serial electrocardiograms after myocardial infarction. Am Heart J 1964;60:430.

145. Anderssen N, Skjaeggestad O. The electrocardiogram in patients with previous myocardial infarction. Acta Med Scand 1964;176:123.

146. Shanoff HM, Little JA. Studies of male survivors of myocardial infarction: VI. The electrocardiogram. Can Med Assoc J 1965;93:1049-1052.

147. Cox CJB. Return to normal of the electrocardiogram after myocardial infarction. Lancet 1967;1:1194-1197.

148. Pyorala K, Kentala E. Disappearance of Minnesota Code Q-QS patterns in the first year after myocardial infarction. Ann Clin Res 1974;6:137-141.

149. Wasserman AG, Bren GB. Ross AM, et al. Prognostic implications of diagnostic Q waves after myocardial infarction. Circulation 1982;65:1451-1455.

150. Kalbfleisch JM, Shadaksharappa KS, Conrad LL, et al. Disappearance of the Q-deflection following myocardial infarction. Am Heart J 1968;76:193-198.

151. Theroux P, Ross J Jr, Franklin D, et al. Coronary arterial reperfusion. III. Early and late effects on regional myocardial function and dimensions in conscious dogs. Am J Cardiol 1976; 38:599-606.

152. Fibrinolytic Therapy Trialists (FTT) Collaborative Group. Indications for fibrinolytic therapy in suspected acute myocardial infarction: Collaborative overview of early mortality and major morbidity results from all randomised trials of more than 1000 patients. Lancet 1994;343:311-322.

153. Neuhaus KL, Tebbe U, Sauer G, et al. High-dose intravenous streptokinase infusion in acute myocardial infarction. Clin Cardiol 1983;6:426-434.

154. Loukinen KL, O'Neill W, Laufer N, et al. Myocardial rupture complicating tissue plasminogen activator therapy of acute myocardial infarction. JACC 1989;13:94A.

155. Honan MB, Harrell FE, Reimer KA, et al. Cardiac rupture, mortality and the timing of thrombolytic therapy: A meta-analysis. JACC 1990;16:359-367.

156. Leinbach RC, Gold HK, Harper RW, et al. Early intraaortic balloon pumping for anterior myocardial infarction without shock. Circulation 1978; 58:201-210.

157. Gold HK, Leinbach RC, Harper RW. Usefulness of intravenous propranolol in predicting left anterior descending blood flow during anterior myocardial infarction. Am J Cardiol 1984;54:264-268.

158. Rogers WJ, Hood WP Jr, Mantle JA, et al. Return of left ventricular function after reperfusion in patients with myocardidal infarction: Importance of subtotal stenosis or intact collaterals. Ciculation 1984;69:338-349.

159. Blanke H, Cohen M, Karsch KR, et al. Prevalence and significance of residual flow to the infarct zone during the acute phase of mycoardial infarction. JACC1985;5:827-831.

160. Fulton WFM. The time factor in the enlargement of anastomoses in coronary artery disease. Scott Med J 1964;9:18-23.

161. Rude RE, Poole WK, Muller JE, et al. Electrocardiographic and clinical criteria for recognition of acute myocardial infarction based on analysis of 3,697 patients. Am J Cardiol 1983; 52:936-942.

162. Sullivan W, Vlodover Z, Tuna N, et al. Correlation of electrocardiographic and pathophysiologic findings in healed myocardial infarction. Am J Cardiol 1978;42:724-732.

163. Ward RM, Ideker RE, Wagner GS, et al. Myocardial infarcts in the lateral third of the left ventricle: Size and ECG recognition. (abstract) Am J Cardiol 1980;45:473.

164. Williams RA, Cohn PF, Vokonas PS, et al. Electrocardiographic, arteriographic and ventriculographic correlations in transmural myocardial infarction. Am J Cardiol 1973; 31:595-599.

165. Hamby RI, Hoffman I, Hilsenrath J, et al. Clinical, hemodynamic and angiographic aspects of inferior and anterior myocardial infarctions in patients with angina pectoris. Am J Cardiol 1974;34:513-519.

166. Lee GB, Wilson WJ, Amplatz K, et al. Correlation of the vectorcardiogram and electrocardiogram with coronary arteriogram. Circulation 1968;38:190-200.

167. McConahay DR, McCallister BD, Hallerman FJ, et al. Comparative quantitative analysis of the electrocardiogram and the vectorcardiogram: Correlations with the coronary arteriogram. Circulation 1970;42:245-259.

168. Fuchs RM, Achuff SC, Grunwald L, et al. Electrocardiographic localization of coronary artery narrowings: Studies during myocardial ischemia and infarction in patients with one vessel disease. Circulation 1982;66:1168-1176.

169. Serruys PW, van den Brand M, Hooghoudt TEH, et al. Coronary recanalization in acute myocardial infarction: Immediate results and potential risks. Eur Heart J 1982;3:404-415.

170. Blanke H, Schicha H, Cohen M, et al. Long-term follow-up after intracoronary streptokinase therapy for acute myocarial infarction. Am Heart J 1985;110:736-742.

171. Sanz G, Castaner A, Betriu A, et al. Determinants of prognosis in survivors of myocardial infarction: A prospective clinical angiographic study. N Engl J Med 1982;306:1065-1070

Development and Pathophysiological Basis of Thrombolytic Therapy in Acute Myocardial Infarction: Part IV

K. Peter Rentrop, M.D.

From St. Vincent's Hospital and Medical Center and Columbia-Presbyterian Medical Center, New York, New York

Acute and day 10 to 14 recanalization rates with intracoronary thrombolytic and/or spasmolytic therapy were determined in the First Mt. Sinai-N.Y.U. Reperfusion Trial (1984). Recanalization of total occlusion was accelerated by intracoronary streptokinase, the first proven potentially beneficial effect of thrombolytic therapy. Intravenous administration of thrombolytic agents, including t-PA, was less effective in accelerating recanalization than intracoronary streptokinase as assessed by 90-minute rates of TIMI-III flow. In clinical practice the greater ease of intravenous administration outweighed this disadvantage, but intracoronary administration was uniquely suited to analyze the pathophysiological principles of reverfusion therapy. The first randomized trial (n = 533) to establish the benefits of early reperfusion achieved infarct vessel patency in 85% of patients within 200 minutes of symptom onset by administering intracoronary streptokinase alone or following a rapid intravenous infusion of streptokinase (Simoons, 1985). Ejection fraction improved significantly and mortality at 28 days was reduced (6% vs 12%). The ISIS-2 Trial (1988) showed mortality reduction with intravenous thrombolytic therapy up to 24 hours after infarct onset, but did not explain the benefit of late reperfusion. In the Second Mt. Sinai-N.Y.U. Reperfusion Trial (1989; n = 393), intracoronary streptokinase administered 4 to 14 hours after infarct onset increased thallium uptake. Streptokinase improved ejection fraction in patients with collateralized total occlusion but not in those with noncollateralized total occlusion. Preintervention antegrade flow was associated with ejection fraction improvement regardless of treatment assignment. We concluded that thrombolytic therapy after > 4 hours of infarction salvages myocardium in patients with collateralized total coronary artery occlusion. Total coronary occlusion was associated with collateral flow in 33% at acute angiography, but in 90% at day 10 to 14 angiography, indicating a second phase of collateral growth. An angioplasty model was developed to assess appearance and disappearance of collateral flow immediately after controlled coronary occlusion and reflow in humans. Using this model we demonstrated limitation of ischemia by collateral recruitment prospectively. (J Interven Cardiol 1999;12:XX-XX)

I. Coronary Artery Recanalization: The First Mount Sinai-N.Y.U. Reperfusion Trial: Acceleration of Coronary Artery Recanalization

Several groups published randomized trials that assessed the angiographic outcomes of intracoronary thrombolytic therapy in 1983 and 1984.[122,172-174] The First Mount Sinai-N.Y.U. Reperfusion Trial, for which this author served with Drs. F. Feit and R. Gorlin as Principal Investigator, was performed between April 1, 1981 and October 31, 1982 at four New York City hospitals.[173] The factorial trial design was suggested by Dr. T. Chalmers, President and Dean of The Mount Sinai Medical Center.

One hundred twenty-four patients were randomly assigned to one of four treatment groups: intracoronary streptokinase, intracoronary nitroglycerin, intracoronary streptokinase plus intracoronary nitroglycerin, or conventional therapy without initial angiography.

Recanalization occurred during intracoronary streptokinase infusion in 74% (32 of 43) of patients, a result similar to that obtained in other trials.[122,172,174] Acute recanalization rates associated with intracoronary administration of nitroglycerin were significantly lower, ranging between 6% in our trial and 17% in Lieboff's study,[174] and were comparable to the 10% recanalization rate reported with intracoronary infusion of dextrose.[172] These findings confirmed the results of our early nonrandomized studies. We concluded that the only important factor causing recanalization during interventional angiography is lysis of an occlusive thrombus by the administration of a thrombolytic agent.[173]

Our trial differed from all others by including a predischarge angiogram performed on day 10 to 14 in, not only streptokinase-treated patients, but also in control patients. The predischarge angiograms revealed patency of the infarct related artery in 77% of all patients (71 of 92);

there was no significant difference among groups: streptokinase, 73% (16 of 22) ; streptokinasenitroglycerin 88% (21 of 25); nitroglycerin, 81% (17 of 21); and controls, 67% (16 of 24). This finding suggested that recanalization occurred, albeit with delay, in nearly the same proportion of patients not treated with streptokinase as did acute recanalization in patients treated with streptokinase.

Delayed recanalization rates not related to thrombolytic therapy could be assessed directly in the nitroglycerin group based on paired angiograms that had been obtained at the time of intervention and on day 10 to 14. Antegrade flow at day 10 to 14 angiography was found in 77% (10 of 13) of vessels that were completely obstructed initially and had failed to recanalize during the infusion of nitroglycerin alone. This finding directly proved delayed recanalization in 75% of patients not treated with a thrombolytic agent. It expanded the results of our early, nonrandomized serial angiographic study, which had demonstrated spontaneous recanalization in four of nine patients in whom recanalization had not been attempted.[50]

We hypothesized that delayed recanalization in the nitroglycerin group was due to gradual endogenous thrombolysis, possibly enhanced by administration of anticoagulants during the hospital stay. The idea that prolonged anticoagulation could enhance spontaneous thrombolysis was indirectly supported by a prospective study by Betriu[175] involving 259 consecutive survivors of acute myocardial infarction who were not routinely treated with anticoagulation.Coronary angiography 1 month after the acute event revealed total occlusion of the infarct related artery in 45% of Betriu's patients as compared with 27% of our patients after 2 weeks of continuous anticoagulation.

None of the trials published by the end of 1984 was sufficiently powered to unequivocally assess changes in ejection fraction or mortality associated with intracoronary streptokinase.[176] We therefore concluded at the time that acceleration of recanalization of total coronary artery obstruction was the only proven, potentially beneficial effect of intracoronary streptokinase during acute myocardial infarction. In the 33% of our study patients with incomplete obstruction initially, the effects of intracoronary streptokinase infusion were yet to be assessed.[173]

Coronary Artery Recanalization with Intravenous Versus Intracoronary Application of Thrombolytic Agents

Our initial demonstration of rapid coronary artery recanalization by intracoronary infusion of streptokinase soon prompted West German hematologists and cardiologists to reconsider their belief that intravenous thrombolytic therapy could not achieve coronary artery recanalization rapidly enough to salvage myocardium. Dr. H. Koestering, the hematologist of our Goettingen group, argued that the standard intravenous infusion of 1.45 million units of streptokinase over 12 hours had been designed to achieve a prolonged lytic state and not to dissolve the obstructing coronary thrombus as quickly as possible. He proposed rapid intravenous infusion of a high dose of streptokinase.

Koestering and Neuhaus, also at the University of Goettingen, tested this concept in a pilot study in which they administered 1.5 million units of streptokinase intravenously over the course of 1 hour to 38 patients with acute myocardial infarction. They demonstrated angiographically that recanalization of a total coronary artery occlusion occurred in 68% of the study patients within 30 to 80 minutes.[177] Similar results were reported by Schroeder[178] in Berlin who infused 500,000 units of streptokinase intravenously within 30 minutes and documented recanalization of total coronary artery occlusion within 1 hour in 8 of 15 patients with acute myocardial infarction. Rapid restoration of antegrade flow

offered a more plausible explanation for any clinical benefit of intravenous thrombolytic therapy than reduction in blood viscosity or improvement of the microcirculation, and these concepts were discarded.[177,178]

Schroeder concluded that the acute recanalization rates achieved with intravenous infusion of streptokinase are comparable to those achieved with intracoronary administration.[178] This conclusion was not supported by a study published by this author in 1985, which pooled the angiographic data of the first five studies of high dose intravenous streptokinase and the first ten studies of intracoronary streptokinase.[179] The acute recanalization rate (1 hour to 90 minutes) for intravenous streptokinase was only 45% (range 10%-62%), a result subsequently confirmed prospectively in the TIMI I Trial,[180] compared to 74% (range 60%-94%) for intracoronary streptokinase.[179]

Angiograms performed several hours or days after intravenous infusion of streptokinase revealed a mean patency rate of 84% (range 73%-97%) in another analysis of pooled data performed by this author.[179] This late patency rate was comparable to that observed in studies using intracoronary streptokinase. This author concluded that intravenous infusion of streptokinase did not accelerate coronary artery recanalization in acute myocardial infarction as effectively as intracoronary streptokinase. However, it was suggested that the delay in recanalization could be offset by the time saved in initiation of therapy because intravenous administration does not require antecedent coronary angiography.[181]

Preliminary reports published in the mid-1980s suggested that the new clot-selective thrombolytic agent rt-PA recanalized acute total coronary artery occlusions more rapidly than intravenous streptokinase.[180] In 1989, this author concluded that the 90-minute recanalization rates achieved with intravenous rt-PA were comparable to those achieved with intracoronary streptokinase.[182] However, it became apparent that the researchers investigating rt-PA and those studying intracoronary streptokinase defined the term "recanalization" differently. To assess the results of intracoronary streptokinase infusion, we introduced a classification of antegrade flow that was identical to that subsequently adopted by the TIMI investigators, some of whom served on our Data Monitoring Committee at the National Institutes of Health (NIH). Our protocols specified that intracoronary drug infusion had to be continued for up to 90 minutes until brisk antegrade flow ("TIMI" grade III in today's terminology) was achieved. In the Second Mount Sinai-N.Y.U. Reperfusion Trial, intracoronary drug infusions were double-blinded and recanalization rates were assessed in a core laboratory by observers blinded to treatment assignment. Brisk antegrade flow ("TIMI" grade III) was seen after a 90-minute intracoronary infusion of streptokinase in 75% (48 of 64) of patients with initial total occlusion who were treated within 6 hours.[182] In the GUSTO I Trial, the 90-minute patency rate among patients assigned to the accelerated t-PA regimen within 6 hours was reported as 81%. However, TIMI grade III perfusion was seen only in 54%, the remainder of the "patent" vessels exhibiting TIMI grade II flow.[182] The physiological importance of TIMI grade III flow was understood and spelled out by the GUSTO investigators in that study.[183] Furthermore, it must be emphasized that baseline angiography was not performed in the GUSTO Trial. Therefore the 90-minute patency rate quoted included patients with antegrade flow prior to administration of t-PA, i.e., approximately 15% to 20% of patients in most trials.[179]

Thus, intracoronary thrombolytic therapy remains superior to intravenous administration of even clot-specific agents in achieving a physiologically meaningful degree of antegrade flow within 90 minutes among patients presenting with total coronary occlusion in the first 6 hours of infarction. Even if the use of intracoronary thrombolysis was limited by practical considerations, it was a research tool of unparalleled usefulness for the analysis of the pathophysiology of acute myocardial infarction and reperfusion.

II. Proving the Benefits of Early Thrombolytic Therapy (1985-1986)

The first randomized trials published in 1983/84[86, 122, 172-174] all performed in the United States, failed to unequivocally prove that intracoronary streptokinase therapy confers a mortality benefit or improves left ventricular function because they were too small[176] and therapy was initiated too late. The Western Washington Trial,[86] the largest of the early studies enrolling 250 patients, reported a significant decrease in 30-day mortality following intracoronary streptokinase therapy (3.7% vs 11.2%), but this benefit was lost at 1-year follow-up.[184] Furthermore, the 30-day mortality reduction was not paralleled by an improvement in ejection fraction. Our first trial (n = 124) showed a trend towards an increase in 6-month mortality among streptokinase-treated patients (21% vs 10%), which appears related to an uneven distribution of baseline variables associated with high risk.[173]

The delay from onset of symptoms to initiation of therapy was at least 4 hours in all trials published in 1983/84. Our ejection fraction model predicted that the functional benefit of reperfusion decreases rapidly with delays in treatment and becomes small after 3 hours (Fig. 14).

The first randomized trial that was appropriately designed to assess the effects of early coronary artery recanalization on mortality and left ventricular function was performed in the Netherlands and published in 1985.[185] A total of 533 patients presenting < 4 hours after symptom onset (median = 90 minutes) were enrolled. Rapid recanalization was initially achieved with an intracoronary streptokinase infusion alone. In a second phase of the trial, an intravenous infusion of 500,000 units of streptokinase was initiated immediately after randomization followed by angiography and intracoronary administration of streptokinase. Combining patients who had been treated with intracoronary streptokinase alone and those who had received both intravenous and intracoronary streptokinase, the investigators documented an infarct vessel patency rate of 85% within 200 minutes of symptom onset. The rapid recanalization strategy resulted in a significant reduction in 28-day mortality (6% vs 12%; P = 0.03) and 1-year mortality (9% vs 16%; P = 0.01) as well as a higher left ventricular ejection fraction at predischarge angiography (53% ± 13% vs 47% ± 14%; P = 0.0001).

In the United States and England our demonstration of rapid recanalization by intracoronary thrombolytic therapy led to a comprehensive review of all randomized trials of prolonged intravenous streptokinase infusion for acute myocardial infarction conducted during the 1960s and 1970s.[186] Although these trials had reported contradictory mortality results, pooling of all the data indicated a significant mortality reduction of approximately 20%. The finding of a mortality benefit among patients treated up to 24 hours after symptom onset suggested that the time window for thrombolytic interventions was not as limited as was believed.

This meta-analysis, published in 1982, prompted Italian investigators in 1983 to design the first prospective randomized trial, the GISSI Trial, which was to assess the mortality benefit of intravenous thrombolytic therapy and to analyze the importance of time to therapy,.[187] For this landmark study, published in 1986, the short-term, high dose intravenous streptokinase regimen introduced by Neuhaus and Schroeder was selected.[188] As detailed by the GISSI investigators in another issue of *The Journal for Interventional Cardiology*, nearly 12, 000 patients admitted within 12 hours of symptom onset were enrolled, and a highly significant, 18% mortality reduc-

tion was found in patients treated with streptokinase. The mortality reduction decreased rapidly with time from onset of pain to initiation of therapy. It was 47% for patients treated within 1 hour, 23% for those treated within 3 hours, and lost statistical significance for those treated after 6 hours. The rapid, nonlinear decrease in mortality benefit over time paralleled the rapid decrease in improvement of left ventricular function as suggested by our ejection fraction model (Fig. 15). Lack of a statistically significant mortality benefit in patients treated after 6 hours was seen by some as confirmation that late therapy does not salvage myocardium; however, it was noted by others that the mortality of patients treated between 6 and 9 hours was lower than that of controls, although the sample size of this subgroup was relatively small. It became apparent that the GISSI Trial could not assess late reperfusion with intravenous streptokinase.

III. Proving the Benefit of Late Thrombolytic Therapy: ISIS-2 and the Second Mt. Sinai-N.Y.U. Reperfusion Trial (1986-1989)

Reduction in Mortality:

ISIS-2. In 1988, the ISIS-2 study, which enrolled 17,187 patients presenting up to 24 hours after the onset of suspected acute myocardial infarction, was published.[189] This study, which confirmed the mortality benefit of early thrombolytic therapy demonstrated in the Netherlands Randomized Trial[185] and the GISSI Trial[187] was large enough to assess the effects of late therapy. Among patients allocated to receive intravenous streptokinase 5 to 24 hours after symptom onset a 17% reduction in 5-week cardiovascular mortality was found. This mortality reduction was smaller than that seen among patients treated within 4 hours (35%), but it was highly significant (P = 0.004).

The results of the ISIS-2 Trial were initially received with skepticism in the United States, in part because a plausible mechanism for benefit from late thrombolytic therapy was not known. Some speculated that late therapy might have benefitted primarily the subgroup with preinfarction angina and not patients with evolving infarction. Since ECG changes at entry were not required, it was suspected that the group with preinfarction angina was larger in the ISIS Trial than in U.S. studies of thrombolytic therapy.

Improvement in Thallium Uptake: The Second Mt. Sinai-N.Y.U. Reperfusion Trial

In 1989 we published results from the Second Mount Sinai-N.Y.U. Reperfusion Trial in which we assessed the effects of intracoronary and spasmolytic interventions initiated up to 14 hours after infarct onset on left ventricular function, coronary anatomy, and thallium uptake.[182,190,191] The primary end point, change in ejection fraction from preintervention to day 10 to 14, and the angiographic results have been presented in formal papers. Changes in thallium uptake have been published in abstract form only[191]; these results will be presented in detail in this article because they clarify the mechanisms of benefit from late reperfusion.

Trial Design and Patients.

The Second Mt. Sinai-N.Y.U. Reperfusion Trial was conducted at three New York City hospitals from 1982 to 1985 and supported by an NHLBI R01 grant to this author. A total of 399 patients were enrolled up to 12 hours (mean = 6.3 ± 2.4 hours) and treated up to 14 hours after symptom onset. At the time of enrollment patients were prospectively stratified into an early intervention trial if they had infarct pain for < 2 hours ("Trial A", n = 78) and a late trial ("Trial B", n = 315) if they had in-farct symptoms for 2 to 12 hours. In both trials, patients were randomly assigned to intracoronary streptokinase, intracoronary nitroglycerin, a combination of intracoronary streptokinase and nitroglycerin, or conventional therapy without acute angiography.[190] Time from onset of infarction to interventional angiography was $3.2 + 0.7$ hours in "Trial A" and 7.1 ± 2.4 hours (range = 4 to 14 hours) in "Trial B."

Acquisition and Analysis of Thallium Scintigrams.

In "Trial B" planar thallium scintigraphy was performed in two planes (anterior/posterior and 606° left anterior oblique), using standard techniques, before interventional angiography and on day 10 to 14. Since the benefit of reperfusion therapy was expected to decrease rapidly within the first 3 hours of infarction, the delay in therapy that would have been associated with preintervention thallium scintigraphy was felt to be unacceptable in "Trial A" patients.

Thallium scintigrams were assessed in a core laboratory by readers blinded to treatment assignment using a quantitative and two qualitative methods. For all analyses the left ventricle was divided into five segments per view, i.e., ten segments per study.

A quantitative thallium score was generated by expressing average thallium activity in each segment as percent of thallium activity in the segment with the greatest thallium uptake and calculating the average score of the ten segments.[192,193] Thus a higher quantitative score indicated a greater average uptake of thallium; the maximum possible score was 100.

In the first qualitative analysis, thallium uptake within each of the ten segments of a single study was assessed using a 4-point scale ranging from normal to "no thallium uptake." These readings were subsequently dichotomized into "normal" or "abnormal" uptake. A qualitative score was generated by adding the number of seg-

Table 2

Change in Quantitative Thallium Score from Preintervention to End Point by Treatment Arm

Arm		Preintervention			Change		
	N	Mean	SD		Mean	SEM	
SK	60	72.1	6.0		4.9	0.8	**
SK-NTG	69	72.6	6.1		4.5	0.6	**
NTG	59	74.4	8.7		2.1	0.8	**
Control	57	72.8	10.1		3.7	0.8	**

**The change is significantly different from zero with the following P value: $P < 0.0001$.

ments with abnormal uptake in each study. Thus, a higher qualitative score indicated more extensive abnormal thallium uptake.

The second qualitative analysis determined the percentage of patients, by infarct location, in whom the day 10 to 14 study revealed improved thallium uptake. The images were read in a side-by-side fashion. The preintervention or end point study was randomly assigned a status of "reference study" and each segment of the paired study was scored as "worse," "same," or "improved" in relation to the corresponding region of the reference study. Uptake in the infarct region was considered "improved" if more infarct related segments had improved rather than worsened at end point study.[193]

The trial was analyzed by intention to treat. The statistical methods used have been described.[182,190] The null hypothesis that change in thallium score was the same for the four treatment arms was tested by analysis of covariance.

Results.

Paired studies from preintervention and end point were available in 235 patients. There were significant streptokinase effects for all three analyses but no interactions.

Quantitative thallium scores were not different at baseline between groups. At day 10 to 14 we found a significant im-

provement in quantitative thallium score in all treatment arms (Table 2). Improvement was significantly greater in patients assigned to the streptokinase arms than in those who were not ($P = 0.03$).

Qualitative analysis of baseline thallium scintigrams showed an abnormal thallium uptake in 3.3 ± 1.8 of ten segments/patient without significant difference between treatment arms. There was a significantly greater net improvement in patients in the streptokinase arms (1.5 ± 2.6 segments/patient) than in patients not assigned to streptokinase (0.8 ± 2.2 segments/patient) ($P = 0.03$).

Side-by-side analysis (n = 199) revealed improved thallium uptake in 67% (29 of 43) of patients with anterior wall infarction who were assigned to the streptokinase arms as compared with 47% (23 of 49) of those who were not ($P < 0.05$). Among patients with inferior wall infarction, thallium uptake improved in 54% (30 of 56) if they had been assigned to the streptokinase groups and in 31% (16 of 51) if they had not ($P = 0.02$)

Conclusion.

We concluded that thrombolytic therapy 4 to 14 hours after infarct onset improves thallium uptake independent of infarct location. This finding strongly suggests that late reperfusion results in salvage of jeopardized myocardium. The mortality benefit of thrombolytic therapy up to 24 hours after infarct onset documented in ISIS-2[189] can be explained, at least in part, by this mechanism.

Changes in Ejection Fraction: The Second Mt. Sinai-N.Y.U. Reperfusion Trial

The analysis of the primary end point results of the Second Mt. Sinai-N.Y.U. Reperfusion Trial, change of ejection fraction, led to a more detailed understanding of the mechanisms responsible for myocardial salvage by late thrombolytic therapy. The ejection fraction results that have been published in detail[182] will be summarized briefly.

Left ventricular ejection fraction was determined by radionuclide left ventriculography prior to intervention and on day 10 to 14. Change in ejection fraction was prospectively related to the preintervention angiographic subsets defined in our previous studies: total occlusion of the infarct artery without collateral flow (90 patients); total occlusion with collateral flow (52 patients); subtotal occlusion without collateral flow (48 patients).

There were interactions between baseline angiographic patterns and treatment effects. Ejection fraction did not improve among patients with noncollateralized total occlusion regardless of treatment arm. Patients with collateral flow showed a significant improvement over those without collateral flow in the streptokinase (5.4% ± 2.5%) and the streptokinase-nitroglycerin arms (10.6% ± 2. 7%) , but not in the nitroglycerin arm (Fig. 19A). In patients with initial subtotal occlusion, ejection fraction increased by approximately 6% in all three intervention arms (Fig. 19B). We drew four conclusions from these findings.

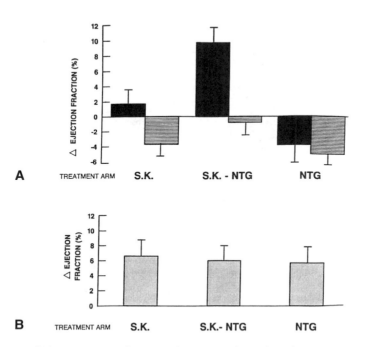

Figure 19. Change (△) in ejection fraction (expressed as the change in percentage units) from preintervention to day 10 to 14 study by treatment arm. SK = intracoronary streptokinase; SK-NTG = intracoronary streptokinase + nitroglycerin; NTG = intracoronary nitroglycerine. (A) (Left panel) In patients with total occlusion of the infarct-related coronary artery before therapy. Closed bars = collateral channels present; striped bar = no collateral channels. (B) (Right panel) In patients with subtotal obstruction of the infarct-related artery before therapy.

First, lack of improvement of left ventricular function among patients with total, noncollateralized occlusions who received intracoronary streptokinase after 6.3 ± 2.4 hours indicated that the 4- to 6-hour "time window" for myocardial salvage by reperfusion, established by Reimer in the experimental animal, applies in this angiographic subset.

Second, the finding that among patients with collateral flow, left ventricular function improved following streptokinase therapy but failed to improve in the absence of streptokinase therapy indicated that collateral flow extends the time window for thrombolytic therapy to at least 14 hours by slowing the progression of myocardial necrosis. Because collateralized total occlusion was found in only 25% of the patients in our trials, whereas 50% of the patients had noncollateralized total occlusion, the overall benefit of late thrombolytic therapy would be expected to be smaller than that of early therapy. This finding provided a pathophysiological basis for the significant, albeit small, survival benefit of thrombolytic therapy initiated more than 5 hours after onset of infarct symptoms demonstrated in the ISIS-2 Trial.[189]

Third, our finding of significant improvement of left ventricular function among patients with antegrade flow at baseline who did not receive thrombolytic therapy confirmed earlier uncontrolled observations.[174] We suggested that this improvement in function indicated recovery of stunned myocardium. Failure of thrombolytic therapy to augment the functional improvement among patients with antegrade flow at baseline led us to conclude that coronary flow was not critically impaired by fibrin-containing thrombus in this angiographic subset.

It had been suggested that antegrade residual flow to the infarct area extends the time window for myocardial salvage by thrombolytic therapy in a similar way to residual flow through collateral channels.[158,174] However, the ejection fraction findings of the Second Mt. Sinai-N.Y.U.

Reperfusion Trial indicate that late thrombolytic therapy effects myocardial salvage only in the subgroup with collateralized total occlusions. It appeared likely that the survival benefit of late thrombolytic therapy demonstrated in the ISIS-2 Trial was due to reperfusion in patients with total occlusion and collateral flow and was not related to resolution of residual thrombus in vessels with antegrade flow prior to therapy.

Growth and Recruitment of Collateral Channels: The Second Mt. Sinai-N.Y.U. Reperfusion Trial

The angiographic findings of the Second Mt. Sinai-N.Y.U. Reperfusion Trial published in 1989 provided important insights into the development and recruitment of collateral channels.[182] We prospectively assessed the prevalence of angiographically demonstrable collateral vessels to the infarct related artery. Collateral vessels were determined to be present if any segment of the infarct related artery filled in any way other than a continuous antegrade manner. At preintervention angiography, collaterals to the infarct related artery were observed in 27% (74 of 274) of the study patients. Among patients with complete occlusion of the infarct related vessel, they were seen in 33% (66 of 199), significantly more frequently than among patients with antegrade flow (11%; 8 of 73) (P < 0.001). The prevalence of collaterals was not related to the time interval from infarct onset to angiography (Table 3).

We concluded that the collaterals demonstrated at acute angiography developed before the acute thrombotic occlusion and not in response to it. We hypothesized that collateral vessels visible at baseline angiography had grown in response to a chronic, high grade lesion present in the infarct vessel prior to the infarct. They were recruited due to an increase in the pressure gradient across the collateral circuit when the epicardial vessel was totally occluded by thrombus.[182]

Table 3

Prevalence of Collateral Flow to a Totally Occluded Infarct Artery at Baseline Angiography* in the Second Mount Sinai-N.Y.U. Reperfusion Trial

	Time to Angiography (Hours)				
	2–4	4–6	6–8	8–14	All
Patients with total occlusion studied (n)	40	56	48	52	196
Collaterals (%)	33	30	29	38	33

*As a function of time interval from onset of pain to angiography (time to angiography).

We assessed the evolution of collaterals further in those patients with complete obstruction at baseline angiography in whom day 10 to14 angiography was performed. Persistent occlusion in 42 patients, i.e., occlusion of the infarct artery at pre- and post intervention angiography as well as on day 10 to14, was associated with an increase in the prevalence of collaterals from 33% at baseline to 90% at day 10 to14 angiography. This finding demonstrated a second distinct phase of collateral growth. The exact time frame of growth of new collateral channels after abrupt coronary closure could not be surmised from our data. Schaper had observed in the experimental animal that the first cellular mitoses occur 24 hours after coronary obstruction.[194] We concluded that growth of collateral channels occurs nearly uniformly in humans within 10 to 14 days of sustained coronary occlusion. Among the 56 patients who experienced acute reperfusion that was sustained at day 10 to 14 angiography, the prevalence of angiographically demonstrable collaterals decreased from 38% to 7%.[182]

These observations prompted this author to develop an angioplasty model that facilitated the angiographic assessment of the appearance and disappearance of collateral flow immediately after controlled coronary artery occlusion and reflow in humans during elective angioplasty.[195] Collateral filling to the index artery was visualized via control injection into the contralateral artery using a second catheter in patients with isolated left anterior descend-

ing or right coronary artery disease and normal left ventricular function. The following grading system of collateral filling was thus introduced and subsequently universally adopted: 0 = none; 1 = filling of side branches of the artery to be dilated via collateral channels without visualization of the epicardial segment; 2 = partial filling of the epicardial segment of the artery being dilated via collateral channels; 3 = complete filling of the epicardial segment via collateral channels.

Improvement of collateral filling by one grade occurred in 8 of 16 study patients, a two grade improvement occurred in 5 patients, and a three grade improvement in 2 patients. After completion of angioplasty, all patients had grade 0 collateral filling.

We used this model to prospectively study the impact of collateral recruitment on the severity of myocardial ischemia as assessed by chest pain, electrocardiographic changes, the extent of new left ventricular asynergy, and decrease in left ventricular ejection fraction during coronary occlusion.[196,197] We found that grade 2 and 3 collateral channels limited acute ischemia, as assessed by all four indexes immediately following abrupt coronary occlusion, whereas grade 0 or 1 collateral filling conferred a negligible degree of protection.

The beneficial effects of collateral recruitment immediately following coronary occlusion cannot be appreciated when coronary angiography is performed only days or weeks after infarction. At this time, persistent coronary occlusion has triggered the growth of collateral channels that were not available at the time of acute occlusion. Lack of acute angiographic data explains the many contradictions in the literature regarding the protective potential of collateral flow. Our studies provided a strong rationale to test therapeutic modalities, which augment the growth of collateral channels.

Appendix: Investigators

I. Goettingen Pilot Studies
   Supported by the Deutsche Forschungsgemeinschaft Grant SFB 89.
   Chairman: Bretschneider H
   Principal Investigator: Rentrop KP
   Coinvestigators:
   Cardiology: Blanke H, Karsch Kr, Kaiser H, Wiegand V, Graf M
   Cardiovascular surgery: Leitz K, Oster H, DeVivie ER
   Physiology: Hellige G, Zipfel J, Baller D, Bretschneider H
   Hematology: Koestering H
   Pathology: Sinapius D
   Nuclear medicine: Schicha H, Emrich D
   Max Plank Institut, Bad Nauheim: Hofman M, Schaper W
II. West German Registry
   Supported by the Deutsche Forschungsgemeinschaft Grant
   Chairman: Bretschneider H
   Chairman: Rentrop KP
   Clinical Units, Principal Investigators: Berlin: Rutsch W; Aachen: Merx W; Hamburg: Mathey DG; Goettingen: Rentrop KP
   Coinvestigators:
   Cardiology: Blanke H, Doerr R, Karsch KR, Kremer P, Kuck K, Schartl M, Schmutzler H
   Surgery: Leitz K, Messmer BJ, Rodewald G, Burcel ES
III. Registry of the European Society of Cardiology
   Supported in part by the Heart Research Foundation, The New York Cardiac Center, The Heineman Foundation, and the Thea Brothers Fund.
   Chairman: Rentrop KP
   Coordinating Center: Rentrop KP, Karsch KR, Painter L. Mount Sinai Medical Center, New York, NY
   Biostatistics: Smith H, Holt J. Mount Sinai Medical Center, New York, NY
   Collaborating Centers and Principal Investigators:
   France: Valeix B, Centre Jules Cantini, Marseille; Guarino L, Hopital Pasteur, Nice; Brochier M, Tours Centre Hospitalier Regional
   Germany: Merx W, RWT Hochschule, Aachen; Rutsch W, Klinikum Charlottenburg, Berlin; Rentrop KP, University Hospital, Goettingen; Mathey DG, University Hospital, Hamburg
   Italy: Camerini F, Hospidale Maggiore, Trieste
   Netherlands: Dohmen, Groot-Zienken-Gasthuis, Den Bosch; Serruys PW, Thoraxcenter, Rotterdam
   Switzerland: Kappenberger L, Zuerich Universitaetsspital, Zurich
   United States: Feit F, Bellevue-New York University Hospital, New York, NY; Schweitzer P, Bronx Veterans' Administration Medical Center, Bronx, NY; Schneider RR, City Hospital Center at Elmhurst, NY; Rentrop KP, Mount Sinai Medical Center, New York, NY
IV. Goettingen Registry
   Supported in part by the Deutsche Forschungsgemeinschaft, Grant SFB 89.
   Chairman: Bretschneider H
   Co-Chairmen: Blanke H; Rentrop KP
   Coinvestigators: Cohen M, Kaiser H, Karsch KR, Levine RA, Neumann P, Scherff F, Schicha H, Schlueter GU, von Hardenberg D
   Biostatistics: Smith H, Holt J, Mount Sinai Medical Center, New York, NY
V. First Mt. Sinai-N.Y.U. Reperfusion Trial
   Supported in part by the Heart Research Foundation, the New York Cardiac Center, the Heineman Foundation, and the Thea Brothers Fund
   Principal Investigators: Rentrop KP, Feit

F, Gorlin R

Trial Design: Chalmers T, Smith H, Gorlin R, Feit F, Fox A, Teicholtz L, Rentrop KP

Monitoring Committee: Chalmers T, Kupfer S, Gorlin R, Wittes J, Goldberg J

Clinical Units:

Mt. Sinai Hospital: Rentrop P, Blanke H, Horowitz S, Karsch K, Goldman M, Cohen M, Pichard A, Gorlin R

Bellevue Hospital: Feit F, Stecy P, Rey M, Meilman H, Siegel S, Slater J, Ehrich M, Nachamie M, Politzer F, Cole W, Fox A

City Hospital at Elmhurst: Schneider R, Lane F, Lee H, Rhee J

Bronx Veterans' Administration: Schweitzer P, Stern E

Data Center: Smith H, Calhoun F, Fagerstrom R, Holt J Data Managers: Painter L, Hosat S, Matheson MA, Napoli S, Hill N, Felton H

Nuclear Core Laboratory: Sanger J, Horowitz S, Goldsmith S

Electrocardiographic Core Laboratory: Rey M, Nachamie M, Ehrich M, Siegel S

Angiographic Core Laboratory: Blanke H, Feit F, Rentrop KP

Creatine Kinase Core Laboratory: Litwak R, Handke B

VI. Second Mount Sinai-New York University Reperfusion Trial

Supported by the Cardiac Diseases Branch, Division of Heart and Vascular Diseases. National Heart, Lung, and Blood Institute. National Institutes of Health Bethesda, MD (Grant R01HL28843).

Steering Committee: Rentrop KP (Chairman), Feit F (Secretary), Sherman W, Fox A, Gorlin R, McKusick K, Cameron A, Goldsmith S, Rey M

Clinical Units, Principal Investigators:

Mt. Sinai Medical Center New York, NY: Rentrop KP (Principal Investigator),

Cohen M, Ambrose J, Blanke H. Cohen B, Milner M, Cowen J, Arora R, Winters S, Phillips R, Reichstein R, Levine R, Rao B, Hosat S

Bellevue Hospital, New York, NY: Feit F (Principal Investigator) , Stecy P, Rey M, Nachamie M, Cole W, Politzer F, Kramer J, Ehrich M, Friedman G, Siegel S, Prior F, Attubato M, Slater J, Gindea A, Napoli S, Harty S, Bernardin V

City Hospital, Elmhurst, NY: Sherman W (Principal Investigator), Schneider R (former Principal Investigator), Perdoncin R, Schwartz W, Lane F, Lee H, Patel R, Hill N

Data Coordinating Center: Thornton J (Principal Investigator), Calhoun F, Smith H, Fagerstrom R, Holt J, Berkowitz-Rudolph L, Fisher J, VanBuskirk M, McAvay G

Radionuclide Ventriculography Core Laboratory: *Harvard University School of Medicine, Boston MA: McKusick K (Principal Investigator), Yasuda T*

Angiography Core Laboratory: St. Luke's Hospital, New York, NY: Cameron A (Principal Investigator), Kemp H

Electrocardiography Core Laboratory: *New York University Hospital School of Medicine, New York, NY:* Rey M (Principal Investigator).

Thallium Scintigraphy Core Laboratory: *Mount Sinai and New York University Schools of Medicine, New York, NY: Goldsmith S (Principal Investigator), Sanger J, Horowitz S, Farrell M*

Hematology Core Laboratory: Mount Sinai Medical Center, New York, NY: Rand J (Principal Investigator)

Safety and Data Monitoring Committee: Hood Jr WB (Chairman), Becker LC, Canner P, Cohn JH, Halperin M, Killip III T, Marder VJ, Rapaport E, Smith H, Robertson TL (Ex Officio Member).

References

172. Khaja F, Walton JA, Brymer JF, et al. Intracoronary fibrinolytic therapy in acute myocardial infarction. Report of a prospective randomized trial. N Engl J Med 1983;308:1305-1311.

173. Rentrop KP, Feit F, Blanke H, et al. Effects of intracoronary streptokinase and intracoronary nitroglycerin infusion on coronary angiographic patterns and mortality in patients with acute myocardial infarction. N Engl J Med 1984;311:1457-1463.

174. Leiboff RH, Katz RJ, Wasserman AG, et al. A randomized angiographically controlled trial of intracoronary streptokinase in acute myocardial infarction. Am J Cardiol 1984;53:404-407.

175. Betriu A, Castaner A, Sanz GA, et al. Angiographic findings 1 month after myocardial infarction: A prospective study of 259 survivors. Circulation 1982;65:1099-1105.

176. Furberg CD. Clinical value of intracoronary streptokinase. Am J Cardiol 1984;53:626-627.

177. Neuhaus KL, Koestering H, Tebbe U, et al. High-dose intravenous streptokinase infusion in acute myocardial infarction. Z Kardiol 1981;70:791-796.

178. Schroeder R, Biamino G, von Leitner ER, et al. Intravenoese streptokinase-Infusion bei akutem Myokardinfarkt. Dtsch med Wschr 1981;106:294-301.

179. Rentrop KP. Thrombolytic therapy in patients with acute myocardial infarction. Circulation 1985;71:627-631.

180. Chesebro JH, Knatterud G, Roberts R, et al. Thrombolysis in myocardial infarction (TIMI) trial, phase I: A comparison between intravenous tissue plasminogen activator and intravenous streptokinase. Circulation 1987;76:142-154.

181. Schroeder R, Biamino G, von Leitner ER, et al. Intravenous short-term infusion of streptokinase in acute myocardial infarction. Circulation 1983;67:536-548.

182. Rentrop KP, Feit F, Sherman W, et al. Serial angiographic assessment of coronary artery obstruction and collateral flow in acute myocardial infarction. Report from the Second Mount Sinai-New York University Reperfusion Trial. Circulation 1989;80:1166-1175.

183. The GUSTO Angiographic Investigators. The effects of tissue plasminogen activator, streptokinase, or both on coronary artery patency, ventricular function, and survival after acute myocardial infarction. N Engl J Med 1993;329:1615-1622.

184. Kennedy JW, Ritchie JL, Davis KB, et al. The Western Washington Randomized Trial of intracoronary streptokinase in acute myocardial infarction. A 12-month follow-up report. N Engl J Med 1985;312:1073-1078.

185. Simoons ML, Serruys PW, v/d Brand M, et al. Improved survival after early thrombolysis in acute myocardial infarction. A randomized trial by the Interuniversity Cardiology Institute in The Netherlands. Lancet 1985;2:578-582.

186. Stampfer MJ, Goldhaber SZ, Yusuf S, et al. Effect of intravenous streptokinase on acute myocardial infarction. Pooled results from randomized trials. N Engl J Med 1982;307: 1180-1182.

187. Gruppo Italiano per lo Studio della Streptochinasi nell'Infarto Miocardico (GISSI). Effectiveness of intravenous thrombolytic treatment in acute myocardial infarction. Lancet 1986;1: 397-402.

188. The ISAM Study Group. A prospective trial of intravenous streptokinase in acute myocardial infarction (I.S.A.M.). N Engl J Med 1986;314:1465-1471.

189. ISIS-2 (Second International Study of Infarct Survival) Collaborative Group. Randomised trial of intravenous streptokinase, oral aspirin, both, or neither among 17,187 cases of suspected acute myocardial infarction: ISIS-2. Lancet 1988;2:349-360.

190. Rentrop KP, Feit F, Sherman W, et al. Late thrombolytic therapy preserves left ventricular function in patients with collateralized total coronary occlusion: Primary end point findings of the Second Mount Sinai-New York University Reperfusion Trial. JACC 1989;14:58-64.

191. Feit F, Rey MJ, Sherman W, et al. Late thrombolytic therapy improves thallium uptake in acute myocardial infarction: A report from the Second Mt. Sinai-N.Y.U. Reperfusion Trial. (abstract) JACC 1990;15:221A.

192. Watson DD, Campbell NP, Read EK, et al. Spatial and temporal quantitation of plane thallium myocardial images. J Nucl Med 1981;22:577.

193. Lim YL, Okada RD, Chesler DA, et al. A new approach to quantitation of exercise thallium-201 scintigraphy before and after an intervention: Application to define the impact of coronary angioplasty on regional myocardial perfusion. Am Heart J 1984; 108:917.

194. Schaper W. Pathophysiology of coronary circulation. Prog Cardiovasc Dis 1971;14:275-296.

195. Rentrop KP, Cohen M, Blanke H, et al. Changes in collateral channel filling immediately after controlled coronary artery occlusion by an angioplasty balloon in human subjects. JACC 1985;5: 587-592.

196. Cohen M, Rentrop KP. Limitation of myocardial ischemia by collateral circulation during sudden controlled coronary artery occlusion in human subjects: A prospective study. Circulation 1986;74:469-476.

197. Rentrop KP, Thornton JC, Feit F, et al. Determinants and protective potential of coronary arterial collaterals as assessed by an angioplasty model. Am J Cardiol 1988;61:677-684.

Chapter 2

Trials of the European Working Party on Streptokinase and of the European Cooperative Study Group on Alteplase in Patients with Acute Myocardial Infarction

Marc Verstraete, M.D. for the European Investigators

From the Center for Molecular and Vascular Biology, University of Leuven, Belgium

Trials of the European Working Party on Streptokinase and of the European Cooperative Working Group on tPA in Patients with Acute Myocardial Infarction

The first trial of the European Working Party was commenced in 1962 at a time when no controlled, strictly randomized, large scale trials on the clinical use of thrombolytic drugs in patients with recent myocardial infarction (MI) were available.

At that time, the frequency with which a fresh thrombus complicates the coronary atheromatous lesion in acute MI was derived from autopsy studies and reported to vary from 13%–74%.[1] This disparity was doubtless due in part to the selection of the patient samples (sudden, early, late deaths), to types of infarctions (transmural, subendocardial), and to the methods of postmortem study (dissection or angiography). The prevailing hypothesis that a coronary thrombus was often *secondary* to a MI was based, among other things, on the fact that at autopsy a thrombus was found more frequently in the older infarcts, after cardiac shock, or after severe heart failure.[2] The finding that radioactive fibrinogen, given in the acute phase of MI, has been recovered in the coronary thrombus at autopsy was wrongly considered as an argument in favor of the thesis that the thrombus follows the MI. In fact, thrombi that are already old may still extend and continue to take up radioactive fibrinogen. New opportunities available 20 years later presented by coronary angiography and performed during the first hours after the initial symptoms of acute MI have brought this long debate to a halt; it is now clear that there is an 85% chance of finding in vivo an occlusion in the coronary artery near the infarcted zone in the first hours after acute MI.

The following considerations, although essentially speculative, appeared to provide in the early 1960s a rational basis for controlled trials with thrombolytic drugs in patients with acute MI. Associated with MI, fibrin had been observed not only in the occluded coronary artery, but also in the collateral circulation in the myocardium, in thrombi forming in the cavity of the ventricle—perhaps provoking peripheral emboli—and in peripheral veins, where deep venous thrombosis, possibly complicated by pulmonary embolism, can occur. At that time, one could question the wisdom to lyse intraventricular clots. It was indeed conceivable that lysis may be incomplete, and fragmentation with resultant arterial embolism might occur. Second, what would be the fate of thrombi which may form during the period of severe plasminogen depletion associated with the administration of high doses of urokinase or streptokinase?

Trials of the European Working Party on Streptokinase in MI

EWP-1: Single-Blind Randomized Trial Comparing Intravenous Streptokinase and Heparin (72-Hour Infusion) in Patients with Recent MI (Less than 72 Hours)

Patients diagnosed in different centers as having, according to the criteria of each center—a MI of < 72 hours' duration—were preselected for this first study, after exclusion of those patients where heparin or streptokinase treatment was considered contraindicated. All patients received the standard general treatment for recent MI appropriate to each center.[3]

Using a sealed envelope system, the candidates for the study were allocated at random in a heparin and streptokinase group. The patients of the heparin group received an initial dose of 10,000 IU heparin over a 30-minute period and 1,250 IU per hour during 72 hours thereafter. The patients belonging to the streptokinase group received an initial dose of 1,250,000 IU streptokinase within 30 minutes, and during the next 72 hours, 100,000 units streptokinase per hour. Twenty-five mg prednisolone was injected intravenously to all patients just before the initial dose of hep-

arin or streptokinase, and daily during the first 3 days.

Of 167 patients, 84 patients were treated with heparin and 83 with streptokinase. On retrospective analysis, the two treatment groups were homogeneous at the time of admission into the study in parameters which might influence the course of a MI.

In an intention-to-treat analysis, no significant difference could be found between these two groups as a whole in the hospital mortality and serum transaminases at different intervals after the start of infusion.

In a secondary analysis, patients of both groups were divided into subgroups, according to several parameters: for example, age; the interval between the onset of the acute retrosternal pain; the start of the heparin respectively streptokinase infusion; and the presence of definite ECG signs of MI (central blind analysis). No significant difference in hospital mortality was found between the two treatment groups of these subgroups. This small trial can be criticized because the minimum criteria for MI were not defined in the protocol, and particularly because very late entry of patients was allowed.

EWP-2: Single-Blind Randomized Trial Comparing Intravenous Streptokinase and Heparin (24-Hour infusion) in Patients with Acute MI (Less than 24 Hours)

Although no significant difference in outcome was obtained in the previous study, this does not exclude the possibility that a favorable result could be reached by streptokinase, administered using another dosage scheme in more selected patient groups. Therefore, a new trial was organized in patients suffering from MI of < 24 hours' duration. This time interval was selected because in the meantime the results of another study in patients with an evolving MI of < 12 hours' duration became available.[4] The overall mortality over the first 40 days in the latter study was 14.1% in the streptokinase-treated patients and 21% in the heparin-treated group (P = 0.031). Excluding the first 24 hours in hospital, the mortality was 8.7% and 16.1%, respectively (P = 0.021).

In the second multicenter trial of the European Working Party, a lower initial dose of streptokinase was used (250,000 compared to 1,250,000 IU in the first study) with the same maintenance dose (100,000 IU hourly), but for a shorter duration (24 hours instead of 72 hours). In the control group, the initial dose of heparin was 10,000 IU over a 20-minute period, followed by 30,000 IU over the next 24 hours. Coumarin was commenced in both at the start of thrombolytic treatment.[5] Both groups received oral anticoagulants, and special attention was paid to the transition period between the trial infusion and the effect of the coumarin treatment, which was covered with repeated heparin injections.

Out of 764 patients who entered in the study, 28 from one center were excluded from the analysis because they were not treated in accordance with the system of serially numbered envelopes. Six other patients also had to be excluded, as in 4 the charts were lost and in 2, the treatment code was not followed. Thus, 730 patients were included in the first analysis: 373 treated with streptokinase and 357 with heparin. Eight centers cooperated in the trial. In this study conducted at the end of the 1960s, only about one-third of the patients were treated in a coronary care unit.

The cases in the two groups did not differ appreciably in those factors which are considered to influence the risks associated with MI, nor in several other ways. The number of patients who had already suffered two or more MIs was only slightly higher in the heparin-treated group (44 out of 344) than in the streptokinase-treated group (35 out of 355). This difference is not significant (P > 0.10), nor is the higher inci-

dence of arrhythmia on admission in patients treated with streptokinase (P = 0.10).

The mean duration of stay in hospital averaged 43 days. The total hospital mortality was 18.5% of 373 patients allotted to streptokinase treatment, and 26.3% of 357 given heparin (P = 0.014). The mortality after infusion (24 hours) was 10.6% of 340 patients treated with streptokinase, and 17.8% of 320 given heparin (P = 0.011). Bleeding from puncture sites and pyrexia occurred more frequently during streptokinase treatment.

After exclusion of those patients whose diagnosis was unconfirmed on blinded retrospective assessment, the total hospital mortality rate was 19.0% of 357 patients treated with streptokinase and 27.4% of 339 treated with heparin (P = 0.011). These results indicate that in acute MI, streptokinase was superior to heparin in reducing hospital mortality and reinfarction rate during an average period of 6 weeks in hospital.

Death was taken as the main yardstick for assessing the effect of treatment, and that meant that only those patients who died contributed directly to the final analysis. No attempt was made to use figures for deaths from specific causes, since a small change in fatality from cardiovascular causes without an overall difference in deaths from all causes may indicate either a diagnostic shift or at most a trivial benefit. It is worth noting, however, that reinfarction while in hospital was less frequent in the streptokinase-treated (6 out of 340) than in the heparin-treated patients (16 out of 320), this difference being significant (P = 0.036).

EWP-3: Single-Blind Randomized Trial Comparing Streptokinase with Glucose (24-Hour Infusion) in Medium Risk Patients with Acute MI (Less than 12 Hours' Duration) Admitted in a Coronary Care Unit

In the second trial of the European Working Party, only one-third of the patients were admitted in a coronary care unit, but in the EWP-3 trial, all patients were. At that time, the value of heparinization in the acute phase of MI had been challenged, as heparin might increase ventricular irritability because of a rise in plasma-free fatty acid. For this reason the comparative arm of streptokinase was a glucose instead of a heparin infusion. The required ECG changes for inclusion of patients in the study were detailed in the protocol, as were the criteria for enzymes creatine kinase; in the previous two EWP trials the minimum criteria for infarction were not defined; however, the diagnosis based on the criteria in use in each participating hospital was retrospectively reviewed by an independent expert, blinded with regard to the treatment given. In EWP-3, patients were stratified according to clinical severity and only high and medium risk patients were randomized.

Five hundred fifteen patients entered the study; 307 were randomized in the medium risk group and the 8 in the high risk group. The 197 low risk patients were not randomized but followed for mortality.[6,7] Randomized patients received either a loading dose of streptokinase (250,000) to overwhelm circulating antistreptokinase antibodies or a placebo; these doses were followed by a 24-hour infusion of streptokinase (100,000 per hour) or glucose. All subjects subsequently received oral anticoagulants. The two treatment groups were roughly comparable, although more patients in the placebo group had frequent ventricular premature beats and more had a history of previous infarction. Various analyses of the role of this accident of randomization did not explain the outcome of the trial.

In contrast to the EWP-2 study, this trial did not reveal a significant difference in mortality rates before the twenty-first hospital day (28 deaths in the control group vs 18 in the streptokinase group), although there was a trend in favor of streptokinase. However, the difference in mortality after the third week was significant ($P < 0.01$). The death rate at 3 weeks of low risk patients (not randomized) was 6.1%. At 6 months, the mortality rate was 30.6% in the control group and 15.6% in the streptokinase-treated group (the survival curves are shown in Fig. 1) The difference in favor of streptokinase was statistically significant ($P < 0.01$). The frequency of sudden arrhythmia as a cause of death was 54% in the control group, but only 36% in the streptokinase group. Reinfarction was the cause in 10% of the patients who died in the streptokinase group, but none in the streptokinase group. As usual, fever, chills, and bleeding complications occurred more frequently in the patients who received streptokinase.[7]

Although the EWP-2 and EWP-3 trials revealed a reduction in total mortality in 40-day of 30% (EWP-2) and at 6-month of 49.3% (EWP-3), these results did not impress cardiologists. As a consequence, in the early 1980s thrombolytic treatment was rarely used in patients with acute MI.

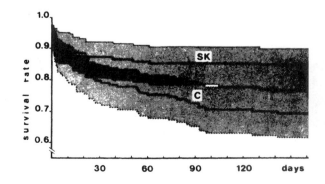

Figure 1. Survival curves with 95% confidence limits in the streptokinase-treated (solid lines) (SK) and the control group (dotted lines) (C).

Table 1

Historical Review of the European Cooperative Study Group for rt-PA

1983	Genentech and the Center for Thrombosis and Vascular Research in Leuven, Belgium reported the cloning of human tPA in *Nature*.
1984	A first meeting was organized in Bad Soden (near Frankfurt), bringing together clinical investigators. The European Cooperative Study Group (ECSG) for Recombinant Tissue-type Plasminogen Activator was established. Prof. Dr. M. Verstraete, head of the Center for Thrombosis and Vascular Research in Leuven, Belgium, was appointed as chairman. The data center was established at the Thoraxcenter in Rotterdam headed by Prof. Dr. J. Lubsen.
1985	Within 1 year after the inaugural meeting, the first two ECSG trials were published in *Lancet*.
1987	ECSG-3, the "Reocclusion study," assessing coronary patency and reocclusion with and without a second tPA infusion of 6 hours in duration, was published in the *American Journal of Cardiology*.
1988	ECSG-4, the "rt-PA/placebo trial," was published in the *British Medical Journal*.
1988	ECSG-5, the "rt-PA/PTCA trial," was published in *Lancet*.
1990	ECSG-6, the "Heparin trial," assessing coronary patency after tPA and aspirin with and without intravenous heparin was presented at the European Congress of Cardiology in Stockholm. Publication occurred in 1992 in the *British Heart Journal*.

Trials of the European Cooperative Study Group for tPA in Acute MI (Table 1)

ECSG-1: Double-Blind Randomized Trial of Intravenous tPA Versus Placebo

In a double-blind randomized trial, 129 patients with first MI of < 6 hours' duration received a bolus of heparin (5,000 IU) intravenously and were allocated to treatment with human recombinant double-chain tissue type plasminogen activator (tPA) (0.75 mg/kg body weight) given intravenously over 90 minutes, or to placebo infusion.[8] Coronary angiography at the end of this infusion showed that the infarct related vessel was patent in 61% of 62 assessable coronary angiograms in the tPA-treated group, compared with 21% in the control group (2P = 0.0001). Treatment with tPA was not accompanied by major complications; minor bleeding was noted in 11 patients after tPA, and in 5 patients treated with placebo. In the tPA group, the circulating fibrinogen level at the end of drug infusion was 52% ± 29% (mean ± SD)

of the starting value.

ECSG-2: Single-Blind Randomized Trial of Intravenous tPA Versus Intravenous Streptokinase

Patients with acute MI of < 6 hours in duration received a bolus injection of 10,000 IU heparin and were randomized to double-chain tPA or streptokinase only; the latter group also received aspirin (0.5 g) and methylprednisolone (0.25 g).[9] Sixty-four patients were assigned 0.75 mg tPA/kg over 90 minutes, and the infarct related coronary artery was patent in 70% of 61 assessable coronary angiograms taken 75–90 minutes after the start of infusion; 65 patients were allocated to 1,500,000 IU streptokinase over 60 minutes, and the infarct related vessel was patent in 55% of 62 assessable angiograms. The 95% confidence interval of the difference ranges from ± 30 to −2% (P = 0.054). Bleeding episodes and other complications were less common in the tPA patients than in the streptokinase group. Hospital mortality was identical in the two treatment groups. At the end of the tPA infusion, the circulating fibrinogen level was 61% ± 35% of the starting value, as measured by a coagulation rate assay, and 69% ± 25% as measured by sodium sulphite precipitation. After streptokinase infusion, corresponding fibrinogen levels were 12% ± 18% and 20% ± 11%. In the tPA group, only 4.5% of the fibrinogen was measured as incoagulable fibrinogen degradation products, compared with 30% in the streptokinase group. Activation of the systemic fibrinolytic system was thus far less pronounced with tPA than with streptokinase.

Quantitative analysis of the coronary stenosis both immediately after thrombolysis and at 3 weeks' follow-up was possible in 33 cases.[10] Residual stenosis (percentage narrowing of diameter) decreased from 74% ± 14% to 56% ± 17% (P < 0.05). No difference was observed between the groups of patients treated with streptokinase (74% ± 9% to 57% ± 12%, n = 17) and with tPA (74% ± 17% to 56% ± 21%, n = 16). Despite the significant regression, a coronary stenosis of > 50% of the diameter persisted in 82% of the patients 3 weeks after the infarction.

ECSG-3: Effect of Prolonged tPA Infusion on Early Reocclusion and Residual Stenosis

To be clinically relevant, thrombolysis requires not only early recanalization, but also long-term maintenance of patency of the infarct related artery. Different studies had shown that coronary reocclusion occurred in circa one-third of patients during the first hours or days after thrombolysis as documented by repeat angiography.[11] The ECSG-3 trial was performed to determine early and late predischarge reocclusion, after patency of the infarct related artery had been shown by coronary angiography in patients with acute MI treated with intravenous tPA. Because reocclusion was reported to occur within 1 hour after cessation of the tPA infusion,[11] an early repeat catheterization was planned at the end of the second infusion: 6 hours after start of the second infusion; the latest after 24 hours

(Fig. 2). A second aim was to assess whether a continued infusion with tPA over 6 hours could prevent early and late reocclusion and further reduce residual stenosis as measured by quantitative coronary angiography.

An intravenous infusion of 40 mg of recombinant double-chain tPA was given intravenously over 90 minutes to 123 patients with acute MI of < 4 hours' duration.[12] A coronary angiogram was recorded at the end of the infusion in 119 patients (Fig. 2). Central assessment of the angiograms revealed a patent infarct related artery in 78 patients (patency rate 66%, 95% confidence limits 57 to 74%). Patients with a patent infarct related artery at the first angiogram were randomized in a double-blind manner to receive a subsequent 6-hour infusion of either 30 mg of double-chain tPA or placebo. All patients had received an initial bolus of 5,000 IU of heparin and then 1,000 IU/hour until a second angiogram was recorded 6–24 hours after the start of the second perfusion. At central assessment of the second coronary angiogram, the reocclusion rate was 2 of 36 patients who received tPA at the second infusion, and 3 of 37 patients not receiving this drug (or the two groups combined: 7%, 95% confidence limits 2 to 15%). Three of 69 patients (5%, 95% confidence limits 1 to 14%) with patent arteries on both previous angiograms had a later occlusion as judged on the angiogram recorded at hospital discharge. No difference in late reocclusion rates between the two treatment groups was observed.

Quantitative angiography was performed with a computer-assisted cardiovascular angiography analysis system (CAAS).[13] A persistent trend of improvement in minimal lumen diameter was found from 90 minutes to 6–24 hours and predischarge. A reduction in "plaque area," the area between the detected and the reference contours of the infarct related segment, was more frequently seen in patients receiving a second infusion of tPA than in patients with no prolonged thrombolytic therapy (83% vs 57%, 2P < 0.025).

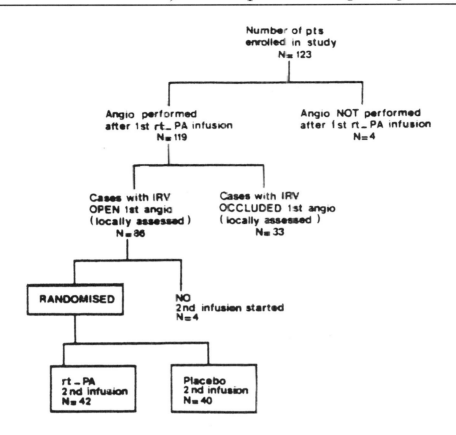

Figure 2. Flow diagram of patients in whom tPA infusion was given. Subsequent randomization based on local assessment of the patency of the infarct related artery at first angiogram. The second angiogram was read blindly by the care laboratory. IRV = infarct related vessel.

ECSG-4: Double-Blind Placebo-Controlled Randomized Trial on the Effect of Alteplase on Enzymatic Infarct Size, Left Ventricular (LV) Function, and Mortality

The aim of this trial was to assess the effect of intravenous alteplase (single-chain tPA) on size of infarct, LV function, and mortality in patients with MI of < 5 hours' duration.[14] Seven hundred and twenty-one patients were enrolled, and 355 patients were allocated to receive intravenous alteplase. Controls comprised 366 similar patients randomized to receive placebo. All patients were given aspirin 250 mg and bolus injection of 5,000 IU heparin immediately before the start of the trial. Patients in the treatment group were given 100 mg alteplase over 3 hours (10 mg intravenous bolus, 50 mg during 1 hour, and 40 mg during next 2 hours) by infusion. Controls were given placebo intravenously. Full anticoagulation treatment and aspirin were given to both groups until angiography (10–22 days after admission); β-blockers were given at discharge.

Compared to controls, mortality was reduced by 51% (95% confidence interval: −76 to 1) in treated patients at 14 days after start of treatment and by 36% (confidence interval [CI] −63 to 13) at 3 months. In patients who had treatment within 3 hours after MI, the mortality was reduced by 82% (CI −95 to −31) at 14 days, and by 59% (CI −83 to −2) at 3 months. During hospital stay (14 days) the incidence of cardiac complications was lower in treated patients than controls (cardiogenic shock, 2.5% vs

6.0%; ventricular fibrillation, 3.4% vs 6.3%; pericarditis, 6.2% vs 11.0%, respectively), but that of coronary angioplasty or artery bypass, or both, was higher (15.8% vs 9.6%) during the first 3 months. Bleeding complications were more common in treated than in untreated patients. Most bleeding was minor, but 1.4% of treated patients had intracranial hemorrhage within 3 days after the start of infusion.

Enzymatic size of infarct, determined by α-hydroxybutyrate dehydrogenase (HBDH) concentrations, was less (20%, 2P = 0.0018) in treated patients than in controls. Left ventricular ejection fraction (LVEF) was 2.2% higher (CI 0.3 to 0.4) and end-diastolic and end-systolic volumes smaller by 6.0 mL (CI −0.2 to −11.9) and 5.8 mL (CI −0.9 to −10.6), respectively, in treated patients.

One-year mortality was reduced from 9.3% to 5.6% (difference 8.7, 95% CI −0.2 to 7.5%) in patients treated with alteplase, aspirin, and intravenous heparin, in comparison with a strategy of aspirin and intravenous heparin alone.[15] Bleeding complications were more common in patients treated with alteplase, with intracranial bleeding in 1.4% of patients. The results of this trial indicate that survival after hospital discharge in patients with completed MI is determined by the remaining LV function, the extent of coronary artery disease, and by the degree of infarct related residual coronary artery narrowing.

ECSG-5: Randomized Trial Comparing the Combined Thrombolytic Treatment with Alteplase, Aspirin, and Intravenous Heparin Plus Percutaneous Transluminal Coronary Angioplasty (PTCA) Versus a Noninvasive Strategy with the Same Drugs but Without Immediate Angiography and PTCA

Three hundred and sixty-seven MI patients were randomly allocated to an invasive strategy of alteplase, aspirin, and intravenous heparin (bolus followed by maintenance infusion), combined with immediate coronary angiography and balloon dilatation of narrowings in the infarct related vessel or to a noninvasive strategy with alteplase, aspirin, and intravenous heparin.[16] Intravenous infusion of 100 mg alteplase was started within 5 hours after onset of symptoms (median 156 min). Angiography was performed 6–165 minutes later in 180 of 183 patients allocated to the invasive strategy, and immediate angioplasty was attempted in 168 patients (92%); 184 patients were allocated to the noninvasive strategy. Coronary angiography was done before discharge in all patients. Immediate PTCA reduced the percentage stenosis of the infarct related segment, but this was offset by a high rate of transient (16%) and sustained (7%) reocclusion during the procedure and recurrent ischemia during the first 24 hours (17%). The clinical course was more favorable after noninvasive therapy, with a lower incidence of recurrent ischemia within 24 hours (30%), bleeding complications, hypotension, and ventricular fibrillation. Mortality at 14 days was lower in patients allocated to noninvasive treatment (3%) than in the group allocated to invasive treatment (7%). No difference between the treatment groups was observed in infarct size estimated from myocardial release of HBDH or in LVEF after 10–22 days. Thus, since immediate PTCA does not provide additional benefit, there seems to be no need for immediate angiography and PTCA in patients with acute MI treated with alteplase, aspirin, and heparin.

The failure of the invasive/intervention treatment strategy can be explained by more frequent coronary reocclusion and reinfarction in the invasive treatment.[17] After exclusion of patients with these events, and after adjustment for other determinants of regional wall motion by multivariate regression analysis, a small benefit in parameters of regional wall motion was found similar to the benefit in the alteplase placebo trial. This suggests that an invasive strategy might be beneficial in selected patients, when additional treatment modalities to prevent reocclusion and reinfarction become available.

The high proportion of patients in whom angioplasty was attempted in the invasive strategy group must be viewed in the context of the underlying philosophy, based on laboratory studies, that maximal myocardial salvage would be achieved by the earliest and most complete myocardial reperfusion, even the initiation of nearly half (43%) of the immediate angioplasty procedures in a vessel not yet reperfused, as was done in this trial. It is important to appreciate that this is a totally different philosophy from that of the TAMI and TIMI-IIB trials, where the question was, having achieved coronary vessel patency, how best to maintain it.

ECSG-6: Double-Blind Randomized Trial of Intravenous Heparin Versus Placebo in Patients Treated with Alteplase and Aspirin

This trial was designed to determine whether concomitant treatment with intravenous heparin affects coronary patency and outcome in patients treated with alteplase for acute MI.[18] Patients aged 21–70 years with clinical and ECG features of infarcting myocardium in whom thrombolytic therapy could be started within 6 hours of the onset of major symptoms were selected. Six hundred and fifty-two patients were randomly allocated either to receive heparin (n = 328) or heparin placebo (n = 324). The treatment regimens were alteplase 100 mg (not weight adjusted) plus aspirin (250 mg intravenously followed by 75–125 mg on alternate days) plus heparin (5,000 units intravenously followed by 1,000 units hourly, without dose adjustment) compared with alteplase plus aspirin plus placebo for heparin. Coronary patency (TIMI grades 2 or 3) at 48–120 hours (mean 81 hours) was 83.4% in the heparin group and 74.7% in the group given placebo for heparin (Fig. 3). The relative risk of an occluded vessel in the heparin tested group

was 0.66 (95% CI 0.47 to 0.93). Mortality was the same, with trends towards a smaller enzymatic infarct size and a higher incidence of bleeding complications in the group treated with heparin.

Plasma fibrinopeptide A levels, as a marker of ongoing in vivo fibrin formation, increased from 21 ng/ml (80%, range 2–390) at baseline to 30 ng/ml (3–390) at 36 hours in patients without intravenous heparin, but decreased in the heparin group from 18 ng/ml (2–210) at baseline to 10 ng/ml (1–170) (2P = 0.0001) (Table 2).[19] Thus, administration of intravenous heparin reduced ongoing fibrin formation. In 48 patients in the heparin group with adequate anticoagulation defined as no activated partial thromboplastin time (aPTT) below twice the baseline value, the plasma fibrinopeptide A levels remained normal (< 4 ng/ml), while in 102 patients allocated to intravenous heparin, but without adequate anticoagulation the plasma fibrinopeptide A levels at 12, 24, and 36 hours were 12 (2–80), 16 (2–240), and 15 (2–240) ng/ml (2P = 0.001). With these findings, the need for individual titration of intravenous heparinization is illustrated.

In a subgroup of patients pertaining to ECSG-6 trial, the relation between the level of anticoagulation and sustained coronary patency was studied.[20] This analysis comprises 149 of 324 patients allocated to heparin therapy and 132 of 320 patients allocated to placebo administration; in both groups an interpretable coronary angiogram was obtained within 6 days of treatment and there were sufficient plasma samples to assess the level of anticoagulation. aPTTs, fibrinogen and D-dimer levels were determined on plasma samples at baseline and at 45 minutes and 3, 12, 24 and 36 hours after the start of alteplase administration.

The coronary artery patency rate in this subgroup of patients who entered the ECSG-6 trial was higher in patients allocated to heparin therapy than in those allocated to placebo (80% and 71%, respectively, P = 0.05). Patients allocated to

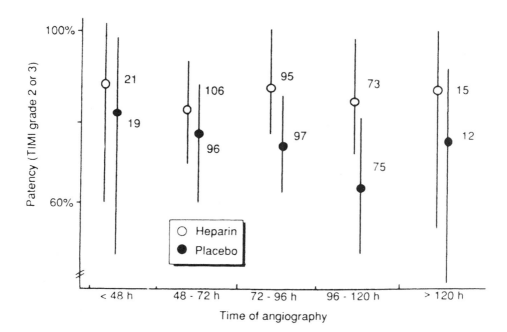

Figure 3. Means and 95% confidence intervals for TIMI grade 2 or 3 perfusion in angiograms performed at different times in heparin and placebo groups.

Table 2

Correlation Between FPA Levels at 24 Hours and Subsequent Coronary Artery Patency in Patients with FPA Data at 24 Hours

| | | FPA Concentration | | |
| | | > 50 ng/ml | < 50 ng/ml | P |
Patient Group	Patency			
Heparin (n = 148)	Occluded	13	14	< 0.0001
	Patent	17	104	
Placebo (n = 139)	Occluded	14	26	0.99
	Patent	33	66	
Adequate Anticoagulation (n = 43)	Occluded	2	1	0.01
	Patent	1	39	

---

heparin were classified into three groups: 48 patients (32%) with all aPTTs prolonged to at least twice their own baseline value (optimal anticoagulation), 40 patients (27%) with the lowest aPPT at 3, 12, 24, or 36 hours between 130% and 200% of the baseline value (suboptimal anticoagulation), and 61 patients with at least one aPTT < 130% of baseline (inadequate anticoagulation). In the heparin group, coronary artery patency correlated with the level of anticoagulation: 90%, 80%, and 72%, respectively, in patients with optimal, suboptimal, and inadequate anticoagulation (P = 0.02, optimal vs inadequate anticoagulation) (Fig. 4). Heparin administration was associated with a smaller reduction in fibrinogen and a smaller increase in D-dimer level during

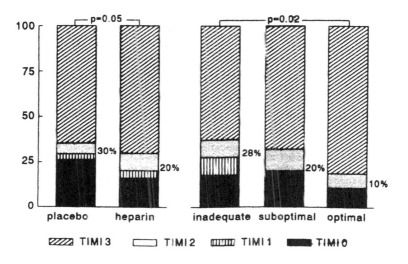

Figure 4. Coronary reperfusion status (TIMI grades 0–3) at angiography within 144 hours in both treatment groups (heparin [n = 149], placebo [n = 132]), and in the heparin subgroups classified on the basis of aPTT into those with optimal (n = 48), suboptimal (n = 40), and inadequate (n = 61) anticoagulation. The figures next to the bars present the percent of occluded vessels (TIMI grade 0 and 1). P values are for differences in TIMI grades 0 and 1 versus TIMI grades 2 and 3.

and after alteplase administration. No correlation was found between fibrinogen or D-dimer levels and coronary artery patency. No intracerebral bleeding occurred in these patients; however, bleeding was more frequent in the subgroup with optimal anticoagulation (P = 0.05).

The conclusion of the ECSG-6 trial is that intravenous heparin improves coronary patency in patients with alteplase, provided the anticoagulation is intensive enough. Whether this can be translated into improved clinical benefit had to be tested in a much larger trial, as was later done in GUSTO-1.

Ancillary Studies in the ECSG Trials

Risk Stratification Before Hospital Discharge

The question whether coronary angiography before hospital discharge is needed for the identification of high risk

patients after thrombolytic treatment was addressed in 1,043 hospital survivors studied in the ECSG-4 and ECSG-5 trials.[21] Coronary angiography was not useful in patients without symptoms of recurrent ischemia and without risk factors such as a previous infarction, use of diuretics and/or digitalis, or an inadequate systolic blood pressure response to exercise (at least 30 mmHg). These patients (47% of the study population) have a very good prognosis (98.6% 1-year survival); prediction of mortality was not improved by knowledge of the coronary anatomy.

The ECG and Thrombolytic Therapy

The value of the Selvester and Cardiac Infarction Injury Scores was assessed in the 721 patients of the ECSG-4 trial with acute MI.[22] ECGs obtained at admission, 6 hours, and 10–22 days after the start of therapy were analyzed. Patients with prior MI or QRS duration ≥ 120 msec were excluded, leaving 322 in the alteplase group and 33 in the placebo group. Cumulative 72-hour release of HBDH and global EF derived from angiography and nuclear scintigraphy were used as independent measures of infarct size. Predischarge results demonstrated a net benefit of alteplase therapy, with the Selvester Score 11% lower (P < 0.01) and the Cardiac Infarction Injury Score 5.4% lower (P = NS) in the alteplase than the control group. Total enzyme release was reduced by 19.2% (P < 0.001) in the alteplase group. In patients with inferior infarction, neither enzyme release (r = 0.30 to 0.40) nor EF (r = 0.22 to 0.31) correlated well with the ECG indices of infarct size. In anterior infarction, the correlations were better, especially between the Selvester Score and enzyme release (r = 0.40 to 0.48), as well as EF (r = −0.48 to −0.67). It is concluded that ECG scoring systems, especially the Selvester Score, although imperfect, are useful to assess thrombolytic therapy in clinical trials. However, their value for the management and assessment of thrombolytic therapy in individual patients is still limited.

In 655 patients without previous infarction and with narrow QRS complexes from the ECSG-4 trial, the initial sum of ST segment elevation was related to infarct size, mortality, and the treatment effect of thrombolytic therapy with alteplase. Reciprocal ST segment depression was also related to infarct size and mortality, based on ST segment elevation, both in patients with anterior and inferior infarctions.[23]

Evaluation of the Effect of Thrombolytic Treatment on Infarct Size and LV function by Enzymatic, Scintigraphic, and Angiographic Methods

In a subset of 312 patients of the ECSG-4 trial, infarct size was assessed by the cumulative myocardial release of HBDH during the first 72 hours and by planar thallium scintigraphy (index of hypoperfu-

sion) performed 10–22 days after the acute event.[24] LVEF was determined by contrast and nuclear angiography. The median values of HBDH during the first 72 hours were 20% lower, and the median values of thallium-201 28% smaller in the tPA group in comparison with controls. A significant but limited improvement of angiographic LVEF (2 absolute percentage points) was also shown in the patients treated with alteplase. A moderate but statistically significant linear association between both measurements of infarct size and LVEF was found.

Early and Late Effects of Thrombolysis on LV Function Measured by Nuclear Ventriculography

The aim of this study was the functional reevaluation of 296 patients pertaining to the ECSG-4 trial, 12–18 months after a double-blind trial evaluating the effect of alteplase versus placebo given within 5 hours of onset of symptoms caused by an acute MI.[25] All patients underwent rest-stress radionuclide angiography (Egna). For each exercise level, the global LVEF was calculated together with an estimate of regional wall motion abnormalities (RWMA). A clear difference of the total workload and the peak workload was found between both therapeutic groups. Discriminant analysis evaluating four parameters (LVEF at peak exercise and at the end point and the workload at those levels) revealed a beneficial therapeutic effect. The RWM at rest showed only a difference in the apicoinferior region. There were less wall motion abnormalities in the treated group. Radionuclide analysis demonstrated a larger functional capacity and a better coordination of myocardial contractility during stress radionuclide angiography 1 year after thrombolytic therapy. At rest, no major differences were found between the hospital stage and the follow-up in both therapeutic groups 1 year later.

Effect of Open Versus Closed Infarct Related Coronary Artery After Thrombolytic Therapy on Serum C-Reactive Protein and Infarct Size

Serum C-reactive protein rises in acute MI, correlating positively with infarct size if thrombolytic treatment is not given. This correlation disappears if thrombolytic treatment is given, although the serum C-reactive protein concentration is still associated with the clinical outcome of the patient. The effect of early coronary recanalization induced by thrombolytic treatment alone or combined with coronary angioplasty on the infarct related rise in serum C-reactive protein concentration was investigated.[26]

The C-reactive protein response caused by the myocardial infarct was lower in patients with an open infarct related coronary artery than in patients with a closed infarct related coronary artery, or in control patients who did not receive thrombolytic therapy. In control patients the expected strong positive correlation between infarct size and serum C-reactive protein ($r = 0.58$; $P < 0.001$, $n = 48$) was found, which was similar to that in patients with a closed infarct related coronary artery ($r = 0.58$; $P < 0.001$, $n = 17$), or in control patients who did not receive thrombolytic therapy. In patients with an open infarct related coronary artery, the correlation between infarct size and serum C-reactive protein was much weaker ($r = 30$; $P < 0.01$, $n = 91$). Consequently, infarct size explained approximately 35% of the variation in serum C-reactive protein values in the control patients and 36% in the patients with a closed infarct related coronary artery, but only 9% of the variation in patients with an open infarct related artery. EF correlated negatively with serum C-reactive protein in both control and recanalized patients. The association was again much stronger in the control patients. EF explained 27% (28% if only the first infarctions were considered) of the variation in serum C-reactive protein

in the control patients and 8% (6%) in the recanalized patients.

The results of this analysis show that coronary recanalization variably reduces the infarct associated rise in serum C-reactive protein. This explains the weaker association between serum C-reactive protein and infarct size in the patients receiving thrombolytic treatment when compared to those treated without thrombolytic drugs, and may have clinical implications.

Long-Term (5 Years') Mortality is Related to TIMI Perfusion grade 3 Flow at Discharge

Long-term follow-up in patients treated with thrombolysis for acute MI thus far has been reported in a few studies only, and no long-term follow-up is available for patients who underwent additional PTCA. This report describes 5-year survival as collected in patients who received placebo, recombinant tissue plasminogen activator (alteplase), or alteplase with additional immediate PTCA in two European Study Group trials.[27–28] Determinants for long-term survival were assessed in 1,043 patients discharged alive. Five-year follow-up information on mortality was collected. Hospital mortality was lower after alteplase than placebo (2.5% vs 5.7%, $P = 0.04$) and higher after alteplase without additional intervention (6.0% vs 2.2%, $P = 0.07$). Of the 1,043 hospital survivors, data were available for 923 patients, of whom 109 died. In the placebo group, mortality after hospital discharge was 10.7% versus 11.0% in the comparative placebo group. The patients treated with alteplase and immediate PTCA had a mortality rate of 10.5% versus 8.9% in the alteplase group without PTCA (all $P = NS$). Significant determinants of mortality in multivariate proportional hazards analysis were enzymatic infarct size, indicators of residual LV function, number of diseased vessels, and TIMI perfusion grade at discharge. Patients with TIMI grade 2 flow had mortality rates similar to those with TIMI flow grades 0 and 1, while prognosis was better in patients with TIMI flow grade 3.

In conclusion, the initial in-hospital benefit of thrombolysis with intravenous tPA is maintained throughout 5 years, with no early or late beneficial effect of systematic immediate PTCA. Enzymatic infarct size, LV function, and extent of coronary artery disease are predictors for long-term survival. TIMI perfusion grade 2 at discharge should be considered as an inadequate result of therapy.

Conclusions

As was recently summarized[26] the ECSG trials provided evidence that treatment with tPA results in early patency of the infarct related coronary artery (ECSG-1 trial), reduces enzymatic infarct size, preserves LV function, and reduces mortality (ECSC-4 trial). Early (90 min) coronary patency after tPA was superior to patency after intravenous streptokinase (ECSG-2 trial). Reocclusion of the infarct related coronary artery was infrequent after tPA (ECSG-3 trial), provided that full intravenous heparinization was applied during the first days (ECSG-6 trial). The superiority of alteplase in comparison to intravenous streptokinase in terms of mortality was confirmed in the GUSTO-1 trial. An invasive strategy of alteplase followed by immediate angioplasty was not superior in terms of enzymatic infarct size reduction and preservation of LV function, probably due to early reocclusion and reinfarction (ECSG-5 trial).

References

1. Van de Loo J. Möglichkeiten und grenzen der kombinierten fibrinolyse-antikoagulantien-therapie des myokardinfarktes. Med Klin 1963; 58:1527-1529.
2. Roberts WC, Buja LM. The frequency and significance of coronary arterial thrombi and other observations after acute myocardial infarction. Am J Med 1972;52:425-443.
3. Amery A, Roeber G, Vermeulen HJ, et al. Single-blind randomised multicentre trial of comparing heparin and streptokinase in recent myocardial infarction. Acta Med Scand 1969;505:1-35.
4. Schmutzler R, Heckner F, Körtge P, et al. Zur thrombolytischen therapie des frischen herzinfarktes. 1. Einführung, behandlungspläne, klinische ergebnisse. Dtsch Med Wschr 1966;91:581-587.
5. European Working Party. Streptokinase in recent myocardial infarction: A controlled multicentre trial. Br Med J 1971;3:325-331.
6. European Cooperative Study Group for Streptokinase Treatment in Acute Myocardial Infarction. Streptokinase in acute myocardial infarction. N Engl J Med 1979;301:797-837.
7. Verstraete M, Van de Loo J, Jesdinsky HJ. Streptokinase in acute myocardial infarction. Acta Med Scand 1981; 648:1-117.
8. Verstraete M, Bleifeld W, Brower RW, et al. Double-blind randomised trial of intravenous tissue-type plasminogen activator versus placebo in acute myocardial infarction. Lancet 1985; 2:965-969.
9. Verstraete M, Bernard R, Bory M, et al. Randomised trial of intravenous recombinant tissue-type plasminogen activator versus intravenous streptokinase in acute myocardial infarction. Lancet 1985;1:842-847.
10. Schmidt WG, Uebis R, von Essen R, et al. Residual coronary stenosis after thrombolysis with rt-PA or streptokinase: Acute results and 3 weeks follow-up. Eur Heart J 1987;8:1182-1188.
11. Gold HK, Leinbach RC, Garabedian HD, et al. Acute coronary reocclusion after thrombolysis with recombinant human tissue-type plasminogen activator: Prevention by a maintenance in-

fusion. Circulation 1986;73:347-352.

12. Verstraete M, Arnold AER, Brower RW, et al. Acute coronary thrombolysis with rt-PA: Initial patency and influence of maintained infusion on reocclusion rate. Am J Cardiol 1987; 60:231-237.

13. Serruys PW, Arnold AER, Brower RW, et al. for the European Cooperative Study Group for rt-PA. Effect of continued rt-PA administration on the residual stenosis after initial successful recanalization in acute myocardial infarction-a quantitative coronary angiography study of a randomized trial. Eur Heart J 1987;8:1172-1181.

14. Van de Werf F, Arnold AER, and the European Cooperative Study Group for rt-PA. Effect of intravenous tissue-type plasminogen activator on infarct size, left ventricular function and survival in patients with acute myocardial infarction. Br Med J 1988;297:1374-1379.

15. Arnold AER, Simoons ML, Van de Werf F, et al. for the European Cooperative Study Group. Recombinant tissue-type plasminogen activator and immediate angioplasty in acute myocardial infarction: One year follow up. Circulation 1992;86:111-120.

16. Simoons ML, Arnold AER, Betriu A, et al. Thrombolysis with rt-PA in acute myocardial infarction: No additional benefit of immediate PTCA. Lancet 1988;1:197-202.

17. Arnold AER, Serruys PW, Rutsch W, et al. for the European Cooperative Study Group for rt-PA. Reasons for no additional benefit of angioplasty immediately after recombinant tissue plasminogen activator for acute myocardial infarction: A regional wall motion analysis. JACC 1991;17:11-21.

18. de Bono DP, Simoons ML, Tijssen JGP, et al. Effect of early intravenous heparin on coronary patency, infarct size and bleeding complications after alteplase thrombolysis: Results of a randomised double blind European Cooperative Study Group trial. Br Heart J 1992;67:122-128.

19. Rapold HJ, de Bono DP, Arnold AER, et al. for the European Cooperative Study Group. Plasma fibrinopeptide A levels in patients with acute myocardial infarction treated with alteplase: Correlation with concomitant heparin, coronary artery patency, and recurrent ischemia. Circulation 1992;85:928-934.

20. Arnout J, Simoons M, de Bono DP, et al. Correlation between level of heparinization and patency of the infarct-related coronary artery after treatment of acute myocardial infarction with alteplase (rt-PA). JACC 1992;20:513-519.

21. Arnold AER, Simoons ML, Detry JMR, et al. for the European Cooperative Study Group. Prediction of mortality after hospital discharge in patients treated with and without recombinant tissue plasminogen activator for myocardial infarction: Is there a need for coronary angiography? Eur Heart J 1993;14:306-315.

22. Willems JL, Willems RJ, Bijnens I, et al. Value of electrocardiographic scoring systems for the assessment of thrombolytic therapy in acute myocardial infarction. Eur Heart J 1991; 12:378-388.

23. Willems JL, Willems RJ, Willems GM, et al. for the European Cooperative Study Group for rt-PA. The significance of initial ST-segment elevation and depression for the management of thrombolytic therapy in acute myocardial infarction. Circulation 1990; 82:1147-1158.

24. Mortelmans L, Vanhaecke J, Lesaffre E, et al. Evaluation of the effect of thrombolytic treatment on infarct size and left ventricular function by enzymatic, scintigraphic, and angiographic methods. Am Heart J 1990;119:1231-1236.

25. Mortelmans L, Scheys I, Brzostek T, et al. Early and late effects of rt-PA vs placebo on left ventricular function measured by nuclear ventriculography. Nucl Med 1993;32:120-127.

26. Pietilä K, Harmoinen A, Hermens W, et al. Serum C-reactive protein and infarct size in myocardial infarct patients with a closed versus an open infarct related coronary artery after thrombolytic therapy. Eur Heart J 1993;14:915-919.

27. Lenderink T, Simoons ML, Van Es GA, et al. for the European Cooperative Study Group. Benefit of thrombolytic therapy is sustained throughout five years and is related to TIMI perfusion garde 3 but not grade 2 flow at dis-

charge. Circulation 1995;92:1110-1116.

28. Arnold AER, de Bono DP, Lubsen J, et al. The clinical trials of the European Cooperative Study for recombinant tissue-type plasminogen activator (rt-PA). In: Becker RC, ed. The Modern Era of Coronary Thrombolysis. Kluwer Academic Publishers, 1994, pp. 69-71.

EWP steering committee: A. Amery; J. Vermylen; and M. Verstraete. ECSG steering committee: M. Verstraete (chairman); D.P. de Bono; R.J. Lennane; J. Lubsen; D. Mathey; P. Raynaud; W. Rutsch; W. Schmidt; P. Serruys; M.L. Simoons; R. Uebis; A. Vahanian; F. Van de Werf; and R. von Essen. The ECSG was founded in 1984 and has conducted six trials between 1984 and 1991.

Address for reprints: Marc Verstraete, M.D., Center for Molecular and Vascular Biology, University of Leuven, Campus Gasthuisberg, Herestraat 49, B-3000 Leven, Belgium. Fax: 32-16-345990.

Chapter 3

Thrombolysis in Acute Myocardial Infarction:
The German Experience

K.-L. Neuhaus, M.D., R. von Essen, M.D., U. Tebbe, M.D., and R. Schroeder, M.D.

From Städt Kliniken Kassel, Kassel, Germany

Introduction

The German experience with thrombolytic treatment of patients with acute myocardial infarction (AMI) dates back to the early 1960s, when Polivoda et al.[1] infused streptokinase (SK) intravenously (I.V.) in 20 patients with AMI of < 4 hours' duration. A loading dose of 300,000 U of SK was given over 30 minutes, followed by a maintenance dose of 700,000 U over 7 hours. One patient who had been treated in < 1 hour from symptom onset did not develop an infarct; five others had only non-Q wave infarctions, but one patient suffered nonfatal intracranial bleeding.[1]

Over the next 15 years, > 20 randomized trials of I.V. thrombolysis have been done, mainly in Europe, but for two main reasons there was no general acceptance of thrombolysis for the treatment of AMI patients. First, the pathophysiological rationale was not very suggestive for most physicians. It was believed that fibrinolytics acted through an improved blood viscosity and restoration of microcirculatory flow, especially in the border zones of the ischemic myocardium. The concept of early reperfusion of major epicardial coronary arteries could not yet have been developed because most scientists regarded the postmortem thrombus in infarct related coronary arteries of AMI patients as a consequence rather than a cause of the acute ischemic event. Second, there was no direct proof of efficacy, either in terms of angiographic evidence or as a significant clinical benefit (especially an improved survival). Nevertheless, there were both pathologists who did demonstrate the right cause and effect relationship between coronary thrombosis and myocardial ischemia[2] long before the pioneering angiographic work of Wood,[3] and clinicians who demonstrated rapid resolution of transmural myocardial ischemia in the ECG during SK infusion, which could not be readily explained by rheologic effects of fibrinolysis.

After the introduction of the reperfusion concept by Chazov et al. in 1976[4] and Rentrop et al. in 1979[5] using intracoronary application of fibrinolytics, the short-term high dose I.V. infusion of SK was the logical next step to promote the widespread use of reperfusion therapy for patients with evolving myocardial infarction.[6,7] In 1981, the authors of this article[8] met in Goettingen to design a randomized multi-

Table 1

Infarct Size, LVEF After 21 Days, Regional Wall Abnormalities, and 21-Day Mortality After Streptokinase and Placebo in the ISAM Study

	Streptokinase	*Placebo*	*P Value*
Area under CK-MB curve (IU/1 × h)	1701 ± 48	1869 ± 51	<0.02
LVEF (%)	56.8 ± 0.7	53.9 ± 0.7	<0.005
Dyssynergy index	226 ± 9	265 ± 10	<0.005
Mortality (%)	6.3	7.1	NS

ISAM = Intravenous Streptokinase in Acute Myocardial Infarction; LVEF = left ventricular ejection fraction.

center trial, the ISAM study (a Prospective Trial of Intravenous Streptokinase in Acute Myocardial Infarction), to test the efficacy of a 1-hour high dose infusion of SK on left ventricular function, infarct size, and mortality in patients with AMI of recent onset. At that time, no dose finding studies had been done, and since one of us had used much higher doses of up to 2.8 million U of SK than the other who had used only 0.5 to 1 million U, we arbitrarily chose a compromise of 1.5 million U over 1 hour for the ISAM study, which is still the standard dose for SK worldwide.[8]

Recruitment for the ISAM study was begun in 1982, but it turned out during the course of the study that the overall mortality rate was much lower than anticipated, probably in part due to the concomitant use of 500-mg aspirin I.V. Therefore, the size of the trial was too small to demonstrate a significant survival benefit, but it did show a significant improvement in LV function and a reduction of infarct size in the SK-treated patients (Table 1). Meanwhile, the GISSI (Gruppo Italiano per lo Studio della Streptochinasi nell'Infarto Miocardio) study group had started the GISSI 1 study,[9] which, on the basis of the early ISAM experience, had been adequately powered to prove the significant impact of I.V. thrombolysis on survival in AMI, and thus became the real landmark study in this field.

With the advent of new thrombolytic drugs, which was greatly influenced by Collen and co-workers, our group[10] fo-

cused its interest on comparative angiographic trials. The first of these trials was the GAUS study (German Activator Urokinase Study), which compared the efficacy of tPA and urokinase (UK) on 90-minute patency of the infarct related artery in patients with evolving myocardial infarction.[10] Although the sponsoring company wanted to test SK versus tPA, we felt that UK would be the scientifically more attractive choice for comparison, since it does not have some of the inherent disadvantages of SK, such as antigenicity and immediate side effects. Again, like in the situation with SK some years ago, dose ranging studies for UK were not available, and an arbitrary regimen of a bolus of 1.5 million U followed by an I.V. infusion of another 1.5 MU over 90 minutes was chosen, based on considerations about plasma concentrations and half-lives. The basic finding of the GAUS study was a virtually equivalent efficacy of UK and tPA given in the standard dose up to the 90-minute angiogram on infarct artery patency in 239 patients (Fig. 1), who, with one single exception, all had had their primary end point angiograms. Beyond this quite surprising equivalent efficacy (for many investigators at that time), the rate of early reocclusions was much lower with UK than with the new fibrin specific compound. In spite of the favorable efficacy profile in GAUS and the inherent advantages over SK, UK has never been tested in a large scale clinical trial, probably because there is no big company selling it in

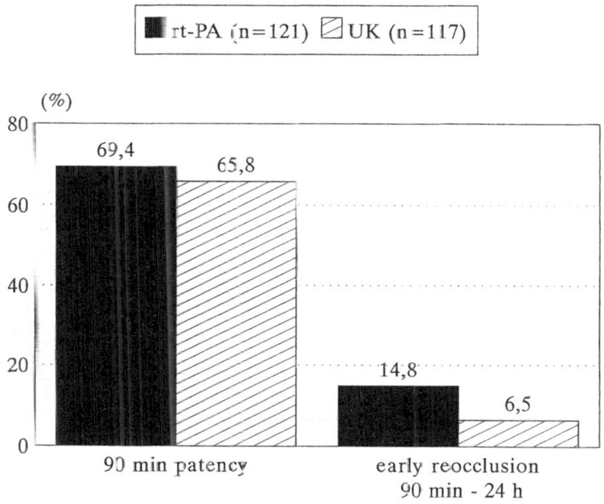

rt-PA (n=121) UK (n=117)

Figure 1. Early TIMI II/III patency and rate of early reocclusions in GAUS, comparing urokinase (1.5 Mio Bolus and 1.5 Mio over 90 min) and the standard regimen tPA (70 mg over 90 min). GAUS = German Activator Urokinase Study; TIMI = Thrombolysis in Myocardial Infarction.

Europe (where UK is cheap), and its tremendous price in the U.S., where it is even more expensive than tPA. Nevertheless, on both sides of the Atlantic, UK is still given in nearly 10% of all AMI patients treated with fibrinolytics.

When it became clear that (even with the presumably more potent tPA) a significant proportion of patients was left with an occluded infarct vessel after I.V. thrombolysis, and that reocclusions were encountered even more often than with conventional fibrinolytics, improvements were tried by increasing dose and duration of the tPA infusion. As a result, the 90-minute patency indeed was increased, but at the cost of unacceptable bleeding risks, especially intracranial hemorrhage.[11] We therefore tried to design a tPA regimen that would retain the improved early patency of high dose tPA by increasing the loading bolus dose and the infusion rate early on, but which at the same time would avoid the prohibitive bleeding risk by restricting the total dose to the standard 100 mg. This regimen of 100 mg over 90 minutes has later been termed "front-loaded tPA." After a most promising pilot study,[12] the front-loaded regimen has been tested in a randomized direct comparison versus anistreplase in > 400 patients,[13] where the pilot data were confirmed. The improved early patency (Fig. 2) without any indication of

an increased bleeding risk in TAPS (rt-PA-APSAC Patency Study) led the GUSTO (Global Use of Strategies to Open Occluded Coronary Arteries) study group to reassess the question whether there was any relevant difference between thrombolytics in terms of clinical end points. This question seemingly had been answered with a definite "no" at that time by two megatrials, GISSI-2 and ISIS-3 (International Study Groups of Infarct Survival). The GUSTO-1 study demonstrated a significant difference in favor of front-loaded tPA, which has been attributed to the improved early patency as compared to SK or a combination of SK and tPA.[14]

The rather complicated dosing schedule for the front-loaded application of tPA prompted the development of mutants with a prolonged plasma half-life in an attempt to enable bolus application, which would be much easier and safer in the clinical setting of acute coronary care. The first such compound, which was viable for clinical investigation, was a deletion mutant of wild type tPA called "reteplase." This drug has been tested by our group in dose ranging studies,[15,16] which again were angiographic studies because 90-minute patency was considered to be the best surrogate for clinical end points. In an attempt to reduce the number of patients needed for an adequately robust definition of a near optimal

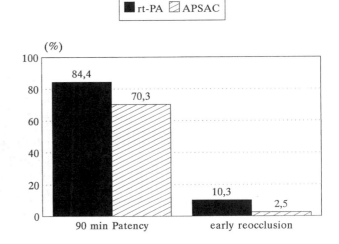

Figure 2. Comparison of early TIMI II/III patency and rate of reocclusions between 90 minutes and 36 hours after the front-loaded tPA regimen (100 mg over 90 min) and APSAC (30-mg bolus) in TAPS. TAPS = rt-PA-APSAC Patency Study; TIMI = Thrombolysis in Myocardial Infarction.

dose, we chose a sequential design with predefined limits of efficacy and safety to decide upon dose escalation (Fig. 3). The sequential approach is quite effective for the early rejection of low doses, and therefore avoids treatment of too many patients with an inappropriate regimen during early phase II. At near optimal doses, however, a parallel group design may be preferable. In the GRECO studies, a single bolus of 15 MU has been shown to yield an early infarct artery patency comparable to standard tPA, anistreplase, or UK (Fig. 4). A further increase in patency has been achieved by an increase in dosing to 20 MU and dividing the total dose in two boluses of 10 MU given 30 minutes apart.[17] The very promising patency profile of this regimen, how-

ever, has not fully translated into survival benefit in a major clinical trial comparing reteplase and SK.[18]

Some years ago, concern was raised about the usefulness of the 90-minute patency as a surrogate for the clinical efficacy of thrombolytics. We therefore have analyzed all the patency data from our angiographic trials and found that 90-minute patency indeed does strongly correlate to mortality. TIMI (Thrombolysis in Myocardial Infarction) grade II flow, however, which had been regarded as successful reperfusion, was associated with a mortality very close to TIMI grade 0 or I flow (Fig. 5).[19] This correlation has been confirmed by the TAMI data and in GUSTO 1, and the rating of angiographic patency has

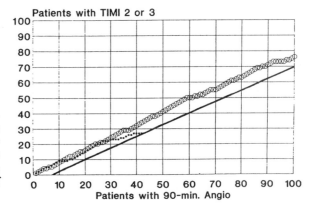

Figure 3. Diagram of sequential patency monitoring showing 90-minute patency plotted sequentially patient by patient. The initial dose of 10 MU (○) had to be increased after 42 patients when the preset lower efficacy limit of 70% (-) had been approached.

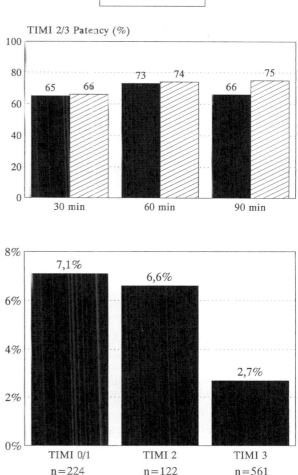

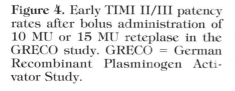

Figure 4. Early TIMI II/III patency rates after bolus administration of 10 MU or 15 MU reteplase in the GRECO study. GRECO = German Recombinant Plasminogen Activator Study.

Figure 5. In-hospital mortality according to the perfusion status of the infarct related artery 90 minutes after the start of thrombolytic therapy. Metaanalysis of four German thrombolytic trials.

been changed accordingly; only a TIMI grade III flow is now considered as a truly successful reperfusion.

Two aspects in thrombolysis for AMI that came up rather early, but never gained appropriate attention, were the different efficacy of thrombolytics with regard to time to treatment, and the effects of body weight on early patency after thrombolysis. In the GAUS trial we observed a lower patency in patients treated with UK and a time to treatment of > 3 hours from symptom onset as compared to treatment within 3 hours (Fig. 6). This different efficacy has not

been found for tPA. A distinct drop in patency rates, especially for TIMI-III flow grade, has been seen in the TAPS trial in heavier patients (Fig. 7), but an adjustment of dose for heavy weight patients has never been seriously considered.

Since the common mode of action of all thrombolytics is the activation of plasminogen to plasmin, it has been questioned whether there is much room for improvement only by modifications of available compounds (e.g., by enhanced fibrin specificity). Optimization of concomitant treatment by better thrombin and platelet inhi-

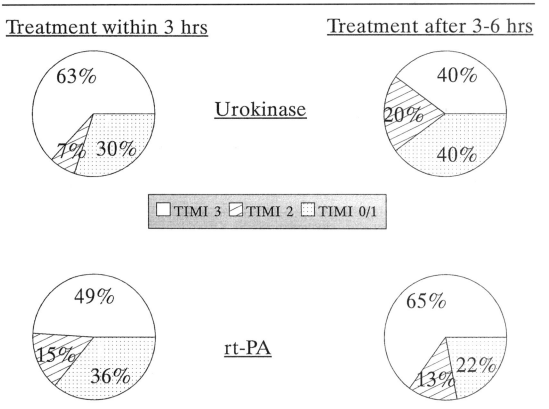

Figure 6. Influence of time-to-treatment on 90-minute patency in GAUS after standard tPA and urokinase. GAUS = German Activator Urokinase Study.

bition, therefore, has gained increasing interest.

Most promising experimental and clinical data regarding specific fibrinogen receptor blockers inhibiting platelets much more effectively than with aspirin, and specific thrombin inhibitors has already been published. One of the latter, a recombinant hirudin, has been compared to heparin in our most recent series of trials. Dose finding has been done by dose escalation trials,[20] which had a design similar to the GRECO studies. A moderate increase in patency and a reduced reocclusion rate have been observed (Table 2), but the clinical trial HIT III (Hirudin for the Improvement of Thrombolysis) had to be terminated early because of an unacceptable high rate of intracranial bleeding.[21] Similar trials with a slightly different recombinant hirudin, GUSTO IIA[22] and TIMI 9A,[23]

which had used a higher dose of hirudin suffered the same problem. Because of the apparently narrow therapeutic window, at least in combination with thrombolytics, the hirudin dose has been drastically reduced by all study groups. In our ongoing trial, HIT IV, we have restricted the thrombolytic drug to SK because we felt that a significant improvement in early patency might be easier to demonstrate for a thrombolytic with a comparatively poor patency profile. HIT IV has a specific design in that it has an angiographic arm with 400 patients to assess the effect of concomitant hirudin on patency and reocclusion, and a safety arm of 800 patients without angiography to detect potential bleeding hazards before a large scale phase III trial is started. Attempting to summarize where we are after > 10 years of intense basic and clinical research to improve reperfusion strategies

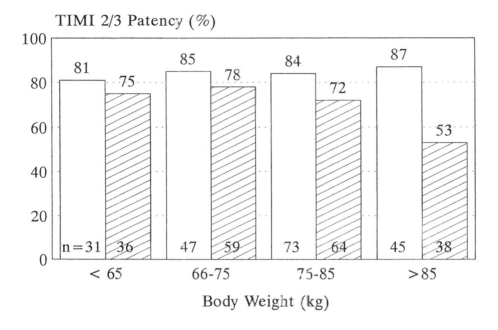

Figure 7. Influence of body weight on 90-minute TIMI II/III patency after front-loaded tPA and APSAC in TAPS. TAPS = rt-PA-APSAC Patency Study; TIMI = Thrombolysis in Myocardial Infarction.

in AMI, one may say that the major steps forward in terms of saving patients' lives have been achieved in the 1980s. Interest for further improvement at present is focused in four areas: (1) better thrombolytics; (2) more potent platelet receptor blockers; (3) more specific thrombin inhibition; and (4) mechanical reperfusion by direct angioplasty. None of these strategies is supposed to, individually, have as big an impact on in-hospital mortality from AMI as standard thrombolytics or aspirin.

Table 2.

Early TIMI-3 Patency Rates and Reocclusions After Thrombolysis with Front-Loaded rt-PA and Conjunctive Therapy with Three Ascending Doses of r-Hirudin in the HIT-II Study

Dose Group	Patients (n)	60-min TIMI-3	90-min TIMI-3	Reocclusions 90 min–48 hrs
B 0.1 mg/kg I 0.06 mg/kg/hr	18	50%	66.7%	0%
B 0.2 mg/kg I 0.1 mg/kg/hr	43	57.5%	70.7%	5.6%
B 0.4 mg/kg 82 I 0.15 mg/kg/hr	63%	76.3%	1.4%	

B = bolus; HIT-II = Hirudin for the Improvement of Thrombolysis; I = infusion.

References

1. Polivoda H, Schröder R, Heckner S. Erste Erfahrungen mit der fibrinolytischen therapie des akuten herzinfarkts. Dtsch Med Wschr 1963;88: 218–224.

2. Sinapius D. Die beziehung zwischen koronarthrombose und myokardinfarkten. Dtsch Med Wschr 1972;97:443–448.

3. De Wood MA, Spores J, Notske RN, et al. Prevalence of total coronary occlusion during the early hours of transmural myocardial infarction. N Engl J Med 1980;303:897–902.

4. Chazov EL, Mateeva LS, Mazev AV, et al. Intracoronary administration of fibrinolysin in acute myocardial infarction. Ter Arkh 1976;48:8–19.

5. Rentrop KP, Blanke H, Karsch KR, et al. Acute myocardial infarction: Intracoronary application of nitroglycerin and streptokinase. Clin Cardiol 1979;2:354–363.

6. Neuhaus KL, Köstering H, Tebbe U, et al. Intravenöse kurzzeit-streptokinase-therapie beim frischen myokardinfarkt. Z Kardiol 1981;70:791–796.

7. Schröder R, Biamino G, von Leitner ER, et al. Intravenous short-term infusion of streptokinase in acute myocardial infarction. Circulation 1983;67:536–548.

8. The ISAM Study Group. A prospective trial of intravenous streptokinase in acute myocardial infarction (I.S.A.M.). N Engl J Med 1986;314:1465–1471.

9. GISSI. Effectiveness of intravenous thrombolytic therapy in acute myocardial infarction. Lancet 1986;1:397–401.

10. Neuhaus KL, Tebbe U, Gottwick M, et al. Intravenous recombinant tissue-plasminogen activator and urokinase in acute myocardial infarction: Results of the German Activator Urokinase Study (GAUS). JACC 1988;12:581–587.

11. The TIMI Study Group. Comparison of invasive and conservative strategies after treatment with intravenous tissue plasminogen activator in acute myocardial infarction. Results of the Thrombolysis in Myocardial Infarction (TIMI) Phase II Trial. N Engl J Med 1989;320:618–627.

12. Neuhaus KL, Feuerer W, Jeep-Tebbe S, et al. Improved thrombolysis with a modified dose regimen of recombinant tissue-type plasminogen activator. JACC 1989;14:1566–1569.

13. Neuhaus KL, von Essen R, Tebbe U, et al. Improved thrombolysis in acute myocardial infarction with front-loaded administration of alteplase: Results of the rt-PA-APSAC Patency Study (TAPS). JACC 1992;19:885–891.

14. The GUSTO Angiographic Investigators. The effects of tissue plasminogen activator, streptokinase, or both on coronary-artery patency, ventricular function and survival after acute myocardial infarction. N Engl J Med 1993;329:1615–1622.

15. Neuhaus KL, von Essen R, Vogt A, et al. Dose finding with a novel recombinant plasminogen activator (BM 06.022) in patients with acute myocardial infarction: Results of the German Recombinant Plasminogen Activator Study. JACC 1994;24:55–60.

16. Tebbe U, von Essen R, Smolarz A, et al. Open, noncontrolled dose-finding study with a novel recombinant plasminogen activator (BM 06.022) given as a double bolus in patients with acute myocardial infarction. Am J Cardiol 1993;72:518–524.

17. Smalling RW, Bode C, Kalbfleisch J, et al. More rapid, complete, and stable coronary thrombolysis with bolus administration of reteplase compared with alteplase infusion in acute myocardial infarction. Circulation 1995;91:2725–2732.

18. International Joint Efficacy Comparison of Thrombolytics (INJECT). Randomized, double blind-blind comparison of reteplase double-bolus administration with streptokinase in acute myocardial infarction (INJECT): Trial to investigate equivalence. Lancet 1995;346:329–336.

19. Vogt A, Von Essen R, Tebbe U, et al. Impact of early perfusion status of the infarct-related artery on short-term mortality after thrombolysis for acute myocardial infarction: Retrospective analysis of four German Multicenter Studies. JACC 1993;21:1391–1395.

20. Neuhaus KL, Niederer W, Wagner J, et al. HIT (hirudin for the improvement of thrombolysis): Results of a dose es-

calation study. Circulation 1993;88:I-292.

21. Neuhaus KL, von Essen R, Tebbe U, et al. Safety observations from the pilot phase of the randomized r-hirudin for improvement of thrombolysis (HIT III) study. Circulation 1994;90: 1638–1642.

22. The GUSTO IIA Investigators. Randomized trial of intravenous heparin versus recombinant hirudin for acute coronary syndromes. Circulation 1994;90:1631–1637.

23. Antman EM for the TIMI 9A Investigators. Hirudin in acute myocardial infarction. Circulation 1994; 90:1624–1630.

Address for reprints: K.-L. Neuhaus, M.D., Städt Kliniken Kassel, Mönchebergstr. 41-43, D-34125 Kassel, Germany. Fax: 49-5-61-980-6980.

Chapter 4

The Western Washington and Myocardial Infarction Triage and Intervention Trials of Thrombolytic Therapy:
15 Years of Collaboration in the Pacific Northwest

Charles Maynard, PH.D., Nathan R. Every, M.D., Jenny S. Martin, R.N., Alfred P. Hallstrom, PH.D., J. Ward Kennedy, M.D., and W. Douglas Weaver, M.D.

From the University of Washington School of Medicine, Department of Medicine and the University of Washington School of Public Health and Community Medicine, Department of Biostatistics, Seattle, Washington.

Beginning in 1981, collaborative efforts developed between the University of Washington and community hospitals in Washington, British Columbia, Canada, and later outside the Pacific Northwest, have generated important findings about the treatment and outcome of acute myocardial infarction (AMI). These efforts, collectively known as the Western Washington and Myocardial Infarction Triage and Intervention Project trials, have included randomized trials of thrombolytic drugs, direct antithrombins, platelet receptors, antagonists, and cell adhesion blockers, as well as the formation of registries of consecutive patients admitted to coronary care units with the diagnosis of suspected AMI. Results of these trials have demonstrated that thrombolytic therapy significantly reduces mortality and morbidity from AMI with minimal risk to patients, and that early treatment is associated with improved infarct size and better left ventricular function. The efforts of the next decade should be focused on the further removal of barriers to rapid treatment and to the evaluation of new agents, so that the devastating effects of myocardial infarction are minimized to the fullest extent. (J Interven Cardiol 1997; 10:171–182)

Introduction

Thrombolytic therapy has been the most important advance in the treatment of acute myocardial infarction (AMI) in the last 15 years. Thrombolytic drugs such as streptokinase, recombinant tissue plasminogen activator (rt-PA) , and now reteplase (r-PA) have dramatically reduced mortality and morbidity from AMI by reperfusing occluded coronary arteries and halting the process of ischemic necrosis. Beginning in 1981, collaborative efforts developed between the University of Washington School of Medicine and community hospitals in Washington, Idaho, Oregon, British Columbia, Canada, and later outside the Pacific Northwest (Table 1) and have generated important new findings about the treatment and outcome of AMI. These efforts have included randomized trials of thrombolytic agents, direct antithrombins, platelet receptors, antagonists, and cell adhesion blockers, as well as the formation of registries of consecutive pa-

Table 1

Western Washington and Myocardial Infarction Triage and Intervention Trials and Registries

Trial	Years	Comparison	Number of Patients	Endpoint
WWIC	1981–83	IC SK vs. control	250	30 day mortality
WWIV	1983–86	IV SK vs. control	368	14 day mortality
WW ED rt-PA	1987–88	rt-PA	160	14 day mortality
WW rt-PA Registry	1987–88		1,028	
MITI	1988–91	Prehospital- vs. hospital-initiated rt-PA	360	Composite endpoint*
MITI registry	1988–94		12,331	

*Composite score combining death, stroke, major bleeding, and infarct size.
ED = emergency department; IC = intracoronary; IV = intravenous; MITI = Myocardial Infarction Triage and Intervention; rt-PA = recombinant tissue plasminogen activator; WW = Western Washington; SK = streptokinase.

tients admitted to coronary care units with the diagnosis of suspected AMI.

Although conducted over a 10-year period, these trials have several factors in common. First, the implementation and successful completion of these trials were dependent upon the efforts of investigators, nurses, paramedics, and other personnel at the University of Washington and other medical centers and hospitals, and the Seattle and King County emergency medical services. Second, over the years of the early trials, there were national and particularly regional efforts to reduce the time from symptom onset to treatment for AMI, so as to better understand the obstacles to seeking emergency medical care. Third, in addition to assessing conventional clinical and angiographic end points, many trials also used quantitative radionuclide methods to measure ventricular function and infarct size in survivors of the index hospitalization at the Seattle Department of Veterans Affairs Medical Center and later at the Georgetown University Medical Center. Finally, to better understand the long-term effects of thrombolytic therapy, long-term follow-up of patients enrolled in all four trials was conducted.

Western Washington Intracoronary Streptokinase Trial

Under the leadership of J. Ward Kennedy, MD, the Western Washington Intracoronary Streptokinase Trial began in July 1981 in 14 hospitals in Western Washington and British Columbia. It ended in February 1983.[1–8] This trial, which was supported in part by the W.M. Keck Foundation and the Medical Research Service of the Veterans Administration, was a randomized comparison of intracoronary streptokinase versus standard therapy, with all patients undergoing coronary angiography prior to randomization. The trial enrolled 250 patients who were ≤ 75 years of age, arrived at the hospital ≤ 12 hours from symptom onset, had appropriate electrocardiographic changes, and did not have contraindications to anticoagulation therapy. Patients who had treatment of congestive heart failure prior to the onset of AMI were not eligible for randomization.

The two groups were similar with respect to baseline characteristics (Table 2). The time from symptom onset to hospital arrival was 2.2 hours for 134 treatment pa-

Table 2

Characteristics of Patients Enrolled in the Western Washington and Myocardial Infarction Triage and Intervention Trials

Characteristic	WWIC	WWIV	rt-PA	MITI
Age	56 ± 10	57 ± 11	58 ± 10	58 ± 10
Women	15%	18%	19%	18%
History MI	13%	14%	16%	20%
Anterior MI	46%	36%	38%	39%
Delay time (hrs)	2.2 ± 2.4	1.9 ± 1.4	1.6 ± 1.1	1.1 ± 0.8
Time from symptom onset to treatment (hrs)	4.6 ± 2.2	3.5 ± 1.4	2.3 ± 2.8	1.8 ± 0.9
Infarct size (treated patients only)	19 ± 13	15 ± 13	13 = 11	6.4 ± 8.8
Radionuclide EF (treated patients only)	46 ± 14	51 ± 15	51 ± 15	54 ± 12

EF = ejection fraction; IC = intracoronary; IV = intravenous; MI = myocardial infarction; MITI = Myocardial Infarction Triage and Intervention; rt-PA = recombinant tissue plasminogen activator; WW = Western Washington.

tients and 2.3 hours for 116 controls, and the time from symptom onset to treatment was 4.6 hours (Fig. 1, Table 2). The remarkable finding of this study was a threefold reduction in mortality for patients receiving intracoronary streptokinase; 30-day mortality was 3.7% in the treatment group and 11.2% in the control group (P = 0.02).[2] It was the first trial of thrombolytic therapy to show a mortality reduction due to treatment. Treatment patients also had better angina and functional class at discharge than did control patients. However, radionuclide ejection fraction at discharge was similar in the two groups.

Follow-up studies were unable to demonstrate differences in key end points that were consistent with the observed mortality difference. For example, radionuclide ejection fraction and thallium infarct size measured approximately 2 months after treatment were similar in treatment and control patients (Fig. 2).[3] Analysis of echocardiograms performed 2 months after treatment also showed similar outcomes for treatment and control patients.[6] The results

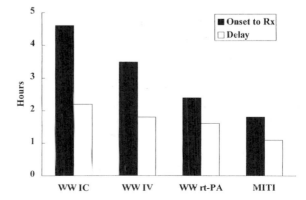

Figure 1. Time from symptom onset to treatment and delay time in patients receiving thrombolytic therapy (1981–1991). IC = intracoronary; IV = intravenous; MITI = Myocardial Infarction Triage and Intervention; rt-PA = recombinant tissue plasminogen activator; WW = western Washington.

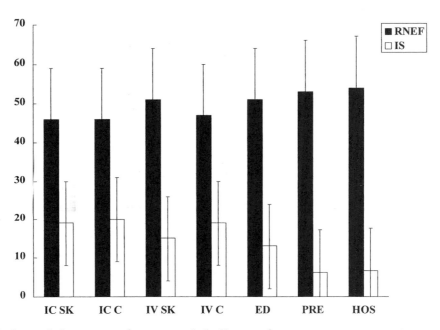

Figure 2. Radionuclide ejection fraction and thallium infarct size measurements in patients receiving thrombolytic therapy (1981–1991). The error bars represent one standard deviation from the mean. ED = emergency department rt-PA trial; HOS = MITI hospital initiated therapy; IC SK = intracoronary streptokinase; IC C = intracoronary control; IS = infarct size; IV SK = intravenous streptokinase; IV C = intravenous control; PRE = MITI prehospital initiated therapy; RNEF = radionuclide ejection fraction.

of a 1-year follow-up study demonstrated that intracoronary streptokinase reduced one year mortality, but only in patients with complete coronary artery reperfusion.[4] One-year survival was 98% in 80 patients with complete reperfusion, 77% in 14 individuals with partial reperfusion, and 85% in 41 patients with no reperfusion. In comparison, 85% of control patients were alive at 1 year. However, follow-up infarct size and ejection fraction did not differ according to reperfusion status. Again, one is left with the puzzling result of a marked reduction in mortality far greater than expected from a small reduction in infarct size. It is likely that this result is a function of late reperfusion achieved by intracoronary streptokinase; that is, mortality was reduced, but reperfusion was too late to bring about significant reductions in infarct size. From this and other observations has been borne the "open artery hypothesis"

that the benefit of coronary artery patency seems to transcend what can be explained by myocardial salvage alone.

In addition to these findings, several other analyses utilizing information from the intracoronary trial have produced important findings concerning coronary anatomy and function and risk stratification, as well as the comparability of methods for measuring infarct size and left ventricular function.[5,7,8] Since all patients enrolled in the trial had baseline angiograms performed prior to the administration of streptokinase, it was possible to obtain baseline information about infarct location and left ventricular function. All available angiograms were read centrally by a panel of cardiologists, and when possible, quantitative analyses of left ventricular angiograms were performed. An important finding of these analyses was that location of the infarct related occlusion was the most important determinant of global and regional left ventricular function.[5] In addition, the baseline angiographic ejection fraction was an important predictor of 1-year survival.[7] These two papers, published over 10 years ago, have contributed to our understanding of the natural history and pathology of AMI.

Western Washington Intravenous Streptokinase Trial

While intracoronary streptokinase reduced hospital mortality, its method of administration has two major limitations. First, it has to be delivered in a cardiac catheterization lab, which is not present in every hospital, and second, the time required to give the drug once the patient arrives at the hospital is frequently too long, particularly during the late evening or early morning hours. In order to achieve the full benefits of reperfusion, the drug must be given to more eligible patients, and it must be given more rapidly than can be done in most cardiac catheterization facilities. As a result, interest shifted to intravenous administration of thrombolytic therapy.

The Western Washington Intravenous Streptokinase Trial began in September 1983 and ended July 31, 1986, after enrolling 368 patients in 27 hospitals in Washington, Idaho, and Vancouver, British Columbia.[9–13] The trial was a randomized comparison of intravenous streptokinase versus standard therapy; it was supported in part by the W.M. Keck Foundation, the National Heart Lung and Blood Institute, and the Seattle Veterans Administration Medical Center. Entry criteria were similar to those used in the intracoronary trial, although arrival < 6 hours from symptom onset was required. Patients with history of congestive heart failure were included, although those with prior coronary artery bypass surgery were excluded.

Both groups had similar baseline characteristics, although the mean delay time for the streptokinase group was slightly less (1.8 vs 2.1 hours).[9] The time from symptom onset to treatment was 3.5 hours, 1 hour less than in the intracoronary trial. Mortality at 14 days was 6.3% in 191 treatment patients and 9.6% in 177 control patients (P = 0.23). There appeared to be no survival benefit for those patients with inferior infarction; 14 day mortality was actually higher in treated patients (4.0% vs 1.8%), although this difference was not statistically significant (P = 0.32). However, for patients with anterior AMI, mortality was worse for control patients (10.4% vs 22.4%, P = 0.06). Other measures of outcome (including length of stay, angina class, and the presence of congestive heart failure) were similar in treatment and control patients. Intracerebral hemorrhage occurred in one (0.5%) patient randomized to streptokinase.

The major conclusion of the trial was that patients with anterior AMI treated within 6 hours of symptom onset had improved survival. It was also the case that a higher proportion of treatment patients received coronary angioplasty (6.3% vs 2.8%) and/or coronary artery bypass graft surgery (6.8% vs 5.6%) within 14 days of randomization. The trial was one of many confirming the benefit of intravenous thrombolytic therapy. As in the intracoronary trial, surviving patients underwent radionuclide and thallium infarct size testing 2 months after infarction.[11] In contrast to findings from the intracoronary trial, where treatment was instituted one hour later, in the intravenous trial the treatment group exhibited both smaller infarct size (19% ± 13% vs 15 ± 13%, P = 0.03) and improved left ventricular function (51% ± 15% vs 47% ± 15%, P = 0.08). This improvement was evident only for patients with anterior infarction who arrived at the hospital within 3 hours of symptom onset. There was no benefit for patients with inferior infarction or for those with anterior infarction of > three hours duration. These results again emphasized the need for early treatment.

Long-term survival was similar for treatment and control patients in the intravenous trial. However, for anterior infarction, 2-year survival was 81% for patients receiving streptokinase and only 65% for those receiving standard therapy (P = 0.05).[9] By one year, 27% and 19% of treatment and control patients, respectively, had undergone a revascularization procedure.

As in the first trial, considerable effort was given to examination of coronary anatomy and left ventricular function and comparability of methods for measuring infarct size.[10,12] Overall, 68% of patients underwent coronary angiography at an average of 10 days after randomization; 170 films were adequate for analysis of global and regional left ventricular function. Streptokinase resulted in better infarct artery patency, better global function as measured by angiographic ejection fraction, and better wall motion in the infarct zone as well as noninfarct areas.[10]

In a report which combined data from both trials, a higher proportion of streptokinase patients underwent coronary angioplasty within 1 year of randomization (7% vs 3%), but the use of coronary artery bypass surgery was similar as was the use of angioplasty for all years after randomization.[13] Further follow-up of patients in the two trials was accomplished; the mean time to follow-up was almost 5 years for the 618 patients; only 3% were lost to follow-up. Three-year survival was 84% for treated patients and 82% for controls (P = 0.16); for patients with inferior infarction, 3-year survival was 89% and 91% for treatment and control patients, respectively (P = 0.63). For anterior AMI, 3 year survival was 76% for the streptokinase group and 67% for the control group (P = 0.14).

The Western Washington Emergency Department Tissue Plasminogen Activator Treatment Trial and Registry

Although the time from symptom onset to treatment was reduced by 1 hour to 3.5 hours in the intravenous trial, this was still considered too long to realize the full benefits of early reperfusion. The Western Washington Emergency Department Tissue Plasminogen Activator Treatment Trial was designed to reduce time to treatment by making the emergency department the locus of diagnosis and treatment activities. In addition, a new thrombolytic agent, rt-PA, was used in this nonrandomized trial, which was supported by Genentech, Inc. of South San Francisco, CA. The primary objective of the trial was to evaluate initiating administration of rt-PA in the emergency department. A randomized trial was not performed because clear evidence favoring thrombolytic therapy made a placebo controlled trial unethical. Second, there were insufficient resources to enroll the large numbers of patients required for a head-to-head comparison of thrombolytic agents. Entry criteria were similar to those used in the intravenous trial. In a departure from previous Western Washington trials, a registry of all patients with documented AMI was established to determine the proportion of eligible patients who actually received thrombolytic therapy.

Between January 1987 and January 1988, 160 patients received rt-PA in eight hospitals in Seattle and Tacoma, Washington.[14-18] Characteristics of patients treated with rt-PA were very similar to those of patients enrolled in the intravenous trial.[14] The average delay time was 1.6 hours, and the time from symptom onset to treatment was 2.3 hours, approximately 1 hour shorter than in the intravenous trial, where treatment was started in the coronary care unit. Mortality at 14 days was 5.6%, and 1-year survival was 92% (85% anterior and 96% inferior). Intracerebral hemorrhage occurred in three patients (1.9%). In comparison to the intravenous trial, a much higher proportion of patients underwent coronary angiography, doing so earlier in the course of hospitalization (Table 3). Furthermore, the proportion of patients undergoing revascularization

Table 3

Cardiac Procedure Utilization Prior to Hospital Discharge (Treated Patients Only)

Procedure	WWIC	WWIV	rt-PA	MITI
Coronary angiography	—	72%	91%	73%
Days to angiography	—	10 ± 7	5 ± 3	2 ± 2
Coronary angioplasty	2%	6%	19%	27%
Coronary artery bypass surgery	10%	7%	21%	14%

IC = intracoronary; IV = intravenous; MI = myocardial infarction; MITI = Myocardial Infarction Triage and Intervention; rt-PA = recombinant tissue plasminogen activator; WW = Western Washington.

procedures prior to hospital discharge increased dramatically in the emergency department trial.

At the eight participating hospitals, the medical records of all patients who developed AMI during the course of the trial were reviewed. Of the 1,028 patients with documented AMI, 22% were eligible for thrombolytic therapy under study criteria, and of those eligible, 79% were offered therapy, with 72% enrolled in the trial. Women were less likely to meet eligibility criteria than men, but even among eligible patients, women were less likely to receive thrombolytic therapy.[18]

As in the previous two trials, patients enrolled in the emergency department rt-PA trial had radionuclide ejection fraction and infarct size measurements performed 11 weeks after infarction, as well as echocardiographic evaluation of segmental wall motion at 11 hours, and again at 13 weeks after infarction.[14,15] The results of the first two trials demonstrated a trend toward a reduction in infarct size, with shorter time to treatment. However, in the emergency department rt-PA trial there was no association between infarct size or ejection fraction and time to treatment.[17] Echocardiographic analysis did demonstrate improvement in regional wall motion after early treatment with rt-PA.[15]

The emergency department rt-PA trial documented that thrombolytic therapy could be delivered in a safe and effective manner in the emergency department.

Treatment times were reduced by beginning diagnosis and treatment in the emergency department, as opposed to the coronary care unit. In the eight hospitals that participated in both the intravenous and emergency department rt-PA trials, the time from hospital arrival to treatment was reduced from 91 to 52 minutes.[16] The trial also showed that the proportion of patients treated could be significantly increased if age restrictions were removed or if patients arriving > 6 hours from symptom onset were offered treatment.[14]

The Myocardial Infarction Triage and Intervention Prehospital Treatment Trial (MITI) and Registry

MITI Prehospital Treatment Trial

During the seven years of the Western Washington trials, the time from symptom onset to treatment was reduced by 50% from 4.6 hours in the intracoronary trial to 2.3 hours in the emergency department rt-PA trial. While it was a significant reduction, this time greatly exceeded the first hour from symptom onset, where the most dramatic reductions in mortality and infarct size were expected to be achieved. Even with the best emergency medical system and the fastest emergency department, achieving the 1-hour goal is very difficult, since most patients delay at least 30 minutes prior to seeking help for their symptoms. However, identifying and treating patients either at home or at the place of symptom onset could result in shorter treatment times and improved outcomes for patients with AMI. The trial and registry were supported by the National Heart Lung and Blood Institute and by a grant from Genentech Inc., Marquette Electronics (Milwaukee, WI), and Pharmacia Deltec (St. Paul, MN).

The logistical challenges to developing a program for identifying AMI in the field and for delivering thrombolytic therapy in the prehospital setting are considerable.[19] As in the previous Western Washington trials, the cooperation of the academic group and community hospitals was critical, but in the MITI trial, the Seattle and King County emergency medical system had significant roles. Whereas previously it was primarily responsible for transporting patients from the place of symptom onset to the hospital, the emergency medical system and its paramedics, under the remote guidance of an emergency physician, were now sharing responsibility for identifying and treating patients with suspected AMI. In this sense, the MITI trial represented a distinct departure from the previous trials.

Under the leadership of W. Douglas Weaver, M.D., the MITI prehospital treatment trial of prehospital versus hospital initiated thrombolytic therapy (rt-PA) was designed to assess the feasibility and efficacy of prehospital thrombolytic therapy.[20,21] The trial began in 1988 involving 19 hospitals and all 15 paramedic units in Seattle, and suburban King County, Washington. Paramedics evaluated 8,863 patients who complained of chest pain and were considered for inclusion in the trial. This evaluation involved obtaining clinical findings, performing a prehospital ECG (which was transmitted to the hospital), and informing the patient about participation in the trial. The effort was aided in great part by engineers who developed a 12-lead ECG that could be transmitted by cellular telephone to the hospital, and by the Cellular One Division of McCaw

Communications (Seattle, WA). The decision to randomize was made by a physician who reviewed clinical findings and results of the ECG. The drug was delivered by an infusion pump developed by Pharmacia Deltec. Over a 3-year period, the study enrolled and randomized 360 patients (175 prehospital, 185 in-hospital) who were 75 years of age or younger, had ST segment elevation, symptom duration ≤ 6 hours, and no risk factors for serious bleeding.

The primary end point of the trial was a composite score, which included death, stroke, serious bleeding, and tomographic thallium infarct size measured 30 days after infarction. The two groups were similar with respect to composite score (406 prehospital vs 400 in-hospital, $P = 0.64$), mortality (5.7% vs 8.1%, $P = 0.49$), radionuclide ejection fraction (53 vs 54, $P = 0.34$), and infarct size (6.1 vs 6.6, $P = 0.72$). Hemorrhagic stroke occurred in six patients (1.7%). A secondary analysis showed that treatment within 70 minutes of symptom onset was associated with a reduction in the in-hospital mortality rate from 8.7% to 1.2% ($P = 0.04$), a reduction in infarct size from 11.2% to 4.9% ($P < 0.001$), and an increase in ejection fraction from 49% to 53% ($P = 0.03$). This finding showed that treatment in the first, or "golden," hour could essentially abort the infarct; in fact, 40% of the patients treated in the MITI prehospital thrombolytic trial had no measurable infarct by quantitative thallium imaging.

In the MITI trial, the mean time from symptom onset to treatment was 92 ± 58 minutes (median, 77 min) in the prehospital group and 120 ± 49 minutes (median, 110 min) in the hospital group; thus, prehospital therapy resulted in a 33-minute reduction in time to treatment. The time to treatment in the hospital group was more rapid than expected, resulting in minimal variation in treatment time. Virtually all patients were treated within three hours of symptom onset. These rapid treatment times resulted in very small infarct sizes; the overall infarct size was 6% and was approximately 10% for anterior AMI and

3% for inferior infarcts. These results are vastly different from the much larger infarct sizes obtained in the Western Washington trials (Fig. 2, Table 2).

As in the previous trials, the influence of thrombolytic therapy on long-term survival was examined in the MITI trial.[21] Two-year survival was 89% for prehospital and 91% (P = 0.46) for hospital-treated patients. Two-year survival (free of death or readmission to the hospital for angina, myocardial infarction, congestive heart failure, or revascularization) was 56% and 64% for prehospital and hospital patients, respectively (P = 0.42). For patients treated < 70 minutes from symptom onset, 2-year survival was 98%, and it was 88% for those treated later (P = 0.12). Two-year event-free survival was 65% for the early group and 59% for the late group (P = 0.80). Poorer long-term survival was associated with advanced age, history of congestive heart failure, and coronary artery bypass surgery performed before the index hospitalization, but not with time from symptom onset to treatment. Finally, the utilization of cardiac procedures both prior to and after hospital discharge was similar in both randomization groups. In comparison to previous trials, there was an increase in the use of coronary angioplasty prior to hospital discharge (Table 3). This finding is most likely related to advances in the use of angioplasty in patients with AMI.

MITI Registry

The MITI registry, which lists all patients admitted to Seattle metropolitan area hospitals with the diagnosis of suspected AMI, was implemented in part to add perspective to the randomized trial.[22–47] Since the trial evaluated only those patients considered to be candidates for thrombolytic therapy (20%–40% of all patients with AMI), study investigators believed it was essential to collect information on patients who were not eligible for thrombolytic therapy, as well as those who were eligible but were not enrolled in the trial. This reg-

istry was much more extensive than the emergency department rt-PA registry, in that much more detail was collected on each patient, and the accrual period was 6.5 years as compared to 1 year. The successful implementation of the registry was due to the efforts of Dr. Mickey Eisenberg, a co-investigator in the MITI prehospital trial, Sherry Schaeffer, the supervisor of individuals who abstracted information from the hospital chart to data collection forms, and Diana Caldwell, who was the lead abstractor.

Accrual of patients in the registry began in January 1988 and ended in June 1994, when funding for the registry ceased. Patients were identified from coronary care unit logs as well as hospital discharge listings with appropriate ICD-9 codes. Patients who developed chest pain while admitted to the hospital for another medical condition were not included in the registry. As of June 1994, the registry contained 45,260 patients with suspected AMI. Demographic and outcome data have been abstracted for all patients.

More detailed information was abstracted for the 12,331 patients who developed AMI during the course of hospitalization. Variable collection for these patients has changed over the years of the registry. Initially, a six-page form with information about prior medical conditions, symptoms on admission to the hospital, laboratory data, resource utilization, and outcomes was used for all patients with AMI. In 1991, a more detailed data collection form was instituted for select subsets of patients, including those receiving thrombolytic therapy or primary coronary angioplasty within 6 hours of hospital admission. In 1993, data collection using a simplified form for all admissions was implemented. Most recently, there has been interest in evaluating the long-term outcomes of patients in the MITI registry. This has been accomplished by linking the MITI database to the National Death Index and the state of Washington episode of illness file, which contains information on rehospitalizations in Washington state as well as current vital status from state death records. In addition, socio-economic characteristics of the registry have been obtained by linking patient addresses to 1990 census block data.

Using data from the MITI registry, study investigators have published manuscripts on a variety of topics related to AMI. The effects of age,[25,28] gender,[26,27,44] race,[22,37] prior coronary bypass surgery,[24] cardiac catheterization,[31] primary coronary angioplasty,[30] clinical risk factors,[41] and coronary artery bypass surgery[46] on outcomes have been examined. In addition, reports on hospital mortality rates[29] and time to treatment,[32,40,43] have been published, as have an evaluation of computer-interpreted electrocardiography[23] and several manuscripts examining the ECG as a predictive tool for estimating infarct size and guiding decisions for reperfusion therapy.[34,35,38] Additional work has focused on a comparison of the epidemiology of AMI in Girona, Spain, and Seattle,[33] and temporal changes in the use of thrombolytic therapy in Seattle.[36] In addition, treatment for AMI in St. Petersburg, Russia and Seattle have also been compared.[42] In topics related to health services research, papers on the effect of cardiac catheterization facilities and health care organization on cardiac procedure utilization[31,39] have been published, as has a recent analysis of hospital length of stay.[43] Current activities with respect to the registry are focused on analysis of long-term outcomes, including survival and rehospitalization.[47]

Activities Following the MITI Prehospital Treatment Trial

Following the completion of the MITI prehospital thrombolytic trial, there have been investigations of new thrombolytic agents, direct antithrombins, platelet receptors, antagonists, and cell adhesion blockers, as well as efforts to evaluate the prehospital ECG in a wider group of patients than those eligible for thrombolytic therapy.[48–54] The more recent efforts of MITI have included key investigators in Canada as well as the United States. Investigators at Vancouver General Hospital and St. Paul's Hospital in Vancouver, British Columbia, have been extremely important in recent efforts. The purpose of these efforts, as well as those of the past, has been to implement and test strategies for improving the treatment and outcome of AMI.

Prourokinase trials

The MITI group has done two trials evaluating two separate formulations of prourokinase. In the first study, a new recombinant glycosylated prourokinase (A-74187) was evaluated by studying coronary artery patency and TIMI III flow rates at 90 minutes in patients with AMI. Plasma was collected serially to measure fibrinogen, plasminogen, antithrombin III, and fibrinopeptide A. The drug was given as either 60 or 80 mg of monotherapy or as 60 mg and "primed" with a bolus of 250,000 IU of recombinant urokinase. Experimental studies have suggested that prourokinase can be "activated" by giving small doses of a second, nonspecific thrombolytic drug which in turn enhances the number of plasminogen molecules on the clot surface, thus speeding the conversion of prourokinase to clot-sound urokinase. The first study showed that prourokinase in all three dosages resulted in TIMI III flow rates of approximately 50%–60%. Unlike the earlier experimental studies, there was no further enhancement of lytic activity with priming.[48]

A second trial studied an unglycosylated formulation of prourokinase, evaluating the "priming" concept by using an initial bolus of rt-PA (5–10 mg) followed by a 90 minute infusion of prourokinase (40 mg/hour). Coronary angiography was performed at 90 minutes, and central assessment of patency and flow rates was accomplished. Patency was achieved in 77% of patients, while TIMI III flow rates were evident in 60% of patients. The incidence of the reocclusion was almost zero. This study, like many others, suggested that prourokinase in conjunction with another thrombolytic agent may result in lower rates of reocclusion.[49] These two studies have provided a rationale for large comparative studies of prourokinase. Unfortunately, because of commercial concerns about the varied mutations of prourokinase and the possible inability to have a single market presence for one formulation, commercialization of prourokinase has been delayed.

RheothRx Trial

Early results from the MITI registry indicated that thrombolytic therapy and primary angioplasty were used in a relatively small proportion of patients. No more than half of patients with AMI have ST segment elevation or new bundle branch block on the admission electrocardiogram. Clinical trials and registries have shown that patients with nondiagnostic electrocardiographic changes, particularly ST segment depression, have an equally poor, if not worse, prognosis. Although aspirin and heparin are used commonly in these patients, the support for this approach comes primarily from experience in patients with unstable angina.

RheothRx® or poloxamer 188, is a surfactant which has been experimentally shown to enhance the rate of clot lysis and to attenuate size, possibly by modifying white cell adhesion to damaged microvasculature. It also can change red cell permeability in ischemic tissue. In an effort to determine whether RheothRx reduces infarct size and improves the outcome of patients with nondiagnostic electrocardiographic changes, 196 patients were enrolled and randomized to placebo or RheothRx.[50] Two thirds of the patients developed evidence of acute injury by enzyme testing. Infarct size was determined prior to discharge by using tomographic thallium imaging, which was

interpreted at a core laboratory. Dr. Manual Cerqueira has played the key role in assessing infarct size after AMI; first at the Department of Veterans Affairs Medical Center in Seattle and then at Georgetown University.

The trial was terminated because of evidence of increased transient renal dysfunction in the RheothRx group. Nonetheless, much was learned about the characteristics of patients with nondiagnostic electrocardiographic changes. These patients were older (mean age 67 years) and had more hypertension, diabetes mellitus, and prior cigarette smoking than typical in patients with ST elevation or new bundle branch block on the admission ECG. The average duration of symptoms was 6.2 hours. Infarct size averaged 15% of the left ventricle and was not changed by RheothRx treatment. Mortality rates were 11.3% in the RheothRx group and 7.1% in control patients ($P = 0.30$). Treatment of this patient population is challenging and will be the subject of future investigations.

r-PA and AMI (RAPID Trial)

A third-generation plasminogen activator, r-PA, is a nonglycosylated deletion mutant of wild type tissue plasminogen activator (t-PA) that is expressed in *Escherichia coli*. The structural changes of the molecule result in properties markedly different from that of rt-PA. The mutant has less affinity with fibrin, a longer half-life, and a greater thrombolytic potency. RAPID II was an angiographic trial evaluating 90-minute patency for double bolus r-PA, compared with a 90-minute or "accelerated" infusion of rt-PA.[51,52] Three hundred twenty-four patients were enrolled in the trial and angiographic patency was determined at 30, 60, and 90 minutes. The TIMI III flow rate was 60% for r-PA compared to 45% for rt-PA ($P < 0.05$). Treatment with r-PA is convenient, simple to administer, and has minimal complications.

Efegateran and streptokinase can accelerate patency like accelerated rt-PA (ESCALAT trial)

ESCALAT was designed to evaluate whether a direct antithrombin, efegateran, could overcome the initial lag phase of lysis associated with streptokinase. Efegateran is a small, direct thrombin inhibitor produced by chemical synthesis. Experimental evidence suggests that efegateran has a greater effect on clot lysis initiated by streptokinase than for rt-PA. The design of this dose ranging study was to determine whether the combination of efegateran and streptokinase could achieve TIMI III flow rates equivalent to those using accelerated rt-PA and heparin.

Two hundred thirty patients were enrolled in the study at medical centers across the United States and Canada.[53] Angiograms were obtained at 90 minutes, and coagulation parameters and clinical events were monitored for 30 days. After exploring four doses ranging from 0.3 mg/kg to 1.0 mg/kg, a dose of 0.5 mg/kg per hour was chosen. The 90-minute patency rate for efegateran and streptokinase was 73% versus 79% for rt-PA and heparin (P = 0.54). TIMI III flow rates, although enhanced at 40%, were not as high as those seen with rt-PA and heparin (53%, P = 0.085). Significantly, there were no cases of intracranial hemorrhage. The result of this trial, similar to those reported for other antithrombins, has confirmed that the addition of direct antithrombins appears to enhance patency achieved by streptokinase alone. The therapeutic range of dose appears narrow if one is to avoid excessive hemorrhage.

Optimal stent trial (OPUS 1)

OPUS is an ongoing study evaluating the strategy of optimal balloon angioplasty versus the strategy of primary stenting in patients who are candidates for both. Earlier trials demonstrated that there was less angiographic and clinical restenosis in patients treated with stents compared to balloon angioplasty. However, in a secondary analysis of the studies, coronary arteries of > 3.0 mm with good angioplasty results showed no differences in restenosis compared to the stent strategy. A second limitation of the earlier studies is that obligatory follow-up angiograms can lead to repeat procedures that may not be driven totally by clinical indications. The OPUS trial is the first effort by the MITI group to collaborate with interested interventionalists in the United States and Canada. The hypothesis of the trial is that optimal angioplasty (results of < 20% visual stenosis or < 30% stenosis by quantitative coronary angiography) can be achieved in 80% of those undergoing balloon angioplasty and is equivalent to stenting. In the 20% of patients with suboptimal balloon angioplasty results or in those with significant dissection, stents are recommended. In the primary stent strategy, "optimal" stent placement is accomplished without prior balloon angioplasty in order to minimize external injury and to reduce the number of ancillary balloons and use of other equipment. The trial will enroll 2,200 patients, and will evaluate clinical restenosis rates in the two treatment groups. In addition, postprocedure utilization and quality of life will be measured. Completion of the trial is expected in 1997.

Conclusion

In the 10 years from the beginning of the intracoronary trial to the end of the MITI prehospital treatment trial, the time from symptom onset to treatment dropped from 4.6 hours to 1.8 hours (Fig. 1). This remarkable reduction of 60% resulted in improved left ventricular function and infarct size (Fig. 3); the findings for infarct size in the MITI trial were particularly striking, as many patients had no detectable defects. It is important to recognize that patients in the MITI trial were highly selected, and that their treatment times were not representative of the overall community. In 1992 in metropolitan Seattle,

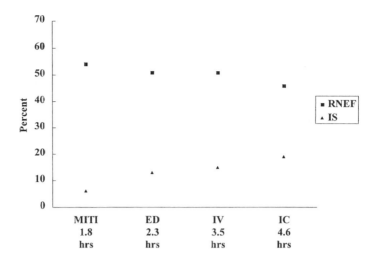

Figure 3. Ejection fraction and infarct size by trial. This figure displays the reduction in infarct size and increase in ejection fraction with decreasing time from symptom onset to treatment in each trial. This figure includes only patients who received thrombolytic therapy. ED = emergency department rt-PA trial; IC = western Washington intracoronary trial; IS = infarct size; IV = western Washington intravenous trial; MITI = Myocardial Infarction Triage and Intervention; RNEF = radionuclide ejection fraction.

60% of patients received thrombolytic therapy within 3 hours of symptom onset, in comparison to *all* trial patients. Much of this discrepancy is due to differences in patient delay, which is the most significant barrier to rapid treatment. Yet, in the group randomized to hospital therapy, the time from hospital arrival to treatment was 20 minutes, considerably less than the median of 47 minutes in all Seattle area hospitals. The rapid treatment time achieved for hospital initiated therapy in the MITI trial is a goal which must be attained to reduce mortality and morbidity from AMI.

The Western Washington and MITI trials have proven that thrombolytic therapy significantly reduces morbidity and mortality from AMI with minimal risk to patients. Moreover, these trials have clearly indicated that early treatment is associated with improved infarct size and better left ventricular function; in short, this translates to better lives for those who are affected by this all too pervasive condition. The efforts of the next decade should be focused on further removal of barriers to rapid treatment and the evaluation of new agents, so that the devastating effects of myocardial infarction can be minimized to the fullest extent.

References

1. Kennedy JW, Fritz JK, Ritchie JL. Streptokinase in Acute Myocardial Infarction: Western Washington Randomized Trial: Protocol and progress report. Am Heart J 1982; 104:899-911.
2. Kennedy JW, Ritchie JL, Davis KB, et al. Western Washington Randomized Trial of Intracoronary Streptokinase in Acute Myocardial Infarction. N Engl J Med 1983;309:1477-1482.
3. Ritchie J, Davis K, Williams D, et al. Global and Regional Left Ventricular Function and Tomographic Radionuclide Perfusion: The Western Washington Streptokinase in Myocardial Infarction Trial. Circulation 1984; 70:867-875.
4. Kennedy JW, Ritchie JL, Davis KB, et al. Western Washington Randomized Trial of Intracoronary Streptokinase in Acute Myocardial Infarction: 12 month

follow-up report. N Engl J Med 1985; 312:1073-1078.

5. Stadius ML, Maynard C, Fritz JK, et al. Coronary anatomy and left ventricular function in the first twelve hours of acute myocardial infarction. Circulation 1985;72:292-301.

6. Stratton JR, Speck SM, Caldwell JH, et al. Late effects of intracoronary streptokinase on regional wall motion, ventricular aneurysm, and left ventricular thrombus in myocardial infarction: Results from the Western Washington Randomized Trial. JACC 1985;5:1023-1028.

7. Stadius ML, Davis K, Maynard C, et al. Risk sratification for one year survival based on characteristics identified in the early hours of acute myocardial infarction. Circulation 1986;74:703-711.

8. Stratton JR, Speck SM, Caldwell JH, et al. The Relationship of global and regional left ventricular function to tomographic thallium-201 myocardial perfusion in patients with prior myocardial infarction. JACC 1988;12:71-77.

9. Kennedy JW, Martin GV, Davis KB, et al. The Western Washington Intravenous Streptokinase in Acute Myocardial Infarction Randomized Trial. Circulation 1988;77:345-352.

10. Martin GV, Sheehan FL, Stadius M, et al. Intravenous Streptokinase for Acute Myocardial Infarction: Effects on global and regional systolic function. Circulation 1988;78:258-266.

11. Ritchie JL, Cerqueira M, Maynard C, et al. Ventricular function and infarct size: The Western Washington Intravenous Streptokinase in Myocardial Infarction Trial. JACC 1988;11:689-697.

12. Cowan M, Hindman N, Wagner G, et al. Estimation of myocardial infarct size by electrocardiographic and radionuclide techniques. J Electrocardiol 1987;20:78-81.

13. Cerqueira MD, Maynard C, Ritchie JL, et al. Long-term survival in 618 patients from the Western Washington Streptokinase in Myocardial Infarction Trials. JACC 1992;20:1452-1459.

14. Althouse R, Maynard C, Cerqueira MD, et al. The Western Washington Myocardial Infarction Registry and Emergency Department Tissue Plasminogen Activator Treatment Trial. Am J Cardiol 1990;66:1298-1303.

15. Otto CM, Stratton JR, Maynard C, et al. Echocardiographic evaluation of segmental wall motion early and late after thrombolytic therapy in acute myocardial infarction. Am J Cardiol 1990;65:132-138.

16. Maynard C, Althouse R, Olsufka M, et al. Early versus late hospital arrival for acute myocardial infarction in the western washington thrombolytic therapy trials. Am J Cardiol 1989; 63:1296-1300.

17. Cerqueira M, Maynard C, Ritchie JL. Radionuclide assessment of infarct size and left ventricular function in clinical trials of thrombolysis. Circulation 1991;84(supp.1 I):I100-I108.

18. Maynard C, Althouse R, Cerqueira M, et al. Underutilization of thrombolytic therapy in eligible women with acute myocardial infarction. Am J Cardiol 1991;68:529-530.

19. Weaver WD, Eisenberg MS, Martin JS, et al. Myocardial Infarction Triage and Intervention Project, Phase I: Patient characteristics and feasibility of prehospital initiation of thrombolytic therapy. JACC 1990;15:925-931.

20. Weaver WD, Cerqueira M, Hallstrom AP, et al. for the MITI Project Investigators. Prehospital initiated vs hospital initiated thrombolytic therapy. JAMA 1993;270:1211-1216.

21. Brouwer MA, Martin JS, Maynard C, et al. Influence of early prehospital thrombolysis on mortality and event-free survival. Am J Cardiol 1996; 78:497-502.

22. Maynard C, Litwin PE, Martin JS, et al. Characteristics of black patients admitted to coronary care units in metropolitan Seattle. Am J Cardiol 1991;67:18-23.

23. Kudenchuk P, Ho MT, Weaver WD, et al. Accuracy of computer-interpreted electrocardiography in selecting patients for thrombolytic therapy. JACC 1991;17:1486-1491.

24. Maynard C, Weaver WD, Litwin PE, et al. Acute myocardial infarction and prior coronary artery surgery in the Myocardial Infarction Triage and Intervention Registry. Cor Art Dis 1991;2:443-448.

25. Weaver WD, Litwin PE, Martin JS, et al. Effect of age on the use of thrombolytic therapy and mortality in acute myocardial infarction. JACC 1991; 18:657-662.

26. Maynard C, Litwin PE, Martin JS, et al. Gender differences in the treatment of acute myocardial infarction. Arch Intern Med 1992;152:972-976.

27. Maynard C, Weaver WD. Treatment of women with acute myocardial infarction: New findings from the MITI Registry. J Myocard Ischemia 1992; 4:27-37.

28. Maynard C, Litwin PE, Martin JS, et al. Treatment and outcome of acute myocardial infarction in women 75 years and older. Cardiol Elderly 1993; 1:121-125.

29. Maynard C, Weaver WD, Litwin PE, et al. Hospital mortality in acute myocardial infarction in the era of reperfusion therapy. Am J Cardiol 1993;72:877-882.

30. Weaver WD, Litwin PE, Martin JS. The Use of direct angioplasty for treatment of patients with acute myocardial infarction in hospitals with and without on-site cardiac surgery. Circulation 1993;88:2067-2075.

31. Every NR, Larson E, Fihn S, et al. The Effect of on-site catheterization facilities on utilization of cardiac procedures and mortality after acute myocardial infarction. N Engl J Med 1993;329:546-551.

32. Martin JS, Marriott LL, Smith DD. Early thrombolytic therapy in acute MI. Heartbeat 1993;3:1-8.

33. Hallstrom AP, Marrugat J, Perez G, et al. Characteristics of myocardial infarction episodes in two distant communities: from the REGICOR Registry in Girona, Spain and the MITI Registry in greater Seattle, USA. J Thromb Thrombolysis 1994;1:85-93.

34. Wilkins ML, Anderson ST, Pryor AD, et al. Variability of acute ST-segment predicted myocardial infarct size in the absence of thrombolytic therapy. Am J Cardiol 1994;74:174-177.

35. Wilkins ML, Pryor AD, Maynard C, et al. An electrocardiographic acuteness score for quantifying the timing of a myocardial infarction to guide decisions regarding reperfusion therapy. Am J Cardiol 1995;75:617-620.

36. Maynard C, Litwin PE, Martin JS, et al. Changes in the use of thrombolytic therapy in Seattle area hospitals from 1988 to 1992. J Thromb Thrombolysis 1995;1:195-199.

37. Maynard C, Every NR, Litwin PE, et al. Outcomes in African American women with suspected acute myocardial infarction. J Natl Med Assoc 1995; 87:339-344.

38. Raitt MH, Maynard C, Wagner GS, et al. The appearance of abnormal Q waves early in the course of acute myocardial infarction: Implications for the efficacy of thrombolytic therapy. JACC 1995;25:1084-1088.

39. Every NR, Fihn SD, Maynard C, et al. Resource utilization in the treatment of acute myocardial infarction: Staff model HMO versus fee for service hospitals. JACC 1995;26:401-406.

40. Maynard C, Weaver WD. Streamlining the triage system for acute myocardial infarction. Cardiol Clin 1995;13:311-320.

41. Spertus JA, Weiss NS, Every NR, et al. The influence of clinical risk factors on the use of angiography and revascularization after acute myocardial infarction. Arch Intern Med 1995;155:2309-2316.

42. Reiss JA, Every N, Weaver WD. A comparison of the treatment of acute myocardial infarction between St. Petersburg, Russia and Seattle, Washington. Int J Cardiol 1996;53:29-36.

43. Raitt MH, Maynard C, Wagner GS, et al. Relation between symptom duration before thrombolytic therapy and final myocardial infarct size. Circulation 1996;93:48-53.

44. Kudenchuk PJ, Maynard, C Martin JS, et al. Women with acute myocardial infarction: Presentation, treatment, and outcome. Am J Cardiol 1996;78:9-14.

45. Every NR, Spertus J, Fihn SD, et al. Length of hospital stay after acute myocardial infarction in the Myocardial Infarction Triage and Intervention (MITI) Project Registry. JACC 1996; 28:287-293.

46. Every NR, Maynard C, Cochran RP, et al. for the MITI Investigators. Characteristics, management, and outcome of acute myocardial infarction treated with bypass surgery. Circulation 1996;94:II-81-II-96.

47. Every NR, Parsons LP, Hlatky M, et al. for the MITI Investigators. Hospital and long-term outcome in acute myocardial infarction patients treated with thrombolytic therapy versus primary angioplasty: Results from a large community experience. N Engl J Med 1996;335:1253-1260.

48. Weaver WD, Hartmann JR, Anderson

JL, et al. New recombinant glycosated prourokinase for treatment of patients with acute myocardial infarction. JACC 1994;24:1242-1248.

49. Zarich SW, Kowalchuk GJ, Weaver WD, et al for the PATENT study group. Sequential combination thrombolytic therapy for acute myocardial infarction: Results of the pro-urokinase and t-PA enhancement of thrombolysis (PATENT) trial. JACC 1995;26:374-379.

50. Weaver WD, for the Myocardial Infarction Study Group. Randomized, placebo-controlled trial of RheothRx® (poloaxmer 188) injection in patients with suspected acute myocardial infarction. (abstract) Circulation 1995;92:I-24.

51. Bode C, Smalling RW, Berg G, et al. Randomized comparison of coronary thrombolysis achieved with double-bolus reteplase (recombinant plasminogen activator) and frontl-loaded, accelerated alteplase (recombinant tissue plasminogen activator) in patients with acute myocardial infarction. Circulation 1996;94:891-898.

52. Weaver WD. Results of the RAPID 1 and RAPID 2 Thrombolytic Trials in acute myocardial infarction. Eur Heart J 1996;17(suppl. E):14-20.

53. Weaver WD, Fung A, Lorch G, et al. Efegatran and streptokinase vs tPA and heparin for treatment of AMI. (abstract) Circulation 1996;94:I-430.

54. Aufderheide TP, Kereiakes DJ, Weaver WD, et al. Planning, implementation, and process monitoring for 12-lead ECG diagnostic programs. Prehospital and Disaster Medicine 1996;11:162-171.

Address for reprints: Charles Maynard, Ph. D., MITI Coordinating Center, 1910 Fairview Ave E #204, Seattle, WA 98102. Fax: (206) 543-1690. E-mail: cmaynard@u.washington.edu

Chapter 5

Trials of Thrombolytic Therapy: The International Studies of Infarct Survival Experience

Charles H. Hennekens, M.D.

From the Harvard Medical School, Division of Preventive Medicine, Brigham and Women's Hospital, Boston, Massachusetts

Introduction

The International Studies of Infarct Survival (ISIS) represent a worldwide collaborative effort to identify widely available, beneficial, and practical treatments for acute myocardial infarction (MI). Begun in 1981 and coordinated by a team of research scientists based in Oxford, England, including Peter Sleight (chairman of the steering committee), Rory Collins, (coordinator), and Richard Peto (statistician), the four ISIS trials that have been completed to date have enlisted the collaboration of physicians and nurses in hospitals in over 20 countries and have randomized more than 130,000 patients with suspected acute MI. My colleagues and I at Brigham and Women's Hospital have had the honor and pleasure to serve as the US national coordinators.

The completed ISIS trials have evaluated the effects of beta-blocker therapy, aspirin, thrombolytic agents, converting enzyme inhibitors, nitrates, and magnesium in the treatment of acute evolving MI. The hallmark of the ISIS trials has been to develop extremely streamlined, simple study protocols, which minimize the overall costs of the trial and the demands of participation that are placed on busy clinicians. These features, in turn, have allowed each of the ISIS trials to successfully randomize within a relatively short timespan the tens of thousands of patients necessary to detect reliably the effects of each of the various interventions that have been evaluated.[1]

Because of their simple design, large sample size, and use of mortality as the primary outcome, the ISIS trials have played a crucial role in providing some of the most reliable evidence concerning therapies of acute MI. Perhaps not surprisingly, therapies that have been demonstrated to be beneficial have rapidly been incorporated into the standard of care for patients with acute MI. The ISIS trials have also served as a model of the utility of large, simple, randomized trials to answer important medical questions.

There have been three fundamental premises guiding the design and conduct of the ISIS trials. The first is a belief that the greatest overall public health benefit will result from the identification of effective, widely practical treatment regimens that can be used in most medical settings rather than those that can be administered only at specialized tertiary care facilities. For this reason, the ISIS investigations have focused on strategies to decrease mortality in acute MI, which, in and of themselves, do not require cardiac catheterization or other invasive procedures for either diagnostic or therapeutic purposes.

Second, benefits of truly effective therapies are likely to occur in a wide spectrum of patients with diverse clinical presentations. For this reason, the entry criteria for the ISIS trials are intentionally broad and are designed to mimic the reality physicians must face when deciding whether or not to initiate a given treatment plan in a patient with suspected evolving MI.

Third, and perhaps most important, the ISIS collaboration clearly recognizes the fact that most new therapies are likely to confer benefits that are only small to moderate in size, on the order of 10%-30% reductions in risk. Such benefits on mortality are clinically extremely worthwhile, but can be detected reliably only by randomizing some tens of thousands of patients. The ISIS protocols, therefore, are streamlined to maximize randomization and minimize interference with the responsible physician's individual choice of adjunctive therapies and interventions. Nonetheless, by selectively collecting the most important entry and follow-up variables that relate directly to the efficacy or adverse effects of the treatment in question, the ISIS trials have been able to yield reliable data that have provided a rational basis for clinical decisions for individual patients and policy decisions for the health of the general public. Further, by limiting paperwork and not mandating protocol-driven interventions, the ISIS approach has proven remarkably cost-effective. Indeed, the large ISIS trials have been conducted at a small fraction of the cost of other smaller trials, which, because of their inadequate sample sizes, have failed to demonstrate either statistically significant effects or informative null findings.

The First International Study of Infarct Survival

Beta-blocking agents reduce the heart rate and blood pressure product, inhibit the effects of catecholamines, and increase thresholds for ventricular fibrillation. It is not surprising, therefore, that beta blockers were among the first agents to be evaluated in randomized clinical trials of evolving MI. In 1981, when ISIS-1 began, the available trials of beta-blocking agents for acute infarction were all too small to demonstrate the observed small to moderate clinical benefit with statistical significance. However, it was judged that the prevention of even 1 death per 200 patients treated with beta blockade would represent a worthwhile addition to usual care. However, to detect such an effect reliably would require the randomization of more than 15,000 patients.

In a collaborative effort involving 245 coronary care units in 11 countries, the ISIS-1 trial randomized 16,027 patients with suspected acute MI to a regimen of either intravenous atenolol or no beta-blocker therapy.[2] Patients assigned to active treatment received an immediate intravenous injection of 5-10 mg atenolol, followed by 100 mg/day orally for 7 days. Beta-blocking agents were avoided in those assigned at random to no beta-blocker therapy unless believed medically indicated. As in the subsequent ISIS collaborations, all other treatment decisions were at the discretion of the treating physician.

In the 7-day treatment period during which atenolol was given, there was a statistically significant 15% reduction in mortality in the treated group (3.89% vs 4.57%, $P < 0.04$). Almost all of the benefit was observed in days 0 to 1, during which there were 121 deaths in the atenolol and 171 deaths in the control group. The early mortality benefit attributable to atenolol was maintained at 14 days (Fig. 1) and at the end of 1 year of follow-up (10.7% vs 12.0%).

Despite its large size, the 95% confidence limits of the risk reduction associated

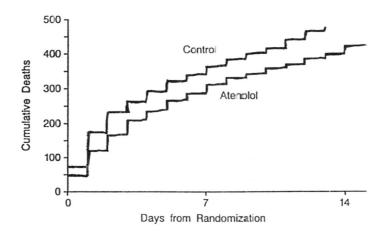

Figure 1. Cumulative 14-day mortality among patients allocated to atenolol versus control in ISIS-1. ISIS 5 International Study of Infarct Survival.

with atenolol in ISIS-1 were wide, ranging from 1% to 25%. However, an overview that included ISIS-1 and 27 smaller completed trials suggested a similar sized mortality reduction from beta-blockade (14%), and when a combined outcome of mortality, nonfatal cardiac arrest, and nonfatal reinfarction was considered from all available trials, the 10%-15% reduction persisted with far narrower confidence limits. Taken together, these data suggest that early treatment of 200 acute MI patients with beta-blocker therapy would lead to avoidance of 1 reinfarction, 1 cardiac arrest, and 1 death during the initial 7-day period.

The Second International Study of Infarct Survival.

As with beta blockers, data from randomized trials of thrombolytic therapy completed prior to 1985 did not yield truly reliable results. Indeed, the largest of the early trials enrolled 750 patients, an inadequate sample in which to detect the most plausible 20%-25% reduction in mortality.

ISIS-2 was designed to test directly in a randomized, double-blind, placebo-controlled trial the benefits and risks of thrombolytic therapy with streptokinase and antithrombotic therapy with aspirin in acute

MI. Using a 2×2 factorial design, the ISIS-2 collaborative group randomized 17,187 patients presenting within 24 hours of symptom onset to one of four treatment groups: 1.5 million units of intravenous streptokinase over 60 minutes; 162.5 mg/day of oral aspirin for 30 days; both active treatments; or both placebos.[3]

The principal findings of ISIS-2 are presented in Figure 2. For the primary end point of total vascular mortality, there were statistically significant reductions of 25% for streptokinase alone (95% confidence interval [CI] − 32% to − 18%, P < 0.0001) and 23% for aspirin alone (95% CI − 30% to − 15%, P < 0.00001). Patients allocated to both agents had a 42% reduction in vascular mortality (95% CI − 50% to − 34%, P < 0.00001), indicating that the effects of streptokinase and aspirin in acute MI are largely additive. For the subgroup of patients treated within 6 hours of symptom onset, the reductions in vascular mortality were 30% for streptokinase, 23% for aspirin, and 53% for both agents.

For aspirin, the mortality benefit was similar when the drug was started 0 to 4 hours (25%), 5 to 12 hours (21%), or 13 to 24 hours (21%) after the onset of clinical symptoms. Aspirin use also resulted in highly significant reductions in nonfatal reinfarction

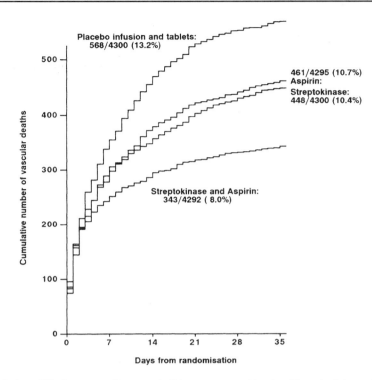

Figure 2. Cumulative 35-day vascular mortality among patients allocated to active streptokinase only, active aspirin only, both active treatments, and neither treatment in ISIS-2. ISIS 5 International Study of Infarct Survival.

(49%) and nonfatal stroke (46%). As regards side effects, for bleeds requiring transfusion, there was no significant difference between the aspirin and placebo groups (0.4% vs 0.4%), although there was a small 0.6% excess (P < 0.01) of minor bleeds among those allocated to aspirin. For cerebral hemorrhage, there was no difference between the aspirin and placebo groups.

For streptokinase, those randomized within 4 hours of symptom onset experienced the greatest mortality reduction, although statistically significant benefits were observed for patients randomized throughout the 24-hour period. As expected, there was an excess of confirmed cerebral hemorrhage with streptokinase (7 events vs 0, P < 0.02), all of which occurred within 1 day of randomization. Reinfarction was also slightly more common among those assigned streptokinase, but this increase was not statistically significant. Furthermore, aspirin appeared to abolish the excess reinfarction attributable to streptokinase.

In addition to demonstrating the independent and additive effects of streptokinase and aspirin, ISIS-2 also supplied important information concerning which patients to treat. Because the ISIS-2 entry criteria were broad, the trial included elderly patients, those with bundle branch block, and patients with inferior as well as anterior infarctions. In each of these subgroups, clear mortality reductions were demonstrated for both agents.

Thus, in addition to providing definitive evidence of the benefit of aspirin in acute MI and refuting the existing clinical impression that thrombolysis should be avoided in patients already on aspirin, ISIS-2 also made a significant contribution to the treatment of acute MI by demonstrating clear benefits of streptokinase and widening the eligibility criteria for thrombolytic therapy.

The Third International Study of Infarct Survival

While ISIS-2 (streptokinase), Gruppo Italiano per lo Studio Della Sopravvivenza Nell'Infarto Miocardico (GISSI-1, streptokinase), APSAC Intervention Mortality Study (AIMS), and Anglo-Scandinavian Study of Early Thrombolysis (ASSET, tissue plasminogen activator [tPA]) all documented clear mortality benefits for each of the various thrombolytic agents, these trials could not provide direct evidence to compare these agents. It was also still unclear following completion of these trials whether acute MI patients treated with aspirin would benefit further from the addition of heparin. These questions formed the basis for ISIS-3.

The ISIS-3 collaborative group randomized 41,299 patients to thrombolytic therapy with streptokinase, APSAC, or tPA.[4] Patients presenting within 24 hours of onset of suspected acute infarction and with no clear contraindications for thrombolysis were assigned at random to IV streptokinase (1.5 MU over 1 hour), IV tPA (duteplase, 0.50 million U/kg over 4 hours), or IV APSAC (30 U over 3 min). All patients received daily aspirin (162.5 mg), with the first dose crushed or chewed to achieve a rapid clinical antithrombotic effect. In addition, half were randomly assigned to receive subcutaneous heparin (12,500 IU twice daily for 7 days), beginning 4 hours after randomization.

As shown in Figure 3, ISIS-3 demonstrated no differences in mortality between the three thrombolytic agents. Specifically, among the 13,780 patients randomized to streptokinase, there were 1,455 deaths (10.5%) within the initial 35-day follow-up period as compared to 1,448 deaths (10.6%) among the 13,773 patients randomized to APSAC and 1,418 deaths (10.3%) among the 13,746 randomized to tPA.

Long-term survival was also virtually identical for the three agents at both 3 and 6 months. In-hospital clinical events were similar for the three agents regarding cardiac rupture, cardiogenic shock, heart failure requiring treatment, and ventricular fibrillation. For nonfatal reinfarction, there was a greater reduction with tPA, while patients allocated to the bacterial proteins streptokinase and APSAC had higher rates of allergy and hypotension requiring treat-

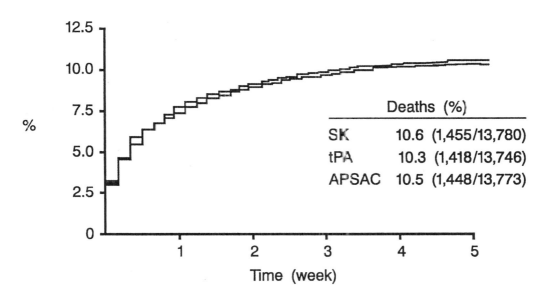

Deaths (%)	
SK	10.6 (1,455/13,780)
tPA	10.3 (1,418/13,746)
APSAC	10.5 (1,448/13,773)

Figure 3. Cumulative 35-day mortality among patients allocated to streptokinase, tPA, and APSAC in ISIS-3. APSAC 5 anisoylated plasminogen streptokinase activator complex; ISIS 5 International Study of Infarct Survival; tPA 5 tissue plasminogen activator.

ment. Streptokinase produced fewer non-cerebral bleeds than either APSAC or tPA.

While there were no major differences between thrombolytic agents in terms of lives saved or serious in-hospital clinical events, significant differences were found in ISIS-3 for rates of total stroke and cerebral hemorrhage. Specifically, there were 141 total strokes in the streptokinase group as compared to 172 and 188 in the APSAC and tPA groups, respectively. For cerebral hemorrhage there were 32 events (2/1,000) in the streptokinase group as compared to 75 (5/1,000) in the APSAC group and 89 (7/1,000) in the tPA group. While the absolute rates for cerebral hemorrhage for all three agents were low, this apparent advantage for streptokinase was statistically significant ($P < 0.0001$ for streptokinase vs APSAC; $P < 0.00001$ for streptokinase vs tPA).

With regard to the addition of delayed subcutaneous heparin to thrombolytics and aspirin, there was no reduction in the pre-specified end point of 35-day mortality. During the scheduled 7-day period of heparin use, there were slightly fewer deaths in the aspirin plus heparin group compared to the aspirin group alone, but this difference was of borderline significance. There was, however, a small but significant excess of strokes deemed definite or probable cerebral hemorrhages among those allocated aspirin plus heparin (0.56% vs 0.40%, $P < 0.05$). In contrast, reinfarction was more common among those randomized to aspirin alone as compared to those receiving aspirin plus delayed subcutaneous heparin.

The Fourth International Study of Infarct Survival

In 1991, the ISIS collaborative group chose to investigate several other promising but unproved approaches to the treatment of acute MI. In identifying agents for study, it was considered important to examine treatment strategies that might benefit both high and low risk patients present-ing with acute MI and not simply those who are eligible for thrombolysis.

With this in mind, the ISIS-4 collaborative group chose to study three promising drug regimens: a twice-daily dose of the angiotensin converting enzyme (ACE) inhibitor captopril for 30 days; a once-daily dose of controlled release mononitrate for 30 days; and a 24-hour infusion of intravenous magnesium.[5] As was true in each of the preceding ISIS trials, the available data were far too limited to allow reliable clinical recommendations concerning these therapies. For example, while ACE inhibiting agents had been shown to be successful in reducing mortality in patients with clinical congestive heart failure and in patients a week or two out from acute infarction, it was unclear whether these agents provided a net benefit in the acute setting. Similarly, while nitrates had often been used in evolving MI because of their ability to reduce myocardial loading conditions and to potentially limit infarct size, barely 3,000 total patients had received intravenous nitroglycerin in previous randomized trials, and even fewer patients had been studied on oral nitrate preparations. Finally, because of its effect on calcium regulation, arrhythmia thresholds, and tissue preservation, magnesium therapy had often been considered as an adjunctive therapy for acute infarction, although until recently no data from a randomized trial of even modest size had been available.

In ISIS-4, which randomized 58,050 patients, there was a significant 7% (SD = 3) proportional reduction in 5-week mortality in the ACE inhibitor group ($P = 0.02$), which corresponds to an absolute difference of 4.9 (SD = 2.2) fewer deaths per 1,000 patients treated for 1 month (Fig. 4). The absolute benefits appeared to be larger (perhaps about 10 fewer deaths per 1,000) in certain higher risk groups, such as those presenting with a history of previous MI or with heart failure. The survival advantage appeared to be maintained in the longer term (5.4 [SD = 2.8] fewer deaths per 1,000

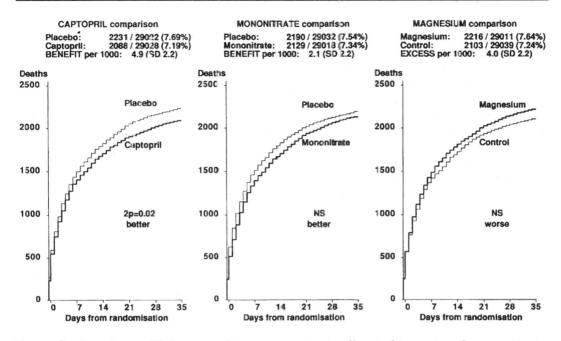

Figure 4. Cumulative 35-day mortality among patients allocated to captopril, mononitrate, and magnesium in ISIS-4. ISIS 5 International Study of Infarct Survival

at 12 months). The ACE inhibition was associated with an increase of 52/1,000 patients (SD = 2) in hypotension considered severe enough to require termination of study treatment, of 5/1,000 (SD = 2) in reported cardiogenic shock, and of 5/1,000 (SD = 1) in some degree of renal dysfunction. ACE inhibition produced no excess of deaths on days 0-1, even among patients with low blood pressure at entry.

For mononitrate, there was no significant reduction in 5-week vascular mortality, either overall or in any subgroup examined. Further follow-up did not indicate any later survival advantage. The only significant side-effect of the mononitrate regimen studied was an increase of 15/1,000 (SD = 2) in hypotension. Those allocated active treatment had somewhat fewer deaths on days 0-1, which is reassuring about the safety of using nitrates early in acute MI.

There was also no significant mortality reduction for magnesium, either overall or in any subgroup that was examined.

Further follow-up did not indicate any later survival advantage. In contrast to some previous smaller trials, there was a significant excess with magnesium of 12/1,000 (SD = 3) in heart failure and of 5/1,000 (SD = 2) in reported cardiogenic shock during or just after the infusion period. Magnesium was also associated with an increase of 11/1,000 (SD = 2) in hypotension considered severe enough to require termination of study treatment, of 3/1,000 (SD = 0.6) in bradycardia, and of 3/1,000 (SD = 0.4) in a cutaneous flushing or burning sensation (but assessment of magnesium involved open control). There was no evidence of a net adverse effect on mortality on days 0-1.

Because of its size, ISIS-4 provides reliable evidence about the effects of adding each of these three treatments to established treatments for acute MI. ACE inhibition was effective, intravenous magnesium was ineffective, and although oral nitrate therapy appeared safe, it did not produce a clear reduction in 1-month mortality. Other trials have shown that starting long-term converting enzyme inhibitor in the weeks or months after MI in patients with impaired ventricular function avoids about 2 deaths per 1,000 patients per month of treatment. Data from ISIS-4, as well as other trials, now collectively demonstrate that for a wide range of patients without clear contraindications, converting enzyme inhibitor therapy started early in acute MI prevents about 5 deaths per 1,000 in the first month (P = 0.006), with somewhat greater benefits in higher-risk patients. This benefit from 1 month of early treatment seems to persist for at least the first year.

Summary

The ISIS trials have made substantial contributions to clinical knowledge concerning a range of promising treatments for evolving acute infarction. Because of their simple design, the ISIS trials have been able to enroll the large number of patients needed to detect reliably the most plausible effects of acute MI interventions. Their simple design has also made the ISIS trials extremely cost-efficient, and the testing of treatments that can be administered in a wide range of medical settings has meant that the ISIS findings can have an extremely broad public health impact. The ISIS trials are a model of international cooperation in identifying effective treatments for acute MI, which is the leading cause of death in the US and most developed countries and which is rapidly becoming the leading cause of death worldwide.[6] With the continued cooperation of physicians and nurses in dozens of countries, future ISIS trials may provide further valuable evidence concerning effective treatment strategies for acute MI.

References

1. Ridker PM, Hennekens CH. The International Studies of Infarct Survival. In: Becker RC, ed. The Modern Era of Coronary Thrombolysis. Boston: Kluwer Academic Publishers, 1994, pp. 81-90.
2. ISIS-1 (First International Study of Infarct Survival) Collaborative Group. Randomised trial of intravenous atenolol among 16027 cases of suspected acute myocardial infarction: ISIS-1. Lancet 1986;2:57-65.
3. ISIS-2 (Second International Study of Infarct Survival) Collaborative Group. Randomised trial of intravenous streptokinase, oral aspirin, both, or neither among 17187 cases of suspected acute myocardial infarction: ISIS-2. Lancet 1988;2:349-360.
4. ISIS-3 (Third International Study of Infarct Survival) Collaborative Group. ISIS-3: A randomised comparison of streptokinase vs tissue plasminogen activator vs antistreplase and of aspirin plus heparin vs aspirin alone among 41299 cases of suspected acute myocardial infarction. Lancet 1992;339:753-770.
5. ISIS-4 (Fourth International Study of Infarct Survival) Collaborative Group. ISIS-4: A randomised factorial trial assessing early oral captopril, oral mononitrate, and intravenous magnesium sulphate in 58050 patients with suspected acute myocardial infarction. Lancet 1995;345:669-685.
6. Hennekens CH. The increasing burden of cardiovascular disease: Current knowledge and future directions for research on risk factors. Circulation 1998; in press.

Chapter 6

The GISSI Story (1983–1996):
A Comprehensive Review

Gianni Tognoni, M.D., Claudio Fresco, M.D., Aldo P. Maggioni, M.D., and Fabio M. Turazza, M.D., on behalf of
The Gissi Investigators

Introduction

A written history of GISSI (Gruppo Italiano per lo Studio della Sopravvivenza nell'Infarto Miocardico) activity and results has been proposed in so many oral and written contributions dispersed in most of the opinion-making contexts over the last 10 years, that the preparation of this overview has raised the question on how to avoid being too repetitive. The material has been organized in such a way that the account of what has been achieved in terms of technical results is framed and commented from the standpoint of the GISSI investigators.

The conception and organization of developing trials is rarely discussed, though it could be as informative as what is reported in scientific publications. This presentation of the GISSI experience is an attempt to fill this gap.

1. Some Prehistoric Notes

Everything started back in late 1983, while the Italian arm of the ISIS-1[1] was closing its randomization into the early β-blockade trial. Professor Rovelli, a true pioneer and leader in Italian cardiology (but who had never been associated with a major controlled trial) approached his senior colleague, Professor Selvini (who had been the principal clinical investigator for the Italian arm of ISIS-1, and an enthusiastic promoter of cooperation and controlled experimentation in cardiology), to explore the possibility of redirecting the ISIS-linked network (30 centers) to a trial as large as the ISAM (Intravenous Streptokinase in Acute Myocardial Infarction),[2] which had recently started. The discussion with the group at the M. Negri Institute immediately faced the true challenge of a trial on thrombolysis: the size of the population had to be one order of magnitude greater; the possibility of reaching the numbers requested in a reasonable time span was conceivable only through a new participation in the planned ISIS-2[3] or by risking an exclusively Italian trial. Making a decision on this latter direction was not easy: a body of data had to be gathered, and it was necessary to create an autonomous coordinating office for the overall management of the study and the huge amount of data that was expected.

The risk was taken, and the enthusiasm of the National Health Service (NHS) cardiologists was increased by the formal adhesion of their society (the Associazione Nazionale Medici Cardiologi Ospedalieri [ANMCO]). The commitment was maintained even when it had become clear that no substantial funds were available (nothing from industry; minor sums were granted by public sources). Less than 2 years later, following the presentation to the Italian investigators in September, the results of the GISSI[4] were requested by Dr. Braunwald as the closing slide of his main lecture at the 1985 American Heart Association meeting. These data, which were presented publicly following a last minute invitation at a satellite symposium, had been discussed 3 days before in a closed meeting with the TIMI (Thrombolysis in Myocardial Infarction) investigators.

Some key features that can be seen in this review of GISSI's entrance into the international scene should be emphasized, as they have since characterized the "internal" life of the group. The trial was born as a highly participatory activity, as it was proposed and very soon perceived as a collective identity card of a whole professional society. As a result of the "extreme" degree of autonomy due to the absence of even an ad hoc financial support, the trial could be realized only if the routine clinical activity was transformed into an experimental exercise.

The drafting and the discussion of the protocol profoundly revised the heterogeneity of individual practices into a common core of recommended behaviors to be adopted in the data collection, and accepted a central coordination and quality control. This was done to assure the consistency of the information, but at the same time transformed the individual clinical settings into a cooperative, public health-oriented network.

The experiment on thrombolysis became a permanent training opportunity for the participants, and the tiny group in charge of the methodological coordination was expanded to include clinicians ready to play an even more active role in the discussion of methodological and organizational problems, thus bridging the traditional

"separateness" of investigators versus care providers.

It is interesting to reread the texts published in Italian before the results of the first GISSI, to feel the essence of a season of cultural creativity, which was felt as a result in itself (see a brief account in a publication certainly not routinely accessible to cardiologists).[5,6]

The collective planning of the protocols, and the attention to link the specific goal of the trial to broader scientific and organizational interests of the Italian cardiology working in the NHS, remained the permanent and most deeply rooted trait of the GISSI experience also for the subsequent trials. The transformation of the first acronym with the substitution of the "s" for "streptokinase" with the "s" from "survival" was in this sense less than a material change, and more the recognition that a longer term project had started with the creation of a nationwide research group: randomized clinical trials became the occasion for revising the ongoing practices; to promote what was felt "recommended" in the diagnostic, monitoring, therapeutic behavior; to assess how the results pursued and obtained were transferable into the current patterns of care.

Let us see whether this openly formulated (as documented in "internal" documents and publications in Italian) comprehensive cultural project can be recognized through the revisiting of at least some of the results. The brief "chapters" that follow have been conceived as preselected, but independent pieces, meant to allow at the end the appearance of a reasonably consistent mosaic (Fig. 1).

2. The Main General Results: 2.1 Continuity

It is tempting to suggest that the main overall (cultural and institutional) result of GISSI is the one summarized in Table 1.[4,7,8] Over more than a 10-year period, a whole cardiological community of a country has

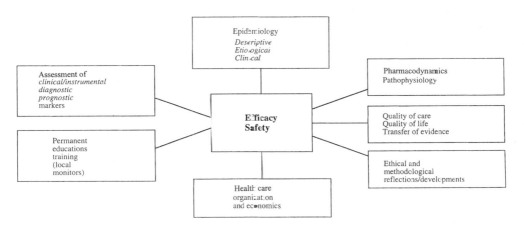

Figure 1. The results and by-products of the GISSI experience.

Table 1.

Continuity and Consistency A Principal Result of GISSI

	GISSI-1	*GISSI-2*	*GISSI-3*	*GISSI-Prevention*
Timing				
1st pt.	Feb. 84	Feb. 88	June 91	Oct. 93
last pt.	June 85	July 89	July 93	Ongoing
Presentation to investigators	Sept. 85	March 90	Nov. 93	For 3.5 yrs following-up
Publication	March 86	July 90	May 94	
Setting				
no. CCUs	176	223	200	172
no. pts.	11,806	12,490	19,394	11,379
Costs (U.S. $)				
Overall	350,000	4,000,000	6,000,000	4,000,000
$/pt.	29.6	320	309	350
Scientific productivity *	7	36	19	—

*No. of papers published in major refereed journals (+ presentation at ACC/AHA/ECC).
CCU = Coronary care unit; GISSI = Gruppo Italiano per lo Studio della Sopravvivenza nell'Infarto Miocardico Acuto.

been acting as an experimental research group.

2.2 Drug Efficacy Testing

The principal results are recalled and briefly commented on in the three "profiles" that reproduce the protocols, the main findings, and implications of the individual trials.

It is interesting to note that:

1. All the messages on the profile of thrombolysis as it has more recently and convincingly been described by the Fibrinolytic Therapy Trialists (FTT) Collaborative Group[9] were already well-identified in the first GISSI population: the early hazard was specifically discussed by the Data Monitoring Committee in the interim analysis made after 7,000 randomized

patients; the strong time dependence of the size of the effect was so suggestive that it had to be underplayed in the public presentation to avoid exclusion of patients arriving after 6 hours from the benefits of thrombolysis; it was clear that patients with ST depression were a different population; the overall safety profile was extremely reassuring.

2. Symmetrically the last "acute" phase trial, GISSI-3, with its underlining and unexpected important benefit of ACE-I (angiotensin converting enzyme) in the first days following acute myocardial infarction (AMI), becomes the point of departure of a strategy of (meta)-analysis of the role of ACE-I in terms of "early" and "late" interventions, which coincides with a revision of the hypothetical mechanism(s) of action of the same drugs.

3. The history of GISSI, with its open design, has always run strictly in parallel to and consistent with the blinded ISIS protocols, thus further supporting the fact that the hard end-points evaluated in very large scale trials are protected from confounding.

4. The combined end-point adopted (not without controversy) in the GISSI-2[10] protocol anticipated a tendency that was later more widely accepted.

5. The "continuity" of the involvement of the same cardiological community translated into the effective incorporation in the subsequent trials of all the treatments documented as "recommended" (e.g., aspirin, beta-blockade, thrombolysis), and to the timely withdrawal of those without evidence of benefit (e.g., calcium channel blockers, heparin).

6. The original "participatory" commitment has always been given priority, also by presenting first the results to the assembly of investigators, having their comments, submitting for publication within the shortest delays.

7. Concluded trials, though conducted without the "formal" monitoring rules of industry supported protocols, have been pivotal in the approval process of their tested treatments, also in the U.S.

Profile 1: GISSI (1984–1985)[4]

Questions

1. Does intravenous streptokinase (SK) infusion produce a clinically relevant benefit in terms of reduction of in-hospital and 1-year mortality?

2. Is the effect, if any, dependent on the interval from onset of pain to SK administration?

3. Are the risks associated with the treatment acceptable?

Setting

One hundred seventy-six of 200 of the coronary care units (CCUs) distributed across the whole country randomized 11,806 patients over a 17-month period.

Protocol

Figure 2 summarizes the main features of the unblinded protocol with central randomization. Patients were eligible: (1) if they had chest pain accompanied by significant ST segment elevation or depression (1 mm or more in any limb lead and/or 2 mm or more in any precordial lead); and (2) if they were admitted to the CCU within 12 hours from the onset of symptoms.

Results

Table 2 summarizes the main results of the study (with the principal causes of death), while Table 3 gives results for the whole population stratified by hours elapsed from symptoms onset. Streptokinase administration produced a statistically highly significant 18% decrease in the overall mortality of the whole population, and the beneficial effect was even more impressive in the predefined subpopulation treated soon after onset of pain. In fact in those treated within 3 hours, overall mortality was reduced by 23%. Further, a data generated analysis of the 1,277 patients randomized within 1 hour after onset of pain

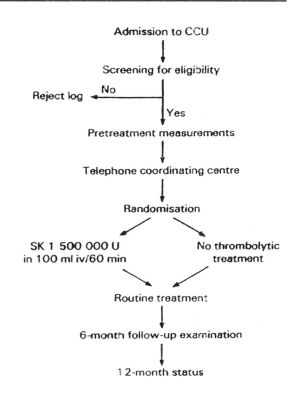

Figure 2. GISSI protocol. © The Lancet Ltd., 1986.

Table 2.

GISSI-1: Overall Mortality and Causes of Death

—	SK	C	P	RR (95% CI)	Total
Percent mortality	10.7	13.0	0.0002	0.81 (0.72–0.90)	11.6
Deaths/no. of patients	628/5860	758/5852	—	—	1386/11,712
Causes of death					
CV	588	696	—	—	1284
Non-CV	32	45	—	—	77
Undefined	8	17	—	—	25

CI = confidence interval; CV = cardiovascular; RR = risk ratio; SK = streptokinase. Other abbreviations as in Table 1.

Table 3.

GISSI-1: Mortality by Hours from Onset of Symptoms

Hours	SK % (deaths/n)	C % (deaths/n)	P	RR (95% CI)	Total % (deaths/n)
≤ 3	9.2 (278/3016)	12.0 (369/3078)	0.0005	0.74 (0.63–0.87)	10.6 (647/6094)
> 3–6	11.7 (217/1849)	14.1 (254/1800)	0.03	0.80 (0.66–0.98)	12.9 (474/3649)
> 6–9	12.6 (87/693)	14.1 (93/659)	NS	0.87 (0.64–1.19)	13.3 (180/1352)
> 9–12	15.8 (46/292)	13.6 (41/302)	NS	1.19 (0.75–1.87)	14.6 (87/594)
< 1	8.2 (52/635)	15.4 (99/642)	0.0001	0.49 (0.34–0.69)	11.8 (151/1277)

Abbreviations as in Tables 1 and 2. n = no. of patients; NS = not significant.

suggests that very early treatment could reduce the in-hospital mortality by about 47%. The in-hospital reinfarction rate was almost double between the patients given SK: in the next few years, this difference will be canceled by the widespread diffusion of aspirin.[3] Long-term follow-up of > 98% of the patients recruited in the GISSI-1 trial showed persistence of the beneficial effect observed during the hospital phase.[11]

Implications

GISSI is hailed as a landmark trial and regarded as the beginning of a new era, because systemic thrombolysis is shown to be not only effective, but remarkably safe in routine conditions of care: for example, the incidence of the feared cerebrovascular events (defined as the sum of ischemic and hemorrhagic episodes) in the SK and control group was very low (< 1%) and comparable in the two groups.

Profile 2: GISSI-2 (1988–1989)[7]

Questions

1. Does the pharmacologically more promising profile of alteplase translate into a clinically relevant advantage (higher efficacy, lower hemorrhagic risk) once compared directly with SK?

2. Does an anticoagulant prophylactic regimen with subcutaneous heparin add to the effect of aspirin, with respect to the incidence of early postinfarction ischemic events (and thus on the overall outcome)?

3. What is the yield of different prognostic tests at discharge?

Setting

Two hundred thirty-three of 250 of the Italian CCUs randomized 12,490 patients over 17 months, while 8,000 additional patients were included by an International arm.[12]

Protocol

Figure 3 summarizes the features of the 2×2 factorially designed study. Patients were eligible: (1) if they had chest pain accompanied by ST segment elevation of 1 mm or more in any limb lead of the ECG and/or of 2 mm or more in any precordial lead; (2) if they had been admitted to the CCU within 6 hours from the onset of symptoms; and (3) if they had no clear contraindication to the fibrinolytic treatments or to heparin.

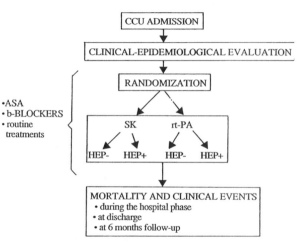

Figure 3. GISSI-2 protocol. GISSI, October 1987.

Half of all patients were randomly allocated to receive SK (1.5 million U infused over 30–60 min) and half to receive tPA (100 mg infused IV over 3 hours). Half of all patients were also allocated randomly to receive 12,500 U subcutaneous heparin twice daily, starting 12 hours after the beginning of the tPA or SK infusion and to be continued until hospital discharge. It was decided in advance that a combined end-point of mortality and severe left ventricular (LV) dysfunction would be the best indicator of the patients' clinical status.[10]

Results

Table 4 shows the main results with respect to the tested treatments. There were no differences in any of the four treatment groups (SK vs tPA, heparin vs no heparin) as regards to the combined end-point or its individual components. Overall mortality was 8.8%. The overall stroke rate was 1.1% in the tPA group and 0.9% in the SK group.

Implications

The overall in-hospital mortality (8.8%) was much lower than in the corresponding control cohort of GISSI-1 (about 13%). This improvement shows that, over 5 years, the results of large scale trials can be directly transferred to routine clinical practice countrywide and produce epidemiologically and clinically relevant benefits.

Despite the pharmacological differences between tPA and SK, the lack of clinical evidence of different benefits was observed in all subgroups analyzed and was supported by similar effects on clinical and laboratory indicators of LV damage. The absence of a heparin specific effect on reinfarction is probably explained by the underlying aspirin effect: the low incidence rates closely match ISIS-2 data.[3]

The publication of the GISSI-2 study marked the beginning of the so-called "heparin controversy." Some authors[13,14] claimed that the expression of the full thrombolytic potential of tPA necessitated concomitant intravenous heparin, rather than twice daily subcutaneous treatment beginning after 12 hours. Data supporting such claims, however, derived from small series, where results regarding patency rates were clearly conflicting; one factor in this may be the various time intervals set for coronary angiography after thrombolysis.[15–17] Anyway, the "heparin controversy" was solved neither from the various "position papers," nor from the recently published GUSTO-I (Global Use of Strategies to Open Occluded Coronary Arteries) trial,[18] as in this trial a tPA (conventional administration) plus intravenous heparin arm versus tPA without intravenous heparin was absent.

The adoption of a combined end-point (mortality plus severe LV dysfunction) appears to have been satisfactory from a methodological point of view, since it bridges two usually separate lines of evaluation of acute treatments in evolving myocardial infarction (MI)[10]; in fact, the GISSI-2 results, encouraging with respect to total in-hospital mortality rate, reliably documented the burden of chronic or long-term consequences of AMI, a problem faced by the subsequent GISSI-3 study.[8]

Profile 3: GISSI-3 (1991–1993)[8]

Background and Questions

LV dysfunction was well-known as the strongest indicator of poor prognosis in MI.[19–21]

The possibility of preventing such deterioration through very early intervention with ACE inhibitors,[22,23] or nitrates[24] had been repeatedly emphasized, mainly in relation to the theory of LV remodeling.[25,26] However, most studies on ACE inhibitors concentrated on selected groups of patients at higher risk of LV dilation and dysfunction.[27,28]

The results of a controversial meta-analysis[29] strongly supported a life-saving

Table 4.
GISSI-2: Effects of Randomized Treatment on Combined End Point

	tPA n = 6182	SK n = 6199	RR (95% CI)	Hep n = 6175	No Hep n = 6206	RR (95% CI)	Total n = 12,381
Total events (%)	1428 (23.1)	1394 (22.5)	1.04 (0.95–1.13)	1403 (22.7)	1419 (22.9)	0.99 (0.91–1.08)	2822 (22.8)
Deaths	556 (9.0)	536 (8.6)		518 (8.3)	574 (9.3)		1092 (8.8)
Clinical heart failure	478 (7.7)	502 (8.1)		494 (8.0)	486 (7.8)		980 (7.9)
EF ≤ 35%	153 (2.5)	137 (2.2)		141 (2.3)	149 (2.4)		290 (2.4)
Myocardial segments injured ≤ 45%	106 (1.7)	90 (1.5)		108 (1.8)	87 (1.4)		196 (1.6)
QRS score > 10	135 (2.2)	129 (2.1)		141 (2.3)	123 (2.0)		264 (2.1)

EF = ejection fraction; Hep = heparin. Other abbreviations as in Tables 1 and 2.

role for nitrates in patients with AMI: the widespread use of nitrates in CCUs in the absence of definite data on their effects suggested the need for a formal evaluation. On the other hand, the unexpected and enforced termination of the CONSENSUS II trial[30] suggested that early ACE inhibition was ineffective and possibly carried an excess risk for elderly patients.

Setting

Between June 1991 and July 1993, a total of 43,047 patients were admitted to the 200 participating CCUs (about two thirds of such units in Italy). Nineteen thousand three hundred and ninety-four (45%) of the patients were randomized.

Protocol

The GISSI-3 protocol[31] was explicitly designed not only to test the drug effects of ACE inhibitors and transdermal glyceryl trinitrate (GTN), but also to assess formally, with a classic 2×2 factorial design, the benefit-to-risk ratio of the combination of these drugs on the whole population of AMI patients and on elderly patients and women, who are at higher risk of AMI mortality, despite intensive use of recommended treatments. As in GISSI-2,[7] the main end-point of the study included the combined outcome measure of mortality and severe ventricular dysfunction,[10] which is highly predictive of poor outcome over the medium term (6 months).[32]

Figure 4 shows the study protocol. Patients were eligible: (1) if they had chest pain accompanied by elevation or depression of the ST segment of at least 1 mm in one or more peripheral leads of the ECG, or of at least 2 mm in one or more precordial leads; (2) if they had been admitted to the participating CCU within 24 hours of

GISSI-3 PROTOCOL

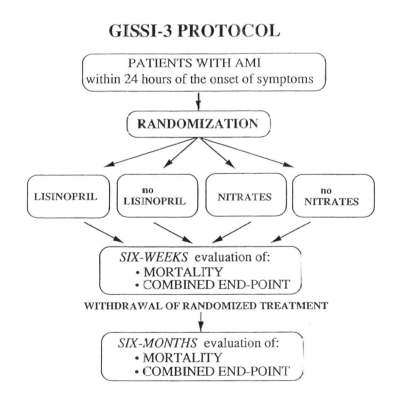

Figure 4. GISSI-3 protocol. (Reproduced with permission from Am J Cardiol 1992;70 : 62C-69C).

symptom onset; and (3) if they had no clear contraindications to the study treatments. The four treatment groups received lisinopril alone, transdermal GTN alone, combined therapy with lisinopril and transdermal GTN, or no trial medication. Study treatment was withdrawn at 6 weeks, if there were no specific indications to continue, and patients were followed-up for 6 months from randomization.

Results

Lisinopril versus control

Patients allocated lisinopril had an 11% lower risk of death than the controls (6.3 vs 7.1%). The survival curves of lisinopril-treated patients and controls separated early (day 0–1) and continue to diverge throughout the next 6 weeks (Fig. 5).

Lisinopril also reduced the rate of the other main outcome measure, the combined endpoint (Table 5). In addition to the smaller number of deaths in the lisinopril group, there was a smaller proportion of patients with a left ventricular ejection fraction (LVEF) of 35% or less, but no differences were observed between lisinopril and control groups in akinetic/dyskinetic score or clinical heart failure rates.

Among patients > 70 years of age, there was a significant reduction in the combined end-point rate with lisinopril (12%; $2P = 0.0039$). There was a similar pattern for women: the combined end-point rate was 11% lower ($2P = 0.039$). Rates of reinfarction, postinfarction angina, cardiogenic shock, and stroke did not differ significantly between lisinopril patients and controls. As expected, persistent hypotension and renal dysfunction were signifi-

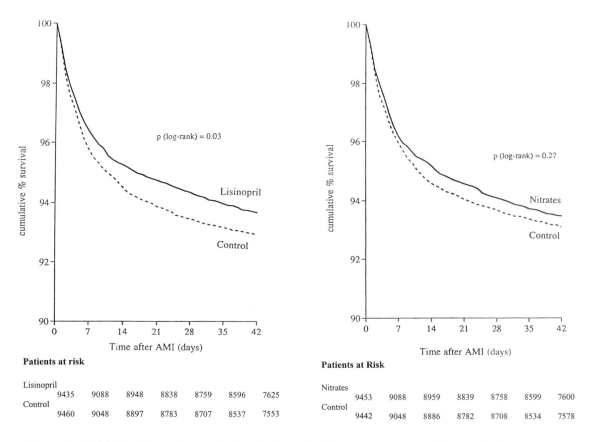

Figure 5. GISSI-3: Six-week survival in lisinopril, nitrates, and respective control groups.

Table 5.

GISSI-3: Six-Week Mortality and Combined End Point Rates in Lisinopril and Control Groups

	Lisinopril (n = 9435)	Controls (n = 9460)	OR (95% CI)	2P*
No. of deaths (%)	597 (6.3)	673 (7.1)	0.88 (0.79–0.99)	0.03
Combined end point events (%)	1473 (15.6)	1609 (17.0)	0.90 (0.84–0.98)	0.009
Deaths	597 (6.3)	673 (7.1)	—	—
Clinical heart failure	366 (3.9)	354 (3.7)	—	—
EF ≤ 35 %	451 (4.8)	530 (5.3)	—	—
α-dyskinetic score ≤ 45%	59 (0.6)	52 (0.6)	—	—

*Two-tailed P value for difference between groups.
AD = akinesis/dyskinesis; EF = ejection fraction; GISSI = same as in Table 1; OR = odds ratio.

cantly more common among lisinopril-treated patients than among controls, even if the higher rates of these complications did not result in an increase in mortality or in severe renal failure.

Transdermal GTN versus control

Systematic 6-week treatment with transdermal GTN did not produce a significant benefit in terms of total mortality rate or combined end-point rate. The survival curves showed a small, but not significant, benefit for GTN treatment (Fig. 5, right). There were no significant differences between GTN allocated and control patients in rate of reinfarction, revascularization procedures, persistent hypotension, or renal dysfunction. The nitrate group had a slightly lower rate of postinfarction angina (2P = 0.033).

Implications

The overall 11% mortality reduction with lisinopril was obtained in a context of an already low baseline mortality, reflecting the hemodynamic stability of the patients and their exposure to the best recommended treatments for the acute phase of AMI. The GISSI-3 findings may be seen as completing the range of indications for the use of ACE inhibitors in cardiac patients. While the results of the AIRE study[33] clearly showed the need to treat cardiac failure as soon as it becomes clinically evident, the GISSI-3 data extended the indication for starting ACE inhibitor treatment to all patients with documented AMI starting within 24 hours. Against the expectation from SOLVD and SAVE[34–36] that a beneficial effect of ACE inhibitors would appear only after a long period of treatment, the GISSI-3 study showed for the first time that early administration of lisinopril can produce clinically relevant benefits within the first few days from the start of treatment. This point, together with the safety of lisinopril and other ACE inhibitors used in AMI patients, was the most powerful argument against the authors that claimed in favor of the so-called "delayed, selective approach," with ACE inhibitors used only in patients with signs or symptoms of LV dysfunction.[37]

The absence of a statistically significant effect of transdermal GTN was probably unexpected by comparison with the available data on which the protocol was planned.[29] The consistency of the GISSI-3 and ISIS-4 results[38] clearly showed that the systematic administration of transdermal GTN alone for 6 weeks after AMI does not produce any clinically relevant beneficial effect. However, these findings do not rule out the benefits of transdermal GTN for the treatment of anginal pain and/or cardiac failure in AMI.

2.3. The Contribution of GISSI to the Safety Profile of Thrombolysis: The Case of Stroke

Comparison Between Thrombolytic and Conventional Treatment in Terms of Total Stroke

With respect to the incidence of total stroke, GISSI-1, comparing SK versus conventional treatment, have consistently shown that the total rate of cerebrovascular events was not different between the control group and the patients treated with thrombolytic agents[4] (Table 6). These data have been confirmed by the other trials that tested different thrombolytic agents versus control.[3,39,40] In each one of these trials, taken separately, the incidence of stroke in the treated groups is absolutely comparable with that of control groups, irrespective of the fibrinolytic agent used in the trial.

When all the trials comparing thrombolytic versus conventional treatment are considered together in an overview, it appears that, in the group of patients treated with a thrombolytic agent, there is an excess of one nonfatal disabling stroke in every 1,000 treated patients. However, this excess of risk of stroke must be considered in the context of the 19 fewer deaths from every 1,000 treated patients. These data are derived from the FTT overview.[9]

Comparison Among Thrombolytics in Terms of Total and Hemorrhagic Stroke (Table 7)

The results derived from GISSI-2 and the International Study trials will first be taken into consideration.[7,12] The definite diagnosis of ischemic and hemorrhagic stroke was made on the basis of computed tomographic scan or autopsy results and available for about 74% of the total stroke events. Patients treated with tPA showed a higher number of total and of hemorrhagic events compared to patients treated with SK. The difference in terms of hemorrhagic strokes did not reach the level of statistical significance due to the low number of events, but when the incidence of total stroke was considered, the difference was statistically significant. The treatment with

---

Table 6.

Incidence of Stroke in Large Scale Randomized Clinical Trials on Thrombolytic Agents in Patients with Acute Myocardial Infarction

| | | Events/Patients % | | RR |
		Treated	Controls	(95% CI)
Trial	Drug			
GISSI-1	SK	54/5860	45/5852	1.20
		0.9	0.8	(0.81–1.78)
ISIS-2	SK	61/8490	67/8491	0.91
		0.7	0.8	(0.64–1.29)
AIMS	APSAC	8/624	4/634	1.99
		1.3	0.6	(0.64–6.20)
ASSET	tPA	28/2515	26/2493	1.07
		1.1	1.0	(0.62–1.83)

AIMS = Anistreplase Intervention Mortality Study; APSAC = anisoylated plasminogen-streptokinase activator complex; ASSET = Anglo-Scandinavian Study of Early Thrombosis; GISSI = same as in Table 1; ISIS-2 = International Study Groups of Infarct Survival. Other abbreviations as in Table 2.

Table 7.

Stroke Events: Comparison Between the Different Thrombolytic Agents

GISSI-2/International Study

	SK (10,396)	tPA (10,372)	OR (95% CI)	RRCox (95% CI)
		Events (%)		
Etiology				
Overall	98 (0.94)	138 (1.33)	1.41 (1.09–1.83)	1.40 (1.08–1.82)
Hemorrhagic	30 (0.29)	44 (0.42)	1.47 (0.93–2.31)	1.39 (0.87–1.99)

ISIS-3 Study

	SK (13,607)	tPA (13,569)	OR (95% CI)	
Overall	141 (1.0)	188 (1.4)	1.34 (1.08–1.66)	
Hemorrhagic	32 (0.2)	89 (0.7)	2.58 (1.81–3.69)	

GUSTO Study

	SK + SQ Hep (9709)	tPA + IVHep (10,268)	OR (95% CI)	
Overall	118 (1.22)	159 (1.55)	1.28 (1.01–1.62)	
Hemorrhagic	48 (0.49)	75 (0.72)	1.33 (0.94–1.87)	

Overview of GISSI-2, International Study, ISIS-3 and GUSTO-1

	SK (33,712)	tPA (34,209)	ORMHP (95% CI)	
Overall	357 (1.05)	485 (1.41)	1.34 (1.17–1.54)	
Hemorrhagic	110 (0.32)	207 (0.61)	1.82 (1.46–2.27)	

GUSTO = Global Use of Streptokinase and tPA for Occluded Coronary Arteries; OR = odds ratio. Other abbreviations as in Tables 2 and 5.

tPA remained significantly associated with an increased risk of stroke, even in the adjusted analysis.

The findings derived from GISSI-2 and the International Study have been completely confirmed by the ISIS-3 study.[41] A significant excess of total (1.4% vs 1.0%) and hemorrhagic stroke (0.7% vs 0.2%) was confirmed in the patients allocated to tPA treatment and, more recently, by the results of the GUSTO trial.[18]

In order to more reliably compare the excess rate of stroke in the tPA group, a meta-analysis of these three large scale randomized trials (GISSI-2, ISIS-3, and GUSTO) was done on about 68,000 patients. The excess rate of total and hemorrhagic stroke for the tPA-treated patients is highly statistically significant and it is quantifiable in 4 total events per 1,000 treated patients and in 3 hemorrhagic strokes per 1,000 treated patients.

Clinical/Epidemiological Indicators of Risk for Total Stroke

The large number of patients and stroke events we studied in GISSI-1, GISSI-2, and the International Study allowed us to analyze the effect of the possible risk factors for total stroke.[42,43] Multiple logistic regression was used to assess the independent association between the more relevant clinical/epidemiological variables and the occurrence of total stroke.

Beside the already quoted excess of stroke in the tPA-treated patients, older patients appeared to be strongly related to the occurrence of stroke. Patients with anterior AMI were more likely to suffer a stroke. Total stroke occurred more often also in patients with more extensive cardiac impairment: Killip Class 2 or 3+4 at entry. No relationship was found between hemorrhagic stroke and anterior site of MI or cardiac impairment, suggesting that the excess rate of stroke in these two populations of patients is mainly due to the ischemic etiology of the event. Patients with increased risk for ischemic stroke, particularly those with anterior infarction or LV impairment, should not be denied thrombolytic therapy. On the contrary, in such patients thrombolysis is specifically indicated since such therapy can reduce the risk of LV thrombi, either for the favorable effect on hemostasis or the limitation of infarct size.

Clinical/Epidemiological Indicators of Risk for Hemorrhagic Stroke

When a decision to administer a thrombolytic drug should be taken, the possibility of defining a risk profile for intracranial hemorrhage could be even more interesting. For this purpose, a model was developed for the assessment of the risk for intracranial hemorrhage during thrombolytic therapy using data from different studies: the Netherland Registry, GISSI-2 and the International Study, TAMI (Thrombolysis and Angioplasty in Myocardial Infarction), ISAM, and TIMI tri-

als on a total of > 30,000 patients.[44] Data were available from 150 patients with documented intracranial hemorrhage (cases) and 294 matched controls. Logistic regression analysis revealed four factors known at hospital admission that appeared independently related to hemorrhagic stroke: advanced age (> 65 years) (OR [odds ratio] 2.2); low body weight (< 70 kg) (OR 2.1); hypertension upon admission (systolic blood pressure $\geq$ 170 and/or diastolic blood pressure $\geq$ 95) (OR 2.0); and a drug regimen with tPA, using current therapeutical dosage (100 mg over 3 hours) (OR 1.6).

Thus, from this analysis there is a further confirmation that a fibrinolytic treatment with tPA is less safe (in terms of stroke) than SK, in particular in the subgroups of patients at higher risk of intracranial hemorrhage. In fact, if we stratify the risk of hemorrhagic stroke by age and kind of thrombolytic agent, the excess of stroke increases significantly with increasing age only for tPA, whereas there was not such an increasing trend with SK (Fig. 6).

3. The GISSI Database(s) as Epidemiological Observatory

The findings in the first GISSI trial that, contrary to the traditional fears, age was not a specific risk factor, and that female sex appeared for the first time in the cardiological literature as exposed to an "excess risk of death," led to a protocol for GISSI-2 where the purpose of a formal epidemiological use of the database was at least as important as the testing of the treatment. Data to be collected were specifically chosen to allow an analysis of the baseline and clinical variables whose impact on the outcome was suspected to be specifically relevant.

The "chapters" that follow highlight some of the main findings, which could be derived from the whole database, once it was clear that the tested treatments were strictly equivalent. We recall first the results related to some baseline characteris-

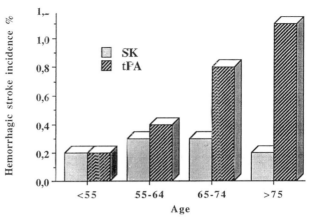

Figure 6. Direct comparison of streptokinase versus tPA: hemorrhagic stroke subdivided by age.

tics of the patients (sex, age, smoking); then concentrate on the presentation of the findings on the clinical epidemiology of some key cardiological variables, on the evaluation of diagnostic tests at discharge, and on pharmacoepidemiology.

3.1. The Epidemiology of Baseline Characteristics in the Thrombolytic Era: 3.1.1. Age

Mortality for ischemic heart disease (IHD) increases progressively with age, and about 80% of total mortality for IHD in the U.S. occurs in individuals > 65 years of age. However, it was unclear whether the increased incidence of fatal outcome in the elderly was the result of more severe atherosclerosis and larger infarct size, or whether it was due to a greater vulnerability to myocardial necrosis of the aging heart. We assessed the impact of clinical and epidemiological variables on in-hospital and 6-month mortality as a function of age in patients who entered the GISSI-2 study with their first confirmed MI.[45]

Patients and Results

Of the total number of randomized patients, 9,720 (78.5%) were cases of first confirmed MI. Among these patients, there was a total mortality of 10.6% at 6 months postdischarge: 7.9% died during hospitalization; and 2.9% during the 6-month pe-

riod following discharge. Total in-hospital mortality was 1.9% in cases up to the age of 40 and increase up to 31.8% in cases 80 years of age and over (Fig. 7). Conversely, indicators of infarct size did not show the same trend.

In-hospital mortality

Age resulted to be a very powerful predictor of in-hospital death, with an OR of 3.1 for the patients 61–70 years of age and 13.1 for the patients > 70 years of age. Very strong association (OR > 2) was evident for age, female sex, Killip Class at admission, insulin dependent diabetes, anterior wall infarction, heart failure after the fourth day from admission, and number of leads with ST segment elevation on the admission ECG. After multivariate analysis, advanced age was confirmed to be an independent predictor of adverse outcome.

Postdischarge findings

Age also maintained its ability to predict adverse outcome after the discharge, with a risk ratio of 2.0 for the patients 61–70 years of age and 3.9 for the patients > 70 years of age.

Causes of death

Half of the deaths in each age group occurred in days 0 and 1: 70 (56%) of 125 patients < 60 years of age; 112 (46%) of 244

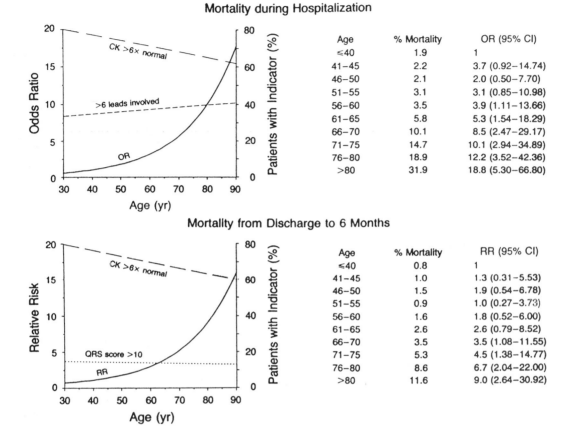

Figure 7. Mortality among patients with first myocardial infarctions, according to age and indicators of infarct size. Age was considered a continuous variable, with 40 years of age as the reference value. Values for the indicators of the size of the myocardial infarction did not show any increase with age. Mortality during hospitalization increased exponentially with age: it is shown as an odds ratio (OR, calculated with the formula $x = 0.1002588 \times e^{0.0575x}$) and 95% confidence interval (CI). The curves for the indicators of infarct size show the percentage of patients with peak creatinine kinase (CK) ratios more than six times the upper normal value of the study-center laboratory (CK > 6x normal) and the percentage with involvement of > 6 ECG leads at entry. Mortality during the interval from discharge to 6 months after discharge also increased exponentially with age; it is shown as a relative risk (RR, calculated with the formula $x = 0.1094814 \times e^{0.0553x}$). The curves for the indicators of infarct size show the percentage of patients with peak CK ratios > 6 times normal and the percentage with QRS scores above 10.

60–70 years of age; and 210 (52%) of 403 > 70 years of age. Among the causes of in-hospital cardiac death, cardiac rupture found at autopsy increased progressively from 5.2% in patients < 60 years of age to 11.1% of the patients 61–70 years of age, and to 19.6% in the oldest strata. At least two coronary arteries with significant stenoses were found in 40% of the patients < 60 years of age, in 35% of the patients 61–70 years of age, and in 32% of the patients > 70 years of age. Infarcts involving < 10% of the LV were found in 20% of the patients ≤ 60 years of age, in 22.5% of the patients 61–70 years of age, and in 31.5% of the patients > 70 years of age.

Comments

This study has allowed us to make two important new observations: (1) the age related increase of both in-hospital and 6-month mortality; and (2) the dramatic age related increase of mortality appears not to be related to a larger infarct size or to detectable accumulated IHD, but to a greater vulnerability of the heart to the infarction. In 65% of cases, AMI, independent of age, occurred unheralded as the very first manifestation of IHD. Despite data documenting similar infarct sizes among different age groups, the impairment of LV function assessed at admission by the Killip classification was progressively worse in older patients. Moreover, the number of patients who developed clinical LV failure was higher, and mean ejection fraction (EF) was lower in older patients. Cardiac rupture, seen as a major expression of vulnerability, also rose continuously as a function of age, contributing for almost 20% of cardiac deaths in patients older than 70. Despite the fact that in-hospital survivors had a similar degree of estimated myocardial damage across all age groups, postdischarge mortality increased exponentially and was 15-fold higher in patients older than 80, compared to those younger than 40 years. The possibility that a greater myocardial vulnerability to necrosis is responsible for the dramatic increase of mortality during the acute phase of infarction in elderly patients has considerable theoretical and practical implications. First, old age appears to be an independent major determinant of survival besides infarct size. Second, if the relation between MI and IHD mortality in the elderly is as age dependent as our findings suggest, they ought to be considered separately, both in epidemiological studies and in preventive intervention trials, because they reflect different types of events.

The exponential increase of the incidence of MI with age, both in males and females, and the exponential increase of mortality with age after MI found in our study strongly support the strategy of not having an age limit in RCT enrollment (an idea adopted by recent large population clinical trials and pioneered by GISSI group).

Our study shows that Killip class and age are the strongest independent predictors of adverse outcome, either in the acute phase or in the 6-month postdischarge follow-up period. One possible explanation is that the aging heart is more vulnerable to MIs.

3.1.2. Sex

Many reports indicated that women had a higher mortality rate than men after AMI, but the reasons for this apparently worse prognosis in women appeared not clear.

Women usually develop AMI less often and at a more advanced age than men. The co-existing illnesses associated with older age may, in part, complicate prognosis and medical decision making for women with AMI and explain some of the observed gender differences with respect to outcome. It was still debated whether female sex per se was an independent negative prognostic factor or the higher mortality rate reported among women reflects only the differences in the epidemiological and clinical history related variables and in the therapeutic interventions, generally less aggressive in women than in men.

The setting of the GISSI-2 study provided the opportunity to reevaluate, in a large population of patients, all managed with the same baseline treatments: (1) the differences in the baseline characteristics between males and females; and (2) the independence of the association between female sex and 6-month mortality in a large population of patients with AMI.

Patients and Results

The data are derived from the analysis of the 10,219 hospital survivors with confirmed AMI. The assessment of the prognostic significance of female sex was part of a wider evaluation conducted of the whole GISSI-2 database[46]: as previously mentioned, within this framework, a prognostic study was planned to reassess the determinants of 6-month mortality in survivors of AMI in the thrombolytic era.

Women enrolled in the GISSI-2 trial were 9 years older than men (on average), and had a significantly higher rate of prior MI, diabetes, hypertension, and angina. At entry, women presented with significantly higher Killip class, higher systolic blood pressure, higher heart rate, and lower body mass index. Infarct site was similar.

While at univariate analysis female sex was shown as an independent predictor of a fatal outcome (OR 1.70, 95% CI [confidence interval] 1.29–2.23), at multivariate analysis (Cox model) female sex was not confirmed to be an independent risk factor for 6-month mortality.

Comments

The GISSI data confirmed the higher risk profile of women with AMI. Interestingly, female sex did not make an independent contribution to the 6-month mortality risk. Although this finding is in disagreement with the conclusions of two other recent studies,[47,48] it is fair to recall that with regard to long-term outcome after hospital discharge, the majority of available studies either did not indicate female sex as an independent predictor of mortality[49–51] or showed an even better prognosis in women.[52–55]

3.1.3. Smoking

Over the last few years, some studies, utilizing data derived from retrospective subgroup analysis, have suggested that active smokers who suffer an AMI paradoxically show an improved short-term survival or a lesser incidence of in-hospital reinfarction when compared with nonsmokers.[56–58]

Furthermore, more recently it was suggested that smokers have a significantly greater chance of achieving a TIMI grade III patency after thrombolytic treatment, possibly due to a more active thrombogenic mechanism operative in smokers, leading to a larger thrombus component and a greater susceptibility to lytic therapy.[59]

The purpose of the analysis of the GISSI-2 database was to evaluate the effect of smoking on in-hospital mortality, reinfarction, and stroke rates. The relationship between noninvasive markers of reperfusion and smoking history have been also evaluated.

Patients and Results

Of the 9,720 patients with a first confirmed MI, 2,611 (26.9%) were nonsmokers, 1,932 (19.9%) ex-smokers, and 5,151 (53.0%) were active smokers.

Significant differences emerged in the clinical histories of the three groups of patients stratified by smoking habits. Nonsmokers presented consistently worse baseline characteristics than active smokers or ex-smokers. A history of active or past smoking was significantly more common among younger patients, while nonsmokers were generally older and more often females.

Reinfarction, stroke, and postinfarction angina rates were significantly lower among active smokers than among ex-smokers or nonsmokers, while ventricular fibrillation (VF) was more frequent in smokers than in the other two groups. No significant differences emerged among the three groups in the distribution of the predictors of poor predischarge prognosis. Once the confounding variables were adjusted for smoking, no longer did it appear to protect against reinfarction and stroke: OR 1.35 (95% CI 0.91–2.02) and 0.79 (95% CI 0.58–1.06), respectively.

Of the 9,720 patients, 772 (7.9%) died during the hospital stay. A history of smoking was found to be protective with respect to the outcome of the first infarction: in-hospital mortality significantly increased from 4.7% among active smokers, to 7.6%

among ex-smokers, and to 13.8% among nonsmoking patients. This difference may be due to the different characteristics of smokers, particularly to their being younger than nonsmokers.

To assess the independent contribution of the smoking history, the same variables were introduced in a multivariate model. The apparently strong protective effect of active smoking was not confirmed once the other variables, particularly age, were taken into account.

Comments

Although the GISSI-2 study does not provide data on mortality prior to hospital admission, and although the study population represents a selected group of patients with AMI with ST segment elevation at entry and eligible for thrombolysis, it nonetheless allows some general conclusions regarding the relationship between smoking history and outcome. The apparently strong protective effect of a smoking history must be read as a confounding variable, as statistical significance disappeared when data were simply adjusted for age, considered as a continuous variable. This observation applies equally to mortality, reinfarction, and stroke during the hospital stay.

3.2. Clinical Epidemiology of Key Clinical Variables: 3.2.1. Primary and Secondary VF

VF, both primary and secondary, is relatively common in patients with AMI. The impact of thrombolytic therapy on the incidence and the outcome after these arrhythmias have been evaluated by GISSI investigators.[60–62] The GISSI-1 study, which tested SK versus standard therapy, has been analyzed to address these issues. In this trial, which was run in the mid-1980s, intravenous beta-blockers were very rarely used by Italian cardiologists.

Patients and Results

Primary VF was considered present when the arrhythmia occurred in a patient with first MI within 48 hours from symptom onset and in the absence of heart failure or shock. All the other episodes of VF were considered secondary.

The incidences were 2.8% and 2.7% for primary and secondary VF, respectively, in the 11,712 patients admitted to GISSI-1 study. Primary VF was associated with a significant excess of in-hospital death (10.8% vs 5.9%; RR [risk ratio] 1.94; 95% CI 1.35–2.78). A significant excess of in-hospital death was also evident in patients with secondary VF (38% vs 24%; RR 1.98; 95% CI 1.56–2.52). Thrombolytic therapy with intravenous SK did not reduce the incidence of primary VF, but significantly reduced the incidence of secondary VF (2.4% vs 2.9%; RR 0.80; 95% CI 0.64–1.00). This reduction was particularly large in patients treated within 3 hours of symptom onset (2.6% vs 3.7%; RR 0.71; 95% CI 0.53–0.95). Both primary and secondary VF do not increase mortality after discharge (to 1 year). Patients > 65 years of age were significantly protected from primary VF (RR 0.6; 95% CI 0.45–0.80), but at the same time had significantly more episodes of secondary VF (3.3% vs 2.3%). Infarct site was not associated with the incidence of both types of ventricular arrhythmias.

Comments

Our data show that VF, primary or secondary, is a negative predictor of in-hospital survival in patients with AMI. The impact of a wide adoption of thrombolytic therapy seems not to affect the incidence of primary VF, but do exert a positive effect on the incidence of secondary VF. This protection appeared to be due to a reduction of late VF occurring beyond day 1 and probably reflects the positive effect of thrombolytic therapy on infarct size.

3.2.2 Ventricular Arrhythmias

Several studies over the last 15 years have shown that the presence of frequent and/or complex ventricular arrhythmias was an independent risk factor for subsequent mortality in patients recovering from an AMI.[63–65] At the same time, a growing body of evidence has accumulated on the effects of thrombolysis on the natural history of infarction and on the prevalence and the clinical relevance of different risk factors known to play an important role in terms of mortality risk of post-MI patients. The aim of the analysis of the GISSI-2 database was to evaluate the prevalence and the prognostic value of ventricular arrhythmias in Holter recordings of 8,676 patients recovering from an AMI.

Patients and Results

Of the total 8,676 patients with 24-hour Holter monitoring data available, 3,112 (35.9%) were free from ventricular arrhythmias, while 1,712 patients presented with > 10 premature ventricular beats (PVBs)/hour (19.7%); 2,892 patients (33.3%) presented with complex ventricular arrhythmias and nonsustained ventricular tachycardia was observed in 586 patients (6.8% of the recordings).

Signs or symptoms of severe LV damage were determinants of occurrence and severity of ventricular arrhythmias. Thirty-six and seven tenths percent of the patients without clinical symptoms of congestive heart failure were free of arrhythmias versus 26.8% of those with patent clinical congestive heart failure (P < 0.001); similarly, 36.3% of patients with an EF > 35% and 25.1% of those with an EF ≤ 35% (P < 0.002), and 36.2% of patients with < 45% of myocardial segment injured versus 26.3% of those with ≥ 45% (P < 0.0001) did not show arrhythmias before hospital discharge.

Figure 8 shows the 6-month survival curves of patients without arrhythmias, of those with 1–10 PVBs/hour and of those with more than 10 PVBs/hour. Increasing risks of mortality were experienced by the subgroups with more frequent arrhythmias: compared to the mortality rate of patients without ventricular arrhythmias (2.0%), those with 1–10 PVBs/hour have a risk 1.33 times higher (95% CI 0.97–1.81), while > 10 PVBs/hour the ORMHP increased to 2.98 (95% CI 2.13–4.17).

As expected, mortality rates were consistently higher among patients with clinical signs of congestive heart failure or with echocardiographic evidence of extensive LV damage. However, in each subgroup of patients the presence of > 10 PVBs/hour or of complex ventricular arrhythmias was significantly associated to a higher mortality regardless of depressed LV function.

Comments

Our analysis[66] showed that, despite a decrease in mortality after infarction in patients treated with thrombolytic agents, ventricular arrhythmias were still a marker of electrical instability that could help to identify subjects at risk of death in the first 6 months following the acute event. The higher prevalence of ventricular arrhythmias in patients with signs or symptoms of LV damage implies a wide overlap between the populations with these two independent, negative post-AMI prognostic factors. For this reason, therapeutic strategies oriented to prevent or treat LV dysfunction might represent the most important tools to obtain further relevant improvements in survival of post-AMI patients.

3.2.3. Pericardial Involvement

Prior the advent of thrombolysis, the reported incidence rate of clinical infarction associated pericardial involvement varied from 7%–23%[67–69]; a much higher incidence is detected at autopsy. Since thrombolysis determines an early restoration of the coronary flow leading to a smaller infarct size

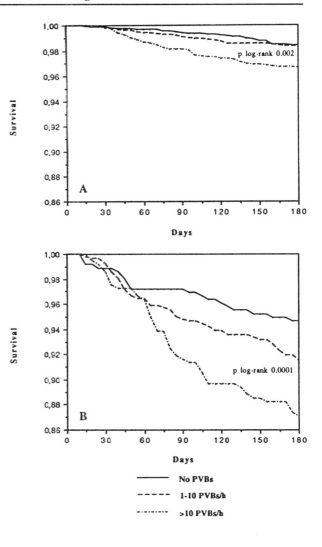

Figure 8. Plots of 6-month survival of patients by frequency of premature ventricular beats (PVBs) according to ventricular function. (A) Patients without left ventricular (LV) dysfunction. (B) Patients with LV dysfunction. In each subgroup of patients, the presence of > 10 PVBs/hour is significantly associated with a higher mortality rate.

and to better ventricular function and survival, it is expected that thrombolytic treatment can also reduce the occurrence of pericardial involvement.

The two large databases of the GISSI-1 and GISSI-2 trials relative, respectively, to 11,806 and 12,381 patients, were reviewed: (1) to describe the epidemiology of pericardial involvement in thrombolyzed and nonthrombolyzed patients; (2) to assess whether pericardial involvement is a marker of infarct size; and (3) to evaluate if pericardial involvement is an independent prognostic risk factor for in-hospital and long-term mortality.

Patients and Results

The major finding of GISSI-1 has been the drop in the incidence of pericardial involvement in thrombolyzed patients (6.7% vs 12%). This incidence rate has been confirmed by GISSI-2, in which all patients were thrombolyzed either with SK (5.6%) or with tPA (6.3%), and by other studies in which pericardial involvement was diagnosed in 6.8% and 6.2% of the patients treated, respectively, with anistreplase or with tPA (Table 8).

The review of the GISSI-1 data has provided direct and indirect evidence indicat-

Table 8.

Incidence of Pericardial Involvement by Treatment

	Events/Pts. (%)	OR (95% CI)
Patients Within 6 Hours from Onset of Symptoms		
GISSI-1		
Standard treatment	562/4619 (12.2)	1
SK	297/4577 (6.5)	0.51 (0.44–0.59)
GISSI-2		
SK	318/5719 (5.6)	1
tPA	363/5764 (6.3)	1.14 (0.98–1.33)
No heparin	338/5770 (5.9)	1
Heparin	343/5713 (6)	1.03 (0.88–1.20)
Patients > 6 to 12 Hours from Onset of Symptoms		
GISSI-1		
Standard treatment	97/895 (10.9)	1
SK	73/929 (7.9)	0.7 (0.51–0.96)

Abbreviations as in Tables 1 and 2.

ing that pericardial involvement in the acute phase of MI is a sign of greater infarct size. The most convincing evidence is the increasing incidence of pericardial involvement as the number of leads presenting ST elevation increases; the incidence of pericardial involvement in anterior and multisite MI and in inferior wall infarction with ST precordial depression is higher in comparison with that occurring when precordial ST depression is absent. The very low incidence of pericardial involvement among patients with MI and ST depression at entry (GISSI-1) and among those with non-Q wave MI (GISSI-2) compared to those with infarction and ST elevation at onset further proves the smaller extent of infarction in the absence of pericardial involvement, since among the former patients transmural infarctions are known to be less frequent than among the latter. Indirect elements of greater infarct size are the higher incidence of pericardial involvement in patients: (1) in Killip Classes 2–4 at entry compared to those in Killip Class 1; (2) with clinical signs of heart failure during hospital stay; (3) with depressed LVEF; and (4) with greater dyskinetic-akinetic score.

With respect to in-hospital mortality, no significant difference was apparent by presence/absence of pericardial involvement. In GISSI-1, mortality among SK-treated patients was 11.3% and 11.6%, respectively, in the absence and in the presence of pericardial involvement. The mortality rates in the control group were, respectively, 14.4% and 13.2% among patients with and without pericardial involvement. In GISSI-2, in-hospital mortality was 9.4% and 9.0%, respectively, with and without pericardial involvement.

In GISSI-1, 1-year mortality was significantly higher among patients with pericardial involvement; the association was significant both in the univariate analysis and in the adjusted analysis. In GISSI-2, however, pericardial involvement did not retain its prognostic significance as an independent risk factor for long-term mortality once the data were adjusted by more specific indicators of ventricular status (LV echo EF, echo akinetic-dyskinetic score, QRS score, peak creatine kinase) (Table 9).

Table 9.

Relation Between Pericardial Involvement and Long-Term Mortality

| | GISSI-1 (1 year)* | | | |
	SK (n = 5505)		Control (n = 5521)	
	Deaths (%)	RR (95% CI)	Deaths (%)	RR (95% CI)
	Deaths (%)	RR (95% CI)	(n = 11,483)†	
	GISSI-2 (6 months)			
Pericarditis				
No	17.1	1	18.8	1 12.4 1
Yes	20.3	1.58 (1.25–2.00)	23	1.57 (1.33–1.58)
14.2	1.02 (0.82–1.26)			

*Adjusted for age, sex, Killip class, previous infarction, hours from symptom onset, electrocardiographic extension and infarct site; †adjusted for age, sex, Killip class, previous infarction, hours from symptom onset, electrocardiographic extension, infarct site, clinical LVF, ejection fraction, echo a-dyskinetic score, QRS score and peak creatine kinase.
LVF = left ventricular function. Other abbreviations as in Tables 1 and 2.

Comments

Our analysis of the GISSI-1 and GISSI-2 studies[70] confirms that pericardial involvement is a reliable bedside, cost-free marker of infarct size and outcome, and should therefore be sought with great attention and lead to a closer follow-up.

3.2.4. Hypertension

Hypertension has been recognized as a major coronary risk factor for many years[71–73]; however, the prognostic value of a history of hypertension in post-AMI patients is still doubtful. We assessed the impact on short (in-hospital) and medium term (6 months) morbidity and mortality of a history of hypertension[74] in patients admitted to the CCU for AMI and treated with a thrombolytic drug and, when not contraindicated, with aspirin and beta-blockers.

Patients and Results

Of the 12,381 patients randomized in GISSI-2 study, the 11,483 patients (92.7%) with a confirmed AMI were selected. The study population was divided into two groups: 3,306 patients with and 7,406 without a history of treated hypertension (28.8% and 64.5% of the whole population, respectively). Patients for whom blood pressure status prior to the index infarction was unknown, or for whom the relevant data were missing because they died before the information could be collected (6.7% of the total population), were excluded. Hypertension was classified as present if subjects were on antihypertensive therapy at the time of the AMI.

Hypertensives presented a significantly higher mortality, both in-hospital (crude OR 1.62; 95% CI 1.40–1.88) and during the following 6 months (crude RR 1.69; 95% CI 1.33–2.14). The difference persisted also after an adjusted analysis including all major prognostic factors: OR 1.50 (95% CI 1.26–1.79) and RR 1.36 (95% CI 1.08–1.71) for in-hospital and 6-month mortality, respectively. LV failure and recurrent ischemic events (angina and reinfarction) were significantly more frequent in hypertensives, both during hospitalization and follow-up. Rupture of the interventricular septum and/or of the papillary muscle were more frequent in hypertensives. With respect to cardiac deaths, no specific cause was significantly more frequent among hypertensives compared with normotensives. After taking into account all the variables, history of hypertension retained its negative prognostic significance with an OR of 1.30 (95% CI 1.10–1.54). The prevalence of echocardiographically determined LV dysfunction was similar in the two groups. Frequent ventricular premature beats or complex ventricular arrhythmias at Holter monitoring were more common among hypertensives. Significantly more hypertensives could not undergo the exercise test, both for cardiac and for noncardiac reasons, and a greater proportion of negative tests was observed among normotensives. Six-month mortality was significantly higher among hypertensives compared to normotensives (RR 1.69; 95% CI 1.33–2.14, for total mortality and 1.54; 95% CI 1.16–2.03, for cardiac mortality). Reinfarction, angina, and LV failure were also significantly more frequent in hypertensives. The multivariate analysis showed that the history of treated hypertension maintained its independent negative prognostic effect also in the follow-up period, with a mortality risk of 1.40 (95% CI 1.11–1.75). The relationship remained virtually unchanged (RR 1.36; CI 1.08–1.71) after the inclusion of prescriptions of hypotensive agents, digitalis, and aspirin at discharge (significantly differently distributed between groups).

Comments

These results document the negative prognostic impact on the short- and medium-term of a history of hypertension in patients with AMI also in the thrombolytic era. The data derived from the GISSI-2 study indicates that patients with a history of hypertension had higher mortality rates than normotensives during hospitalization, also after controlling for major confounders. Moreover, several other major clinical events were more frequent in the hypertensive group. During the 6-month period between hospital discharge and the clinical follow-up visit, a significant excess of mortality and of other major clinical events was found in hypertensives, which persisted after controlling for all major clinical or instrumental confounders.

Our study confirms the negative prognostic significance of a history of hypertension in a large population of patients with AMI in the thrombolytic era.

3.3. Diagnostic-Prognostic Tests: 3.3.1. Stress Test

Exercise testing can provide valuable and inexpensive information on survivors of AMI. The importance of this technique began to emerge in the 1970s.[75] The test provides information on myocardial ischemia and LV function, two major pathophysiological determinants of the clinical outcome. The data available from the prethrombolytic era showed that patients with the highest mortality were those who could not perform an exercise test. Only small series of low risk patients were tested, and the predictive value of the test from these highly selected populations was generally unreliable.[76]

Over the past decade, the treatment of AMI has changed dramatically because of the introduction of systemic thrombolytic treatment, and consequently the value of exercise testing is under debate. The first aim of the analysis of the GISSI-2 database was to reassess the prognostic role of exercise testing in a large population of MI survivors treated acutely following all available recommended treatments (thrombolysis in all patients, aspirin in 84%, intravenous beta-blockers in 48%).[77] To clarify the issue of whether exercise testing is of value for risk stratification of patients with recent AMI who have received thrombolytic therapy, the exercise tests were evaluated by splitting the results in the three categories commonly used in clinical practice: negative; not diagnostic (negative but submaximal); and positive results.

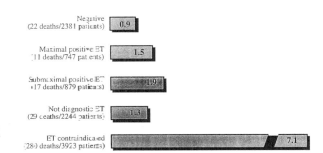

Figure 9. GISSI-2: Six-month total mortality by exercise test results.

Patients and Results

The exercise test was performed in 6,296 patients of the 10,407 patients discharged from the hospital with a diagnosis of AMI, on average 28 days (range 7–57) after randomization. The test was not performed in 3,923 subjects, because of cardiac (1,037 patients) or other (2,886) reasons. Patients excluded from exercise testing were significantly older, often females, had a history of MI, hypertension, or diabetes, or had anterior wall MI; this is the picture of a high risk population.

Among the 6,251 patients who had had exercise tests and had complete survival data (because of missing data in 45 forms, the analysis was restricted to 99.3% of the 6,296 patients who had an exercise test) there were 79 deaths (1.3%). Among the 3,923 patients who did not have exercise tests, there were 280 deaths (7.1%). As previously reported,[46] ineligibility for exercise testing was by multivariate analysis the strongest factor among the seven independent predictors of 6-month mortality in the GISSI-2 study. The test was judged positive for residual ischemia in 1,626 patients (26.0%), negative in 2,381 (38.1%), and nondiagnostic in 2,244 (35.9%).

The mortality rate was 1.7% in patients with a positive test, 0.9% for those with a negative test, and 1.3% for those with a nondiagnostic test. In the adjusted analysis, a positive response to exercise testing was confirmed to be an independent predictor of total 6-month mortality (RR 1.90; 95% CI 1.07–3.39). However, when the patients with a positive test result were stratified by maximal or submaximal exercise, only submaximal positive tests gave predictors of mortality (RR 2.28; 95% CI 1.17–4.45). In Figure 9, the 6-month total mortality data by exercise test results are reported. The 6-month mortality rate was 1.9% in patients with submaximal test and 1.5% in patients with maximal positive test.

Another important finding concerned the silent versus symptomatic exercise-induced ischemia issue. Among the patients with a positive stress test result, 537 (33.0%) had symptomatic myocardial ischemia, while 1,089 (67.0%) had silent myocardial ischemia. Mortality was higher among patients with symptomatic ischemia than among those with silent ischemia (2.6% vs 1.3%). In the adjusted analysis, symptomatic-induced myocardial ischemia was significantly associated with an increased risk of 6-month mortality, although silent-induced myocardial ischemia was not. Even after splitting the population with silent ischemia by the occurrence of ST segment depression at maximal or submaximal level of exercise or by the degree of ST segment depression, the exercise-induced silent myocardial ischemia was not significantly associated with a higher risk of death compared to an exercise stress testing with negative results (Figure 10).

A low work capacity (< 100 W/< 0.6 min) appeared to have a negative independent prognostic significance (OR 2.05; 95% CI 1.23–3.43), and the same was true for an inadequate (≤ 28 mmHg) blood pressure response during exercise (OR 1.86; 95% CI 1.05–3.31).

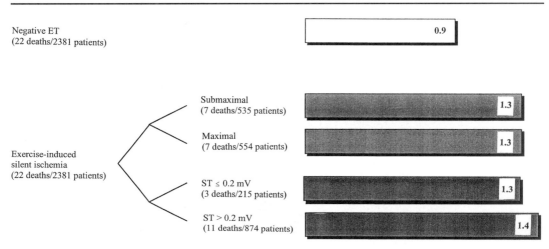

Negative ET
(22 deaths/2381 patients) — 0.9

Exercise-induced
silent ischemia
(22 deaths/2381 patients)

Submaximal
(7 deaths/535 patients) — 1.3

Maximal
(7 deaths/554 patients) — 1.3

ST ≤ 0.2 mV
(3 deaths/215 patients) — 1.3

ST > 0.2 mV
(11 deaths/874 patients) — 1.4

Figure 10. GISSI-2: Six-month total mortality of patients with silent ischemia by heart rate achieved and ST depression entry.

Comments

In a context in which the association between the exercise testing results and 6-month mortality are by definition weak (due to the overall low risk of patients who can undergo the test), exercise-induced symptomatic ischemia in the adjusted analysis retains an independent negative prognostic role. However, it is unclear why silent ischemia should entail a better prognosis than symptomatic ischemia. One of the most relevant findings was that being able to undergo exercise testing 1 month after MI is a reliable marker of a favorable prognosis, whatever the test results. As in the prethrombolytic era, exclusion from exercise testing is the strongest negative prognostic indicator. Although exercise-induced symptomatic ischemia and low work capacity resulted as independent prognostic indicators for a higher 6-month mortality, the absolute risk of death is very low even in these subgroups of patients (the highest mortality rate was 2.6% in patients with symptomatic ischemia).

3.3.2. LV Function

In the prethrombolytic era, impaired LV function following AMI was shown to be an independent predictor of mortality.[78,79] Until the early 1990s, knowledge of risk assessment in patients discharged alive after AMI essentially relied on studies carried out before the widespread application of thrombolysis. At the time of GISSI-2's publication, it was to be determined whether and to what extent available information and proposed criteria of the prognostic stratification were applicable in the thrombolytic era. The assessment of the prognostic significance of LV function was part of a wider evaluation conducted of the whole GISSI-2 database.[46] Within this framework, a prognostic study was planned to reassess the determinants of mortality risk in survivors of AMI in the thrombolytic era.

Patients and Results

A two-dimensional echocardiographic examination was performed to assess segmental LV systolic function just before discharge from the hospital (approximately 2 weeks after the onset of infarction). A determination of EF was available in 27.5% of the patients. The variables analyzed included data from the history, ECG, hospital course, and special tests. Enrolled patients were seen during a clinic visit at 6 months

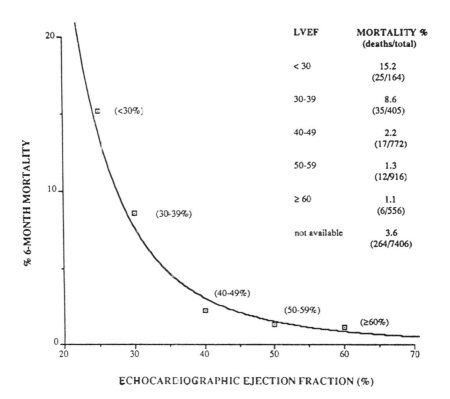

LVEF	MORTALITY % (deaths/total)
< 30	15.2 (25/164)
30-39	8.6 (35/405)
40-49	2.2 (17/772)
50-59	1.3 (12/916)
≥ 60	1.1 (6/556)
not available	3.6 (264/7406)

Figure 11. Plot of 6-month all-cause mortality in five categories of echocardiographic left ventricular ejection fraction (LVEF) The EF-mortality curve exhibits a hyperbolic trend with an upturn in mortality occurring at values of < 40%.

after randomization. In the analysis, risk assessment was based on all-cause mortality, including fatal MI. Among the 10,219 hospital survivors followed-up, 359 death events were observed by 6 months (3.5% mortality rate).

There was a progressive increase in 6-month mortality as the EF declined below 0.40 with the subgroup with the most severe impairment of systolic function exhibiting a 15.2% mortality rate (Fig. 11). On multivariate analysis, performed according to the Cox model, out of the eight variables retained as independent predictors of outcome, three related to the extent of myocardial damage after infarction, namely early and late LV failure and recovery phase LV dysfunction (Table 10).

Comments

After the exclusion from exercise testing for clinical reasons, two variables relating to the extent of postinfarction LV damage (i.e., early LV failure and recovery phase LV dysfunction) were the strongest independent predictors of mortality with relative risks of similar magnitude.

The independent prognostic information carried by clinical or radiographic evidence of early LV failure and an objective measure of LV function, obtained near hospital discharge, confirms the findings of other studies carried out before the use of thrombolytic therapy.[19,78,79] In keeping with current knowledge,[19,80,81] the analysis of LVEFs, available in a representative sam-

Table 10.

GISSI-2: Ranked Independent Predictors and Factors Not Predictive of 6-Month Mortality Among 10,219 Hospital Survivors by the Cox Model

Variable	RR	95% CI
Independent predictors		
Ineligibility for exercise test		
Cardiac reason	3.30	2.36–4.62
Noncardiac reason	3.28	2.23–4.72
Early LV failure	2.41	1.87–3.09
Recovery phase LV dysfunction	2.30	1.78–2.98
Age > 70 years	1.81	1.43–2.30
Electrical instability	1.70	1.32–2.19
Late LV failure	1.54	1.17–2.03
Previous myocardial infarction	1.47	1.14–1.89
History of treated hypertension	1.32	1.05–1.65
Nonpredictive factors		
Female sex	0.92	0.70–1.21
History of angina	1.03	0.80–1.30
History of insulin dependent diabetes	1.17	0.69–1.99
Postinfarction angina	1.09	0.81–1.46
Anterior (Q wave) site	1.14	0.91–1.42
QRS score > 10	0.95	0.73–1.24
Positive exercise test	1.50	0.94 2.38

LV = left ventricular. Other abbreviations as in Tables 1 and 2.

ple of 2,813 patients, showed an inverse curvilinear relation between EF and mortality with an upturn in mortality occurring at values < 40% (Fig. 11).

Surprisingly, in multivariate analysis, a third indicator of LV dysfunction (i.e., late LV failure) was retained as an independent risk predictor even when an echocardiographic measure of LV function was available: notably, nearly 60% of patients with late LV failure did not exhibit the selected echocardiographic marker of LV dysfunction. A possible explanation of this finding could be the well-known high incidence of abnormal diastolic function in these patients.

3.4. GISSI as a Pharmacoepidemiological Observatory

The characteristics of continuity, which has been underlined above, has made the GISSI database a unique opportunity for assessing the evolution of treatments in AMI. The findings presented below on some of the most "recommended" versus "controversial" treatments that had been the object of specific trials are a coherent expression of the broader interest of the GISSI investigators on the timely transferability of controlled evidence into the routine practice.

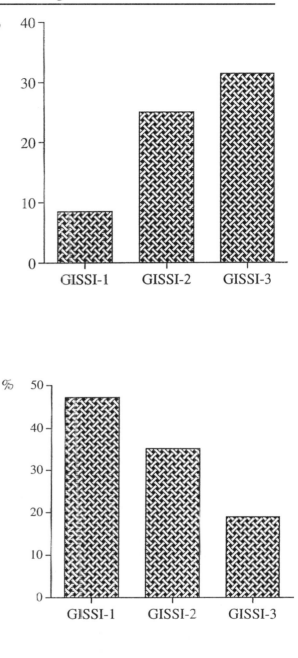

Figure 12. GISSI studies: prescriptions of (A) β-blockers and (B) calcium antagonists at discharge after acute myocardial infarction.

Patients and Results

The rate of prescription of beta-blocker agents at discharge increased from 8.5% in GISSI-1 to 31.4% in GISSI-3 (Fig. 12A). On the contrary, prescription of calcium antagonists at discharge decreased progressively, from 47.2% in GISSI-1 to 35.1% in GISSI-2 to 19.0% in GISSI-3 (P < 0.001) (Fig. 12B). This decrease was most evident for nifedipine (25.1% in GISSI-1, 15.8% in GISSI-2, and 5.8% in GISSI-3; P < 0.01) and verapamil (11.1%, 3.9%, and 1.1%, respectively; P < 0.01) and was less marked for diltiazem (7.3%, 13.5%, and 6.7%, respectively; P = NS).

The percentage of patients discharged after AMI with at least one prescription of a

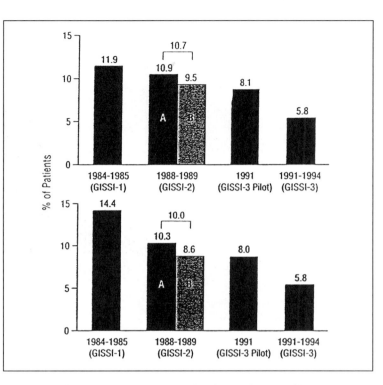

Figure 13. Percentages of patients with antiarrhythmic drugs (Class I and III) prescribed at discharge (top) and being taken at the follow-up visit (6 months after acute myocardial infarction [AMI] in GISSI-1, GISSI-2, and GISSI-3 and 6 weeks after AMI in the GISSI-3 pilot study) (bottom). Panels A and B represent patients discharged before and after May 10, 1989, respectively.

Class I or III antiarrhythmic drug during GISSI-1, GISSI-2, the GISSI-3 pilot study, and GISSI-3 are shown in Figure 13; the percentage decreased progressively and significantly over time, from 11.9% in 1984 to 5.8% in 1991–1994 (P < 0.001). During GISSI-2, antiarrhythmic prescriptions at discharge further decreased after the appearance of results from the CAST trial, from 10.9% to 9.5% (P = 0.09). The figure also shows the same significant trend at follow-up visits (P < 0.001).

public health, and economic reasons. The analysis of the GISSI databases documents the treatment preferences of a population of cardiologists. This collected information was highly representative of the whole country, and was consistent with the results of the available literature. These data show that the main lessons from clinical trials can be rapidly transferred into clinical practice, when the population of cardiologists is directly involved in the planification and conduction of clinical studies.

Comments

The issue of the timeliness and relevance of trial results for setting protocols in routine care has received increasing attention during the last few years for ethical,

4. Further Views

The areas that have been presented so far have been chosen as "models" of: (1) the way epidemiology has interplayed with the experimental setting, both with prospectively planned objectives and through "classic" analysis of the existing databases; (2) the response or the contribution to ongoing debates in the international scene; and (3) the need for an evaluation of the quality of care delivered by those CCUs that were proving to be so efficient in producing experimental data. The picture would be misleading, however, if the model cases were separated from the many other areas of interest and from the tentative "comprehensive mosaic" proposed in Figure 1. The key (apparently methodological) words that are recalled correspond to the GISSI cardiological community's concrete and widespread commitments and involvements. They document that the trial(s) have become the true crossroad of a research group that was the collective responsible for the delivery of care in a country.

5. Concluding Remarks

As recalled in Table 1, with the mention of the ongoing long-term trial of prevention (which, however, belongs to a "new generation" of interests, no more focused on the acute phases of MI), the history of GISSI has not come to an end. More than 10 years is a long time in a changing field like cardiology, where the technology of large scale collaborative trials has become commonplace. The following list of statements (and which, after so many data, do not require further specific comments) could be considered the overall "take home message" or comprehensive result of the GISSI story.

1. Large scale trials are best seen as a "normal" component of routine practice: they are the active and productive "bridge" over uncertainties; they also provide the timely transfer of positive or negative results into the care of patients.

2. An intensive, long-term, diffuse participation of the clinicians who face concrete unresolved questions is the principal determinant of the success of the trial(s),

and at the same time one of the principal and (hopefully) long-lasting outcome of the same trial(s).

3. Population trials are a very effective and powerful "vector" of an epidemiological mentality into the heart of the clinical settings. Even more importantly, the possibility of analyzing epidemiologically the experimentally produced databases allows new insights into the understanding of controversial clinical conditions. An epidemiologically sized experimental setting of the trial is a laboratory for exploring the relevance, the direction, the implications of physiopathological and diagnostic variables.

4. The 10 years of the GISSI history have been the scenario of many, often very harsh, controversies; where the same methodology of large scale trials has been used, the scientific aspects of the problems have prevailed on a priori assumptions or expectations, overemphasized differences, and vested interests.

5. Trials on AMI have become the field test of the degree of reliability of meta-analysis and of the newly emerging "evidence-based medicine." Here again, the continuity of the GISSI studies has proven to be a key factor in imposing a dialogue based on facts, and not on extrapolations and generalization.

6. GISSI has been the product, as well as one of the protagonists, of a broader atmosphere and scenario where the general project of improving survival (a public health oriented goal) in AMI was often contrasted with drug oriented approaches.

7. By definition, this long summary of GISSI has been autofocused. GISSI obviously represents only a small fragment in the mosaic of knowledge produced in the area of thrombolysis. Its very simple, nonpretentious origins recall a message universal to trials: if the simple rules of participation and of simple and rigorous methodology are followed, even the "periphery" can join the "central" dialogue of knowledge.

Appendix

GISSI-1

Steering Committee: Rovelli F (chairman), De Vita C, Feruglio GA, Lotto A, Selvini A, Tognoni G.
Coordination and data monitoring: Farina ML, Foresti A, Franzosi MG, Mauri F, Pampallona S.

GISSI-2

Steering Committee: Feruglio GA, Lotto A, Rovelli F, Solinas P, Tavazzi L, Tognoni G.
Coordination and data monitoring: De Vita C, Franzosi MG, Maggioni AP, Mauri F, Volpi A.

GISSI-3

Steering Committee: De Vita C, Fazzini PF, Geraci E, Tavazzi L, Tognoni G, Vecchio C (chairman).
Scientific and organizing Secretariat: Franzosi MG, Latini R, Maggioni AP, Mauri F, Volpi A.

GISSI-Prevenzione

Steering Committee: Franzosi MG, Geraci E, Nicolosi GL, Tavazzi L, Valagussa F (chairman), Vecchio C.
Scientific and organizing Secretariat: Bomba E, Chieffo C, Maggioni AP, Marchioli R, Schweiger C, Tognoni C.

References

1. ISIS-1 (First International Study of Infarct Survival) Collaborative Group. Randomised trial of intravenous atenolol among 16,027 cases of suspected acute myocardial infarction: ISIS-1. Lancet 1986;ii:57-66.
2. The I.S.A.M. Study Group. A prospective trial of intravenous streptokinase in acute myocardial infarction (I.S.A.M.). N Engl J Med 1986; 314:1465-1471.
3. ISIS-2 (Second International Study of Infarct Survival) Collaborative Group. Randomised trial of intravenous streptokinase, oral aspirin, both, or neither among 17,187 cases of suspected acute myocardial infarction: ISIS-2. Lancet 1988;ii:349-360.
4. Gruppo Italiano per lo Studio della Streptochinasi nell'Infarto Miocardico (GISSI). Effectiveness of intravenous thrombolytic treatment in acute myocardial infarction. Lancet 1986; ii:397-402.
5. Tognoni G, Franzosi MG, Pampallona S. Trombolisi sistemica nell'infarto miocardico acuto: Anticipazioni sullo studio italiano. Cardiologia 1984, 18 Corso di Aggiornamento, Centro A. De Gasperis, Milano, pp. 261-267.
6. Farina ML, Franzosi MG, Pampallona S, et al. Fibrinolisi sistemica nell'infarto miocardico acuto. Casistica, metodo, risultati preliminari del GISSI. Cardiologia 1985, 19 Corso di Aggiornamento, Centro A. De Gasperis, Milano, pp. 290-297.
7. GISSI-2 Gruppo Italiano per lo Studio della Streptokinasi nell'Infarto Miocardico. A factorial randomised trial of alteplase versus streptokinase and heparin versus no heparin among 12490 patients with acute myocardial infarction. Lancet 1990;336:65-71.
8. Gruppo Italiano per lo Studio della Sopravvivenza nell'Infarto Miocardico. GISSI-3: Effects of lisinopril and transdermal glyceryl trinitrate singly and together on 6-week mortality and ventricular function after acute myocardial infarction. Lancet 1994; 343:1115-1122.
9. Fibrinolytic Therapy Trialists' (FTT) Collaborative Group. Indications for fibrinolytic therapy in suspected acute myocardial infarction: Collaborative overview of early mortality and major morbidity results from all randomised trials of more than 1000 patients. Lancet 1994;343:311-322.

10. De Vita C, Franzosi MG, Geraci E, et al. GISSI-2: Mortality plus extensive left ventricular damage as "endpoints." Lancet 1990;335:289.

11. Gruppo Italiano per lo Studio della Streptochinasi nell'Infarto Miocardico (GISSI). Long-term effects of intravenous thrombolysis in acute myocardial infarction: Final report of the GISSI study. Lancet 1987;ii:871-874.

12. International Study Group. In-hospital mortality and clinical course of 20,891 patients with suspected acute myocardial infarction randomised between alteplase and streptokinase with or without heparin. Lancet 1990;336:71-75.

13. White HD. GISSI-2 and the heparin controversy. Lancet 1990;336:297-298.

14. Sobel BE, Hirsh J. Principles and practice of coronary thrombolysis and conjunctive treatment. Am J Cardiol 1991;68:382-388.

15. Ross AM, Hsia J, Hamilton W, et al. Heparin versus aspirin after recombinant tissue plasminogen activator therapy in myocardial infarction: A randomized trial. JACC 1990; 15(Suppl. A):64A.

16. Topol EJ, George BS, Kereiakes DJ, et al. A randomized controlled trial of intravenous tissue plasminogen activator and early intravenous heparin in acute myocardial infarction. Circulation 1989;79:281-286.

17. Bleich SD, Nichols T, Schumacher R, et al. The role of heparin following coronary thrombolysis with tissue plasminogen activator (t-PA). Circulation 1989;80:II-113.

18. The GUSTO Investigators. An international randomized trial comparing four thrombolytic strategies for acute myocardial infarction. N Engl J Med 1993;329:673-682.

19. Multicenter Post-Infarction Research Group. Risk stratification after myocardial infarction. N Engl J Med 1983;309:331-336.

20. Moss AJ, Bigger JT, Odoroff CL. Postinfarct risk stratification. Progr Cardiovasc Dis 1987;29:389-412.

21. White HD, Norris RM, Brown MA, et al. Left ventricular end-systolic volume as the major determinant of survival after recovery from myocardial infarction. Circulation 1987;76:44-51.

22. Oldroyd KG, Pye MP, Ray SG, et al. Effects of early captopril administration on infarct expansion, left ventricular remodeling and exercise capacity after acute myocardial infarction. Am J Cardiol 1991;68:713-718.

23. Sharpe N, Smith H, Murphy J, et al. Early prevention of left ventricular dysfunction after myocardial infarction with angiotensin-converting-enzyme inhibition. Lancet 1991;337:872-876.

24. Jugdutt BI, Warnica JJ. Intravenous nitroglycerin therapy to limit myocardial infarct size, expansion, and complications. Circulation 1988;78:906-919.

25. Eaton LW, Weiss JL, Bulkley BG, et al. Regional cardiac dilation after acute myocardial infarction. N Engl J Med 1979;300:57-62.

26. Pfeffer MA, Braunwald E. Ventricular remodeling after myocardial infarction. Experimental observations and clinical implications. Circulation 1990;81:1161-1172.

27. Pfeffer MA, Kamas GA, Vaughan DE, et al. Effect of captopril on progressive ventricular dilation after anterior myocardial infarction. N Engl J Med 1988;319:80-86.

28. Sharpe N, Murphy J, Smith H, et al. Treatment of patients with symptomless left ventricular dysfunction after myocardial infarction. Lancet 1988; i:255-259.

29. Yusuf S, Collins R, MacMahon S, et al. Effect of intravenous nitrates on mortality in acute myocardial infarction: An overview of the randomised trials. Lancet 1988;i:1088-1092.

30. Swedberg K, Held P, Kjekshus J, et al. Effects of the early administration of enalapril on mortality in patients with acute myocardial infarction: Results of the Cooperative New Scandinavian Enalapril Survival Study II (CONSENSUS II). N Engl J Med 1992;327:678-684.

31. GISSI-3 Gruppo Italiano per lo Studio della Sopravvivenza nell'Infarto Miocardico. GISSI-3 study protocol on the effects of lisinopril, of nitrates, and of their association in patients with acute myocardial infarction. Am J Cardiol 1992;70:62C-69C.

32. Volpi A, De Vita C, Franzosi MG, et al. Determinants of 6-month mortality in survivors of myocardial infarction after thrombolysis: Results of the GISSI-2 data base. Circulation 1993;88:416-429.

33. The Acute Infarction Ramipril Efficacy (AIRE) Study Investigators. Effect of ramipril on mortality and morbidity of survivors of acute myocardial infarction with clinical evidence of heart failure. Lancet 1993;342:821-828.

34. The SOLVD Investigators. Effect of enalapril on survival in patients with reduced left ventricular ejection fractions and congestive heart failure. N Engl J Med 1991;325:293-302.

35. The SOLVD Investigators. Effect of enalapril on mortality and the development of heart failure in asymptomatic patients with reduced left ventricular ejection fractions. N Engl J Med 1992;327:685-691.

36. Pfeffer MA, Braunwald E, Moyé LA, et al. Effect of captopril on mortality and morbidity in patients with left ventricular dysfunction after myocardial infarction. Results of the Survival and Ventricular Enlargement Trial. N Engl J Med 1992;327:669-677.

37. Latini R, Maggioni AP, Flather M, et al. ACE inhibitor use in patients with myocardial infarction. Summary of evidence from clinical trials. Circulation 1995;92:3132-3137.

38. ISIS Collaborative Group, Oxford, UK. ISIS-4: Randomised study of oral isosorbide mononitrate in over 50,000 patients with suspected acute myocardial infarction. Circulation 1993;88:I-394.

39. Wilcox RG, von der Lippe G, Olsson CG, et al., for the ASSET Study Group. Trial of tissue plasminogen activator for mortality reduction in the acute myocardial infarction. Lancet 1988; ii:525-530.

40. AIMS Trial Study Group. Effect of intravenous APSAC on mortality after acute myocardial infarction: Preliminary report of a placebo-controlled clinical trial. Lancet 1988; i:545-549.

41. ISIS-3 (Third International Study of Infarct Survival Collaborative Group). ISIS-3: A randomised comparison of streptokinase vs tissue plasminogen activator vs anistreplase and of aspirin and heparin vs heparin alone among 41299 cases of suspected acute myocardial infarction. Lancet 1992; 339:753-770.

42. Maggioni AP, Franzosi MG, Santoro E, et al., the GISSI-2, and the International Study Group. The risk of stroke in patients with acute myocardial infarction after thrombolytic and antithrombotic treatment. N Engl J Med 1992;327:1-6.

43. Maggioni AP, Franzosi MG, Farina ML, et al. Cerebrovascular events after myocardial infarction: Analysis of the GISSI trial. Br Med J 1991;302:1428-1431.

44. Simoons ML, Maggioni AP, Knatterud G, et al. Individual risk assessment for intracranial haemorrhage during thrombolytic therapy. Lancet 1993; 342:1523-1528.

45. Maggioni AP, Maseri A, Fresco C, et al., on behalf of the Investigators of the Gruppo Italiano per lo Studio della Sopravvivenza nell'Infarto Miocardico (GISSI-2). Age-related increase in mortality among patients with first myocardial infarctions treated with thrombolysis. N Engl J Med 1993;329:1442-1448.

46. Volpi A, De Vita C, Franzosi MG, et al., and the Ad hoc working group of the Gruppo Italiano per lo Studio della Sopravvivenza nell'Infarto Miocardico (GISSI)-2 Data base. Determinants of 6-month mortality in survivors of myocardial infarction after thrombolysis. Results of the GISSI-2 data base. Circulation 1993;88:416-429.

47. Tofler GH, Stone PH, Muller JE, et al., and the MILIS study group. Effect of gender and race on prognosis after myocardial infarction: Adverse prognosis of women, particularly black women. JACC 1987;9:473-482.

48. Greeland P, Reicher-Reiss H, Godbourt U, et al., and the Israeli SPRINT investigator. In-hospital and 1-year mortality in 1,524 women after myocardial infarction: Comparison with 4,315 men. Circulation 1991; 83:484-491.

49. Norris RM, Caughey DE, Deeming LW, et al. Coronary prognostic index for predicting survival after recovery from acute myocardial infarction. Lancet 1970;2:485-487.

50. Henning H, Gilpin EA, Covell JW, et al. Prognosis after acute myocardial infarction: A multivariate analysis of mortality and survival. Circulation 1979;59:1124-1136.

51. Henning R, Wedel H. The long-term prognosis after myocardial infarction: A five-year follow-up study. Eur Heart J 1981;2:65-74.

52. Martin CA, Thompson PL, Armstrong BK, et al. Long-term prognosis after

recovery from myocardial infarction: A nine-year follow-up of the Perth Coronary Register. Circulation 1983; 68:961-969.

53. Weinblatt E, Shapiro S, Frank CW. Prognosis of women with newly diagnosed coronary heart disease: A comparison with course of disease among men. Am J Public Health 1973; 63:577-593.

54. Pohjola S, Siltanen P, Romo M. Five-year survival of 728 patients after myocardial infarction: A community study. Br Heart J 1980;43:176-183.

55. Wong ND, Cupples LA, Ostfeld AM, et al. Risk factors for long-term coronary prognosis after initial myocardial infarction: The Framingham Study. Am J Epidemiol 1989;130:469-480.

56. Rivers JT, White JD, Cross DB, et al. Reinfarction after thrombolysis therapy for acute myocardial infarction followed by conservative management: Incidence and effect of smoking. JACC 1990;16:340-348.

57. Barbash GI, White HD, Modan M, et al. Significance of smoking in patients receiving thrombolytic therapy for acute myocardial infarction. Experience gleaned from the International Tissue Plasminogen Activator/Streptokinase Mortality Trial. Circulation 1993;87:53-58.

58. Mueller HS, Cohen LS, Braunwald E, et al. Predictors of early morbidity and mortality after thrombolytic therapy of acute myocardial infarction. Analyses of patient subgroups in the thrombolysis in myocardial infarction (TIMI) trial, phase II. Circulation 1992; 85:1254-1264.

59. Gomez MA, Karagounis LA, Allen A, et al. Effect of cigarette smoking on coronary patency after thrombolytic therapy for myocardial infarction. Am J Cardiol 1993;72:373-378.

60. Volpi A, Maggioni A, Franzosi MG, et al. In-hospital prognosis of patients with acute myocardial infarction complicated by primary ventricular fibrillation. N Engl J Med 1987;317:257-261.

61. Volpi A, Cavalli A, Franzosi MG, et al., and the GISSI Investigators. One-year prognosis of primary ventricular fibrillation complicating acute myocardial infarction. Am J Cardiol 1989; 63:1174-1178.

62. Volpi A, Cavalli A, Santoro E, et al., and GISSI Investigators. Incidence and prognosis of secondary ventricular fibrillation in acute myocardial infarction. Evidence for a protective effect of Thrombolytic therapy. Circulation 1990;82:1279-1288.

63. The Coronary Drug Project Research Group. Prognostic importance of premature beats following myocardial infarction. Experience in the coronary drug project. JAMA 1973;223:1116-1124.

64. Ruberman W, Weinblatt E, Goldberg JD, et al. Ventricular premature complexes and sudden death after myocardial infarction. Circulation 1981; 64:297-305.

65. Bigger JT, Weld FM, Rolnitzky LM. Prevalence, characteristics and significance of ventricular tachycardia (three or more complexes) detected with ambulatory electrocardiographic recording in the late hospital phase of acute myocardial infarction. Am J Cardiol 1981;48:815-823.

66. Maggioni AP, Zuanetti G, Franzosi MG, et al., on behalf of GISSI-2 Investigators. Prevalence and prognostic significance of ventricular arrhythmias after acute myocardial infarction in the fibrinolytic era. GISSI-2 results. Circulation 1993;87:312-322.

67. Toole JC, Silverman ME. Pericarditis of acute myocardial infarction. Chest 1975;67:647-653.

68. Galve E, Garcia-Del Castillo H, Evangelista A, et al. Pericardial effusion in the course of myocardial infarction: Incidence, natural history, and clinical relevance. Circulation 1986;73:294-299.

69. Krainin FM, Flessas AP, Spodick DH. Infarction-associated pericarditis. N Engl J Med 1984;311:1211-1214.

70. Correale E, Maggioni AP, Romano S, et al., on behalf of the Gruppo Italiano per lo Studio della Sopravvivenza nell'Infarto Miocardico (GISSI). Comparison of frequency, diagnostic and prognostic significance of pericardial involvement in acute myocardial infarction treated with and without thrombolytics. Am J Cardiol 1993; 71:1377-1381.

71. The Pooling Project Research Group. Relationship of blood pressure, serum cholesterol, smoking habit, relative weight and ECG abnormalities to incidence of major coronary events: Final report of the Pooling Project. J Chron Dis 1978;31:201-306.

72. MacMahon S, Peto R, Cutler J, et al. Blood pressure, stroke, and coronary heart disease. Part 1: Prolonged differences in blood pressure: Prospective observational studies corrected for the regression dilution bias. Lancet 1990;335:765-774.

73. Stamler J, Stamler R, Neaton JD. Blood pressure, systolic and diastolic, and cardiovascular risk. US population data. Arch Intern Med 1993; 153:598-615.

74. Fresco C, Avanzini F, Bosi S, et al., on behalf of the GISSI-2 Investigators. Prognostic value of a history of hypertension in 11483 patients with acute myocardial infarction treated with thrombolysis. J Hypertens 1996; 14:743-750.

75. Théroux P, Waters DD, Halphen C, et al. Prognostic value of exercise testing soon after myocardial infarction. N Engl J Med 1979;301:341-345.

76. Froelicher VF, Perdue S, Pewen W, et al. Application of meta-analysis using an electronic spread sheet to exercise testing in patients after myocardial infarction. Am J Med 1987;83:1045-1054.

77. Villella A, Maggioni AP, Villella M, et al., on behalf of the GISSI-2 Investigators. Prognostic significance of maximal exercise testing after myocardial infarction treated with thrombolytic agents: The GISSI-2 data-base. Lancet 1995;346:523-529.

78. Sanz G, Castaner A, Betriu A, et al. Determinants of prognosis in survivors of myocardial infarction. N Engl J Med 1982;306:1065-1070.

79. Nicod P, Gilpin E, Dittrich H, et al. Influence on prognosis and morbidity of left ventricular ejection fraction with and without signs of left ventricular failure after acute myocardial infarction. Am J Cardiol 1988;61:1165-1171.

80. Gadsboll N, Hoilund-Carlsen PF, Madsen EB, et al. Right and left ventricular ejection fractions: Relation to one-year prognosis in acute myocardial infarction. Eur Heart J 1987; 8:1201-1209.

81. Serruys PW, Simoons ML, Suryapranata H, et al., for the Working Group on Thrombolytic Therapy in Acute Myocardial Infarction of The Netherlands Interuniversity Cardiology Institute. Preservation of global and regional left ventricular function after early thrombolysis in acute myocardial infarction. JACC 1986;7:729-742.

GISSI studies (Gruppo Italiano per lo Studio della Sopravvivenza nell'Infarto Miocardico Acuto) are endorsed by Istituto di Ricerche Farmacologiche "Mario Negri" (IRFMN), Milano, and Associazione Nazionale Medici Cardiologi Ospedalieri (ANMCO), Firenze, Italy.

Address for reprints: Gianni Tognoni, M.D., Head, Lab of Clinical Pharmacology, Instituto "Mario Negri," Via Eritrea 62, 20157 Milano, Italy. Fax: 39-2332-00049.

Chapter 7

A Review of Thrombolysis Mortality Trials: ISAM to ASSET

Rolf Schröder, M.D.

From the Department of Cardiology, Klinikum Steglitz, Free University Berlin, Germany

Large controlled mortality studies with streptokinase, APSAC or tissue plasminogen activator (tPA) have conclusively shown that thrombolytic therapy within 6 hours after symptom onset improves survival after acute myocardial infarction. There is evidence of benefit even for patients treated between 7–24 hours after pain onset, suggesting that early recanalization of the infarct-related artery is not the only mechanism by which thrombolysis improves survival. There is no apparent upper age limit for thrombolytic therapy. Serious side effects are generally rare and not age dependent. Inclusion criteria as well as concomittant adjuvant therapy were different in the various trials. Furthermore, the 95% confidence intervals for mortality reduction by different thrombolytic agents are overlapping. To evaluate their relative efficacy and safety direct head-to-head comparison is needed.(J Interven Cardiol 1990:3:3)

Introduction

Within the last 4 years, results from five controlled mortality trials with short-term intravenous infusion of thrombolytic agents in acute myocardial infarction have been reported: ISAM (Intravenous Streptokinase in Acute Myocardial Infarction). GISSI-1 (Gruppo Italiano per lo Studio della Streptochinasi nell'Infarto Miocardico),[2] ISIS-2 Second International Study of Infarct Survival, AIMS (APSAC Intervention Mortality Study, and ASSET (Anglo-Scandinavian Study of Ears Thrombolysis).[6] Table 1 shows data of the study resigns.

In the first three trials, 1.5 million units of streptokinase were given as a 1-hour intravenous infusion: II AIMS, 30 mg of APSAC were injected intravenously; and in ASSET, 100 mg of tPA was given 10 mg as a bolus dose followed by an infusion 50 mg within 1 hour and another 20 mg in each of the next 2 hours. Patients were included within 6 hours after symptom onset in ISAM and AIMS; within 5 hours of symptom onset in ASSET; within 12 hours in GISSI-1; and within the first 24 hours after onset of suspected myocardial infarction in ISIS-2. The age limit was 75 years in ISAM and ASSET; 70 years in AIMS; and there was no upper age limit in GISSI-1 and ISIS-

Table 1.

Study Design of 5 Thrombolysis Mortality Trials

ISAM	n = 1741	STK	≤6 h	≤75 y	ST ↑
GISSI-1	n = 11806	STK	≤12 h	no limit	ST↑ (↓)
ISIS-2	n = 17187	STK	≤24 h	no limit	susp. MI
AIMS	n = 1255	APSAC	≤6 h	≤70 y	ST ↑
ASSET	n = 5009	tPA	≤5 h	≤75 y	susp. MI

2. Inclusion criteria were significant ST segment elevations in the prerandomization ECG in ISAM, GISSI-1, and AIMS. In GISSI-1, a small number of patients with only ST segment depressions were also included. In ISIS-2 and ASSET, patients with clinically suspected acute myocardial infarction were randomized. GISSI-1 was a controlled but open trial, the others were double-blind placebo-controlled trials.

In Table 2 the adjuvant therapy administered to the thrombolysis and control groups are listed. In ISAM, 5,000 IU of heparin were immediately administered intravenously followed by an infusion for at least 72 hours. In addition, 0.5 g of aspirin intravenously, oral phenprocoumon for at least 4 weeks, and in about 75% of patients intravenous nitroglycerin over 24–48 hours was given. In GISSI-1,[7] anticoagulation was optional, only about 20% of patients had intravenous heparin during the acute phase. ISIS-2 had a 2 × 2 factorial design, treatment was either streptokinase, aspirin, both or neither. Anticoagulation was also optional. In AIMS, subsequent anticoagulation began with intravenous heparin after 6 hours and warfarin continued for at least 3 months. In ASSET, after an initial bolus

dose of 5,000 IU, a heparin infusion of 1,000 IU/hour was given for 21 hours after administration of tPA or placebo.

In Figure 1, reduction in mortality during the first 3–5 weeks is shown. In the ISAM trial, mortality in the placebo group was substantially lower than in the other trials. This is not because mainly low risk patients had been included. Except for different age limits, the exclusion and inclusion criteria were the same for all trials. It may be that vigorous anticoagulation and intravenous infusion of nitroglycerin substantially lowered the mortality in the ISAM placebo group. In the other four trials, reduction in mortality was statistically significant, 20% difference in favor of streptokinase in GISSI-1 in patients treated within 12 hours after symptom onset; 23% in ISIS-2 in patients treated within 24 hours after symptom onset; and in those who received streptokinase and aspirin as compared to both placebo, the reduction in mortality was 39%. The largest mortality difference in favor of thrombolysis was noticed with APSAC. However, since only patients 70 years of age or younger were included in AIMS, the placebo group mortality appeared relatively high.

Table 2.

Adjuvant Therapy Administered to Both Treatment Groups

ISAM	Heparin i.v., ASA i.v., coumadin, TNG i.v. (~75%)
GISSI-1	Anticoagulation optional (~20% Heparin i.v.)
ISIS-2	2 × 2 factorial design: STK, ASA, both, or neither
AIMS	Heparin i.v., warfarin, timolol
ASSET	Heparin i.v.

Table 3.

ISIS-2: Mortality with "Proven" Myocardial Infarction

Streptokinase	Placebo	Difference
456/4494 (10.1%)	640/4499 (14.2%)	29%
STK and ASA	Both PLA	Difference
197/2221 (8.9%)	361/2235 (16.2%)	45%

Abbreviations: STK = streptokinase; PLA = placebo; ASA = acetyl salicylic acid.

The results of ISIS-2 and ASSET are debated, because patients with suspected acute myocardial infarction were randomized on the basis of their clinical presentation. Thus, it is suspected that many patients might not have had an acute myocardial infarction, but, for example, unstable angina pectoris. Therefore, prerandomization ECGs were retrospectively analyzed in ISIS-2. In 62% there was either a significant ST segment elevation or, in 6%, a bundle branch block. Eight percent had only ST segment depression; and 27% other abnormalities, mostly Q-waves and/or negative T-waves. Two percent had a normal ECG. The reduction in mortality in patients with proven myocardial infarction was somewhat larger than in the total group (Table 3).

In ASSET, the in-hospital diagnosis in 72% of patients was definite, probable or, in about 6%, possible myocardial infarction.[6] In 17%, an ischemic heart disease was diagnosed, which means previous myocardial infarction or angina pectoris without new ECG, or significant enzyme charges. Eleven percent had chest pain of unknown cause or other diagnoses. In the 72% with an in-hospital diagnosis of myocardial infarction, mortality was reduced by 28% (9.4% tPA vs 13.1% placebo).

In both trials a small number of patients presented with absolutely normal ECGs. Mortality in these patient groups was low, but there was still a difference in favor of thrombolysis (Table 4). Thus, at least these patients suffered no harm from the treatment.

The only subgroup without any beneficial effect were patients who showed only ST segment depression in the prerandomization ECG (Table 5). In the GISSI-1 trial, the in-hospital mortality was higher in those treated with streptokinase as compared to conventional treatment and, during follow-up at 1 year, the difference became conventionally significant. The noticeable findings in both trials were the high mortality in these subgroups—higher than in those with proven transmural myocardial infarction.

Reinfarction

The in-hospital reinfarction rates were higher in the thrombolysis group as compared to control in all trials where data

Table 4.

Mortality in Patients Presenting with "Normal" ECG

	Treatment		Control
ISIS-2	3/160 (1.9%)	vs	6/155 (3.9%)
ASSET	7/443 (1.6%)	vs	13/431 (3.0%)

Table 5.

Mortality with ST-Segment Depression in the Pre-Randomization ECG

	Treatment		Control
GISSI-1	46/224 (20%)	vs	37/227 (16%)
At 1 year	76/223 (34%)	vs	55/227 (24%)
ISIS-2	107/571 (19%)	vs	105/566 (19%)

Table 6.

In-Hospital Reinfarction Rate

	Treatment		Control
ISAM	2.3%	vs	1.1%
GISSI-1	4.1%	vs	2.1%
ISIS-2	3.8%	vs	2.9%
ASSET	4.5%	vs	3.9%

Table 7.

In-Hospital Non-Fatal Reinfarction Rate in ISIS-2 According to Treatment with Streptokinase. Aspirin, Both, or Neither (Abbreviations: See Table 3)

	STK	STK-PLA
ASA	1.8%	1.9%
ASA-PLA	3.8%	2.9%

were provided (Table 6). However, in general, the reinfarction rate was relatively low. Not only the in-hospital reinfarction rate was higher in thrombolysed patients. During the first weeks after hospital discharge the differences in reinfarctions were still continuously increasing: 7.2% versus 4.6% at 6 months after discharge in ISAM;[8] and 7.6% versus 4.6% in the GISSI-1 trial.[7]

In ISIS-2, concomittant treatment with aspirin significantly reduced the rate of nonfatal reinfarction in streptokinase treated patients (Table 7). With aspirin placebo, the in-hospital nonfatal reinfarction rate was 3.8% in streptokinase patients as compared to 2.9% in patients who had neither aspirin nor streptokinase. However, with aspirin the reinfarction rate was the same regardless of whether patients had been treated with streptokinase or not.

Side Effects

In all trials, bleedings occurred significantly more often with thrombolytic therapy, however, serious bleeding complications were rare. The most serious side effect of any thrombolytic therapy is the development of intracranial hemorrhage. Fortunately, the excess of hemorrhagic strokes are outweighed in ISIS-2 and GISSI-1 by less ischemic strokes from cerebral emboli. It is often difficult to clearly differentiate ischemic from hemorrhagic strokes, especially in large trials where not all patients had computer tomography or autopsy. Therefore, it is more appropriate to compare the incidence of strokes of either etiology.

Table 8 shows the time-dependent incidences of stroke in the ISIS-2 trial. During day 0 and 1, i.e., day of randomization and day thereafter—there was an excess of strokes in streptokinase patients as compared with placebo, probably due to cerebral hemorrhages in the streptokinase group. However, after day 1 there were more strokes in the placebo group—most probably because of a lower incidence of ischemic strokes with streptokinase. Aspirin prevents embolic strokes. After day 1 in patients with streptokinase and aspirin there were 0.31% strokes as compared to 0.85% in patients with neither aspirin nor streptokinase. There was also a trend to a lower rate

Table 8.

Time-Dependent Incidence of Strokes in ISIS-2 (Abbreviations: See Table 3)

	STK	PLA	STK + ASA	Both PLA
Day 0–1	0.32%	0.15%	0.28%	0.21%
After day 1	0.40%	0.64%	0.31%	0.85%
Any	0.72%	0.79%	0.59%	1.06%
Fatal	0.28%	0.31%	0.28%	0.42%

Table 9.

Incidence of Fatal Stroke

	Treatment		Control
GISSI-1	15/5860 (0.25%)	vs	11/5852 (0.19%)
ISIS-2	24/8490 (0.28%)	vs	26/8491 (0.31%)
ASSET	11/2512 (0.44%)	vs	6/2493 (0.24%)

of fatal strokes in patients treated with streptokinase and aspirin as compared with both placebos.

Since definition of cerebral events has been different in the various thrombolysis trials, it appears more appropriate to compare the rate of fatal strokes as an unequivocal end point (Table 9). The incidence of fatal strokes in placebo or control groups were similar in GISSI-1, ISIS-2, and in ASSET. With streptokinase treatment in GISSI-1 and ISIS-2 the incidence of fatal strokes was comparable to that in the placebo groups. With tPA, however, there was a trend to a somewhat higher rate of fatal strokes. In the combined GISSI-2 and International Study with direct comparison of tPA and streptokinase there was also a significantly higher total stroke rate with tPA (1.3% tPA vs 0.9% streptokinase).[9]

No Upper Age Limit for Thrombolytic Therapy

In many trials and also in clinical practice in many centers older patients are excluded from thrombolytic therapy because of a suspected increased risk of severe side effects. However, it has been shown in all trials where older patients are included, that there is no such increased risk, especially not for the incidence of stroke. In ISIS-2 (as in other trials), the incidence of stroke in the placebo group was age dependent. However, there was no excess of strokes in either age group in streptokinase treated patients. For patients over 70 years of age, the incidence of stroke in hospital was 1.1% with streptokinase, as compared to 1.3% with placebo. Thus, it comes as no surprise that there also was no difference in the percent mortality reduction by streptokinase when different age groups are compared. Since acute myocardial infarction is associated with a much higher mortality risk in older patients, in absolute terms the survival benefit was somewhat greater among patients over age 70 than among younger patients.[3]

A beneficial mortality effect had been shown in all controlled trials where older patients had been included: In GISSI-1 patients older than 75 years (29% vs 33%); and in ISIS-2 patients over 70 years (18% versus 22%), and in those treated with streptokinase and aspirin (16% versus 24%; i.e., the lives of 8 patients out of 100 treated are saved). Also, in ASSET, where only patients up to 75 years of age were included, the mortality benefit was greatest in patients between 66 and 75 years (11% vs 16%). All these data clearly demonstrates that thrombolytic therapy should not be withheld from older patients. There is no upper age limit for thrombolytic therapy in acute myocardial infarction.

Time Window for Thrombolytic Treatment

In many centers it is common clinical practice to restrict thrombolytic therapy to patients presenting within 3–4 hours after onset of myocardial infarction symptoms. The generally accepted rationale for this is the concept that only early reperfusion is

Table 10.

Reduction in Mortality Subdivided by Time from Pain Onset

	Treatment	*Control*	*Difference*
ISAM			
0–3 h	25/477 (5.2%)	30/463 (6.5%)	20%
>3–6 h	25/365 (6.8%)	31/405 (7.7%)	12%
GISSI-1			
0–3 h	278/3016 (9.2%)	369/3078 (12.0%)	23%
>3–6 h	217/1849 (11.7%)	254/1800 (14.1%)	17%
ISIS-2			
0–3 h	207/2551 (8.1%)	311/2557 (12.2%)	34%
>3–6 h	264/2799 (9.4%)	337/2803 (12.0%)	22%
AIMS			
0–4 h	18/334 (5.4%)	30/326 (9.2%)	41%
>4–6 h	14/168 (8.3%)	31/176 (17.6%)	53%
ASSET			
0–3 h	81/992 (8.1%)	107/979 (10.9%)	26%
>3–5 h	99/1504 (6.5%)	129/1488 (8.6%)	24%

associated with salvage of ischemic myocardium and subsequent attenuation of left ventricular dysfunction. However, the findings from the ISIS-2 study challenge the notion that myocardial salvage is the only mechanism for improved survival. Streptokinase also reduced mortality when given between 7–24 hours after onset of symptoms of myocardial infarction. An overview of the results from all streptokinase trials provides significant confirmation of benefit among patients treated after 6 hours.[10] The reduction in mortality among those ISIS-2 trial patients with ST segment elevation recorded on their pre-randomization ECG 7–24 hours from symptom onset was 22% (2 P < 0.05), which is similar to the 18% (2 P = 0.02) mortality reduction among all patients entered late.[10] This suggests that not only patients with persistent signs of ischemia may benefit from late thrombolysis.

According to animal experiments and clinical findings, salvage of jeopardized ischemic myocardium can only be expected when recanalization of the infarct-related artery occurs within 2–3 hours.[11–13] However, data from all mortality trials do not support the suggestion that the benefit among those treated within the first 3 hours is much greater than among those treated later (Table 10). There is a growing body of evidence that the issue of preservation of myocardium and left ventricular function in patients with acute myocardial infarction is complex and the mechanisms involved are multifactorial.[14] Patency of the infarct-related artery, achieved also beyond the time when actual salvage of ischemic myocardium can be expected, appears to be an important independent factor for preservation of left ventricular function.[14,15] In addition, thrombolytic agents may exert salutary effects on the development of myocardial necrosis by mechanisms that are independent of their ability to lyse occluding coronary artery thrombi.[16–18] We look forward to the results of the ISIS-3 study and other ongoing late thrombolysis trials to confirm the beneficial effects of late thrombolysis in general as well as to provide sufficient data for reasonable subgroup analysis.

References

1. I.S.A.M. Study Group. A prospective trial of intravenous streptokinase in acute myocardial infarction (I.S.A.M.): Mortality, morbidity, and infarct size at 21 days. New Engl J Med 1986; 314:1465–1471.
2. Gruppo Italieno per lo Studio della Strepochinasi nell' Infarto Miocardico. Effectiveness of intravenous thrombolytic treatment in acute myocardial infarction. Lancet 1986; 1:397–402.
3. ISIS-2 (Second International Study of Infarct Survival) Collaborative Group. Randomised trial of intravenous streptokinase, oral aspirin, both, or neither among 17,187 cases of suspected acute myocardial infarction: ISIS-2. Lancet 1988; 1:349–360.
4. AIMS Trial Study Group. Effect of intravenous APSAC on mortality after acute myocardial infarction: Preliminary report of a placebo-controlled clinical trial. Lancet 1988; 1:545–549.
5. AIMS Trial Study Group. Mortality results at 30 days and beyond on all 1,255 patients with acute myocardial infarction. (abstract) Circulation 1988; 78(Suppl II):II–277.
6. Wilcox RG, Olsson CG, von der Lippe G, et al., for the ASSET Study Group. Trial of tissue plasminogen activator for mortality reduction in acute myocardial infarction. Lancet 1988; 1:525–530.
7. Rovelli F, de Vita C, Feruglio GA, et al. GISSI Trial: Early results and late follow-up. J Am Coll Cardiol 1987; 10:33B–39B.
8. Schröder R, Neuhaus KL, Leizorovicz A, et al., for the ISAM Study Group. A prospective placebo-controlled double-blind multicenter trial of intravenous Streptokinase in Acute Myocardial Infarction (ISAM): Long-term mortality and morbidity. J Am Coll Cardiol 1987; 9:197–203.
9. The International Study Group. In-hospital mortality and clinical course of 20,891 patients with suspected acute myocardial infarction randomised between alteplase and streptokinase with or without heparin. Lancet 1990; 2:71–75.
10. ISIS-2 (Second International Study of Infarct Survival) Collaborative Group. Randomized trial of intravenous streptokinase, oral aspirin, both, or neither among 17,187 cases of suspected acute myocardial infarction: ISIS-2. J Am Coll Cardiol 1988; 12:3A–13A.
11. Schaper W. Natural defense mechanisms to ischemia. Eur Heart J 1983; 4(Suppl. D):73–78.
12. Simoons ML, Serruys PW, van den Brand M, et al. Early thrombolysis in acute myocardial infarction: Limitation of infarct size and improved survival. J Am Coll Cardiol 1986; 7:717–728.
13. Schröder R. Mechanisms by which thrombolysis reduces mortality: Limitation of infarct size-what else? In: Sleight P. Chamberlain DA, eds. Thrombolysis: Dawn of a New Era? London: IBC Technical Services Ltd., 1990 (In press).
14. Braunwald E. Myocardial reperfusion, limitation of infarct size, reduction of left ventricular dysfunction, and improved survival. Should the paradigm be expanded? Circulation 1989; 79:441–444.
15. Schröder R, Neuhaus KL, Linderer T, et al. Impact of late coronary artery reperfusion on left ventricular function one month after acute myocardial infarction (Results from the ISAM Study). Am J Cardiol 1989; 64:878–884.
16. Chamberlain DA. Unanswered questions in thrombolysis. Am J Cardiol 1989; 63:34A–40A.
17. Moriarty AJ, Hughes R, Nelson SD, et al. Streptokinase and reduced plasma viscosity: A second benefit. Eur J Haematol 1988; 41:25–36.
18. Kopia GA, Kopaciewicz LJ, Ruffolo RR. Coronary thrombolysis with intravenous streptokinase in the anesthetized dog: A dose-response study. J Cardiovasc Pharmacol 1988; 244:956–962.

Chapter 8

The Thrombolysis In Myocardial Infarction (TIMI) Trials:
The First Decade

*Christopher P. Cannon, M.D., Eugene Braunwald, M.D.,
Carolyn H. McCabe, B.S., and Elliott M. Antman, M.D.,
for the timi investigators*

*From the Cardiovascular Division, Department of Medicine, Brigham and
Women's Hospital and Harvard Medical School, Boston, Massachusetts*

Introduction

The Thrombolysis in Myocardial Infarction (TIMI) trials are a series of studies begun in 1984, initially under the sponsorship of the National Heart, Lung, and Blood Institute and with data coordination in the first three trials expertly supplied by the Maryland Medical Research Institute. These trials have examined thrombolytic and antithrombotic regimens in acute myocardial infarction (MI) and unstable angina (Table 1). The TIMI 1 trial compared the efficacy of intravenous streptokinase and tissue-type plasminogen activator (tPA) in achieving coronary reperfusion. The TIMI 2 trial examined three strategies for acute MI, focusing on the role of adjunctive angioplasty following thrombolytic therapy, either immediately, at 18–48 hours after enrollment, or as warranted clinically by the development of recurrent ischemia. The TIMI 3 trials explored the role of thrombolytic therapy and of an early invasive strategy in patients with the acute ischemic syndromes of unstable angina and non-Q wave MI. TIMI 4 compared three regimens of thrombolytic therapy, front-loaded tPA, anistreplase, and combination thrombolytic therapy. The

TIMI 5 and 6 trials were pilot trials comparing the new thrombin inhibitor hirudin to heparin given in conjunction with aspirin and tPA or streptokinase, respectively. The TIMI 7 trial was a dose ranging trial of the related thrombin inhibitor, hirulog in patients with unstable angina. The TIMI 8 trial, which was discontinued prematurely, was a double blind trial comparing hirulog to heparin in patients with the acute ischemic syndromes of unstable angina and non-Q wave MI. TIMI 9 is a double blind trial comparing hirudin to heparin in conjunction with thrombolytic therapy and aspirin for acute MI. The TIMI 10 trials will be a series of trials evaluating a more fibrin specific variant of tPA, TNK-tPA.

Together, these TIMI trials have both provided insights into the pathophysiology and clinical course, and provided information that is useful in the treatment of acute MI and unstable angina.

TIMI 1

After initial studies demonstrated that intracoronary streptokinase was able to recanalize occluded coronary arteries, the TIMI 1 trial compared the reperfusion rates of intravenous streptokinase and of the

Table 1.

The TIMI Trials

Trial	Syndrome	Comparison
TIMI 1	Acute MI	t-PA vs. Streptokinase
TIMI 2A	Acute MI	Immediate PTCA vs. delayed PTCA vs. PTCA for recurrent ischemia
TIMI 2B	Acute MI	1. Routine PTCA vs. PTCA for recurrent ischemia
		2. Intravenous vs. delayed beta-blockade
TIMI 3A	Unstable Angina/Non-Q Wave MI	Thrombolytic therapy vs. placebo on lesion severity
TIMI 3B	Unstable Angina/Non-Q Wave MI	1. Thrombolytic therapy vs. placebo
		2. Early invasive vs. early conservative strategy
TIMI 3 Registry	Unstable Angina/Non-Q Wave MI	Natural history study
TIMI 4	Acute MI	Front-loaded t-PA, vs. APSAC vs. combination thrombolytic therapy
TIMI 5	Acute MI	Hirudin vs. heparin with t-PA
TIMI 6	Acute MI	Hirudin vs. heparin with streptokinase
TIMI 7	Unstable Angina	Dose ranging trial of hirulog
TIMI 8	Unstable Angina/Non-Q Wave MI	Hirulog vs. heparin
TIMI 9	Acute MI	Hirudin vs. heparin with thrombolytic therapy
TIMI 9 Registry	Acute MI	Prospective registry of non-thrombolytic treated ST elevation MI patients
TIMI 10	Acute MI	Evaluation of a new thrombolytic agent: TNK-t-PA

newly developed agent, tPA. Two hundred and ninety patients with acute MI underwent initial diagnostic coronary arteriography and were then treated with either streptokinase or tPA in addition to intravenous heparin. The primary end point, reperfusion of initially occluded coronary arteries after 90 minutes, was achieved in 62% of tPA-treated patients compared to 31% of streptokinase-treated patients (P < 0.001) (Fig. 1).[1,4] The patency rate at 90 minutes, independent of findings on baseline arteriogram, was 70% for tPA versus 43% for streptokinase (P < 0.001). TIMI 1 was one of the few trials in which patients had a baseline arteriogram prior to thrombolytic therapy, which allowed comparison of actual reperfusion rates of the different thrombolytic regimens. It also suggested that tPA would be a superior agent in im-

proving outcome, as subsequently shown in the GUSTO-I trial[135] and TIMI 4.[103]

The Open Artery Hypothesis

A second major finding of the TIMI 1 trial was that achieving a patent infarct related artery early after acute MI is important for patient survival. For patients with a patent infarct related artery 90 minutes after the start of thrombolytic therapy, regardless of treatment assignment, there was a lower 6-month (5.6% vs 12.5%) and 1-year mortality (8.1% vs 14.8%).[8] Furthermore, for patients with both early and sustained patency through hospital discharge, the subsequent mortality was extremely low, 3.8% at 1 year.[8] These observations gave early support to the open artery hypothesis[113,136,137] that early reper-

TIMI 1: Comparison of t-PA and Streptokinase

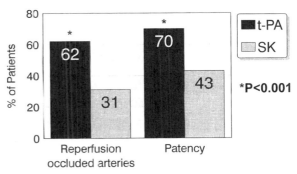

Figure 1. TIMI 1: Rates of coronary reperfusion of initially occluded coronary arteries at 90 minutes and infarct related artery patency for tPA and streptokinase (Data from TIMI Study Group[1]).

fusion decreases infarct size, improves left ventricular function, and improves survival.

TIMI Grade Flow Scoring System

In order to evaluate more carefully the reperfusion achieved by thrombolytic therapy, a grading system of coronary perfusion was developed for use in the TIMI 1 trial,[1] and has subsequently been widely adopted for essentially all angiographic trials of thrombolysis. TIMI grade 0 flow indicates complete occlusion of the coronary artery, while TIMI grade 1 flow denotes some penetration of the obstruction by contrast material, but no perfusion of the distal coronary bed. TIMI grade 2 flow denotes perfusion of the entire coronary artery, but with delayed flow compared to a normal artery; and TIMI grade 3 flow denotes full perfusion with normal flow. The relationship between TIMI flow grade and subsequent mortality was examined in the TIMI 1 trial and it was observed that patients with TIMI grade 3 flow 90 minutes following the onset of thrombolytic therapy had the lowest mortality, 4.7%, compared to 7.0% for patients with TIMI grade 2 flow and 10.6% for patients with TIMI grade 0 or 1 flow (P < 0.005) (Fig. 2).[18] A similar relationship was subsequently observed in the TIMI 4 and 5 trials.[113] In TIMI 4, it was observed that patients with TIMI grade 3 flow 90 minutes following the onset of thrombolytic therapy have a smaller infarct size and a risk of reocclusion one-third that of patients with TIMI grade 2 flow.[105,107] Together with data from other trials,[113,138,139] these findings have helped es-

TIMI 1: Relationship of TIMI Flow Grade at 90 Minutes to 42 Day Mortality

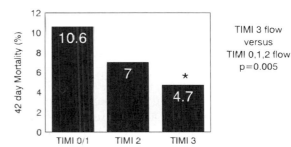

Figure 2. TIMI 1: Relationship of TIMI flow grade 90 minutes following thrombolysis and 42-day mortality (Data from Flygenring BP, et al.[18]).

tablish TIMI grade 3 flow as perhaps the most important end point of thrombolytic efficacy.

TIMI 2: Management Strategies Following Thrombolytic Therapy for Acute MI

In the mid to late 1980s, coronary angioplasty (PTCA) was commonly performed routinely following thrombolytic therapy with the goal of reducing the residual high grade stenosis. The TIMI 2A trial studied 586 patients with acute MI treated with tPA, heparin, and aspirin to evaluate whether an early invasive strategy, involving immediate cardiac catheterization with PTCA when feasible, would be of clinical benefit to patients compared to a delayed invasive strategy with coronary arteriography and PTCA as appropriate at 18–48 hours.[23,48] A third group of patients followed a conservative strategy, with early angiography performed only for recurrent ischemia; all patients underwent follow-up angiography prior to hospital discharge.[48] The TIMI 2B trial treated 3,339 patients with tPA and aspirin who were randomized to either an invasive strategy consisting of coronary arteriography at 18–48 hours followed by PTCA if the anatomy was suitable (i.e., the delayed invasive strategy of TIMI 2A), or to a conservative strategy in which arteriography and PTCA were performed only for recurrent spontaneous ischemia or a positive exercise test.[24,59,63]

TIMI 2A: Immediate Versus Delayed Invasive Strategies

TIMI 2A demonstrated that the outcome, mortality, reinfarction, and patency of the infarct related artery at hospital discharge, following immediate coronary arteriography and PTCA, were no better than those following delayed invasive or conservative strategies.[23,48] Death or reinfarction occurred in 12.8% of the 195 patients in the

early invasive group compared to 8.8% in the 194 patients in the delayed invasive group and 11.7% in the conservative group (P = NS).[23,48] Patency of the infarct related artery at hospital discharge was similar in the three strategies.[48] Complications were higher in the immediate invasive strategy, with a higher rate of emergency coronary artery bypass grafting (CABG) (6.7% vs 1.5%, P = 0.02) and transfusion of ≥ 2 units of blood (20.0% vs 7.2%, P < 0.001) compared to the delayed invasive strategy.[48]

TIMI 2B: Conservative Versus Delayed Invasive Strategies

In TIMI 2B death or recurrent MI through 42 days occurred in 10.9% of patients in the invasive group compared to 9.7% of the conservative group (P = NS).[24] Similarly, no difference between the two strategies was observed through 1 year (Fig. 3A)[59] and then 3 years of follow-up (21.0% death or reinfarction for the invasive strategy vs 20.0% for the conservative strategy, P = NS).[63] In contrast, the rate of revascularization in the two strategies was vastly different: 72.3% of patients in the invasive strategy underwent PTCA or CABG by 1 year, compared to only 35.5% in the conservative strategy (Fig. 3B). Interestingly, this difference was due to more PTCA procedures; the rate of CABG was similar in both groups.

Since approximately 750,000 patients are admitted to an acute care hospital with acute MI, and estimating that two thirds have a Q wave MI, the potential cost savings of following a conservative strategy are astounding. Using a rough estimate of $2,000 for a diagnostic catheterization and $3,000 for a PTCA procedure,[140] this would translate into an annual savings of 2.5 billion dollars. Even when performing a sensitivity analysis and reducing the cost of the procedures by one half, and reducing the estimated number of patients with acute Q wave MI by an additional half, the savings of following a conservative strategy still amounts to $600,000,000.

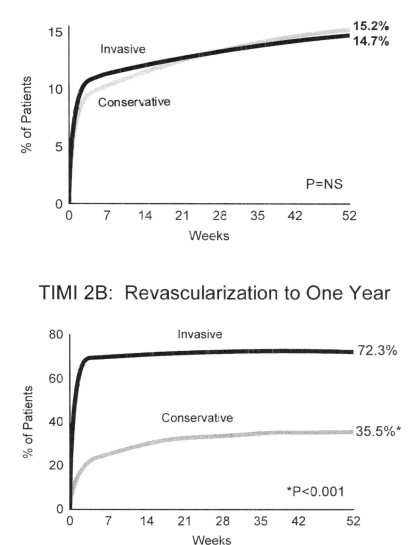

Figure 3. TIMI 2: Rates of death or MI (Panel A) and of revascularization with PTCA or CABG (Panel B) through 1 year of follow-up for patients following an invasive versus conservative strategy. (Adapted from Williams, et al,[59] with permission).

Thus, since both strategies lead to similar long-term outcome, this trial established the "watchful waiting" approach as the preferred strategy for the management of patients treated with thrombolytic therapy for acute MI. This strategy, consisting of initial medical management with the performance of coronary arteriography and revascularization when indicated by recurrent ischemia at rest or on a predischarge exercise test, can be applied to most patients, thereby obviating the need (and cost) of an early invasive strategy for all patients with acute MI.

Early Intravenous Beta-Blockade

The TIMI 2B trial also randomized eligible patients to immediate intravenous followed by oral beta-blockade or to deferred oral beta-blockade.[24] In patients receiving immediate intravenous metoprolol, there was a significant reduction in nonfatal reinfarction (2.3% vs 4.5%, P = 0.02) and recurrent ischemia (15.4% vs 21.2%, P = 0.005) during the first week of therapy, with benefit persisting out to 6 weeks.[54] Intravenous beta-blockade was particularly beneficial in those patients in whom it might be expected to be most effective, i.e., those treated within the first 2 hours of the onset of infarction. In this subgroup, mortality was significantly lower, 5.0% in the intravenous beta-blockade group, compared to 12.1% in the delayed beta-blockade group (P = 0.01).[24] Based on these data, together with the benefit on mortality observed in nonthrombolytic trials, immediate intravenous beta-blockade can be recommended in all patients with acute MI receiving thrombolytic therapy without contraindications.

Intracranial Hemorrhage

Intracranial hemorrhage is one of the most serious complications of thrombolytic therapy. In TIMI 2, a 150-mg dose of tPA was initially given, but this led to a 1.5% rate of intracranial hemorrhage.[24] The dose was then reduced to 100 mg of tPA, which resulted in a 0.5% rate of intracranial hemorrhage.[24,50] Two important risk factors for developing intracranial hemorrhage were identified: age > 60 years (especially > 70 years), and a prior history of neurological disease (either a transient ischemic attack or stroke). When data from TIMI 2 were combined with other major thrombolytic trials,[69] four independent risk factors for intracranial hemorrhage, age > 65, body weight < 70 kg, hypertension at presentation with BP ≥ 170/95, and treatment with tPA.[69] Use of these four risk factors should help identify patients at increased risk for intracranial hemorrhage who might benefit from a less aggressive thrombolytic regimen or an alternate means of reperfusion, e.g., primary angioplasty.

It should be noted, however, that in other thrombolytic trials (e.g., ISIS-2[141] or GUSTO[135]), the overall clinical benefit for the elderly in reduction of cardiovascular mortality outweighs the increased risk of intracranial hemorrhage. In addition, although intracranial hemorrhage is often a devastating complication, it is not uniformly fatal. In TIMI 2, mortality for patients suffering an intracranial hemorrhage was 61% at 1 year, with 31% of patients having either a full recovery or left with only a partial residual neurological deficit.[50]

Relationship of APTT to Patency

Intravenous heparin has been demonstrated in several studies to be important in preventing reocclusion following tPA.[142,143] Because of the known variability of the effect of heparin, the level and consistency of anticoagulation were examined in TIMI 2 with regard to achieving patency of the infarct related artery. The degree of APTT prolongation was important for patency. In patients with a patent infarct related artery at 18–48 hours, the 8-hour mean APTT was higher, 77 seconds, compared to 70 seconds for patients with an occluded artery (P < 0.01).[51] In addition, the stability of the APTT over the first 48 hours was found to be important. Patients with a patent infarct related artery had therapeutic APTT values more frequently than patients with an occluded artery. These data, together with those from TIMI 4,[112] underscore the need for frequent monitoring of the APTT and adjustment of the heparin dose in order to optimize anticoagulation following thrombolytic therapy.[112]

Patient Subgroups and Risk Stratification

The ability to stratify the risk of patients with acute MI may be important in guiding therapy for selected patient subgroups. In TIMI 2, two patient subgroups were prospectively defined, low risk and not low risk, the latter consisting of patients with at least one of the following characteristics: age > 70 years; prior MI; anterior MI; atrial fibrillation/flutter; left bundle branch block; sinus tachycardia and systolic blood pressure < 100 mmHg; pulmonary edema; and cardiogenic shock.[24] Irrespective of treatment assignment, patients with cardiogenic shock or pulmonary edema at presentation, had a six times greater risk of death at 42 days with a mortality of 33.3%.[58] In the remaining patients, the not low risk group had a 42-day mortality of 5.3% compared to 1.5% for low risk patients (P < 0.001). A risk stratification scheme was developed using eight independent risk factors that further defined a patient's risk of mortality: age ≥ 70 years; female gender; diabetes; prior MI; anterior MI; atrial fibrillation; rales > 1/3 lung fields; or hypotension with sinus tachycardia (Fig. 4).[44] Age was observed as a strong individual marker of outcome, with 1-year mortality ranging from 2.8% for patients < 50 years, 6.1% for patients age 50–64, and 13.6% for patients age 65–75 (P = 0.001).[75]

Smokers

A puzzling finding was observed in another subgroup of patients in TIMI 2,

cigarette smokers. Current smokers were found to have a lower mortality, 3.6% compared with 4.8% for ex-smokers, and 8.0% for patients who had never smoked (P < 0.001).[58] Smokers were noted to have a lower risk profile, having their MI at a younger age, and with fewer risk factors (less hypertension, diabetes), but they still had a better outcome after accounting for these differences in a multivariate analysis. In addition, a higher proportion of smokers had the right coronary as the infarct related artery, which could explain part of the better outcome of smokers.[58] A subsequent analysis in the TIMI 4 trial, which included coronary arteriography at 90 minutes, found that current smokers had a higher rate of TIMI grade 3 flow than did ex-smokers and nonsmokers, 55% compared with 43% and 45%, respectively (adjusted P = 0.02).[118] Since a strong relationship exists between early TIMI grade 3 flow and improved survival,[113,137,138] these findings suggest that the lower mortality in current smokers may be related to more complete early reperfusion.[118]

Women

The outcome of acute MI in women has been of great interest in recent years. Studies suggested that an older age at presentation and other co-morbid illness in women with coronary artery disease ac-

Figure 4. TIMI 2: Risk stratification of patients with acute MI. Mortality at 6 weeks could be predicted by number of risk factors present among the following: Age ≥ 70 years, female gender, diabetes, prior MI, anterior MI, atrial fibrillation, rales > 1/3 lung fields, or hypotension with sinus tachycardia.[44] (Data from Hillis, et al.[44]).

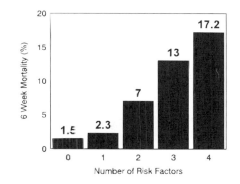

TIMI 2: Risk Factors for Mortality Following Thrombolysis for Acute MI

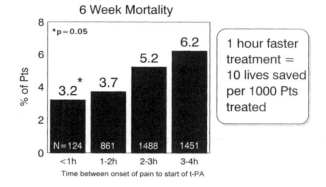

Figure 5. TIMI 2: Effect of time to treatment on 42 day mortality. For each hour earlier that patients were treated, there was an absolute 1% lower mortality, which translates into 10 lives saved for every 1,000 patients treated. (Reproduced from Cannon, et al.[145] with permission).

counted for differences in the outcome in women. In TIMI 2, women had a higher mortality than men at 1 year (12.2% vs 6.1%, P = 0.01) and a higher rate of death or reinfarction at 1 year (21.5% vs 13.5%, P < 0.01).[74] In addition, hemorrhagic complications were higher in women than in men (25.9% vs 13.5%, P < 0.001).[74] Even when correcting for the higher risk baseline characteristics, adjusted mortality remained higher for women (relative risk = 1.54, P = 0.01). Thus, women were found to experience increased mortality and morbidity, with age and other risk factors accounting for a portion, but not all, of the gender related differences in outcome.

Time to Treatment

The importance of early treatment with thrombolytic therapy was first suggested by the GISSI-1 trial, in which patients treated with streptokinase within 1 hour of symptom onset exhibited a 47% reduction in mortality compared with placebo, whereas the entire group of patients in the trial, treated within 12 hours, had a 19% reduction in mortality.[144] The TIMI 2 trial also found a benefit of treatment within the first hour on left ventricular function.[52] More importantly, it was observed in TIMI 2 that for each hour earlier

that a patient received thrombolytic therapy, there was a decrease in the absolute mortality by 1% (Fig. 5).[24,52] These findings have helped focus current attention on developing strategies to rapidly identify and treat patients with acute MI.[145,146]

TIMI 3: Comprehensive Management of Unstable Angina and Non-Q Wave MI

Unstable angina and non-Q wave MI (NQWMI) are at the center of the spectrum of ischemic heart disease, which ranges from stable angina to acute Q wave MI. These two syndromes account for over 1 million hospital admissions in the United States. Because thrombolytic therapy has been shown to be beneficial in the treatment of patients with acute MI presenting with ST elevation, it was hoped that it might play a role in the other acute ischemic syndromes as well. In addition, the appropriate role (and timing) of angiography and revascularization (PTCA or CABG) had not been carefully evaluated in unstable angina and NQWMI. Accordingly, the TIMI 3 trials set out to determine the role of thrombolytic therapy and of an early invasive strategy in these acute ischemic syndromes.

TIMI 3A: Effects of tPA on Coronary Lesions

A total of 391 patients with acute ischemic chest pain and documented coronary artery disease were studied with a baseline coronary arteriogram.[79] Of these, 53 (14%) had no coronary artery with > 60% stenosis,[87] a percentage of patients which has been observed in other trials of acute ischemic syndromes. After 15 patients were excluded because of high risk anatomy, the remaining 306 received heparin and either front-loaded tPA or placebo. Thrombus was visualized definitively in only 35% of patients, a percentage much lower than previously reported, although an additional 40% of patients had mural opacities or eccentric lesions classified as "possible thrombus".[79] Measurable improvement in lesion severity was observed in a similar proportion of patients, 25% following tPA versus 19% following heparin alone (P = 0.25), suggesting that the overall impact of thrombolysis in patients with acute ischemic syndromes would be minimal.[79]

TIMI 3B: Effects of tPA and of an Early Invasive Strategy on Clinical Outcome

In TIMI 3B, 1,473 patients with unstable angina and non-Q wave MI were randomized in a 2 x 2 factorial design to receive either tPA or its placebo and to follow either an early invasive strategy with routine angiography 18–48 hours following randomization with revascularization as appropriate, or an early conservative strategy with angiography and revascularization performed only for recurrent ischemia. All patients received immediate intravenous heparin, aspirin, beta-blockers, calcium antagonists, and nitrates.

Thrombolytic Therapy for Acute Ischemic Syndromes

There was no difference in the primary end point comparing tPA with placebo: the incidence of death; postrandomization infarction; or recurrent, objectively documented ischemia through 6 weeks (54.2% for tPA and 55.5% for placebo, P = NS) (Fig. 6). The incidence of death or MI through 42 days was actually higher (8.8% vs 6.2%, P = 0.05) (Fig. 6).[80] This difference was due to a higher rate of MI in patients with unstable angina, 8.3% for tPA versus 4.6% for placebo (P = 0.01).[80] In addition, tPA was associated with a 0.55% incidence of intracranial hemorrhage.[80] Thus, in the presence of heparin, aspirin, and anti-ischemic therapy, the addition of tPA does not improve clinical outcome, and thus is not indicated in unstable angina or non-Q wave MI.

Figure 6. TIMI 3: Effect of tPA compared with placebo in patients with unstable angina and non-Q wave MI. The incidence of the composite end point (see text) was similar between tPA and placebo. The incidence of death or MI through 42 days was higher in tPA-treated patients. (Data from The TIMI IIIB Investigators[80]).

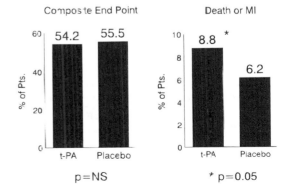

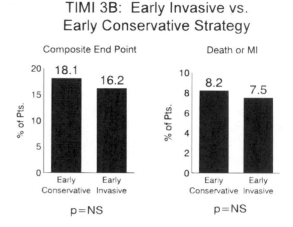

Figure 7. TIMI 3: Comparison of an early invasive vs an early conservative strategy showed no difference in outcome using the prespecified composite end point (see text) or death or MI by 42 days. (Data from The TIMI IIIB Investigators[80]).

Early Invasive Versus Early Conservative Strategy

The primary end point comparing the early invasive and early conservative strategies was the incidence of death, postrandomization infarction, or a positive exercise test at 6 weeks. There was no difference in outcome between the two strategies: 16.2% for the early invasive strategy versus 18.1% for the early conservative strategy (P = NS) (Fig. 7).[80] Similarly, there was no difference in the incidence of death or postrandomization MI (7.5% vs 8.2%, P = NS).[80]

In the early invasive strategy, angiography was carried out 18–48 hours postrandomization in 98% of patients, with revascularization performed in 61% by 6 weeks (38% of the total population had PTCA; 25% had CABG; and 2% had both).[80] In addition, 19% were found not to have a stenosis of > 60% in any coronary artery. In the conservative strategy, catheterization was performed only for recurrent severe ischemia, defined as any one of the following: prolonged ischemia at rest with ECG changes; 20 minutes of ST depression on a Holter monitor; a "high risk" exercise test (early ischemia or ST depression ≥ 0.2 mV); a "high risk" thallium perfusion image; or recurrent unstable angina requiring rehospitalization. Despite this high threshold for recurrent ischemia, 64% of patients underwent cardiac catheterization, with 49% of the total population subsequently undergoing revascularization, evenly split between PTCA and CABG.[80] Posthospital discharge, patients in the early conservative strategy required rehospitalization more frequently and were taking more antianginal medications at the 6-week visit.[80]

At 1 year, the difference in the number of patients who underwent revascularization was even smaller, 6%, with 64% of the early invasive strategy and 58% in the early conservative strategy.[92] Thus, the absolute percentage of patients requiring revascularization was high in the early conservative group, and the relative difference between the two strategies was small.

In summary, TIMI 3B found that in patients with documented unstable angina/non-Q wave infarction, both the early invasive and early conservative strategies led to a similar incidence of serious adverse outcomes, and thus both strategies are suitable for patients with these acute ischemic syndromes. However, since nearly two thirds of patients in the conservative arm required catheterization (despite aggressive [5 drug] medical treatment), the early invasive arm could be viewed as a more expeditious strategy for unstable angina and non-Q wave MI.

Outcome of PTCA

Studies in the 1980s suggested that patients with unstable angina have a worse procedural outcome following PTCA than those with stable angina. However, the results of PTCA in the contemporary era are less clear. In TIMI 3, 444 patients with unstable angina or non-Q wave MI underwent PTCA prior to hospital discharge. The periprocedural complication rate was low: mortality within 24 hours was 0.5%; and the rate of death, MI, CABG, or stroke was 3.8%.[100] Further, pretreatment with tPA did not improve the safety of the procedure, and there was a trend toward increased adverse events.[98] Interestingly, the complication rate was higher in patients with unstable angina than in those with evolving non-Q wave MI.[99] There was no significant difference in outcome between women and men,[102] or between older versus younger patients.[101] While periprocedural outcome was satisfactory, by 1 year, 16.4% of patients in TIMI 3 who underwent PTCA experienced an adverse event,[100] suggesting that more effective medical therapy following PTCA is needed.

TIMI 3 Registry

The TIMI 3 Registry was designed to complement the TIMI 3A and B trials, with the goal of determining the clinical profile and outcome of all patients with unstable angina and non-Q wave MI. Over 9,500 patients with an acute ischemic syndrome were identified and 3,316 patients were enrolled and followed prospectively in the Registry.[81,83,96] To define the natural history, and major predictors of subsequent outcome (death, MI, or recurrent ischemia at 6 weeks), the demographic features of age, gender, and race were examined first. As expected, younger patients (age < 75 years), had a lower rate of adverse events compared to the elderly (age ≥ 75 years; odds ratio = 0.5, P < 0.0001).[83,96] Interestingly, black patients, a high risk

group in acute Q wave MI in the TIMI 2 trial,[65] did not have a higher risk of death, MI, or recurrent ischemia (odds ratio = 0.6, P < 0.001).[83] Women were found to have less severe coronary disease when catheterized, but had a clinical outcome similar to men.[83]

The ECG was also evaluated as a predictor of outcome in unstable angina and non-Q wave MI. Patients presenting with ST depression or transient (reversible) ST elevation on their admission ECG had nearly twice the rate of death or MI at 6 weeks, 9.1%, compared with 4.8% for patients without ST deviation.[88] Patients with T wave inversion did not have a worse prognosis than those without ST or T wave changes (4.8% death or MI at 6 weeks and 4.9%, respectively).[88] Thus, new ST deviation denoted a high risk group of patients with acute ischemic syndromes, but new T wave inversion did not add to the clinical history in predicting outcome.[88]

Two other interesting findings in the TIMI 3 Registry were that women represented 42% of patients with acute ischemic syndromes, a much higher proportion than with acute Q wave MI.[81] When examined in the TIMI 3B and TIMI 2 trials, a clear gradient was observed, with the percentage of women with unstable angina, non-Q wave MI, and Q wave MI being 35%, 27%, and 18%, respectively (P < 0.01).[85] A second observation from the Registry was that, as has been identified in acute MI in the Myocardial Infarction Limitation of Infarct Size (MILIS) trial,[147] and in TIMI 2,[60] a circadian variation exists in the onset of acute ischemic syndromes, with an increase in the number of events occurring between 6:00 am and 12:00 noon (P < 0.0001).[81]

TIMI 4: New Regimens of Thrombolytic Therapy for Acute MI

Although by 1990, thrombolytic therapy had clearly been shown to reduce mortality and morbidity following acute MI, it was uncertain whether more aggressive thrombolytic-antithrombotic therapies could improve outcome compared with standard regimens. Two promising regimens that evolved from pilot studies were front-loaded tPA[148] and combination thrombolytic therapy.[149]

The TIMI 4 trial was a double blind trial of 382 patients with acute MI presenting within 6 hours.[103] Patients were randomized to receive either: front-loaded tPA (15-mg bolus, 50 mg over 30 min, and 35 mg over 60 min)[148]; APSAC (30 U); or combination of tPA (15-mg bolus, and 50 mg over 30 min) and APSAC (20 U), in conjunction with immediate intravenous heparin and aspirin. The primary end point was the "Unsatisfactory Outcome" end point, defined as the occurrence of any of the following events prior to hospital discharge: death; intracranial hemorrhage; severe congestive heart failure or cardiogenic shock; reduced ejection fraction; reinfarction; major spontaneous bleed; TIMI flow < 2 at 90 minutes or 18–36 hours; reocclusion by sestamibi scanning; or anaphylaxis.[103,150]

Patency of the infarct related artery (TIMI grade 2 or 3 flow) at 60 minutes after the start of double blind thrombolytic therapy was significantly higher in tPA-treated patients, 77.8% compared with 59.5% for APSAC-treated patients and 59.3% for combination-treated patients (P = 0.02, tPA vs APSAC; P = 0.03, tPA vs combination) (Fig. 8).[103] At 90 minutes, TIMI grade 3 flow was significantly higher in tPA-treated patients, 60.2%, compared with 42.9% for APSAC and 44.8% for the combination (P < 0.01, tPA vs APSAC; P = 0.02, tPA vs combination). The incidence of Unsatisfactory Outcome was 41.3% for tPA compared with 49.0% for APSAC and 53.6% for the combination (P = 0.19, tPA vs APSAC; P = 0.06, tPA vs combination). Mortality at 1 year was lowest in the tPA-treated patients, 5.3%, compared to 11.0% for APSAC and 10.5% for combination thrombolytic therapy (P = 0.07, tPA vs APSAC; P = 0.13, tPA vs combination).[103]

Thus, front-loaded tPA achieved significantly higher rates of reperfusion at 60 and 90 minutes and was associated with improved overall clinical benefit and survival compared to a standard thrombolytic agent or combination thrombolytic therapy. The findings in this double blind trial are consistent with those observed in the much larger GUSTO-I trial, lending support to the finding of improved outcome with front-loaded tPA. These findings also support the early open artery theory, whereby more rapid reperfusion of the infarct related artery is associated with improved clinical outcome.[113,137] Furthermore, these findings suggest that further improvements in outcome of patients with acute MI might be achieved with more effective thrombolytic-antithrombotic regimens[121] which improve early (and sustained) infarct related artery patency.[103]

Rescue PTCA

Although routine adjunctive PTCA was clearly shown not to be of benefit following thrombolysis in the TIMI 2 trial,[23,24] a strategy of "rescue" PTCA (performed only for persistent occlusion) may be beneficial by establishing early infarct related artery patency. In TIMI 4, the outcome in patients with a patent infarct related artery at 90 minutes following thrombolysis was compared to those with an occluded infarct-related artery at 90 minutes, of whom approximately 50% underwent rescue PTCA at the discretion of the treating physician. In-hospital adverse outcome, defined as death, reinfarction, new onset severe congestive heart failure or cardiogenic shock, or ejection fraction < 40%, was lowest among patients with a patent artery at 90 minutes, 22%, compared with 28.8% for those with an occluded artery at 90 minutes who underwent successful rescue PTCA, and 34.5% in those with an occluded artery at 90 minutes in whom no rescue PTCA was performed.[114] Interestingly, 71% of this latter group had a patent infarct related

TIMI 4: Angiographic Results

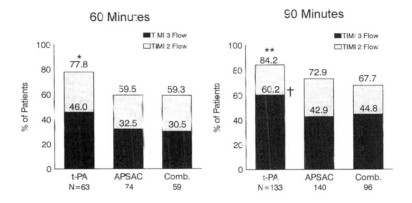

Figure 8. TIMI 4: Angiographic results at 60 and 90 minutes. *P = 0.02, tPA vs APSAC; P = 0.03, tPA vs combination; **P = 0.02, tPA vs APSAC, P < 0.01, tPA vs combination; †P < 0.01, tPA vs APSAC; P = 0.02, tPA vs combination. APSAC = anisoylated plasminogen streptokinase activator complex; Comb = combination thrombolytic therapy; N = number of patients with angiogram performed; TIMI = Thrombolysis in Myocardial Infarction perfusion grade[1]; tPA = tissue-type plasminogen activator. (Reproduced from Cannon, et al.[103], with permission).

artery at the 24-hour follow-up catheterization. Patients with a failed rescue PTCA had a significantly higher adverse outcome, 83.3% (P = 0.01).[114]

These findings are consistent with the open artery hypothesis—both early[113,137,139,151] and late patency being of benefit.[139,152] The patients with patent infarct related arteries at 90 minutes had the best outcome, but those with a successful rescue angioplasty at 120 minutes had the second best outcome (thus, the earlier the reperfusion, the better the improvement). The lack of a greater difference between those with a successful rescue PTCA and those with an occluded artery at 90 minutes in whom PTCA was not performed, was likely due to the high rate of late patency, 71% (i.e., so-called "catch-up") in this group. While myocardial salvage was likely not different between these two groups, both groups derived the later benefits (electrical stability and minimized remodeling)[136,139,152] of a patent infarct related artery.

TIMI Frame Count

To date, the most widely used means of categorizing coronary blood flow in clinical trials has been the TIMI flow grading system, devised in the TIMI 1 trial.[1] However, large interobserver variability in its subjective visual assessment has hampered reproducibility in some trials. In order to provide a more quantitative standardization of coronary blood flow and the TIMI flow grades, Gibson and colleagues developed a new, simple, and objective measure of coronary flow, the so-called TIMI frame count.[115] This method involves counting the number of cineframes for contrast dye to fill the infarct related artery during angiography. The TIMI frame count for patients with TIMI grade 3 flow was 35 ± 13 frames compared to 88 ± 31 frames for TIMI grade 2 flow (P < 0.01).[115] In addition, TIMI frame count correlated with CK determined infarct size, left ventricular function, and most importantly, clinical outcome.[115]

This method offers a means of describing coronary flow as a continuous variable, and allows for standardization of the subjective flow grading, which has been noted to vary between individual observers and even between Core Laboratories.[138,148,153] Use of TIMI frame count should allow a reproducible, quantitative, and clinically relevant measurement of success in clinical trials of thrombolysis.

Noninvasive Assessment of Patency

A third major goal of the TIMI 4 (and TIMI 5) trial was to assess two new, noninvasive tests for determining infarct related artery patency: creatine kinase isoenzyme subforms (CK-MB and CK-MM subforms)[154,155]; and sestamibi radionuclide imaging.[156] The ratio of MB subforms (MB_2/MB_1) and in the rate of rise of MM_3 isoforms were correlated with the angiographic patency at 90 minutes. Preliminary results demonstrated a high sensitivity (up to 91%) for detection of early reperfusion, as well as a high specificity.[104] Since the results of these tests can be obtained within a matter of approximately 30 minutes, it suggests that CK-MM and CK-MB subforms may be a useful noninvasive tool to detect the success or failure of thrombolysis in achieving early reperfusion.

Nonfatal and Composite End Points

Another major goal of the TIMI 4 and TIMI 5 trials was its prospective use of a composite end point to compare new thrombolytic-antithrombotic regimens. While early mortality is obviously the most important end point in thrombolytic trials, its use as the sole end point requires trials of tens of thousands of patients. The use of nonfatal end points in addition to mortality could be used to construct a composite end point that can reduce the sample size of clinical trials.

To address this issue, the nonfatal components of the composite end point, "Unsatisfactory Outcome" was prospec-

tively correlated with 1-year mortality. The unsatisfactory outcome end point was defined as the occurrence of any of the following events prior to hospital discharge: intracranial hemorrhage; severe heart failure/shock; ejection fraction < 40%; reinfarction; major spontaneous bleed; TIMI flow < 2 at 90 minutes or 18–36 hours; reocclusion by sestamibi, or anaphylaxis. A second unsatisfactory outcome end point weights the events according to severity. In TIMI 4, the relative risk of death at 1 year in patients who had a nonfatal component of the unsatisfactory outcome end point prior to discharge was 3.7 (P = 0.002).[109] Results of the weighted end point at hospital discharge also related to 1-year mortality: for scores of 0, 0.1–0.4, > 0.4, the resultant mortality was 7.6%, 18%, and 40%, respectively (P < 0.001).[109] Thus, the nonfatal end point "unsatisfactory outcome" identified patients at high risk for 1-year mortality and can be used as a predictor of survival. Use of composite end points such as the one used in TIMI 4 and 5 should allow evaluation of new thrombolytic-antithrombotic regimens in moderate sized trials, thereby expanding the number of new regimens which can be tested and helping advance progress in the field.

TIMI 5: Hirudin Versus Heparin in Acute MI

Despite the use of aggressive regimens of front-loaded tPA, intravenous heparin and aspirin, failure to achieve initial reperfusion, and reocclusion of the infarct related artery remain major limitations of thrombolytic therapy. Hirudin is a direct thrombin inhibitor which has been shown to be superior to heparin in reducing thrombus formation, enhancing thrombolysis, and reducing reocclusion in experimental models.[157–160] Hirudin selectively binds to thrombin in a 1:1 relationship at two sites: (1) the carboxy-terminus of hirudin binds to the "substrate recognition site" of thrombin—the site where thrombin binds to fibrinogen or the platelet; and (2)

TIMI 5: Angiographic Results

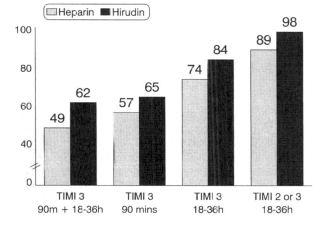

Figure 9. TIMI 5: Angiographic results comparing hirudin and heparin following front-loaded tPA. (Data from Cannon, et al.[121]).

the amino-terminus of hirudin binds to the active catalytic site of thrombin.[161] Recombinant desulfatohirudin (CGP 39393) is identical to hirudin except for a missing sulfate group on the tyrosine 63.[162] The binding of hirudin to thrombin inhibits all of the major actions of thrombin including the cleavage of fibrinogen to fibrin, activation of platelets, and the activation of thrombin's own positive amplification reactions.[162,163] Given the promising experimental results, the TIMI investigators set out to examine the effects of hirudin in patients with acute MI.

The TIMI 5 trial was a randomized, dose ranging, pilot trial of recombinant desulfatohirudin (hirudin) versus heparin given in conjunction with front-loaded tPA and aspirin to 246 patients with acute MI.[121] Patients received a 5-day infusion of either intravenous heparin (5,000-U bolus; 1,000 U/hour titrated to an APTT of 65–90 sec) or hirudin (at 1 of 4 doses ranging from 0.15 mg/kg bolus with a 0.05 mg/kg per hour infusion up to 0.6 mg/kg bolus with a 0.2 mg/kg per hour infusion). Coronary angiography was performed at 90 minutes and 18–36 hours, unless rescue angioplasty was performed.

The primary end point, TIMI grade 3 flow at 90 minutes and 18–36 hours, without death or reinfarction, which could be termed "optimal thrombolysis", was achieved in 61.8% of hirudin patients compared to 49.4% of heparin patients (Fig. 9).[121] There was a trend favoring hirudin for TIMI grade 3 flow at 90 minutes, which was achieved in 64.8% of patients in all hirudin doses combined compared with 57.1% of heparin patients. At 18–36 hours, infarct related artery patency was significantly higher, 98%, in the hirudin-treated patients who underwent follow-up angiography compared with 89% in heparin-treated patients (P = 0.01) (Fig. 9). Importantly, reocclusion by 18–36 hours was only 1.6% for hirudin compared with 6.7% in the heparin group (P = 0.07).[121] The clinical end point of death or recurrent MI during hospitalization followed the same trend, occurring in 6.8% of hirudin-treated patients compared with 16.7% of heparin-treated patients (P = 0.02).[121]

TIMI 5: Variability in APTT

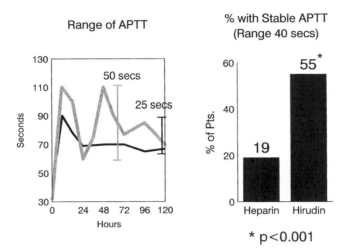

Figure 10. TIMI 5: The stability of APTT in hirudin vs heparin treated patients. Two example patients are shown on the left. The percentage of patients who had a stable APTT during the entire infusion was far greater in the hirudin-treated patients: 55% compared to only 19% of heparin patients ($P < 0.001$). (Data from Cannon, et al.[121]).

Stability of Anticoagulation

One possible explanation of the favorable effects of hirudin observed is that this drug achieved a very consistent level of anticoagulation. Unlike heparin, with which wide fluctuations in APTT are common, hirudin maintained a stable APTT throughout the infusion period in a far greater proportion of patients than did heparin (Fig. 10).[121] With a more stable APTT, hirudin would avoid periods of inadequate anticoagulation, which have been shown to have adverse consequences on patency.[164,165] Interestingly, this stability of anticoagulation may be due, in part, to a lack of circadian variation in the anticoagulant effect,[128] which has been observed to attenuate the effects of heparin.[166]

Major Hemorrhage

Major spontaneous hemorrhage occurred in 1% of hirudin patients versus 5% of heparin patients and major hemorrhage at an instrumented site occurred in 16% of

hirudin versus 19% of heparin patients.[121] There was however, a nonsignificantly higher rate of instrumented site hemorrhage at the highest dose of hirudin (0.2 mg/kg per hour infusion), 29%. Further analysis has demonstrated that the APTT is a good predictor of major hemorrhage, with increased bleeding when the APTT exceeds 100 seconds.[126] This finding, together with the observations in TIMI 9A (see below), the hirudin is now being titrated to avoid excessive APTT values.

TIMI 6: Hirudin with Streptokinase in Acute MI

The TIMI 6 trial was a dose ranging, pilot trial of hirudin given in conjunction with streptokinase and aspirin.[129] In a trial of 193 patients, three doses of hirudin were tested (boluses of 0.15, 0.3–0.6 mg/kg, and infusion rates of 0.05, 0.1, and 0.2 mg/kg per hour) with a heparin comparison group. Although the pilot trial was not sized to detect differences in efficacy, favorable trends were observed (Fig. 11). The in-

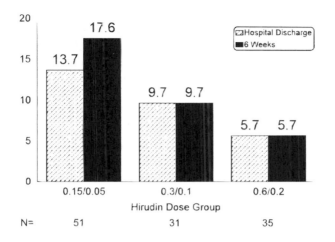

Figure 11. TIMI 6: A pilot trial of hirudin with streptokinase in acute MI. The incidence of death or recurrent MI across the three hirudin dose groups. (Data from Lee, et al.[129]).

hospital incidence of death, MI, or new onset of severe congestive heart failure or cardiogenic shock was 21.6%, 9.7%, and 11.4% of hirudin-treated patients in the three ascending dose groups, respectively, compared with 17.6% of heparin-treated patients.[129] Major hemorrhage, either spontaneous or at an instrumented site, occurred in-hospital in 5.5%, 6.5%, and 5.6% of hirudin-treated patients and 5.6% of heparin-treated patients.[129] Thus, the TIMI 5 and 6 trials suggested favorable initial results with hirudin as adjunctive therapy to thrombolysis.

TIMI 7: Hirulog in Unstable Angina

Because antithrombotic therapy with aspirin and heparin has improved the outcome of patients with unstable angina, the use of the more potent selective thrombin inhibitors is hoped to improve outcome even further. Hirulog is a 20 amino acid, synthetic peptide that, like hirudin, binds selectively to thrombin and is a direct, specific inhibitor of both circulating and clot-bound thrombin.[167] In preliminary testing,

hirulog was found to have a potent yet well-tolerated anticoagulant profile in patients with coronary artery disease.[167]

The TIMI 7 trial was a multicenter, randomized, double blind, dose ranging, trial to compare the safety and efficacy of 72 hours of treatment with four doses of hirulog in patients with unstable angina. Patients received an infusion of one of four doses of hirulog (Hirulog): 0.02, 0.25, 0.5, and 1.0 mg/kg per hour. The incidence of death or MI at hospital discharge was 10.6% in the 160 patients who received the lowest dose group and 3.6% in the 250 who received one of the higher doses (P < 0.004).[130] At 6 weeks, death or MI occurred in 12.5% of the low dose group compared with 5.6% of the higher dose group (P < 0.013).[130] Only 0.2% of patients required discontinuation of hirulog due to a hemorrhagic event.

TIMI 8: Hirulog Versus Heparin in Unstable Angina and Non-Q Wave MI

Based on the favorable findings of the TIMI 7 trial, TIMI 8 was designed as a multicenter, randomized, double blind trial to compare the efficacy and safety of intravenous hirulog with intravenous heparin in patients with unstable angina and non-Q wave MI. It was planned to enroll 5,300 patients with the acute ischemic syndromes. However, soon after enrollment began, the trial was discontinued by the sponsor for business related reasons. Thus, a definitive trial is still needed to evaluate more fully the potential benefit of this direct thrombin inhibitor.

TIMI 9: Hirudin Versus Heparin with Thrombolysis in Acute MI

TIMI 9 is a multicenter, randomized, double blind trial to compare the efficacy and safety of intravenous hirudin to intravenous heparin when given in conjunction with thrombolytic therapy to patients with acute MI. Patients with suspected acute MI presenting within 12 hours of symptom onset who are considered candidates for thrombolytic therapy and meet eligibility criteria are randomized to receive either intravenous hirudin or heparin, given as a bolus followed by a continuous infusion for a minimum of 96 hours. The choice of thrombolytic agent is at the discretion of the investigator, but must be one of the reg-imens specified in the protocol. All patients receive 150–325 mg of aspirin daily.

Safety Observations

Although hirudin appeared to be quite safe in the relatively small phase II trials (TIMI 5 and TIMI 6), a bolus dose of 0.6 mg/kg followed by an infusion of 0.2 mg/kg per hour together with a throm-bolytic agent and aspirin in the TIMI 9A was associated with an excess of bleeding (as was a higher dose of heparin). The incidence of intracranial hemorrhage was 1.7% in hirudin-treated patients and 1.9% in heparin-treated patients (P = NS).[133] Major spontaneous hemorrhage was also higher than expected, 7.0% for hirudin and 3.0% for heparin (P = 0.02).[133] Similar findings were observed in the GUSTO IIa and HIT III trials.[168,169] These findings have led to a reduction of the dose of hirudin in TIMI 9B (and GUSTO IIb) to a bolus of 0.1 mg/kg followed by an infusion of 0.1 mg/kg per hour. Further, because the APTT appears to correlate with hemorrhagic events,[126] the hirudin and heparin infusions are adjusted to maintain an APTT of 55–85 seconds, using the nomogram in Table 2.[133]

The findings of TIMI 9A demonstrated that in patients treated with thrombolytic therapy and aspirin, there appears to be a

Table 2.

Nomogram for Titration of Intravenous Heparin in the TIMI 9 and TIMI 10 Trials

APTT (Secs)	Repeat Bolus Dose	Stop Infusion (Minutes)	Rate Change (cc\hr)*	Rate Change (U/hr)
<55	5000 IU	0	+4	+200
55–85	0	0	0	0
86–95	0	0	−2	−100
96–120	0	30	−2	−100
>120	0	60	−4	−200

*assuming a concentration of 50 units/cc of heparin

APTT is checked at 6, 12, 24 hours post initiation of heparin, daily thereafter, and 4–6 hours following any adjustment in dose. Following thrombolytic therapy, only upward titration is suggested at the 6 hour time point.

safety ceiling for anticoagulation—for both heparin and hirudin. At higher levels of anticoagulation, with either hirudin or heparin, there is an excess of bleeding and intracranial hemorrhage and thus it is especially important to maintain the level of anticoagulation within the therapeutic window, between inadequate[164,165] and excessive anticoagulation. In TIMI 9B, using the lower dose of hirudin, it should be possible to safely test the "thrombin hypothesis": that the benefits of hirudin in inhibiting clot-bound thrombin will translate into improved clinical outcome following acute MI.

TIMI 10: TNK-tPA in Acute MI

A new, modified molecule of tissue plasminogen activator, so called TNK-tPA, has recently been developed, which appears to offer several potential advantages over current thrombolytic agents.[170] First, TNK has an 80-fold higher resistance to inhibition by plasminogen activator inhibitor 1 (PAI-1) than standard tPA (alteplase). In addition, TNK is 10 times more fibrin specific and on a per milligram weight basis, is approximately 8–10 times more potent at fibrinolysis. Finally, TNK has a more prolonged half-life and can be administered as a single intravenous bolus.[170]

In animal testing, TNK compared favorably to front-loaded tPA in achieving early reperfusion.[171] Time to reperfusion in a rabbit carotid occlusion model was 26.6 ± 7.4 minutes for tPA compared with 11.0 ±

1.5 minutes for TNK (P = 0.04).[171] Total duration of reperfusion was also improved, from 65.4 ± 12.9 minutes for tPA to 107 ± 1.4 minutes for TNK (P = 0.01), as was total thrombus weight. There appeared to be less bleeding following TNK compared with tPA.[171] Thus, TNK appears to be a promising new thrombolytic agent for use in treatment of acute MI. The TIMI 10 trials will be a series of trials, beginning with Phase 1, which will examine the effects of TNK in patients with acute MI.

TIMI: The Next Decade

Over the past decade, the TIMI trials have examined many new medical regimens and treatment strategies for acute MI and unstable angina. In addition, many new insights into the pathophysiology and prognosis of patients of these syndromes have emerged from the trials. The current and future TIMI trials will hopefully lead to the development of more effective and safer thrombolytic and antithrombotic regimens, with the ultimate goal of continuing to improve the outcome of patients with MI and acute ischemic syndromes.

Acknowledgments: We acknowledge with appreciation the very important contributions made by Dr. Genell Knatterud and her staff at the Maryland Medical Research Institute, as well as Drs Eugene Passamani and Patrice Desvigne-Nickens at the National Heart, Lung, and Blood Institute, to the first three TIMI trials.

References

Comprehensive List of TIMI References

TIMI 1

1. TIMI Study Group. The Thrombolysis in Myocardial Infarction (TIMI) Trial; Phase I findings. N Engl J Med 1985;312:932–936.

2. Hillis LD, Borer J, Braunwald E, et al. High dose intravenous streptokinase for acute myocardial infarction: Preliminary results of a multicenter trial. JACC 1985;6:957–962.

3. Williams DO, Borer J, Braunwald E, et al. Intravenous recombinant tissue-

type plasminogen activator in acute myocardial infarction: A report from the NHLBI thrombolysis in myocardial infarction trial. Circulation 1986;73:338–346.

4. Chesebro JH, Knatterud G, Roberts R, et al. Thrombolysis in Myocardial Infarction (TIMI) Trial, Phase 1: A comparison between intravenous tissue plasminogen activator and intravenous streptokinase. Circulation 1987;76:142–154.

5. Sheehan F, Braunwald E, Canner P, et al. The effect of intravenous thrombolytic therapy on left ventricular function: A report on tissue plasminogen activator and streptokinase from the Thrombolysis in Myocardial Infarction (TIMI Phase I) trial. Circulation 1987;75:817–829.

6. Bennett WR, Yawn DH, Migliore PJ, et al. Activation of the complement system by recombinant tissue plasminogen activator. JACC 1987;10:627–632.

7. Gore JM, Roberts R, Ball SP, et al. Peak creatine kinase as a measure of effectiveness of thrombolytic therapy in acute myocardial infarction. Am J Cardiol 1987;59:1234–1238.

8. Dalen JE, Gore JM, Braunwald E, et al. Six- and twelve-month follow-up of the Phase I Thrombolysis in Myocardial Infarction (TIMI) Trial. Am J Cardiol 1988;62:179–185.

9. Held AC, Gore JM, Paraskos LA, et al. Impact of thrombolytic therapy on left ventricular mural thrombi in acute myocardial infarction. Am J Cardiol 1988;62:310–311.

10. Holmes J D.R., Bove AA, Nishimura RA, et al. Comparison of monoplane and biplane assessment of regional left ventricular wall motion after thrombolytic therapy for acute myocardial infarction. Am J Cardiol 1987;59:793–797.

11. Owen J, Friedman KD, Grossman BA, et al. Quantitation of fragment X formation during thrombolytic therapy with streptokinase and tissue plasminogen activator. J Clin Invest 1987;79:1642–1647.

12. Robertson TL. Myocardial infarction: Systemic thrombolysis in the U.S.A. Eur Heart J 1987;8(Suppl F):67–71.

13. Rao AK, Pratt C, Berke A, et al. Thrombolysis in Myocardial Infarction (TIMI) Trial—Phase I: Hemorrhagic manifestations and changes in plasma fibrinogen and fibrinolytic system in patients treated with recombinant tissue plasminogen activator and streptokinase. JACC 1988;11:1–11.

14. Ong L, Coromilas J, Zimmerman JM, et al. A physiologically based model of creatine kinase-MB release in reperfusion of acute myocardial infarction. Am J Cardiol 1989;64:11–15.

15. Wackers FJT, Terrin ML, Kayden DS, et al. Quantitative radionuclide assessment of regional ventricular function after thrombolytic therapy for acute myocardial infarction: Results of Phase I Thrombolysis in Myocardial Infacrtion (TIMI) Trial. JACC 1989;13:998–1005.

16. Ockene IS, Miner J, Shannon TA, et al. The consent process in the Thrombolysis in Myocardial Infarction (TIMI Phase I) Trial. Clin Res 1991;39:13–17.

17. Habib GB, Heibig J, Forman SA, et al. Influence of coronary collateral vessels on myocardial infarct size in humans. Results of Phase I Thrombolysis in Myocardial Infarction (TIMI) trial. Circulation 1991;83:739–746.

18. Flygenring BP, Sheehan FH, Kennedy JW, et al. for the TIMI Investigators. Does arterial patency 90 minutes following thrombolytic therapy predict 42 day survival? (Abstract) JACC 1991;17(Suppl A):275A.

19. Lenfant C. The rtPA versus streptokinase controversy-I. (Letter) JACC 1992;19:1116.

20. Braunwald E, Knatterud GL, Passamani E. The rtPA versus streptokinase controversy-II. (Letter) JACC 1992;19:1116–1119.

21. Lehmann KG, Francis CK, Dodge HT, et al. Mitral regurgitation in early myocardial infarction: Incidence, clinical detection, and prognostic implications (TIMI I). Ann Intern Med 1992;117:10–17.

22. Lehmann KG, Francis CK, Sheehan FH, et al. Effect of thrombolysis on acute mitral regurgitation during evolving myocardial infarction. Experience from Thrombolysis in Myocardial Infarction (TIMI) Trial. JACC 1993;22:714–719.

TIMI 2

23. TIMI Research Group. Immediate vs delayed catheterization and angioplasty following thrombolytic therapy

for acute myocardial infarction. TIMI II A results. JAMA 1988;260: 2849–2858.

24. TIMI Study Group. Comparison of invasive and conservative strategies after treatment with intravenous tissue plasminogen activator in acute myocardial infarction. Results of the Thrombolysis in Myocardial Infarction (TIMI) Phase II Trial. N Engl J Med 1989;320:618–627.

25. Knatterud GL, Forman SA. Patient recruitment experience in the Thrombolysis in Myocardial Infarction Trial. Control Clin Trials 1987;8:86S–93S.

26. Mueller HS, Rao AK, Forman SA, et al. Thrombolysis in Myocardial Infarction (TIMI): Comparative studies of coronary reperfusion and systemic fibrinogenolysis with two forms of recombinant tissue-type plasminogen activator. JACC 1987;10:479–490.

27. Williams DO, Ruocco NA, Forman S, et al. Coronary angioplasty after recombinant tissue-type plasminogen activator in acute myocardial infarction: A report from the Thrombolysis in Myocardial Infarction (TIMI) Trial. JACC 1987;10:45B–50B.

28. TIMI Operations Committee: Braunwald E, Knatterud GL, Passamani E, et al. Update from the Thrombolysis in Myocardial Infarction Trial. (Letter) JACC 1987;10:970.

29. Passamani E, Hodges M, Grose R, et al. The Thrombolysis and Myocardial Infarction (TIMI) Phase II Pilot Study: Tissue plasminogen activator followed by percutaneous transluminal coronary angioplasty. JACC 1987;10:51B–64B.

30. TIMI Operations Committee: Braunwald E, Knatterud GL, Passamani ER, et al. Announcement of protocol change in Thrombolysis in Myocardial Infarction (TIMI) Trial. (Letter) JACC 1987;9:467.

31. Eisenberg PR, Sobel BE, Jaffe AS. Characterization of vivo of the fibrin specificity of activators of the fibrinolytic system. Circulation 1988;78:592–597.

32. Kayden DS, Mattera JA, Zaret BL, et al. Demonstration of reperfusion after thrombolysis with technetium-99m isonitrile myocardial imaging. J Nucl Med 1988;29:1865–1867.

33. Gibbons RJ, Verani MS, Behrenbeck T, et al. Feasibility of tomographic

99mTc-hexakis-2-methoxy-2-methyl-propyl-isonitrile imaging for the assessment of myocardial area at risk and the effect of treatment in acute myocardial infarction. Circulation 1989;80:1277–1286.

34. Gertz SD, Kalan JM, Kragel AH, et al. Cardiac morphologic findings in patients with acute myocardial infarction treated with recombinant tissue plasminogen activator. Am J Cardiol 1989;65:953–961.

35. Chaitman BR, Thompson B, Wittry MD, et al. The use of tissue type plasminogen activator for acute myocardial infarction in the elderly: Results from Thrombolysis in Myocardial Infarction Phase I, Open Label Studies and the Thrombolysis in Myocardial Infarction Phase II Pilot Study. JACC 1989;65:953–961.

36. Wackers FJT, Gibbons RJ, Verani MS, et al. Serial quantitative planar technetium-99m isonitrile imaging in acute myocardial infarction: Efficacy for noninvasive assessment of thrombolytic therapy. JACC 1989;14:861–873.

37. Gore JM, Corrao JM, Goldberg RJ, et al. Feasibility and safety of emergency interhospital transport of patients during early hours of acute myocardial infarction. Arch Intern Med 1989;149:353–355.

38. Rogers WJ, Bourge RC, Papapietro SE, et al. Variables predictive of good functional outcome following thrombolytic therapy in the Thrombolysis in Myocardial Infarction Phase II (TIMI II) Pilot Study. Am J Cardiol 1989;63:503–512.

39. Sharkey SW, Brunette DD, Ruiz E, et al. An analysis of time delays preceding thrombolysis for acute myocardial infarction. JAMA 1989;262:3171–3174.

40. Feit F, Mueller HS, Braunwald E, et al. Thrombolysis in Myocardial Infarction (TIMI) Phase II Trial: Outcome comparison of a "conservative strategy" in community versus tertiary hospitals. JACC 1990;16:1529–1534.

41. Lawler CM, Bovill EG, Stump DC, et al. Fibrin fragment D-Dimer and fibrinogen B-beta peptides in plasma as markers of clot lysis during thrombolytic therapy in acute myocardial infarction. Blood 1990;76:1341–1348.

42. Gertz SD, Kragel AH, Kalan JM, et al. Comparison of coronary amd myocar-

dial morphologic findings in patients with and without thrombolytic therapy during fatal first acute myocardial infarction. JACC 1990;66:904–909.

43. Baim DS, Braunwald E, Feit F, et al. The Thrombolysis in Myocardial Infarction (TIMI) Trial Phase II: Additional information and perspectives. JACC 1990;15:1188–1192.

44. Hillis LD, Forman S, Braunwald E, et al. Risk stratification before thrombolytic therapy in patients with acute myocardial infarction. JACC 1990;16:313–315.

45. Johnson LL, Seldin DW, Keller AM, et al. Dual isotope thallium and Indium antimyosin SPECT imaging to identify acute infarct patients at further ischemic risk. Circulation 1990;81:37–45.

46. Chaitman BR, Thompson BW, Kern MJ, et al. Tissue plasminogen activator followed by percutaneous transluminal coronary angioplasty: One year TIMI phase II pilot results. Am Heart J 1990;119:213–223.

47. Kayden DS, Wackers FJT, Zaret BL. Silent left ventricular dysfunction during routine activity after thrombolytic therapy for acute myocardial infarction. JACC 1990;15:1500–1507.

48. Rogers WJ, Baim DS, Gore JM, et al. Comparison of immediate invasive, delayed invasive, and conservative strategies after tissue-type plasminogen activator. Results of the Thrombolysis in Myocardial Infarction (TIMI) Phase II-A Trial. Circulation 1990;81:1457–1476.

49. Bovill EG, Terrin ML, Stump DC, et al. Hemorrhagic events during therapy with recombinant tissue-type plasminogen activator, heparin, and aspirin for acute myocardial infarction. Results of the Thrombolysis in Myocardial Infarction (TIMI), Phase II trial. Ann Intern Med 1991;115:256–265.

50. Gore JM, Sloan M, Price T, et al. Intracerebral hemorrhage, cerebral infarction, and subdural hematoma after acute myocardial infarction and thrombolytic therapy in the Thrombolysis in Myocardial Infarction Study. Thrombolysis in Myocardial Infarction, Phase II, pilot and clinical trial. Circulation 1991;83:448–459.

51. Tracy RP, Kleiman N, Thompson BW, et al. Relationship of coagulation parameters to patency at 18–48 hours in the Thrombolysis in Myocardial Infarction Phase II Trial. (Abstract) Clin Res 1991;39:239A.

52. Timm TC, Ross R, McKendall GR, et al. Left ventricular function and early cardiac events as a function of time to treatment with tPA: A report from TIMI II. (Abstract) Circulation 1991;84:II-230.

53. Zaret BL, Wackers FJ, Terrin M, et al. Does left ventricular ejection fraction following thrombolytic therapy have the same prognostic impact described in the prethrombolytic era? Results of the TIMI II trial. (Abstract) JACC 1991;17(2):214A.

54. Roberts R, Rogers WJ, Meuller HS, et al. Immediate versus deferred B-blockade following thrombolytic therapy in patients with acute myocardial infarction: Results of the Thrombolysis in Myocardial Infarction (TIMI) II-B Study. Circulation 1991;83:422–437.

55. Kleiman NS, Terrin M, Mueller H, et al. Mechanism of early death despite thrombolytic therapy: Experience from the Thrombolysis in Myocardial Infarction Investigation Phase II (TIMI II) Study. JACC 1992;19:1129–1135.

56. Zaret BL, Wackers FJT, Terrin ML, et al. Assessment of global and regional left ventricular performance at rest and during exercise following thrombolytic therapy for acute myocardial infarction: Results of the Thrombolysis in Myocardial Infarction (TIMI II) Study. Am J Cardiol 1992;69:1–9.

57. Ruocco NA Jr, Bergelson BA, Jacobs AK, et al. Invasive versus conservative strategy post thrombolytic therapy for acute myocardial infarction in patients with antecedent angina. A report from Thrombolysis in Myocardial Infarction II. JACC 1992;20:1445–1451.

58. Mueller HS, Cohen LS, Braunwald E, et al. Predictors of early morbidity and mortality after thrombolytic therapy of acute myocardial infarction. Analyses of patient subgroups in the Thrombolysis in Myocardial Infarction (TIMI) Trial, Phase II. Circulation 1992;85:1254–1264.

59. Williams DO, Braunwald E, Knatterud G, et al. One-year results of the Thrombolysis in Myocardial Infarction Investigation (TIMI) phase II trial. Circulation 1992;85(2):533–542.

60. Tofler GH, Muller JE, Stone PH, et al. Modifiers of Timing and Possible Triggers of Acute Myocardial Infarction in the Thrombolysis in Myocardial Infarction Phase II (TIMI) Study Group. JACC 1992;20:1049–1055.

61. Baim DS, Diver DJ, Feit F, et al. Coronary angioplasty performed within the Thrombolysis in Myocardial Infarction (TIMI II) Study. Circulation 1992;85:93–105.

62. Berger PB, Ruocco NA Jr, Ryan TJ, et al. The incidence and prognostic implications of heart block complicating inferior myocardial infarction treated with thrombolytic therapy: Results from TIMI II. JACC 1992;20:533–540.

63. Terrin ML, Williams DO, Kleiman NS, et al. Two- and three-year results of the Thrombolysis in Myocardial Infarction (TIMI) Phase II clinical trial. JACC 1993;22:1763–1772

64. Chaitman BR, McMahon RP, Terrin M, et al. Impact of treatment strategy on predischarge exercise test in the thrombolysis in myocardial infarction (TIMI) II trial. Am J Cardiol 1993;71:131–138.

65. Taylor HA, Chaitman BR, Rogers WJ, et al. Race and prognosis after myocardial infarction: Results of the Thrombolysis in Myocardial Infarction (TIMI) Phase II trial. Circulation 1993;88(Part I):1484–1494.

66. Berger PB, Ruocco NA, Ryan TJ, et al. The frequency and significance of right ventricular dysfunction during inferior wall left ventricular myocardial infarction treated with thrombolytic therapy: Results from the Thrombolysis in Myocardial Infarction (TIMI) II Trial. Am J Cardiol 1993;71:1148–1152.

67. Berger PB, Ruocco NA, Ryan TJ, et al. The incidence and significance of ventricular tachycardia and fibrillation in the absence of hypotension or heart failure in acute myocardial infarction treated with rtPA: Results from the TIMI II trial. JACC 1993;22:1773–1779.

68. Mueller HS, Forman SA, Manegus MA, et al. Prognostic significance of nonfatal reinfarction in TIMI II. (Abstract) Circulation 1993;88:I-490.

69. Simoons ML, Maggioni AP, Knatterud G, et al. Individual risk assessment for intracranial hemorrhage during thrombolytic therapy. Lancet 1993;342:1523–1528.

70. McKendall GR, Forman S, Sopko G, et al. The value of rescue PTCA following unsuccessful thrombolytic therapy: A report from TIMI. (Abstract) JACC 1993;21(Suppl A):396A.

71. Schweiger MJ, McMahon RP, Terrin ML, et al. Comparison of patients with < 60% to ≥ 60% diameter narrowing of the myocardial infarct-related artery after thrombolysis. Am J Cardiol 1994;74:105–110.

72. Hall C, Cannon CP, Forman S, et al. Prognostic value of N-terminal proatrial natriuretic factor plasma levels measured within the first 12 hours after myocardial infarction. (Abstract) Circulation 1994;90(Pt. 2):I-110.

73. Cox DA, Rogers WJ, Aguirre FV, et al. Effect on outcome of the presence or absence of chest pain at initiation of tissue plasminogen activator therapy in acute myocardial infarction. Am J Cardiol 1994;73:729–736.

74. Becker RC, Terrin M, Ross R, et al. Comparison of clinical outcomes for women and men after acute myocardial infarction. Ann Intern Med 1994;120:638–645.

75. Aguirre FV, McMahon RP, Mueller H, et al. Impact of age on clinical outcome and postlytic management strategies in patients treated with thrombolytic therapy. Results from the TIMI II study. Circulation 1994;90:78–86.

76. Gersh BJ, Chesebro JH, Braunwald E, et al. Coronary artery bypass surgery after thrombolytic therapy in the Thrombolysis in Myocardial Infarction Trial, Phase II (TIMI II). JACC 1995;25:395–402.

77. Aguirre FV, McMahon RP, Berger P, et al. Clinical characteristics, angiographic findings, and clinical outcome among patients evolving Q wave and non-Q wave myocardial infarction following thrombolysis: Results from the TIMI II Study. Circulation 1995 (in press).

78. Sloan MA, Price TR, Petito CK, et al. Clinical features and pathogenesis of intracerebral hemorrhage after rtPA and heparin therapy for acute myocardial infarction: The TIMI II pilot and randomized trial combined experience. Neurology 1995 (in press).

TIMI 3

79. The TIMI IIIA Investigators. Early effects of tissue-type plasminogen activator added to conventional therapy on the culprit lesion in patients presenting with ischemic cardiac pain at rest. Results of the Thrombolysis in Myocardial Ischemia (TIMI IIIA) Trial. Circulation 1993;87:38–52.

80. The TIMI IIIB Investigators. Effects of tissue plasminogen activator and a comparison of early invasive and conservative strategies in unstable angina and non-Q-wave myocardial infarction: Results of the TIMI IIIB Trial. Circulation 1994;89:1545–1556.

81. Cannon CP, Theroux P, Gibson R, et al. Clinical profile of 4600 patients with unstable angina and non-Q wave MI: Results of the TIMI-3 Registry. (Abstract) Circulation 1992;86(Suppl I):I-387.

82. Cannon CP, Thompson B, McCabe CH, et al. Predictors of non-Q wave myocardial infarction in patients with acute ischemic syndromes: An analysis from the Thrombolysis in Myocardial Ischemia—TIMI III Trials. Am J Cardiol 1995 (in press).

83. Stone P, Kleiman N, Kronenberg M, et al. Effect of gender, race, and age on the natural history of unstable angina and non-Q wave MI: The T3 Registry. (Abstract) JACC 1993;21(Suppl A):453A.

84. Kleiman NS, Anderson HV, Thompson B, et al. Patients with unstable angina and prior bypass grafting have higher rates of death and rehospitalization: Results of the T3 Registry. (Abstract) JACC 1993;21(Suppl A):196A.

85. McCabe CH, Prior MJ, Fraulini T, et al. Gender differences between patients with acute MI, non-Q wave MI, and unstable angina—Results from TIMI II and T3B. (Abstract) JACC 1993;21(Suppl A):271A.

86. Diver DJ, Brown BG, Breall JA, et al. Characterization of patient management and outcome in the TIMI-IIIA trial. (Abstract) JACC 1994;(Special Issue):289A.

87. Diver DJ, Bier JD, Ferreira PE, et al. Clinical and arteriographic characterization of patients with unstable angina without critical coronary arterial narrowing (from the TIMI-IIIA trial). Am J Cardiol 1994;74:531–537.

88. Cannon CP, Stone PH, Rogers WJ, et al. The ECG as a predictor of outcome in acute coronary syndromes. Results of the TIMI III Registry ECG Ancillary Study. (Abstract) JACC 1994;(Special Issue):196A.

89. Becker R, Tracy R, Bovill E, et al. Should aPTT assays be standardized in multicenter clinical trials designed to investigate the benefits of heparin? (Abstract) JACC 1994;(Special Issue):57A.

90. Becker R, Tracy R, Thompson B, et al. Anticoagulation profile in heparinized patients with unstable angina and non-Q wave myocardial infarction experiencing clinical events. (Abstract) Circulation 1994;90(Pt. 2):I-664.

91. Gibson RS, Thompson BW, Buckley RS, et al. Differences in practice patterns between USA and Canada for management of unstable angina and acute non-Q wave infarction. (Abstract) JACC 1994;(Special Issue):288A.

92. Anderson HV, Cannon C, Williams D, et al. One-year results of the TIMI-IIIB clinical trial. (Abstract) Circulation 1994;90(Pt. 2):I-231.

93. Anderson HV, Williams DO, Powers E, et al. Coronary thrombus seen on early angiography in unstable angina/non Q wave MI: TIMI-IIIB results. (Abstract) Circulation 1994;90(Pt. 2):I-664.

94. Becker RC, Bovill EG, Corrao JM, et al. Platelet activation determined by flow cytometry persists despite antithrombotic therapy in patients with unstable angina and non-Q wave myocardial infarction. J Thromb Thrombolysis 1994;1:95–100.

95. Becker RC, Tracy RP, Bovill EG, et al. Surface 12-lead electrocardiogram findings and plasma markers of thrombin activity and generation in patients with myocardial ischemia at rest. J Thromb Thrombolysis 1994;1:101–107.

96. Stone PH, Kleiman N, Kronenberg M, et al. The influence of race and age on the management and outcome of patients with unstable angina and non-Q-wave MI. The TIMI III Registry. (Abstract) Circulation 1994;90(Pt. 2):I-663.

97. Hadjis T, Lam JYT, Theroux P, et al. Interaction between heparin and nitroglycerin: An ancillary TIMI-3 Study. (Abstract) Circulation 1994;90(Pt. 2):I-374.

98. Buller CE, Fung AY, Thompson CR, et

al. Does pre-treatment with tPA improve safety of coronary angioplasty in acute coronary syndromes? Results from TIMI IIIB. (Abstract) Circulation 1994;90(Pt. 2):I-22.

99. Williams DO, Sharaf BL, Braunwald E, et al. Percutaneous transluminal coronary angioplasty (PTCA) for acute myocardial ischemia: A comparison of unstable angina and non-Q wave MI. (Abstract) Circulation 1994;90(Pt. 2):I-433.

100. Williams DO, Sharaf BL, Braunwald E, et al. Percutaneous transluminal coronary angioplasty (PTCA) for acute myocardial ischemia: The TIMI-3 experience. (Abstract) Circulation 1994;90(Pt. 2):I-433.

101. Williams DO, Thompson B, Braunwald E, et al. Advanced age does not diminish the results of PTCA for acute ischemic syndromes. (Abstract) JACC 1995; Special Issue: 346A.

102. Williams DO, Thompson B, Braunwald E, et al. Contemporary PTCA for acute coronary ischemia: Results in women match those of men. (Abstract) JACC 1995; Special Issue: 138A.

TIMI 4

103. Cannon CP, McCabe CH, Diver DJ, et al. Comparison of front-loaded recombinant tissue-type plasminogen activator, anistreplase and combination thrombolytic therapy for acute myocardial infarction: Results of the Thrombolysis in Myocardial Infarction (TIMI) 4 trial. JACC 1994;24: 1602–1610.

104. Abendschein DR, Puleo PR, Cannon CP, et al. Noninvasive detection of early coronary artery patency based on plasma MM and MB creatine kinase (CK) isoforms. (Abstract) Circulation 1992;86(Suppl I):I-266.

105. Gibson CM, Cannon CP, Piana RN, et al. Relationship of coronary flow to myocardial infarction size: Two simple new methods to subclassify TIMI flow grades. (Abstract) Circulation 1992;86 (Suppl I):I-453.

106. Gibson CM, Piana RN, Davis SF, et al. Improvement in minimum lumen diameter during the first day after thrombolysis. (Abstract) Circulation 1992;86(Suppl I):I-453.

107. Gibson CM, Cannon CP, Piana RN, et al. Consequences of TIMI 2 vs 3 flow at 90 minutes following thrombolysis.

(Abstract) JACC 1993;21(Suppl A):348A.

108. Cannon CP, McCabe CH, Diver DJ, et al. Use of a composite end point to evaluate new thrombolytic-antithrombotic regimens for acute myocardial infarction. Results from the TIMI 4 trial. (Abstract) Clin Res 1993;41:199A.

109. Cannon CP, McCabe CH, Schweiger MJ et al. Prospective validation of a composite end point for evaluation of new thrombolytic regimens for acute MI. Results from the TIMI 4 trial. (Abstract) Circulation 1993;88:I-60.

110. Wackers FJT, Cannon CP, McMahon M, et al. Natural history of serial intrahospital quantitative planar Tc-99 sestamibi imaging following thrombolytic therapy for acute myocardial infarction. (Abstract) JACC 1993; 21(Suppl A):249A.

111. Barr SA, Zaret BL, Cannon CP, et al. Does decreasing defect size in serial quantitative planar Tc-99 sestamibi imaging following thrombolytic therapy for acute myocardial infarction correlate with improved left ventricular function? (Abstract) Circulation 1993;88:I-486.

112. Flaker GC, Bartolozzi J, Davis V, et al. Use of a standardized nomogram to achieve therapeutic anticoagulation after thrombolytic therapy in myocardial infarction. Arch Intern Med 1994;154:1492–1496.

113. Cannon CP, Braunwald E. GUSTO, TIMI and the case for rapid reperfusion. Acta Cardiol 1994;49:1–8.

114. Gibson CM, Cannon CP, Piana RN, et al. Rescue PTCA in the TIMI 4 trial. (Abstract) JACC 1994;(Special Issue): 225A.

115. Gibson CM, Cannon CP, Baim DS, et al. TIMI frame count: A new standardization of infarct-related artery flow grade, and its relationship to clinical outcomes in the TIMI-4 trial. (Abstract) Circulation 1994;90(Pt. 2):I-220.

116. Antman EM, Cannon CP, Mueller J, et al. Do clinical trial results influence physician drug use in myocardial infarction? (Abstract) Circulation 1994;90(Pt. 2):I-167.

117. Kloner RA, Shook T, Przyklenk K, et al. Previous angina alters in-hospital outcome in TIMI 4: A clinical correlate to preconditioning? Circulation 1995;91:37–45.

118. Zahger D, Cercek B, Cannon CP, et al.

How do smokers differ from non-smokers in their response to thrombolysis? (The TIMI-4 Trial). Am J Cardiol 1995;75:232–236.

119. Gibson CM, Cannon CP, Piana RN, et al. Angiographic predictors of reocclusion after thrombolysis: Results from the Thrombolysis in Myocardial Infarction (TIMI) 4. JACC 1995;25:582–589.

120. Zahger D, Cercek B, Cannon CP, et al. Reduced efficacy of thrombolytic therapy for acute myocardial infarction in patients with previous coronary bypass surgery. Results from the Thrombolysis in Myocardial Infarction (TIMI) 4 trial. J Thromb Thrombolysis (in press).

TIMI 5

121. Cannon CP, McCabe CH, Henry TD, et al. A pilot trial of recombinant desulfatohirudin compared with heparin in conjunction with tissue-type plasminogen activator and aspirin for acute myocardial infarction: Results of the Thrombolysis in Myocardial Infarction (TIMI) 5 Trial. JACC 1994;23:993–1003.

122. Sharaf BL, Miele N, Ferreira P, et al. Culprit lesion changes in acute myocardial infarction: A TIMI 5 comparison of patients treated with tPA and either heparin or hirudin. (Abstract) JACC 1993;21:419A.

123. Eisenberg PR, Abendschein DR, Becker RC, et al. Lack of suppression of thrombin activity in vivo: A determinant of failure of recanalization. (Abstract) JACC 1993;21(Suppl A):464A.

124. Loscalzo J, Abendschein D, Eisenberg P, et al. Comparative effects of heparin and hirudin on fibrinolytic and thrombotic activities during tissue-type plasminogen activator therapy. (Abstract) Circulation 1993;88(Pt. 2):I-200.

125. Scharfstein JS, George D, Burchenal JEB, et al. Hemostatic markers predict clinical events in patient treated with rtPA and adjunctive antithrombotic therapy. (Abstract) JACC 1994;(Special Issue):56A.

126. Cannon CP, Becker RC, Loscalzo J, et al. Usefulness of APTT to predict bleeding for hirudin (and heparin). (Abstract) Circulation 1994;90(Pt. 2):I-563.

127. Becker R, Cannon C, George D, et al. Toward establishing anticoagulation guidelines for intravenous heparin administration among patients with myocardial infarction given tissue plasminogen activator. (Abstract) JACC 1995;Special Issue:309A.

128. Henry TD, Becker RC, Cannon CP, et al. Is there a circadian variation in anticoagulant response to hirudin following acute myocardial infarction? (Abstract) JACC 1995;Special Issue:310A.

TIMI 6

129. Lee LV, for the TIMI 6 Investigators. Initial experience with hirudin and streptokinase in acute myocardial infarction: Results of the Thrombolysis in Myocardial Infarction (TIMI) 6 trial. Am J Cardiol 1995;75:7–13.

TIMI 7

130. Fuchs J, Cannon CP, and the TIMI 7 Investigators. Hirolog in the treatment of unstable angina: Results of the Thrombin Inhibition in Myocardial Ischemia (TIMI) 7 trial. Circulation (in press).

131. Borzak S, Kraft PL, Douthat L, et al. Prior aspirin use in unstable coronary disease: myth of aspirin resistance? (Abstract) Circulation 1994;90(Pt. 2):I-232.

132. Borzak S, Kraft PL, Douthat L, et al. What beyond aspirin and anticoagulation improves outcome in unstable angina? Effect of medical therapy. (Abstract) JACC 1995;Special Issue:356A.

TIMI 9

133. Antman EM, for the TIMI 9A Investigators. Hirudin in acute myocardial infarction: Safety report from the Thrombolysis and Thrombin Inhibition in Myocardial Infarction (TIMI) 9A trial. Circulation 1994;90:1624–1630.

TIMI 9 Registry

134. Cannon CP, Henry TD, Schweiger MJ, et al. Current management of ST elevation myocardial infarction and out-

come of thrombolytic ineligible patients: Results of the multicenter TIMI 9 Registry. (Abstract) JACC 1995;Special Issue:231A.

Additional References

135. The GUSTO Investigators. An international randomized trial comparing four thrombolytic strategies for acute myocardial infarction. N Engl J Med1993;329:673–682.

136. Braunwald E. Myocardial reperfusion, limitation of infarct size, reduction of left ventricular dysfunction, and improved survival: Should the paradigm be expanded? Circulation 1989;79:441–444.

137. Braunwald E. The open-artery theory is alive and well—again. N Engl J Med 1993;329:1650–1652.

138. The GUSTO Angiographic Investigators. The comparative effects of tissue plasminogen activator, streptokinase, or both on coronary artery patency, ventricular function and survival after acute myocardial infarction. N Engl J Med 1993;329:1615–1622.

139. Gersh BJ, Anderson JL. Thrombolysis and myocardial salvage. Results of clinical trials and the animal paradigm—paradoxic or predictable? Circulation 1993;88:296–306.

140. Goldman L. Cost-effective strategies in cardiology. In: Braunwald E, ed. Heart Disease. A Textbook of Cardiovascular Medicine. Philadelphia: W.B. Saunders Company, 1992, pp. 1694–1707.

141. ISIS-2 (Second International Study of Infarct Survival) Collaborative Group. Randomised trial of intravenous streptokinase, oral aspirin, both, or neither among 17,187 cases of suspected acute myocardial infarction: ISIS-2. Lancet 1988;2:349–360.

142. Hsia J, Hamilton WP, Kleiman N, et al. A comparison between heparin and low-dose aspirin as adjunctive therapy with tissue plasminogen activator for acute myocardial infarction. N Engl J Med 1990;323:1433–1437.

143. de Bono DP, Simoons MI, Tijssen J, et al. Effect of early intravenous heparin on coronary patency, infarct size, and bleeding complications after alteplase thrombolysis: Results of a randomized double blind European Cooperative Study Group trial. Br Heart J 1992;67:122–128.

144. Gruppo Italiano per lo Studio della Streptochinasi nell'Infarto Miocardico (GISSI). Effectiveness of intravenous thrombolytic treatment in acute myocardial infarction. Lancet 1986; 1 397–401.

145. Cannon CP, Antman EM, Walls R, et al. Time as an adjunctive agent to thrombolytic therapy. J Thromb Thrombolysis 1994;1:27–34.

146. National Heart Attack Alert Program Coordinating Committee—60 Minutes to Treatment Working Group. Emergency department: Rapid identification and treatment of patients with acute myocardial infarction. Ann Emerg Med 1994;23:311–329.

147. Muller JE, Stone PH, Turi ZG, et al. Circadian variation in the frequency of onset of acute myocardial infarction. N Engl J Med 1985;313:1315–1322.

148. Neuhaus K-L, Feuerer W, Jeep-Teebe S, et al. Improved thrombolysis with a modified dose regimen of recombinant tissue-type plasminogen activator. JACC 1989;14:1566–1569.

149. Grines CL, Nissen SE, Booth DC, et al. A prospective, randomized trial comparing combination half-dose tissue-type plasminogen activator and streptokinase with full-dose tissue-type plasminogen activator. Circulation 1991;84:540–549.

150. Braunwald E, Cannon CP, McCabe CH. An approach to evaluating thrombolytic therapy in acute myocardial infarction. The "Unsatisfactory Outcome" end point. Circulation 1992; 86:583–687.

151. Califf RM, Topol EJ, Gersh BJ. From myocardial salvage to patient salvage in acute myocardial infarction. The role of reperfusion therapy. JACC 1989;14:1382–1388.

152. Kim CB, Braunwald E. Potential benefits of late reperfusion of infarcted myocardium: The open artery hypothesis. Circulation 1993;88:2426–2436.

153. Weaver WD, Bode C, Burnett C, et al. Reteplase vs. Alteplase Patency Investigation During myocardial infarction trial (RAPID 2). (Abstract) JACC 1995;Special Issue:87A.

154. Puleo PR, Perryman B. Noninvasive detection of reperfusion in acute myocardial infarction based on plasma activity of creatine kinase MB subfractions. JACC 1991;17:1047–1052.

155. Abendschein D, Seacord LM, Nohara R, et al. Prompt detection of myocar-

dial injury by assay of creatine kinase MM isoforms in the presence of high grade stenosis. Clin Cardiol 1988;11:661–664.

156. Wackers FJT, Gibbons RJ, Verani MS, et al. Serial quantitative planar technetium-99m isonitrile imaging in acute myocardial infarction: Efficacy for noninvasive assessment of thrombolytic therapy. JACC 1989;14:861–873.

157. Heras M, Chesebro JH, Penny WJ, et al. Effects of thrombin inhibition on the development of acute platelet-thrombus deposition during angioplasty in pigs. Heparin versus recombinant hirudin, a specific thrombin inhibitor. Circulation 1989;79:657–665.

158. Heras M, Chesebro JH, Webster MWI, et al. Hirudin, heparin and placebo during deep arterial injury in the pig: The in vivo role of thrombin in platelet-mediated thrombosis. Circulation 1990;82:1476–1484.

159. Haskel EJ, Torr SR, Day KC, et al. Prevention of arterial reocclusion after thrombolysis with recombinant lipoprotein-associated coagulation inhibitor. Circulation 1991;84:821–827.

160. Rudd MA, George D, Johnstone MT, et al. Effect of thrombin inhibition on the dynamics of thrombolysis and on platelet function during thrombolytic therapy. Circ Res 1992;70:829–834.

161. Rydel TJ, Ravichandran KG, Tulinsky A, et al. The structure of a complex of recombinant hirudin and human alpha-thrombin. Science 1990;249: 277–280.

162. Talbot M. Biology of recombinant hirudin (CGP 39393): A new prospect in the treatment of thrombosis. Semin Thromb Hemost 1989;15:293–301.

163. Markwardt F, Nowak G, Sturzebecher J, et al. Pharmacokinetics and anticoagulant effect of hirudin in man. Thromb Haemost 1984;52:160–163.

164. Arnout J, Simoons M, de Bono D, et al. Correlation between level of heparinization and patency of the infarct-related coronary artery after treatment of acute myocardial infarction with alteplase (rtPA). JACC 1992;20:513–519.

165. Hsia J, Kleiman N, Aguirre F, et al. Heparin-induced prolongation of partial thromboplastin time after thrombolysis: Relationship to coronary artery patency. JACC 1992;20:31–35.

166. Decousus HA, Croze M, Levi FA, et al. Circadian changes in anticoagulant effect of heparin infused at a constant rate. Br Med J 1985;290:341–344.

167. Cannon CP, Maraganore JM, Loscalzo J, et al. Anticoagulant effects of Hirulog, a novel thrombin inhibitor, in patients with coronary artery disease. Am J Cardiol 1993;71:778–782.

168. The Global Use of Strategies to Open Occluded Coronary Arteries (GUSTO) IIa Investigators. A randomized trial of intravenous heparin versus recombinant hirudin for acute coronary syndromes. Circulation 1994;90:1631–1637.

169. Neuhaus K-L, von Essen R, Tebbe U, et al. Safety observations from the pilot phase of a randomized trial: r-Hirudin for Improvement of Thrombolysis (HIT-III) Study. A study of the Arbeitsgemeinschaft Leitender, Kardiologischer Koinkenhausarzte (ALKK). Circulation 1994;90:1638–1642.

170. Keyt BA, Paoni NF, Refino CJ, et al. A faster-acting and more potent form of tissue plasminogen activator. Proc Natl Acad Sci USA 1994;91: 3670–3674.

171. Benedict CR, Fefino C, Keyt B, et al. A new variant of tissue plasminogen activator with enhanced efficacy and lower incidence of bleeding when compared to recombinant human tissue plasminogen activator (Activase). (Abstract) JACC 1994;(Special Issue): 314A.

Address for reprints: Eugene Braunwald, M.D., Chairman, Department of Medicine, Brigham and Women's Hospital, 75 Francis Street, Boston, MA 02115. Fax: (617) 732-6439.

Chapter 9

The Thrombolysis and Angioplasty in Myocardial Infarction (TAMI) Trials:
A Decade of Reperfusion Strategies

Gregory W. Barsness, M.D., E. Magnus Ohman, M.D.,* Robert M. Califf, M.D.,* Dean J. Kereiakes, M.D.,** Barry S. George, M.D.,†
and Eric J. Topol, M.D.‡*

From **Duke University Medical Center, Durham, North Carolina; **Christ Hospital, Cincinnati, Ohio; †Riverside Methodist Hospital, Columbus, Ohio; and the ‡Cleveland Clinic Foundation, Cleveland, Ohio*

Beginning with its inception in 1985, the TAMI group performed randomized clinical trials in both academic and nonacademic settings. The ten TAMI trials not only proved the viability of clinical research in a nontraditional environment, but also contributed significantly to the clinical investigation of acute myocardial infarction through small mechanistic trials. Despite having insufficient power to address overall survival and clinical outcome measures because of patient enrollments ranging from only 50–575 patients, the trials used similar entry criteria and follow-up measures, which permitted broader analyses of the prospectively collected dataset of randomized patients. This article reviews the history of the TAMI collaboration and discusses the findings of the individual trials as well as the contributions of larger analyses to our understanding of patient selection, prognosis, costs, and outcomes. (J Interven Cardiol 1996;9 : 89–115)

Introduction

The first successful large scale applications of thrombolytic therapy in acute myocardial infarction over 10 years ago[1-3] ushered in a new era of research into aggressive modes of myocardial reperfusion. Despite a prolonged bias against the thrombotic model of acute coronary syndromes,[4] DeWood et al.'s[5] clear demonstration of the occlusive nature of myocardial infarction (MI) served to renew interest in the potential therapeutic role of thrombolysis. In addition, the appreciation that infarct size,[6] and therefore prognosis,[7] could be positively affected by early intervention fueled the search for improved therapeutic strategies.

In an effort to evaluate potential new strategies for the treatment of MI, an assembly of colleagues in medicine and cardiology formed the Thrombolysis and Angioplasty in Myocardial Infarction (TAMI) study group in July 1985. Supported by the expertise in clinical data management and analysis of the Duke Databank for Cardiovascular Disease and the angiographic core laboratory at the University of Michigan, this multicenter group has sought to provide insight into the expanding role of pharmacological and mechanical

Table 1

The TAMI Trials in Myocardial Infarction

Trial	Patients	Comparison
TAMI 1	386	Thrombolysis and immediate vs delayed adjunctive PTCA
TAMI 2	147*	Combination thrombolysis with tPA and UK
TAMI 3	175*	Thrombolysis with immediate vs delayed heparin
TAMI 4	50	Thrombolysis with adjunctive prostacyclin
TAMI UK	102	Efficacy study of high dose UK
TAMI 5	575	1. tPA vs UK vs combination thrombolysis 2. Aggressive vs elective catheterization
TAMI 6	197	Late thrombolysis with tPA vs placebo
TAMI 7	232	Dose ranging trial of accelerated thrombolysis with tPA ± UK
TAMI 8	70	Dose ranging trial of 7E3 as an adjunct to thrombolysis
TAMI 9	430	Thrombolysis and Fluosol vs placebo

tPA = tissue type plasminogen activator; UK = urokinase.
*The original TAMI 2 and TAMI 3 publications reported the results of 146 patients and 134 patients, respectively.

treatment of MI. From the original TAMI group, composed of investigators at Duke University (Durham, NC, USA), the University of Michigan (Ann Arbor, MI, USA), Riverside Methodist Hospital (Columbus, OH, USA), and Christ Hospital (Cincinnati, OH, USA), this collaboration has grown to include many sites from several states (see Appendix).

With the early realization that intravenous thrombolysis would become a standard therapy for MI, the TAMI group has gone on to complete ten studies of various therapeutic regimens in acute MI (Table 1). These trials focused on combination therapies felt to be potentially superior to thrombolysis alone. Recombinant tissue type plasminogen activator (tPA) was the primary thrombolytic agent used due to early demonstrations of greater efficacy.[8-10] Protocols called for the randomization of patients suffering acute MI to tPA plus various adjunctive therapies, including coro-

nary angioplasty, combination therapy with urokinase (UK), early intravenous heparin, prostacyclin, early catheterization, profound platelet inhibition, and fluosol (Tables 2 and 3). Additional studies looked at the efficacy of high dose UK, late thrombolysis, and accelerated dosing of thrombolytics.

TAMI 1

At the inception of the first TAMI trial, investigators were faced with a myriad of questions regarding thrombolytic therapy. Early studies of intracoronary and intravenous thrombolysis in acute MI had clearly demonstrated a reduction in mortality[11] and improvement in left ventricular (LV) function,[12,13] but the benefit of additional early and aggressive mechanical revascularization to improve coronary blood flow remained in question. The TAMI 1 trial was designed to evaluate the

Table 2

Primary Questions Addressed in the TAMI Trials

Trial	Primary Results
TAMI 1	Immediate angioplasty confers no additional benefit following successful thrombolysis.
TAMI 2	Combination thrombolysis is safe and may decrease reocclusion after rescue PTCA.
TAMI 3	Immediate heparinization adds no significant patency benefit at 90 minutes
TAMI 4	Prostacyclin does not improve patency or LV function after thrombolysis.
TAMI UK	High dose UK is safe and effective as monotherapy in thrombolysis.
TAMI 5	1. Combination thrombolytic therapy can safely reduce adverse in-hospital events. 2. Early catheterization may benefit certain patient populations.
TAMI 6	Late thrombolysis improves early IRA patency and prevents cavity dilatation.
TAMI 7	Weight-adjusted, front-loaded tPA provides improved IRA patency.
TAMI 8	Potent platelet inhibition combined with thrombolysis may safely improve patency.
TAMI 9	Fluosol provides no benefit in the setting of thrombolysis.

IRA = infarct related artery; LV = left ventricular; PTCA = percutaneous transluminal coronary angioplasty; tPA = tissue type plasminogen activator; UK = urokinase.

Table 3

Patients Undergoing Acute (90-minute) and Convalescent (5–7 day) Catheterization and Thrombolytic Agent Received

Trial	Acute (90-Minute) Catheterization	Convalescent (5–7 day) Catheterization	tPA	Agent UK	tPA + UK
TAMI 1	384	359	386	—	—
TAMI 2	146	104	—	—	146
TAMI 3	134	111	134	—	—
TAMI 4	50	46	50	—	—
TAMI UK	102	86	—	102	—
TAMI 5	357*	503	191	190	194
TAMI 6	197	125†	96	—	—
TAMI 7	219	181	177	—	42
TAMI 8	—	46	70	—	—
TAMI 9	—	334	430	—	—
Total	1589	1945	1534	292	382

tPA = tissue type plasminogen activator; UK = urokinase.
*Includes 75 cross-over patients from the delayed angiography arm undergoing catheterization ≤ 4 days after randomization. †Convalescent catheterization performed at 4–6 months in TAMI 6.

potential benefit of immediate coronary angioplasty after successful thrombolysis.[14] The TAMI 1 trial sought to capture thrombolytic eligible patients suffering acute MI. Patients were enrolled if they had ischemic symptoms for < 6 hours, had ST segment elevation > 1 mm in two or more contiguous leads, were < 75 years old, had no recent stroke, surgery or trauma, had not had coronary bypass, and were not in cardiogenic shock at the time of enrollment. All patients received intravenous tPA, 150 mg over 6–8 hours, and intravenous heparin at the time of acute catheterization. All patients underwent 90-minute catheterization to assess infarct related artery (IRA) patency. Those with TIMI 2–3 flow and anatomy suitable for angioplasty were randomized to immediate or delayed (elective) IRA percutaneous transluminal coronary angioplasty (PTCA). All patients underwent repeat catheterization at day 7.

A total of 386 patients were enrolled between December 1985 and October 1986. Of the 288 patients with patent IRAs at 90-minute catheterization, 197 were anatomically appropriate for randomization. The primary end point, LV function, was not significantly different between the two groups. There was also no difference in the clinical end points of death, requirement for emergency bypass surgery, or reocclusion at 7 days. There was a greater requirement for emergency PTCA in the delayed angioplasty arm (P = 0.01). Bleeding complications in both arms were primarily associated with the vascular access site. These results indicate that immediate PTCA in the setting of successful thrombolysis (TIMI 2 or 3 flow) offers no particular advantage over an elective approach in this subset of patients.[15,16]

Further analysis of the data shed new light on the pharmacology and efficacy of thrombolytic therapy. Initial trials with tPA raised some questions concerning the optimal dose and rate of administration. Despite the aggressive protocol of thrombolytic administration in the TAMI 1 trial, there remained a 90-minute patency rate of just 75% and a 15% reocclusion rate at 7–10 days. This apparent "ceiling" of thrombolytic efficacy was poorly understood and felt to be multifactorial, related to baseline patient characteristics as well as inadequacies of drug dosing.[15] In the TAMI 1 trial, 150 mg of predominantly single-chain tPA was given according to two dosing schedules. The first 178 patients received 60 mg tPA in the first hour, followed by 20 mg/hour for 2 hours, then 10 mg/hour for 5 hours. The next 208 patients received a weight-adjusted dose of 1 mg/kg for 1 hour and the balance of the 150 mg over the next 5 hours. The selection of two dosing regimens permitted the relative efficacy and complication rates to be compared. The second regimen, with a weight-adjusted first-hour dose and shorter maintenance infusion proved superior with respect to overall efficacy and rapidity of infarct-vessel patency (P = 0.02), with fewer bleeding complications.[17] Scrutiny of the coagulation studies performed on TAMI 1 patients identified the importance of the early phase tPA dose in producing fibrinogenolysis. These data also pointed out the potential adverse effects of aggressive thrombolysis, including the apparent increased risk of hemorrhagic stroke in women and the elderly.[18] Despite the risk of intracerebral hemorrhage, these results, when combined with other reports demonstrating the importance of early aggressive dosing and weight adjustment,[8,19] became the eventual foundation for the development of the highly effective and safe front-loaded regimen used in the GUSTO (Global Use of Strategies to Open Occluded Coronary Arteries) trials.

This trial also demonstrated the poor prognosis of patients requiring emergency PTCA because of thrombolytic failure. In fact, while immediate angioplasty was highly successful at opening occluded infarct vessels after failed thrombolysis, the morbidity and mortality in this group was clearly demonstrated, with a 10.4% in-hospital mortality rate and 29% reocclusion without improvement in LV function.[20]

While the baseline characteristics and clinical courses were similar between those who did and did not achieve pharmacological reperfusion, those patients found to be occluded at 90-minute catheterization had significantly more complications during catheterization, including ventricular fibrillation, severe bradycardia and hypotension.[21] A long-term benefit of "salvage" or "rescue" angioplasty, however, was suggested by a low 6-month out-of-hospital mortality in this group, lending credence to the open artery hypothesis.[15]

The ability to accurately noninvasively identify reperfusion after thrombolytic administration also came under examination in the TAMI 1 trial. By prospectively recording clinical criteria of presumed reperfusion, Califf and colleagues[22] demonstrated that although chest pain amelioration and ST segment resolution on the routine 12-lead electrocardiogram were associated with perfusion, the low incidence of complete resolution of symptoms (29%) or ST segment elevation (6%) makes these markers untenable for clinical management. Even partial resolution of these variables occurred in a minority of those demonstrating reperfusion confirming the failure of these clinical measures to adequately predict perfusion status.

TAMI 2

TAMI 1 demonstrated that a 6–8 hour infusion of tPA failed to achieve IRA recanalization in a significant minority of patients. The reasons for thrombolytic failure were multifactorial, including baseline patient characteristics. However, development of the concept of in-vivo fibrinolytic synergism[23,24] placed emphasis on optimizing the thrombolytic strategy. TAMI 2 was the first clinical trial of combination thrombolytic therapy. In this trial, 146 consecutive patients were treated with one of five escalating dosing regimens of tPA and UK, to a maximum dose of 1.0 mg/kg tPA and 2.0 million units UK. Selection criteria were

similar to TAMI 1. Each patient received thrombolytics over 1 hour and patency was assessed at 90-minute and 7-day catheterization. All patients received intravenous heparin for 72 hours with an activated partial thromboplastin time (aPTT) target of 2–2.5 times control. At initial catheterization, angioplasty was considered only in cases of IRA occlusion (TIMI grade 0 or 1 flow) or with evidence of ongoing ischemia.

In this trial, tPA and UK demonstrated no significant synergism. The 90-minute patency rate for the high dose combination (75%) was virtually identical to tPA monotherapy in TAMI 1, although there was a trend toward decreased reocclusion (9% vs 15%, P = 0.11). There was also no significant increase in bleeding complications compared with the TAMI 1 study. For the small group of patients undergoing rescue angioplasty in this trial, however, there was a substantial and statistically significant improvement in outcome compared with TAMI 1. Among the 27 patients undergoing PTCA for thrombolytic failure, there was no in-hospital mortality, only 4% reocclusion, and a significant five percentage point improvement in LV function.[25] These promising observations prompted the large, randomized trial, the TAMI 5 study.

TAMI 3

Initial studies by Cercek et al.[26] and others[27] indicated a potential role for heparin in facilitating fibrinolysis by tPA. The early administration of heparin was felt to blunt the increase in thrombin activity known to occur during thrombolytic therapy.[28] Despite the use of early heparin in most early clinical trials of tPA, enthusiasm for this approach was tempered by concerns about an increased risk of bleeding, and the benefit of conjunctive heparin remained controversial. TAMI 3 was therefore designed as a randomized controlled trial to evaluate the potential benefit of conjunctive heparin on early patency and reocclusion. Patient selection was similar to TAMI 1 and 2, and 134 patients received a 4-hour infusion of tPA with randomization to immediate intravenous heparin (10,000 unit bolus) or delayed heparin (5,000 unit bolus) at the 90-minute catheterization. Angioplasty was considered only in cases of thrombolytic failure, and all patients went on to receive at least 24 hours of intravenous heparin with a target aPTT of 1.5–2 times control. IRA patency at initial 90-minute angiogram, the primary end point, was not statistically different in the two groups (79% heparin vs. 73% no heparin, P = 0.41). Likewise, reocclusion rates were similar. There was no difference in bleeding complications between the two groups, all of which occurred more than 90 minutes after tPA administration.[29]

While failing to demonstrate a benefit for conjunctive heparin, this trial was powered to detect a 20% difference in 90-minute patency (assuming α = 0.05, power = 0.80, and a control patency of 0.67). It would require several thousand patients to capture a difference in bleeding rates, and it is not surprising that no difference was found between the two strategies. This trial did demonstrate, however, that thrombolysis with early heparinization would likely be associated with only a modest effect on outcome.

TAMI 4

The apparent inability of aggressive thrombolytic administration, with or without adjunctive mechanical strategies, to achieve significantly improved reperfusion results led to experimentation with additional adjunctive pharmacological therapies. Prostacyclin in particular looked promising as an adjunct to an aggressive thrombolytic regimen for a number of reasons. Prostacyclin had been shown to reduce experimental infarct size,[30–32] possibly through inhibition of oxygen derived free radical formation[33] and neutrophil function.[34] Additionally, the strong platelet in-

hibition and systemic and coronary artery vasodilatation properties of this agent promised accelerated thrombolysis,[35] improved IRA patency and blood flow, and improved hemodynamics.

TAMI 4 examined this potential role of prostacyclin as adjunctive therapy in MI thrombolysis.[36] Patient selection was similar to the prior TAMI trials. Twenty-five patients received 100 milligrams of tPA over 3 hours (1 mg/kg for 1 hour, up to 80 mg, with a 10% bolus, then the remainder over 2 hours), in addition to an infusion of Iloprost, a stable analog of prostacyclin. The Iloprost infusion of 0.5 ng/kg/min was gradually increased to a maximum of 2 ng/kg/min as blood pressure allowed and continued for up to 48 hours. Additional therapies included aspirin and a 72-hour heparin infusion. As in previous studies, patients underwent 90-minute and 7-day catheterizations. The primary end point was 90-minute IRA patency.

After review of data from the first 25 patients treated with Iloprost and tPA, concerns regarding an apparently low IRA patency rate, high abrupt closure rate after rescue angioplasty, and poor LV recovery resulted in a decision to treat an additional 25 patients with tPA only. The treatment groups were comparable in all aspects except for a 0.7-hour delay in therapy with the combined tPA and Iloprost arm, felt to be related to the time required for reconstitution of the additional medication. There was no significant difference between 90-minute IRA patency rates in the two groups. Improvement in left ventricular ejection fraction (LVEF), however, was actually greater in patients treated with tPA alone (47.3 ± 11.5 to 50.4 ± 9.8) compared with those receiving combination therapy (51.3 ± 10.1 to 49.0 ± 9.4, P = 0.05). Careful study of hemostatic parameters revealed improved fibrinolysis in the tPA alone group. The greater decrease in fibrinogen (P = 0.001) and increase in fibrin degradation products (P < 0.005) 4 hours after initiation of therapy in the tPA alone arm was felt to be related to the ability of prostacyclin to increase hepatic blood flow and accelerate the clearance of tPA, a finding later demonstrated experimentally in animal models by Kerins et al.[37] Although there was no significant increase in bleeding complications associated with prostacyclin in this study, nausea and vomiting occurred in 76% of those receiving the drug, compared with 26% of those receiving only tPA (P = 0.001). Systolic blood pressure was also significantly lowered by prostacyclin (113 ± 19 mmHg vs 122 ± 21 mmHg, P < 0.001). The poor tolerance and lack of clinical efficacy of prostacyclin found in TAMI 4 pointed out the importance of careful experimental pharmacological testing of new drug combinations contemplated for clinical use. This was the first clinical study of an agent alleged to reduce reperfusion injury. While subsequent small studies have renewed interest in prostacyclin as a therapeutic agent in MI,[38] TAMI 4 failed to demonstrate the potential of prostacyclin to safely improve outcome in this setting.

TAMI UK

Despite evidence of its potential efficacy over more than 20 years, randomized clinical experience with intravenous UK as thrombolytic monotherapy in the setting of acute MI had been limited to five studies including a total of 735 patients.[39–43] These studies had demonstrated the relative safety of UK, with reperfusion rates comparable to that of tPA and a trend toward less recurrent ischemia and reocclusion. Of note, high dose UK had been shown to be safe and effective when given as a bolus,[42] thereby rapidly promoting a thrombolytic state and potentially improving outcome. To build on this preliminary information, TAMI UK was designed as a prospective pilot evaluation of the safety and efficacy of high dose UK in acute MI.[44] Patient selection was similar to previous TAMI studies, but enrollment was limited to centers in North Carolina. Patients received 3 million

units of intravenous UK, initially as a 45–60 minute infusion (61 patients), and later as a 1.5 million unit bolus followed by a 1.5 million unit infusion (41 patients). All patients received aspirin and a 7-day infusion of heparin. As in prior TAMI studies, 90-minute and 7-day catheterizations were performed. Rescue angioplasty was performed in patients with persistent IRA occlusion or ongoing ischemia.

The IRA patency rate was similar between the two treatment strategies of UK infusion (62%) and UK bolus and infusion (63%). These results, while comparable to the patency rates realized in the German Activator UK Study, were lacking in comparison to that found with tPA monotherapy in TAMI 1 and high dose combination therapy in TAMI 2. UK therapy, as delivered in this study, also offered no advantage in lowering reocclusion, with an overall event rate of 7%. In those patients undergoing rescue PTCA, however, the reocclusion rate of 10% was significantly lower than the 29% reocclusion found in TAMI 1, and approaching the 4% reocclusion rate described with combination tPA and UK in TAMI 2. In addition, acute angioplasty was highly successful with this thrombolytic regimen. When used as a rescue procedure, there was a 96% success rate, comparing favorably to success rates of approximately 90% found with tPA in earlier TAMI studies and with streptokinase.[45,46] Thus, while safe, high dose UK demonstrated no clear benefit as monotherapy in acute MI, and this study opened the way for further evaluation of UK and tPA in TAMI 5.

TAMI 5

By 1988, the impressive survival benefit afforded by intravenous thrombolytic therapy was plainly evident. The preferred pharmacological and mechanical reperfusion strategies in acute MI, however, remained equivocal. Differences between early patency with various thrombolytic agents did not appear to be sustained, and clinical outcome measures remained largely equivalent. A combination therapy of UK, with low reocclusion rates, and tPA, with excellent early patency rates, held a theoretical advantage for obtaining early and sustained patency. The TAMI 2 trial, while not demonstrating the superiority of this approach, did affirm the safety and efficacy of combination thrombolysis, as well as denoting some benefit in those patients undergoing rescue PTCA. While it was clear from the TAMI 1 trial that there was no advantage to be gained from immediate adjunctive angioplasty in the setting of successful thrombolysis, the clinical benefit of rescue PTCA in opening persistently occluded vessels remained uncertain.

The TAMI 5 trial[47] was an investigation of both the role of combination thrombolysis as well as the potential benefit of an early diagnostic catheterization strategy. Patient selection was similar to previous TAMI trials. Five hundred seventy-five patients were randomized in a 3×2 factorial design to one of three thrombolytic regimens, and then to either an early or a deferred catheterization strategy. The thrombolytic assignments were to: (1) tPA, 100 mg over 3 hours, including 60 mg over the first hour with 20 mg each additional hour; (2) UK, 1.5 million units over 1 hour; or (3) combination tPA, 1 mg/kg up to 90 mg, and UK, 1.5 million units, each over 1 hour. All patients received aspirin, diltiazem, and intravenous heparin to maintain an aPTT of 1.5–2 times control. The 287 patients randomized to early catheterization underwent 90-minute angiography and rescue PTCA of occluded IRAs. All patients were to undergo 7-day convalescent arteriography.

There was no significant difference in the primary end point of global LV function between groups. Early catheterization, however, was associated with improved regional infarct zone function ($P = 0.004$). The secondary end point, a composite of adverse clinical events ranked in order of importance to the patient (death, stroke, re-

infarction, recurrent ischemia, and heart failure) was reduced in the groups receiving combination therapy (32%) compared to either tPA (40%) or UK (45%) alone ($P = 0.04$). Likewise, an aggressive catheterization strategy produced a similar reduction in adverse outcome, with untoward events occurring in 45% of patients treated with a conservative approach, but only 33% of those treated aggressively ($P = 0.004$). Patients randomized to both an aggressive catheterization strategy and combination thrombolysis had an event rate of 28%, the lowest of any group ($P = 0.009$). Combination therapy also resulted in a significantly lower reocclusion rate (2%) than either tPA (11%) or UK (7%) alone. Bleeding complications were not significantly different between groups. The overall efficacy of these thrombolytic regimens, however, failed to improve on the 70%–80% early patency rates noted in previous studies. Thus, TAMI 5 demonstrated the safety and potential benefit of an early, aggressive pharmacological and mechanical approach to the treatment of acute MI.

TAMI 6

The important benefits of a patent IRA early in MI were established and expanded upon in the early 1980s. Unfortunately, a significant percentage of patients present 6–24 hours after the onset of symptoms. The efficacy and extent of benefit of reperfusion therapy in this group of patients was largely untested. The TAMI 6 trial[48] was designed as a randomized, controlled trial of late thrombolytic therapy to evaluate the benefit of late reperfusion and to help elucidate a potential mechanism. Enrollment differed somewhat from previous TAMI trials in that patients presenting < 6 hours from symptom onset were excluded, although other inclusion and exclusion criteria were similar. One hundred ninety-seven patients presenting 6–24 hours from symptom onset with ST segment elevation were randomized in a 2×2 factorial design to thrombolytic therapy (tPA, 1 mg/kg over 60 minutes, up to 80 mg, and 20 mg over the next hour) or placebo. All patients then underwent 6- to 24-hour catheterization. Patients with persistently occluded IRAs and suitable anatomy were then eligible for further randomization to angioplasty or continued medical therapy. All patients received heparin to maintain an aPTT of 1.5–2 times control for at least 48 hours, as well as aspirin. After hospital discharge, patients were eligible for two follow-up studies, a rest and exercise gated cardiac blood pool scan at 4–6 weeks after infarction, and a convalescent catheterization at 4–6 months. The primary end point was IRA patency at 6–24 hours. There was no significant difference in any of the secondary end points of in-hospital mortality, 6-month reinfarction rate, hospital readmission, coronary bypass grafting, or nonacute PTCA among the groups. The patients treated with tPA, however, had a significantly higher IRA patency than those treated with placebo at acute catheterization (65% and 27%, respectively, P < 0.0001), a difference that was lost at 6-month follow-up (59% patency in both groups). Patients treated with tPA had no increase in the median end-diastolic volume at 6 months (149 mL to 146 mL at follow-up), compared with a 25% increase in placebo-treated patients (127 mL to 159 mL, P = 0.006). The bleeding complications and transfusion requirements were similar between the groups.

A similar long-term benefit of rescue angioplasty was not identified, although infarct-vessel patency was achieved in a significant majority (81%) of patients undergoing this procedure. Randomization to rescue angioplasty was associated with a trend towards improved resting LVEF at 1 month (50.1% vs 42.7%, P = 0.58) compared with patients with an occluded IRA not undergoing rescue angioplasty, but this advantage was lost at 6-month follow-up. Subsequent catheterization also revealed no significant difference between IRA patency rates in these small groups (60% vs 38% in patients with (n = 20) and without

(n = 25) rescue angioplasty, respectively). Likewise, there were no significant differences in clinical event rates at 6 months.

This study demonstrated that thrombolytic therapy was a safe and effective management strategy, despite the late presentation (approximately 15 hours after symptom onset), leading to greater early patency and improved ventricular healing and remodeling. Although without adequate sample size to address the impact on survival or global ejection fraction (EF), this trial cleared the way for further analysis of thrombolysis in this high risk group of patients.

TAMI 7

The success of previous TAMI studies in demonstrating an improved clinical outcome associated with early and sustained IRA patency resulted in further efforts to identify the risks and benefits associated with reperfusion therapy. The apparent patency rate ceiling of approximately 75% for various thrombolytic regimens, in particular, was targeted as an area for improvement. Early studies exploring the feasibility of achieving patency rates in excess of 85% using accelerated dosing regimens of tPA[49,50] provided the impetus for a larger, systematic look at front-loaded tPA therapy for acute MI. Hence, the TAMI 7 trial[51] was designed to evaluate the efficacy of front-loaded tPA in attaining high early patency rates, as well as to assess the reocclusion rates of this new regimen. Participant selection was similar to previous TAMI trials and included 232 patients assigned in a sequential fashion to one of five thrombolytic regimens. These treatment regimens included a high dose, accelerated tPA (1 mg/kg with a 10% bolus over 30 minutes, then 0.25 mg/kg over 30 minutes) arm, as well as an arm with the same total dose of tPA (1.25 mg/kg with a 20 mg bolus) over 90 minutes for comparison. A weight-adjusted, front-loaded tPA regimen (0.75 mg/kg with a 10% bolus over 30 minutes, then 0.5 mg/kg over 1 hour), an arm with a 20 mg bolus of tPA followed by a 30-minute wait and 80 mg over 2 hours, and a combination therapy arm with 1 mg/kg tPA over 30 minutes with 1.5 million units UK over 1 hour were the additional regimens used. This last regimen was modified by the addition of front-loaded tPA to the combination therapy arm used successfully in TAMI 5. As in prior TAMI studies, patients underwent an acute (90-minute) catheterization and received aspirin and intravenous heparin for an aPTT of two times control until the time of convalescent catheterization at 5–10 days. The primary end point was IRA patency. The weight-adjusted, front-loaded strategy of tPA administration provided a 90-minute IRA patency rate of 83%, the highest of the strategies tested (95%, confidence interval [CI] 74%–93%), resembling the findings of Carney et al.,[50] who used a similar, although nonweight-adjusted regimen. In addition, there was a trend toward a decrease in the adverse clinical outcomes of death, reocclusion, reinfarction, and restenosis in this group as well. Bleeding complications were similar among the groups, although there were two intracranial bleeds in the combination therapy arm (5%), the only such events occurring in the trial.

TAMI 7 affirmed the possibility that 90-minute coronary patency rates approaching 85% and reocclusion rates as low as 4% could be safely obtained with a front-loaded tPA regimen. Using a similar front-loaded tPA regimen, Neuhaus and colleagues[52] demonstrated equally encouraging 90-minute patency rates. These trials were too small, however, to adequately ascertain the clinical importance of this finding and any relationship to a survival advantage. The GUSTO-I trial had enough power in its assessment of four separate thrombolytic strategies to eventually verify this, finding a front-loaded, weight-adjusted tPA strategy superior to streptokinase (SK) or combination (SK and tPA) regimens in providing a net benefit of 9–11 lives saved per 1,000 patients treated.[53]

TAMI 8

Despite great strides in the ability to achieve reperfusion in a large majority of thrombolytic treated patients, recurrent ischemia, reocclusion, and reinfarction continued to affect a considerable percentage of them. Platelet rich thrombi contribute to this problem to no small degree, resulting in extension of myocardial necrosis and mortality rates of up to two times those seen in patients spared reocclusion.[54] Several studies pointed to the importance of controlling platelet effects to reduce platelet dependent sequelae. The Second International Study of Infarct Survival (ISIS 2) demonstrated the ability of aspirin, a potent antiplatelet agent, to reduce reinfarction and mortality.[55] The prevention of reocclusion by reducing platelet aggregation promised to be a powerful means of decreasing mortality in acute MI, a position strengthened by the meta-analysis of Roux et al.,[56] which demonstrated a significantly decreased reocclusion rate in patients treated with aspirin. Further study of novel platelet inhibitors indicated a potentially powerful role in reducing serious clinical events associated with vascular reocclusion. Despite the additional support garnered from experimental models of reperfusion demonstrating the value of these powerful platelet inhibitors in accelerating thrombolysis and preventing reocclusion,[57–59] however, concerns about the safety of using potent antiplatelet agents in combination with thrombolytic therapy remained an obstacle to extensive clinical use. TAMI 8[60] was a pilot study of the physiological activity and safety of one of these potent antiplatelet agents, the murine derived chimeric monoclonal antibody 7E3 Fab, which is directed against the glycoprotein IIb/IIIa platelet receptor and had shown promise as an adjunct to thrombolytic therapy in animal models.[61] Patient selection for this study was similar to previous TAMI trials, and 60 patients experiencing acute MI were treated with tPA (100 mg over 3 hours), heparin, aspirin, metoprolol, and escalating doses of 7E3 at 15, 6, or 3 hours after beginning tPA. An additional ten patients served as controls and were treated with tPA alone. Platelet inhibition studies and bleeding times were measured and cardiac catheterization was performed as needed.

This study demonstrated the significant platelet inhibitory effect of 7E3 Fab, while further characterizing the important role for antiplatelet agents in the setting of acute MI. At the highest doses of 7E3 administered (0.02 and 0.25 mg/kg), there was > 90% ex-vivo inhibition of platelet aggregation to 20 μM ADP, with no increase in bleeding complications compared to the control group. Infarct-vessel patency was increased in the treatment group of patients undergoing delayed (average of 5 days after tPA administration) catheterization (92% vs. 56%), with a trend toward decreased recurrent ischemia in this group as well.

TAMI 9

While TAMI 4 had not been able to demonstrate the utility of prostacyclin administration in the setting of acute MI work continued in the arena of limiting reperfusion injury, the process was felt to adversely affect clinical outcome despite, or because of, early reperfusion. Other compounds with the potential to modify this destructive process of neutrophil activation and oxygen derived free radical formation remained under active investigation. Intracoronary administration of Fluosol, a combination of perfluorodecalin and perfluorotripropylamine emulsified in a detergent, poloxamer 188 (RheothRx), and egg-yolk phospholipids, had successfully reduced infarct size and resulted in improved LV function in animal models.[62,63] These results were expanded upon by a

small experience in humans demonstrating similar salutary effects of this compound administered during direct angioplasty.[64] Pathophysiological explanations for benefit were developed, including a role for preserving the coronary microvasculature, enhancing tissue oxygen delivery and allowing significant myocardial salvage, but the proof of significant clinical benefit awaited an expanded clinical evaluation. The TAMI 9 trial[65] examined the safety and potential of intravenous Fluosol, in conjunction with tPA thrombolysis, to limit infarct size or improve systolic function in patients with acute MI. Patient recruitment was similar to previous TAMI trials. All patients received a 3-hour infusion of tPA, along with aspirin, heparin and, if there were no contraindications, atenolol. Patients were then randomized to receive either placebo or open-label Fluosol, administered as 1 mL/min for 5 minutes, then 5 mL/min for 5 minutes, and then 20 mL/min, to a total dose of 15 mL/kg. Patients underwent cardiac catheterization and exercise perfusion scanning at 5–14 days as part of the protocol. The primary end points were global and regional LV function. A secondary clinical end point was the composite of all-cause mortality, stroke, nonfatal reinfarction, emergency revascularization, new heart failure or pulmonary edema, and recurrent ischemia.

No significant difference was found based on treatment assignment in either global or regional LV function of the 430 patients, even when the analysis was confined to patients with anterior MIs. Additionally, there was no improvement in infarct size as assessed by thallium imaging in the Fluosol group, although there was a trend towards smaller infarctions in patients with anterior MI (mean 21.2% of LV affected in placebo group vs mean 18.7% in Fluosol group, P = NS). There was no significant difference between the two treatment groups in regard to the composite clinical end point or bleeding complications, but there was less recurrent ischemia noted in the group receiving Fluosol (6% vs 11%, P = 0.039), as well as a trend toward a reduced reinfarction rate. Unfortunately, there was also a significantly higher incidence of clinically detected heart failure in the Fluosol group (45% vs 31%, P = 0.004), likely reflecting the large volume of fluid required to deliver the medication.

Overall, this trial failed to demonstrate a significant clinical benefit of Fluosol in the treatment of acute MI. However, new-generation compounds, based on perfluorodecalin or perfluorooctylbromide and with higher perfluorocarbon content, have the potential to offer improved safety and oxygen carrying capacity over a wide range of uses.[66] In addition, poloxamer 188 (RheothRx), the nonionic block copolymer surfactant found in Fluosol, has demonstrated beneficial hemorheological properties, the ability to enhance thrombolysis, and a potential role in inhibiting neutrophil chemotaxis and adhesion.[67,68] In animal models, this agent reduced infarct size by as much as 50%,[67,69,70] a trend again demonstrated in a recent multinational dose finding trial of approximately 3,000 patients with acute MI. This promising dose related decrease in infarction size was countered, however, by a similarly dose related increase in renal dysfunction. This trial also failed to demonstrate a benefit of RheothRx on mortality, reinfarction or cardiogenic shock (M. Flather, personal communication). Still, the interesting finding of reduced recurrent ischemia in the TAMI 9 trial begs further investigation of similar agents in MI, particularly with regard to the intracoronary route of administration and use in direct angioplasty.

The TAMI Dataset

While successfully addressing an assortment of questions central to the treatment of MI, the individual TAMI trials often lacked sufficient power to address many overall survival and clinical outcome measures. Fortunately, the similar entry criteria and follow-up measures used throughout the ten TAMI trials provide a large prospectively collected dataset of randomized patients that can be used as a foundation for extensive review of questions not easily studied on a smaller scale.

Patient Selection

Identification of Those at Risk

Despite major advances in the treatment of MI over the last 10 years, including early and aggressive treatment, patients continue to experience significant morbidity and mortality. From the inception of the TAMI trials, there was a strong emphasis on identifying patients at the highest risk for morbidity and mortality after MI. This ability to predict outcome based on clinical and laboratory variables allows the clinician to optimize efforts and target specific medical interventions towards those patients most likely to benefit from aggressive care.

TAMI 1, as a trial of aggressive versus conservative adjunctive PTCA, was instrumental in the development of an early prognostic decision algorithm. Observation of higher in-hospital mortality in patients who failed thrombolysis or angioplasty, as well as the elderly, women, those with impaired LV function at baseline, and those who experienced reocclusion, led to the recommendation to pursue aggressive revascularization in patients at high risk, defined as those with cardiogenic shock, extensive anterior MI, or remote history of MI.[15] Further evaluation of these results corroborated the striking benefit of aggressively treating patients with anterior infarction. Hospital mortality in this group was reduced to about 7% from 12%–18% in historical cohorts treated with a conservative strategy.[71]

Six-month and 1-year follow-up of these patients confirmed that thrombolytic therapy with an appropriate revascularization strategy was associated with a low risk of death. Reinfarction, in particular, was dramatically affected by aggressive therapy. Compared to the previously defined 1-year reinfarction rate of 12% in Duke patients in the prethrombolytic era of the 1970s,[72] the reinfarction rate of 4% at 1 year in TAMI 1 was substantially lower. Likewise, the low postdischarge 1-year mortality rate in this group (1.9%) was striking.[73]

It was after the completion of several more phases of the TAMI studies and with the accumulation of a larger amount of data, however, that significant strides were made towards a better understanding of the prognosis of patients after MI. The cause of early mortality after thrombolytic therapy was evaluated in 810 TAMI patients.[74] In-hospital mortality was 6.8% in the overall group and was similar throughout the four TAMI trials included in the analysis (1,2,3,UK), with 38% of these deaths occurring in the first day. The majority of early deaths were found to result from cardiogenic shock (48%), ventricular arrhythmias (14%), or cardiac rupture (9%), most frequently in patients experiencing an anterior infarction (47%). Late in-hospital deaths were more often due to recurrent ischemia or reinfarction (32%) or noncardiac causes (18%). Intracranial hemorrhage or stroke accounted for 5% of early deaths and 6% of late in-hospital deaths in this group. The lowest patency rate after treatment (45%) was found in patients who died 24 hours after hospital admission, compared with 71% patency in patients who survived (P = 0.003). These results reaffirmed the need to identify strategies for reducing reocclusion and reinfarction, complications identified as leading to more complicated hospital courses with higher in-hospital mortality.[54]

Two-year follow-up of these 810 patients again suggested that the benefits of successful early intervention and follow-up of MI extended beyond the acute phase and provided excellent long-term survival with a low incidence of recurrent ischemic events.[75] The TAMI protocol allowed for widespread use of both emergency and elective revascularization, resulting in a total postdischarge mortality of only 3.3% at an average follow-up of 18.8 months, including just 2.1% cardiovascular mortality. Nonfatal reinfarction occurred in 5.1% of patients.

Criteria for Reperfusion Therapy

The early and accurate identification of patients with MI grew markedly more important as reperfusion strategies were introduced into the paradigm of care. The transformation from a conservative, watchful approach in acute MI to one of active intervention brought new concerns for optimizing the potential benefits of thrombolytic reperfusion while minimizing the risks inherent in such a strategy. Implicit in this approach is the importance of proper patient selection and of avoiding the inappropriate administration of thrombolytic agents to patients with little to gain or at significant risk for harm from such an intervention, especially patients with a mistaken diagnosis of MI.

In evaluating the incidence and outcomes of the misdiagnosis of acute MI for patients given thrombolytic therapy in TAMI 1–3, 5, and UK, Chapman et al.[76] found that the simple algorithm and specific criteria for diagnosing MI used in the TAMI trials led to a low rate of misdiagnosis and few adverse outcomes. The standard historical, clinical, and ECG criteria for thrombolytic therapy used in these trials included symptoms of acute infarction < 6 hours, but > 20 minutes not relieved with nitroglycerin and ST segment elevation > 1 mm in two contiguous leads or ST segment depression of posterior MI in the absence of Q waves in the same distribution. Exclusion criteria felt to reflect an increased risk of bleeding, including age > 75 years, were used as well. The use of these criteria led to the misdiagnosis of MI in 20 (1.4%) of 1,387 consecutive patients given thrombolytic therapy, despite implementation in a variety of clinical settings, including both community hospitals (63% of patients enrolled) and tertiary care centers. The ECG, in particular, was found to be important to the success of this selection strategy, as 55% of the patients misdiagnosed had a nondiagnostic entry ECG on review. No major complications, including death, occurred in any of the misdiagnosed patients.

Clinical and Angiographic Prognostic Variables

Baseline characteristics were found to be helpful in predicting survival after MI in 1,619 patients from six consecutive TAMI trials. In work by Lee and colleagues,[77] advanced age (P = 0.0001), low systolic blood pressure (P = 0.0004), anterior MI (P = 0.0023) and low blood pressure in the setting of anterior MI (P = 0.0031) were all found to be independent predictors of in-hospital mortality. These findings were confirmed in an analysis of 41,021 patients enrolled in the GUSTO-I trial, which demonstrated the significance of advanced age, low systolic blood pressure at presentation, higher Killip class, elevated heart rate, and anterior location of infarction on survival after acute MI treated with thrombolysis.[78] These noninvasive clinical determinants were inferior, however, to the value of acute catheterization for predicting mortality. Investigators found that in 855 patients enrolled in the first five TAMI trials, catheterization data was prognostically important, with multivessel disease, defined as ≥ 75% luminal diameter stenosis in two or more major epicardial vessels, a key predictor of short-term prognosis. Global EF was the most significant predictor of survival (P = 0.00001), with number of diseased vessels and TIMI flow grade also contributing independent prognostic information.[79]

At the same time, cardiac catheterization permitted identification of those patients with minimal atherosclerotic disease and a better in-hospital prognosis. Of a group of 799 patients studied in the TAMI trials, 43 patients had ≤ 50% stenosis on acute selective coronary angiography, while 42 patients had intermediate lesions on acute catheterization that had resolved by follow-up catheterization at 7–10 days to ≤ 50% stenoses. These patients were noted to be significantly younger (52 years vs 56.7 years, P = 0.002), had less multivessel disease (P < 0.001), had better initial ventricular function (mean EF 54% vs 50.2%, P = 0.006) and a lower in-hospital mortality (1% vs 7%, P = 0.04) than did patients with persistent significant disease.[80]

Mark and colleagues[81] used a similar analysis to identify characteristics predictive of postdischarge survival in 580 patients enrolled in the TAMI 1–3 trials. This group found that a combination of clinical variables and early cardiac catheterization results described a low-risk subgroup of acute MI patients who might be suitable for early (day 4) hospital discharge. The independent predictors of freedom from late major complications included absence of early sustained ventricular tachycardia or fibrillation, lack of sustained hypotension or cardiogenic shock, lack of multivessel disease, and better LV function. The 23% of patients who satisfied these criteria in the test sample had only a 3% major complication rate and no deaths or reinfarctions by day 30.

Similar to variables associated with presentation, the prognostic implications of various baseline characteristics in patients treated for acute MI was another area of intense scrutiny by TAMI investigators. The large TAMI database with its systematic collection of both invasive and noninvasive data permitted a reevaluation of prognostic variables, and consequently, cardiovascular risk factors such as diabetes and cigarette smoking, as well as other laboratory and clinical parameters, which were evaluated to determine the strength of association with a poor outcome after thrombolysis.

Gender

Several early reports on the effects of gender on outcome after MI indicated that women appear to be at increased risk for mortality, reinfarction, or congestive heart failure,[82–86] and unadjusted mortality rates for women continue to exceed those for men in the era of thrombolysis. In an effort to identify the significance of gender as a risk factor for poor outcome after thrombolysis, the outcome of 348 women enrolled in TAMI 1–3, 5, and 7 was compared with the 1,271 men who were enrolled.[87] Women were significantly older (61 years vs 55.8 years, $P < 0.0001$) and had more hypertension (55% vs 39%, $P < 0.0001$), diabetes (21% vs 15%, $P = 0.01$), hypercholesterolemia (24% vs 19%, $P = 0.023$), and peripheral vascular disease (9% vs 4%, $P < 0.0001$). Despite similar heart rates, baseline blood pressure and time to thrombolytic therapy, women had higher unadjusted rates of mortality (9.2% vs 5.4%, $P = 0.014$), reinfarction (6.4% vs 2.6%, $P = 0.005$), and hemorrhagic stroke (2.0% vs 0.55%, $P = 0.017$) than men. After adjustment for baseline characteristics, however, only reinfarction rates remained significantly higher in women (odds ratio 1.95, 95% CI 1.01–3.79), confirming that gender differences in mortality are ascribable to baseline characteristics apart from gender alone.

Diabetes

Diabetes has clearly been shown to have a negative impact on the mortality and morbidity associated with coronary arterial disease. In an effort to identify potential mechanisms for this poor outcome, Granger et al.[88] analyzed patient characteristics from TAMI 1–3, 5, and UK. One hundred forty-eight of the 1,071 patients in these studies had a history of diabetes mellitus. The diabetic patients tended to be older (mean age 59 years vs 56 years) with a higher incidence of hypertension (64% vs 40%) and hypercholesterolemia (22% vs 14%), more multivessel disease (66% vs 46%, $P < 0.0001$), worse noninfarct zone function (-0.13 vs 0.32 SD/chord, $P = 0.02$), and more pulmonary edema (11% vs 4%, $P = 0.001$) than nondiabetic patients. Despite a nearly two-fold in-hospital mortality in all diabetics (11% vs 6%) and even higher mortality in female diabetics (21%), however, diabetes was not found to have an independent influence on mortality after adjustment for these baseline characteristics. Importantly, similar baseline EFs in diabetic and nondiabetic patients, 49% and 51% respectively, and similar 90-minute patency (71% and 70%) and reocclusion rates (12% and 11%) indicate that resistance to thrombolysis is not a likely mechanism of the poor outcome in diabetic patients. Similar mortality rates were also observed in diabetic and nondiabetic patients after revascularization, suggesting that diabetic patients, as a high risk group, may benefit from an aggressive strategy of thrombolysis and, when appropriate, early revascularization.

Angina History

A history of angina can be elicited in one- to two-thirds of patients presenting with acute MI, while the importance of symptom status on clinical outcome remains unclear. In an attempt to prospectively evaluate this effect of preinfarction symptom status on clinical outcome, Muller and colleagues[89] examined 775 patients in TAMI 1–3 and UK with the hypothesis that an angina history of > 7 days prior to infarction would be associated with more extensive coronary artery disease and a more complicated hospital course. Unexpectedly, patients with antecedent angina, despite a worse risk factor profile, more multivessel disease and a lower baseline ejection fraction, had a somewhat less complicated in-hospital course, with a trend towards decreased mortality (4.6% vs 7.2%, $P = 0.21$) and less reocclusion (8.2% vs 13.6%, $P = 0.048$) than patients without an angina history. While unable to fully explain these findings, important potential contributing factors included possible myocardial "preconditioning" promoting the formation of collaterals and thereby limiting the infarct size. Patients with less severe fixed coronary obstruction may, in turn, suffer from the presence of a greater component of fresh thrombus and a more significant ongoing prothrombotic milieu after thrombolysis, predisposing them to greater reocclusion and recurrent ischemia. Finally, the greater preinfarction use of beta-blockers as antianginal therapy may have had a positive effect on outcome. While antecedent angina was not associated with a worse short-term prognosis, however, patients without an angina history had a somewhat better 2-year out-of-hospital survival rate (98.5% vs 94.2%), resulting in similar cumulative 2-year survival rates of 89.1% and 90.2% for patients with and without antecedent angina, respectively.

Smoking

A history of cigarette smoking, although a strong risk factor for premature atherosclerosis, MI, and sudden death, had been paradoxically shown[90–92] to be associated with a lower mortality after acute MI. To further evaluate this relationship, 1,619 patients enrolled in TAMI 1–3, UK, 5, and 7 were studied in light of their smoking status.[93] The group of 878 patients who were current smokers at the time of their infarction did, indeed, have lower in-hospital mortality (4% vs 8.9%, P = 0.0001) in univariate analysis, despite similar 90-minute patency rates (73% vs 74%). Careful adjustment for baseline characteristics, however, revealed significant differences between these two groups and suggested that smoking was not an independent predictor of decreased mortality. Active smokers tended to be younger (mean age 54 vs 60, P < 0.0001), have less three-vessel disease (16% vs 22%, P < 0.001) and better EFs at baseline (53% vs 50%, P = 0.0069), and ex-

perience more inferior infarctions (60% vs 53%, P < 0.0001). Baseline hematocrit and fibrinogen levels were higher in smokers, 44% vs 43% (P = 0.0001) and 2.8 vs 2.7 g/dL (P = 0.003), respectively. The greater percentage of smokers achieving TIMI-3 flow acutely (41.1% vs 34.6%, P = 0.03), with an associated larger minimal lumen diameter found acutely (0.82 vs 0.72 mm, P = 0.04) and at follow-up catheterization (1.2 vs 1.0 mm, P = 0.002), supported a possible mechanism of a largely thrombotic occlusion of a less severely stenotic vessel, leading to improved perfusion characteristics after thrombolysis and subsequent better survival.

Pericarditis

In patients not receiving thrombolytic therapy, the incidence of pericarditis may be as high as 20% during hospitalization and is felt to be associated with transmural necrosis leading to pericardial inflammation. Wall and colleagues[94] identified only 40 (4.9%) of 810 patients enrolled in TAMI 1–3 and UK noted to have a pericardial friction rub by auscultation during hospitalization. These patients had lower EF (45% vs 51%, P = 0.002), more three-vessel disease (30% vs 16%) and higher in-hospital mortality (15% vs 6%, P = 0.056), identifying pericarditis as a factor associated with more extensive myocardial damage and a worse clinical outcome. Importantly, the incidence of pericarditis was significantly less than that reported prior to the thrombolytic era, and cardiac tamponade did not occur clinically in any patient who developed a rub, suggesting the safety of continued anticoagulant therapy in the presence of pericarditis.

Belkin and colleagues[95] corroborated the safety of anticoagulation in the setting of a pericardial effusion in a prospective echocardiographic evaluation of 52 patients enrolled in TAMI 1. Acutely, 8% of the patients studied had a pericardial effusion, with a peak incidence of 24% at day 10. In addition to finding no clinical evidence for tamponade in these patients, there were no echocardiographic signs of cardiac tamponade in these postthrombolytic patients, and only one of ten effusions was noted to be large, despite the significant incidence of effusions and the maintenance of aggressive anticoagulation. Thus, although the echocardiographic incidence of pericardial effusion (24%) was consistent with studies in the prethrombolytic era, this study helped to confirm that adverse sequelae after thrombolytic therapy appear to be rare.

ECG Changes

Precordial ST segment depression had been associated with a poor prognosis in inferior MI prior to the advent of thrombolysis. To determine the impact of thrombolytic therapy on the angiographic and clinical outcomes in this group, Bates et al.[96] evaluated 583 patients enrolled in the first three TAMI trials. Of the 294 patients suffering an inferior MI, 135 (46%) had precordial ST segment depression. Despite reperfusion therapy, these patients tended to experience more complications with worse EFs (53% vs 58%) and a higher mortality (6% vs 5%) than patients without precordial ST segment changes.

In studying records from 810 patients from TAMI 1–3 and UK, Clemmensen and colleagues[97] likewise demonstrated the prognostic importance of complete atrioventricular (AV) block complicating inferior MI after thrombolysis. Of 373 patients admitted with an inferior MI, 50 (13%) developed complete AV block, an incidence similar to prethrombolytic studies. In fact, compared with previous reports, the major effect of thrombolytic reperfusion on the progression of complete AV block was to decrease its duration to a median of 2.5 hours, the shortest duration reported in a large series of patients. While acute patency rates were similar between patients with or without complete AV block, patients who suffered AV block had a greater decrease in

LVEF between initial and predischarge catheterization (-3.5% vs -0.4%, $P = 0.03$), higher rates of reocclusion (29% vs 16%, $P = 0.03$), and more ventricular fibrillation or tachycardia (36% vs 14%, $P < 0.001$), sustained hypotension (36% vs 10%, $P < 0.001$), and pulmonary edema (12% vs 4%, $P = 0.02$). These patients also suffered a significantly higher in-hospital mortality rate (20% vs 4%, $P < 0.001$), with multivariate regression analysis demonstrating that complete AV block is a strong independent predictor of in-hospital mortality ($P = 0.0006$).

EF as a Determinant of Improvement

Significant effort went into the evaluation of changes in regional and global LV systolic function in the week following thrombolysis, which was one of the primary end points of the TAMI studies. Animal models of infarction have provided a theoretical basis for the gradual recovery of EF as a marker of myocardial salvage following successful early reperfusion after MI. Thrombolytic trials, however, have failed to establish a consistent significant effect of reperfusion therapy on EF, despite the demonstration of improved survival. Although Grines and colleagues[98] were able to elucidate a relationship between reduced noninfarct zone regional wall motion and both multivessel disease ($P = 0.0001$), possibly as a result of "ischemia at a distance," and mortality ($P = 0.006$), they found no such relationship with infarct zone function in 332 patients enrolled in TAMI 1. Just as in subsequent studies, reduced global EF was found to be associated with greater in-hospital mortality ($P = 0.025$), but the absolute differences in median EF between survivors and nonsurvivors was not striking (53% vs 50%), limiting the prognostic utility of this finding.

Similar results were obtained by Harrison et al.[99] in an analysis of ventriculograms from 542 patients enrolled in

TAMI 1–3 and UK, calling into question the adequacy of LV functional recovery as a surrogate end point in thrombolytic trials. In these patients, there was no overall change in global EF after thrombolytic therapy, and only moderate improvement in infarct zone function during the first week after therapy. Even at 6 months, a separate analysis revealed that there was only minimal further improvement in LV systolic function.[100] Improvement in global and regional systolic function was most closely related to acute impairment of ventricular function and successful reperfusion. Unlike those patients receiving thrombolytic therapy alone, patients undergoing surgical or mechanical revascularization experienced a beneficial effect on both global and regional wall motion.[99] Other investigators noting the apparent inadequacies of an improvement in LV function as a surrogate end point in TAMI and other thrombolytic trials[101,102] prompted a call for the development of alternative surrogates for mortality reduction in trials underpowered to detect mortality differences.

Importance of IRA Patency

Predictors of in-hospital mortality were also evaluated. Early complete reperfusion, represented by TIMI-3 flow, was found to be predictive of survival; while TIMI-2 flow, representing complete, although sluggish, filling of the infarct vessel, did not portend an improved survival. Failure to achieve TIMI-3 flow independently doubled the odds of in-hospital mortality and was found to be equivalent to either an 18-year increase in age, a 19-point decrease in EF, or up to 1 additional diseased vessel.[20,103]

Further analysis of 1,229 patients enrolled in TAMI phases 1–3, 5, and 7 added to these findings, demonstrating that TIMI-2 flow rather than TIMI-3 flow acutely after thrombolysis was associated with significantly greater rates of recurrent ischemia (22.9% vs 16.9%, P = 0.05) and CHF (26.2% vs 19.0%, P = 0.03). In addition, there was a significant gradient of increasing mortality noted in patients with lower TIMI flow (4.3%, 6.1%, and 10.1% with TIMI 3, 2, and 1 or 0 flow, respectively, P = 0.002), adding credence to the "open-artery hypothesis" that early reperfusion offers a survival benefit in acute MI. These outcomes were independent of the use of adjunctive acute coronary angioplasty and, in fact, the group of patients with TIMI-2 flow acutely had significantly decreased LVEF (49% vs 52%, P = 0.004) and poorer infarct zone wall motion (−2.74 vs −2.44, P = 0.002) compared to the TIMI-3 flow group at acute 90-minute catheterization, indicating the importance of very early total reperfusion towards a good clinical outcome.[104]

IRA Occlusion, Reocclusion, and Recurrent Ischemia

The TAMI 5 trial demonstrated the clinical benefit of acute coronary angiography and rescue angioplasty as needed for failed thrombolysis. Early identification of failed reperfusion allows rapid triage to suitable revascularization or supportive measures. Acute coronary angiography, although a proven and reliable method of identifying failed reperfusion after thrombolysis, is simply not routinely possible in many hospitals and may be associated with an increased complication rate. This, coupled with the inability to accurately identify reperfusion based on clinical parameters alone, led to the evaluation of alternative, noninvasive modes of rapidly identifying failed thrombolysis.

Krucoff et al.[105,106] demonstrated in 22 patients enrolled in the TAMI 7 trial that continuous 12-lead ST segment monitoring offers a noninvasive prediction of coronary occlusion and real-time "visualization" of cyclic changes in coronary flow. A subsequent blinded, prospective, angiographically correlated study involving 144 patients enrolled in the TAMI 7 trial confirmed that this device could reliably detect failed reperfusion with a positive predictive value of 71%, negative predictive value of 87%, and a 90% specificity and 64% sensitivity for coronary occlusion.[107]

Veldkamp and colleagues[108] studied the relative benefit of the continuous 12-lead ST segment monitor compared with repeated static 12-lead ECGs in identifying coronary occlusion in 82 patients in the TAMI 7 trial. The ST segment monitor accurately predicted coronary patency status in 85% of cases at the moment of acute angiography. The best of five methods of static ECG analysis, by comparison, accurately predicted reperfusion status in 83% of cases. In addition, the ST segment monitor frequently demonstrates cyclic patterns after thrombolytic therapy, possibly identifying a subset of patients with specific reperfusion characteristics. The importance and reproducibility of these findings in predicting coronary patency status or reocclusion requires further investigation.

A combined clinical and serological approach to the noninvasive detection of reperfusion also demonstrated promise in a study of 207 patients enrolled in the TAMI 7 trial.[109] A rapid creatine kinase (CK)-MB assay, drawn at presentation and 30, 90, and 180 minutes, and selected clinical variables were used to create a predictive model of reperfusion status. The rapid assay for serum CK-MB allowed determination of CK-MB levels within 10–20 minutes. Baseline CK-MB levels were similar in patients regardless of eventual reperfusion status. Ninety-minute values, however, were higher in the 146 patients (71%) with successful reperfusion than in patients with TIMI grade 0 or 1 flow (P = 0.002). The slope of CK-MB changes between baseline and 90-minute values correlated highly with reperfusion status (P = 0.0003). Baseline clinical characteristics analyzed for association with reperfusion status were derived from patients enrolled in the TAMI 1–5 trials. By logistic regression, factors contributing to the combined model included the slope of the CK-MB change, chest pain before acute angiography, and

time from onset of chest pain to thrombolytic therapy, yielding a highly significant association with infarct artery patency (Chi-square = 26.3, P <0.00001). Unlike previous attempts at predicting coronary patency status, this model was developed to generate probabilities of a persistently occluded infarct artery, permitting additional clinical characteristics, such as age or comorbid illness, to be weighed in the decision to proceed with urgent catheterization.

Even after achieving successful reperfusion of an IRA, maintenance of patency is important, as reocclusion is associated with significantly increased morbidity and mortality. In a study of 733 patients successfully reperfused in the TAMI 1–3 and UK trials,[54] 91 patients (12.4%) experienced reocclusion of the IRA as documented by angiography performed an average of 7 days after thrombolytic therapy. Forty-two percent of reoccluded arteries were noted in asymptomatic patients. Patients who suffered reocclusion in this study had more right coronary artery infarctions (65% vs 44%), more TIMI flow 0 or 1 prior to further intervention (21% vs 10%), and worse infarct zone function (−2.7 SD/chord vs −2.4 SD/chord, P = 0.016) at baseline compared to patients with sustained patency. At follow-up, patients with reocclusion had more complicated hospitalizations, with impaired recovery of LV function (median Δ EF −2 vs 1, P = 0.006 and median Δ infarct-zone wall motion −0.10 SD/chord vs 0.34 SD/chord, P = 0.011) and higher in-hospital mortality rates (11% vs 4.5%, P = 0.01) compared to patients without reocclusion.

To illustrate additional costs associated with recurrent ischemia, clinical and economic parameters were analyzed for 1,221 patients enrolled in the TAMI trials.[110] As in previous studies, recurrent ischemia was found to be a common occurrence, both in the setting of recurrent MI (2.5%) and as an isolated event (18.3%). In addition to the excess mortality and heart failure noted in patients experiencing recurrent ischemia, there was a stepwise increase in health-care resource utilization. Patients without recurrent ischemia had the shortest hospital stays (9 days) and the lowest total charges ($19,721). Patients who experienced recurrent ischemia or recurrent ischemia with reinfarction had longer stays and higher hospital charges (10 days and 14 days, and $23,609 and $24,690, respectively).

Thus, reocclusive events after successful reperfusion are associated with excess cost and mortality rates approaching those seen in the absence of reperfusion therapy. The early and accurate identification of patients who will ultimately experience reocclusion could permit triage to definitive coronary revascularization procedures. Unfortunately, identification of patients at risk for recurrent ischemia is distinctly unreliable. In contrast to previous smaller studies, an evaluation of eight prospectively identified angiographic variables failed to identify any association between 90-minute angiographic appearance and recurrent ischemic events. Ellis and colleagues[111] studied 174 patients enrolled in the TAMI 1 and 3 trials who had successful tPA thrombolysis with TIMI flow grade 2 (59.2%) or 3 (40.8%) and did not undergo immediate coronary angioplasty. Forty-one patients (21.3%) experienced recurrent ischemia during the course of hospitalization. There was no significant association between these ischemic events and any combination of the baseline angiographic variables examined: the IRA; TIMI flow grade; percent diameter stenosis; absolute luminal diameter; angiographically defined thrombus; diffuse disease or ectasia in the IRA; or morphology of the infarct related stenosis. In addition, informal evaluation of various demographic and treatment variables failed to clearly identify any association with recurrent ischemia.

A smaller study of 47 patients enrolled in the TAMI 1 trial was able to identify a qualitative association between angiographic morphology and recurrent ischemia.[112] Inclusion criteria for this study were similar to those in the Ellis study, with the additional analysis of a protocol 24-hour catheterization in 31 patients.

Eighteen patients (38%) had recurrent ischemia/reocclusion. While baseline angiographic characteristics were largely unpredictive of recurrent ischemic events, at 24-hour angiography no patient with subsequent ischemia had concentric narrowing, whereas 44% of patients without ischemic events had this lesion morphology (P = 0.016). Thus, in this small study, lesion morphological changes occurring within 24 hours after successful thrombolysis appear to be predictive of subsequent ischemic episodes and provide information not available at acute angiography. The clinical importance of this finding is unclear.

Just as in the previous informal analysis of TAMI 1 and 3 trial data, clinical data in TAMI 5 were not helpful in predicting reocclusion. In a study of 288 patients randomized to a conservative postthrombolytic strategy in TAMI 5, Muller and colleagues[113] corroborated the inadequacy of clinical predictors of recurrent ischemia requiring urgent catheterization. Fifty-four patients (19%) required urgent catheterization within 24 hours and 75 patients (26%) underwent catheterization within 4 days for symptomatic recurrent ischemia, resulting in emergency angioplasty in 49% of these patients and urgent coronary artery bypass in 3%. Only patient age (P = 0.0016) and anterior infarction (P = 0.017) were associated with the need for urgent catheterization. Other presentation variables studied, including coronary disease risk factors, pulse, blood pressure, time to treatment, and thrombolytic used did not demonstrate a similar association. No clinical variables could adequately predict which patients would likely require intervention for recurrent ischemia.

Revascularization

While early patency of an IRA improves clinical outcome, trials of attaining revascularization by angioplasty after thrombolysis have produced mixed results. The potential benefit of successful mechanical reperfusion must be weighed against the risk of complications. As discussed above, evaluation of the TAMI 1 experience suggested that routine immediate angioplasty after thrombolysis offered no clear short-term benefit over delayed elective angioplasty, even after failed thrombolysis. Six-month follow-up, however, revealed a low out-of-hospital mortality in patients undergoing rescue angioplasty for failed thrombolysis (TIMI grade 0–1 flow).[15]

Stack and colleagues[114] studied the 1-year survival and event-free survival rates in 342 patients undergoing thrombolytic therapy followed by emergency coronary angioplasty for MI at Duke University. These investigators noted a low procedural mortality rate (1.2%) and a high success rate (94%), with an in-hospital mortality of 11%. The 1-year postdischarge survival rate was 98%, with an infarct-free survival of 94% in this group. This low out-of-hospital mortality was noted even in high risk groups, such as patients with cardiogenic shock (4%), EFs less than 40% (3%), and for patients > 65 years old (3%), suggesting that routine mechanical revascularization may have a role after thrombolytic therapy, especially in high risk subgroups.

To identify another subgroup of patients who might benefit from early intervention, 108 patients enrolled in the TAMI 1 trial with TIMI grade 2 flow at acute catheterization were studied.[16] Baseline characteristics were similar between the 49 patients randomized to early PTCA and the 59 patients randomized to medical therapy alone. Despite a trend towards greater improvement in LV function in patients undergoing PTCA (51% to 52% vs 55% to 53%, P = 0.06) compared with medically treated patients, in-hospital mortality and heart failure were not significantly different.

To better assess the in-hospital and long-term outcome of rescue angioplasty, Abbottsmith et al.[115] studied 776 patients who achieved successful reperfusion in the TAMI 1–4 and UK trials. Thrombolytic therapy was successful in 607 of these patients, and 169 patients required rescue angioplasty to achieve patency. These groups

had similar baseline characteristics with the exception of higher acute LVEF (51.3% vs 48.2%, P = 0.003) in the thrombolysis group. The in-hospital and long-term (median follow-up 20 months) mortality rates were similar in patients with and without rescue angioplasty (5.9% vs 4.6% and 3% vs 2%, respectively). Patients requiring rescue angioplasty, however, had higher reocclusion rates (21% vs 11%, P < 0.001) and less infarct zone recovery (0.44 vs 0.21 SD/chord, P = 0.001).

As vascular access site bleeding is a prime complication in the use of PTCA in acute MI, George et al.[116] studied the potential benefit of the brachial versus femoral approach. The brachial artery approach was used in 202 of 704 patients enrolled in the TAMI 1–3 trials. There was no significant difference in any measured clinical outcome between the brachial and femoral approaches, including death (6% vs 6%), reocclusion (10% vs 14%), nadir hematocrit (32.9 vs 33.0), and vascular repair (1% vs 3%). The brachial approach did not result in any significant delay to access or vascular compromise, indicating that in experienced hands, the brachial approach can be used in the setting of acute MI without any increased risk or compromise of results.

The role of early coronary bypass surgery after thrombolytic therapy is controversial as well. Kereiakes and colleagues[117] demonstrated the safety and efficacy of coronary bypass in the setting of acute MI in several analyses of the TAMI studies. In the largest study, 303 (22%) of the 1,387 patients enrolled in the TAMI 1–3, UK, and 5 trials underwent bypass surgery prior to discharge as part of a sequential reperfusion strategy that included acute thrombolysis with or without PTCA. Indications for coronary bypass included failed PTCA (12%), left main or equivalent disease (9%), complex multivessel disease (62%), recurrent ischemia (13%), and refractory pump failure, mitral regurgitation, ventricular septal defect, or an abnormal predischarge functional study (1% each). Thirty-six (11.9%) of the bypass operations were performed early after presentation (< 24 hours). Patients undergoing bypass surgery were older (59.5 vs 56 years, P < 0.0001), had more three-vessel disease (46% vs 11%, P < 0.0001), more diabetes (19% vs 15%, P = 0.048), more prior infarctions (24% vs 10%, P < 0.0001), and worse initial LVEF (48% vs 51.8%, P = 0.0002) than patients not undergoing surgery. Despite the worse clinical status, inhospital mortality rates were similar between the surgical and nonsurgical patients (7% vs 6%). Surgical mortality was 3%. In addition, the surgical patients experienced significantly greater improvement in LVEF (3.4% vs 0.16%, P = 0.036) and regional infarct zone function (0.71 vs 0.34 SD/chord, P = 0.001) than nonsurgical patients. At a median follow-up of > 1,090 days, the clinical status secured by the surgical patients persisted, with similar rates of postdischarge mortality (7.2% vs 6.2%), nonfatal reinfarction (5.3% vs 8.4%), and PTCA or CABG (7.4% vs 17.9%) between the surgical and nonsurgical groups. These results confirmed prior evaluations of coronary bypass patients enrolled in the TAMI 1 trial,[118,119] in which bypass surgery patients and nonsurgical patients were found to have similar short- and long-term mortality rates, a similar frequency of cardiac and noncardiac hospitalizations, similar event-free survival rates, and similar general health status.

Adjunctive Therapies

Despite several theoretical advantages of using the intraaortic balloon pump (IABP) in acute MI, the therapeutic potential of this device remained largely unexplored until the late 1980s. While useful in supporting the failing heart as a bridge to definitive therapy, the afterload reduction and augmented coronary artery perfusion pressure the IABP provides also make it an attractive adjunct to reperfusion therapy. To explore the risks and possible benefit of aortic counterpulsation after thrombolytic therapy for acute MI, 810 patients enrolled in the TAMI 1–3 and UK trials were evaluated in an observational fashion with regard to IABP use and clinical

outcome.[120] The 85 patients who received an IABP during hospitalization were older (58 vs 56 years), had more anterior infarctions (62% vs 38%), more multivessel disease (67% vs 43%), less TIMI flow ≥ 2 (56% vs 72%), lower EF (40% vs 52%), and worse infarct zone and noninfarct zone function (−3.2 vs −2.5 SD/chord and −0.67 vs ± 0.36 SD/chord, respectively) than their counterparts who were not treated with aortic counterpulsation. Despite being a sicker group, patients experienced no reinfarction or reocclusion of the IRA while being treated with the IABP. They also showed greater improvement in global EF (Δ: +1.9% vs +0.7%) and noninfarct zone function (Δ SD/chord: +0.11 vs −0.09) than patients not receiving an IABP at follow-up catheterization. Mortality (32% vs 4%) and in-hospital complications, however, were greater in patients treated with IABP.

Additional analysis of 1,331 patients enrolled in the TAMI 1–3, UK, 5, and 7 trials[121] confirmed the utility of IABP in promoting coronary artery patency after thrombolysis. The 112 patients receiving IABP again were older (58 vs 56 years), had more previous infarction (24% vs 12%), more anterior infarction (66% vs 41%), more heart failure (Killip class > 1: 48% vs 18%), more three-vessel disease (44% vs 17%), and were more likely to have failed to reperfuse by the time of acute angiography (46% vs 29%) compared to patients not undergoing counterpulsation. IABP use was significantly associated with lower reocclusion rates (2% vs 11%), especially in patients who had rescue angioplasty (Chi-square = 5.8, P = 0.016). These results suggested a possible therapeutic role for aortic counterpulsation in treating high risk patients after reperfusion therapy for MI.

Coagulation Parameters and Complications of Thrombolytic and Adjunctive Therapy

Integral to the careful selection of thrombolytic eligible patients is avoidance or modification of therapy in patients determined to be at significantly increased risk for complications, such as bleeding and stroke. The TAMI trials provided information not only on the observed incidence of complications, but also on a variety of clinical and laboratory parameters associated with these complications, helping to better understand the underlying pathophysiology of thrombosis and fibrinolytic therapy. In studying hematological parameters to interpret the adverse events associated with thrombolytic therapy in the 386 TAMI 1 patients, including thrombolytic failure, recurrent ischemia, reocclusion and bleeding, Sane et al.[122] confirmed previous findings that plasma activator inhibitor (PAI) levels and PAI-1 antigen levels are elevated in acute MI. PAI is an important regulator of physiological fibrinolysis, behaving much as an acute phase reactant, and was felt to have a potential impact in therapeutic thrombolysis in certain patients. Close review of the data in these patients, however, demonstrated that neither baseline PAI activity or PAI-1 antigen levels correlate strongly with major clinical outcomes, including patency, reocclusion, reinfarction, in-hospital mortality, or bleeding. An earlier analysis using linear regression in this same population did report a significant correlation between bleeding and higher baseline PAI levels (P = 0.03), as well as lower nadir fibrinogen levels (P = 0.005),[123] although the association with fibrinogen levels was not consistent in later analysis.[124]

To identify mechanisms responsible for the apparent beneficial effect of combination UK and tPA therapy seen in the TAMI 5 trial, Popma and colleagues[125] found that hematological factors, rather than angiographic characteristics, may play a central role. IRA characteristics and hematological parameters were evaluated in 287 patients enrolled in the TAMI 5 trial. As described earlier, clinical events and reocclusion rates were less frequent in patients receiving combination thrombolysis, but differences in acute and convalescent coronary dimensions were not able to account for these differences. The hemostatic protein levels were associated with outcome, however. The significantly higher peak fibrin degradation products (P < 0.0001) in patients receiving UK or combination therapy as opposed to tPA monotherapy was associated with less reocclusion (P = 0.004) and fewer in-hospital clinical events.

Cellular components of hemostasis may have an even more important role in clinical outcome after thrombolysis. Harrington and colleagues[126] demonstrated in 1,001 patients enrolled in TAMI 2, 3, UK, and 5 that thrombocytopenia, defined either as <100,000 platelets/μL or < $_{1/2}$ baseline number, is a frequent event, occurring in 16.4% of these patients, and is associated with excess hemorrhage and in-hospital mortality. Even when corrected for confounding variables such as bypass surgery, intraaortic counterpulsation, and age, thrombocytopenia after thrombolysis was still strongly associated with these adverse clinical events. While not demonstrating causality, this study clearly indicated the prognostic importance of platelet count after thrombolysis.

Template bleeding time, however, was not shown to be as prognostically useful a hemostatic index as platelet count in predicting bleeding. In a study of 127 patients enrolled in TAMI 8 and the Systematic Methods to Approach Restenosis Trial (SMART), standard bleeding time measurements at baseline and 2, 6, 12, 24, 48, and 72 hours after initiation of 7E3 glycoprotein IIb/IIIa inhibitor therapy demonstrated no association with clinical bleeding events. There was a significant association again found between a substantial decline in platelet number at 24 hours and bleeding (P = 0.02). Bernardi and colleagues[127] used this information to recommend platelet count, rather than template bleeding time, in the hematological monitoring of patients receiving platelet function antagonists.

Now firmly established, the importance of certain clinical factors in increasing the risk of bleeding, especially with the introduction of fibrin specific therapy, was not at first clear. Analysis of baseline clinical attributes in the 386 TAMI 1 patients clearly demonstrated an increased hemorrhagic risk associated with increased age (P = 0.0001), female gender (P = 0.002), lighter weight (P = 0.007), and a history of hypertension (P = 0.019),[123] and these results were subsequently verified in a larger population of patients enrolled in TAMI 5.[124] These factors did not correlate with risk of hemorrhagic stroke, however.[128] As expected, invasive procedures, such as coronary artery bypass grafting, aortic counterpulsation, and angioplasty were also significantly associated with hemorrhage,[123] although early catheterization alone did not significantly increase clinical bleeding risk.[124] These results led to the weight-based modification of thrombolytic dosing, as well as the adjustment of criteria for transfusion after the demonstration that a lower threshold for administration of blood products (hematocrit of 22%–24%) could safely reduce transfusion requirements.[44,124]

Certain empirically derived contraindications to thrombolytic therapy also underwent close scrutiny by TAMI investigators. Tenaglia and colleagues[129] were able to show, for instance, that cardiopulmonary resuscitation (CPR) of short duration (< 10 minutes) prior to thrombolysis was not associated with any adverse effect. This was notable in that of the 708 patients enrolled in the TAMI 1–3 trials, 59 patients (8%) required CPR for 10 minutes or less prior to thrombolytic therapy, but there were no bleeding complications directly attributable to CPR. Additionally, Granger and colleagues[88] found that although diabetic retinopathy was noted in 7% of patients with diabetes, there were no ocular hemorrhages noted, and the overall incidence of significant bleeding was no different than in nondiabetics.

Regionalization of Care

The introduction of thrombolytic therapy offered the promise of decreased morbidity and mortality in acute MI, but concerns about potential complications and inadequate emergency preparedness delayed its early use in community hospitals. The early TAMI trials relied heavily on the regionalization of MI care to the large clinical sites. In the TAMI 1 trial, 48% of the 386 patients were transferred to one of the four clinical sites by helicopter from local community hospitals. There were no serious complications during transportation of these patients.[15] An analysis of the early Duke University experience with helicopter transport of acute MI patients confirmed that complications are infrequent and are manageable en route.[130,131] These results seemed to support a regional approach to the management of thrombolysis and infarct management. The availability of catheterization laboratories and emergency coronary bypass grafting in large medical centers was deemed necessary due to the high frequency of failed reperfusion or recurrent ischemia.

Many of these concerns were addressed in the intervening years. As thrombolytic protocols were standardized and physician awareness increased, the willingness to provide thrombolytic therapy and care in the community increased as well. A recognition of the relationship between the timing of reperfusion and outcome prompted attempts at providing early thrombolytic therapy in the community. In the UK trial,[132] 87 of 102 patients were enrolled at 11 community hospitals without complications related to misdiagnosis or inappropriate evaluation. Bleeding and other complications were all treated successfully. Importantly, patients treated in the community received thrombolytic therapy a median of 1.8 hours earlier than if they had waited for arrival to a tertiary center. Thus, the way was opened for the widespread community-based use of thrombolytic agents as a safe and more effective treatment for MI.

Conclusion

The Thrombolysis and Angioplasty in MI study group set out in 1985 to perform randomized clinical trials in the traditional academic setting as well as in a nonacademic environment. The studies very clearly showed that it was possible to perform high quality research in a variety of settings including the community hospital. By taking this nontraditional approach, it was possible to provide protocols to the community at large and not only answer important clinical questions but, more importantly, to provide opportunities for clinical research in the broader community in which most patients are treated.

A decade of collaboration among the TAMI investigators has addressed the role of clinical features in evaluating prognosis, the economic and clinical impact of early hospital discharge, and important lessons about optimal reperfusion strategies. The group as a whole charted many uncharted waters while providing new and innovative treatment strategies to the community. Although large randomized mortality trials have by and large superseded the smaller mechanistic trials, the group's work in the formative years of reperfusion strategies paved the way for the design of many new Phase II clinical trials with adjunctive therapies for acute MI. Thus, the work from the TAMI group has branched out not only into survival benefits for patients with acute MI, but also into understanding the pathophysiology of acute ischemic heart disease. The collaborative work by the TAMI investigators thus represents a small piece of history in U.S. clinical investigation of acute MI in the late 1980s and early 1990s, which provides further stepping stones for improved outcomes and better understanding of the pathophysiology of a condition that affects millions of patients worldwide each year.

Appendix

Comprehensive List of TAMI Investigators: The Cast (listed in order of appearance). University of Michigan, Ann Arbor, Michigan

Eric J. Topol, M.D., Bertram Pitt, M.D., William W. O'Neill, M.D., Joseph A. Walton Jr., M.D., Eric R. Bates, M.D., Stephen G. Ellis, M.D., Patrick D.V. Bourdillon, M.D., M. Anthony Schork, Ph.D., Eva M. Kline, R.N., BSN, Laura Gorman, R.N., BSN, Raymond Worden, B.S., Cindy L. Grines, M.D., Mark L. Sanz, M.D., Darrell L. Debowey, MS, Elizabeth G. Nabel, M.D., Barbara Schumaker, HRA, John Kunkel, B.S., Steven Werns, M.D., Peter Thomasma, B.S., Markus Schwaiger, M.D., Keith Aaronson, M.D., Sheila Squicciarini, B.S., RT(N), Diane Bondi, B.S., Jeffrey J. Popma, M.D., Kate Staford, B.S., RT(N), Anita Galeana, R.N. *Collaborating Centers*

Foote Hospital, Jackson, Michigan: Gregory Baumann, M.D., John Maino II, M.D., Mary Ann Mengleson, M.D., Constance Doyle, M.D., Patricia Lamb, M.D., Sid Shah, M.D., Nathan Sherman, M.D., Douglas Salyards, M.D., Nathan Kander, M.D., Kevin Kelly, M.D., Tama Martini, M.D., Rajesh Shah, M.D., Ronald Wainz, M.D. *South Macomb Hospital, Warren, Michigan:* Stanley Wolfe, M.D., Leonard Bayer, DO, Armando Madrazo, M.D., Robert Moore, M.D. *St. Joseph Mercy Hospital, Ann Arbor, Michigan:* Dennis Wahr, M.D., Kurt Holland, M.D., Richard Judge, M.D., Ron Vanderbelt, M.D., Bruce Genovese, M.D., Lorenzo DiCarlo, M.D., Robert Steele, M.D., Stuart Wilson, M.D., Ralph Brandt, M.D., John Fisher, M.D., Frank Smith, M.D., Stephen Rosenblum, M.D., David Zuehlke, M.D., Marty McClain, R.N., Ann Burr, R.N.

Duke University Medical Center, Durham, North Carolina

Robert M. Califf, M.D., Richard S. Stack, M.D., Kerry L. Lee, Ph.D., Harry R. Phillips III, M.D., Tomoaki Hinchara, M.D., Robert H. Peter, M.D., Kenneth Morris, M.D., Victor S. Behar, M.D., Yi-Hong Kong, M.D., Charles A. Simonton, M.D., Thomas M. Bashore, M.D., Eric Carlson, M.D., Susan J. Mantell, R.N., B.S., Lynne Aronson, B.S., Jane M. Boswick, MPH, Mark A. Hlatky, M.D., Daniel B. Mark, M.D., MPH, Kristina N. Sigmon, MS, Joy Miller, R.N., Lynn Harrelson-Woodlief, MS, Thomas C. Wall, M.D., Peter Quigley, M.D., James Bengtson, M.D., Michael

Honan, M.D., Christopher O'Connor, M.D., Robert Bauman, M.D., Eric Berrios, R.N., Linda Sneed, R.N., Cynthia Flanagan, R.N., Margaret Liu, R.N., Sharon Karnash, B.S., Grace Wilson, B.S., Tammy Allen, R.N., Galen Wagner, M.D., Peter Clemmensen, M.D., Laura Stewart, R.Ph., Tom Burrus, R.ph., James Melton, MHA, Joseph C. Greenfield, M.D., Joseph Loscalzo, M.D., David Pryor, M.D., Arthur A. Sasahara, M.D., James Lancaster, Ph.D., Margaret Lui, R.N., Kimberly Klinker, R.N., Hyla Cohen, M.A., Benetta Walker, B.S., Kathi Lucas, R.N., Cheryl Cortright, R.N., Khalid Sheik, M.D., Sheila Kim-Heinle, M.D., Peter Longabaugh, M.D., E. Magnus Ohman, M.D., Mitchell Krucoff, M.D., Karen Pieper, MS, Marty Croll, R.N., Laura Pendley, R.N., Michael Plummer, R.N., Karen Loffler, R.N., Michelle Pulliam, Rob Christenson, Ph.D., Kirby Quinteros, R.N., Jeffrey D. Leimberger, Ph.D., Linda D. Ray, Nancy Clapp-Channing *Collaborating Centers*

Mariah Parham Hospital, Henderson, North Carolina: Depak Pasi, M.D., J. Franklin Mills, M.D., Peggy Piccioli, HN-ER, Nancy Strickland, R.N.-CCU, Steve Potter, Pharmacist

Alamance County and Alamance Memorial Hospitals, Burlington, North Carolina: James Strickland, M.D., Javed Masoud, M.D., Michael DiMeo, M.D., Don Chaplin, M.D., R. Tempest Lowry, M.D., Becky Clemmons, HN-ER, Marion Isley, HN-CCU, Gene Griner, M.D., William Wilcockson, M.D., Carolyn Summers, HN-ER, Gloria Taylor, R.N.-CCU, Stuart Schnider, M.D., Donald Pathman, M.D., Paul Mele, M.D., Wayne Ruth, M.D.

Durham County General Hospital, Durham, North Carolina: Robert Buchanan, M.D., John Baker, M.D.

Granville Medical Center, Oxford, North Carolina: David Whitcomb, M.D., John Anderson, M.D., Stephen Ertischek, M.D., Bonnie Johnson, HN-ER, Phylis Finch, HN-CCU, John Watson, M.D.

Onslow Memorial Hospital, Jacksonville, North Carolina: Andre Tse, M.D., Edgardo Bianchi, M.D., Eleanor Goodrow, HN-CCU, Carla Hogan, HN-CCU

Person County Memorial Hospital, Roxboro, North Carolina: Mark Zawodniak, M.D., Thomas Long, M.D., Wayne Bierbaum, M.D., Patty Reynolds, Director of Nursing, Steve Long, M.D., Jim Winslow, M.D.

Richmond Memorial Hospital, Rockingham, North Carolina: Moosa Hajisheik, M.D., John Vetter, M.D., Josie Singletary, R.N., Anne Singletary, R.N., Michael Hennigan, M.D., John Flannery, M.D., Daniel Hall, M.D.

Sampson County Hospital, Clinton, North Carolina: Jeffrey Margolis, M.D., Frank Leak, M.D., John Nance, M.D., Latham Peak, M.D., John Rouse, M.D., John Smith, M.D.

Southeastern General Hospital, Lumberton, North Carolina: Sadanaud B. Hegde, M.D., John Hoekstra, M.D., David L. Richardson, M.D., Somnath N. Naik, M.D., Edward Bert Knight, M.D., Gerard M. Devine, M.D., Frieda Pittman, HN-ER, C.R. Beasley, M.D., H.N. Lee, M.D., Van Helms, M.D.

Franklin Regional Medical Center, Louisburg, North Carolina: Paul Kile, M.D.

The Memorial Hospital, Danville, Virginia: Syed Ahmed, M.D., Stephen Davis, M.D., Stuart Smith, M.D., Phillip Levin, M.D.

Randolph Hospital, Inc., Asheboro, North Carolina: Milkiat Dhatt, M.D., Shiv Harsh, M.D.

Wilson Memorial Hospital, Inc., Wilson, North Carolina: James Whitaker, M.D., John Lund, M.D., Mitchell Hardison, M.D., Mark Leithe, M.D.

Halifax-South Boston Community Hospital, South Boston, Virginia: Richard Goulah, M.D.

Riverside Methodist Hospital, Columbus, Ohio

Barry S. George, M.D., Richard J. Candela, M.D., Joanne Dillon, R.N., B.S., Ramona Masek, R.N., B.S., Ronald D. Frazier, M.D., Ann Pickel, R.N., Joy Mayo, M.D., Ph.D., Joseph Mayo, M.D., Anthony

Chapekis, M.D., Howard Kander, M.D., Steven J. Yakubov, M.D. *Collaborating Center*

Hardin Memorial Hospital, Kenton, Ohio: Murlidhar Deshmukh, M.D., Adarsh Sharma, M.D., Chung Chang, M.D.

Christ Hospital, Cincinnati, Ohio

Dean J. Kereiakes, M.D., Charles W. Abbottsmith, M.D., Linda Anderson, R.N., BSN, Linda Martin, R.N., BSN, Nancy Higby, R.N., Richard Sieving, M.D., Wendy Howard, R.N., David Lauston, R.N., Thomas M. Broderick, M.D., Robert J. Joltzis, M.D.

Collaborating Centers

Bethesda North Hospital, Cincinnati, Ohio: Pete Caples, M.D., Theodore Waller, M.D.

Fort Hamilton-Hughes Hospital and Mercy Hospital, Hamilton, Ohio: James Scott Jr., M.D., George Manitsas, M.D., Kenneth Wehr, M.D., Richard Willis, M.D.

Middletown Regional Hospital, Middletown, Ohio: Walter Roehll Jr., M.D.

Our Lady of Mercy Hospital-Anderson, Cincinnati, Ohio: Eli Roth, M.D., Michael Smith, M.D., David Drake, M.D., Debbie Boatright, R.N.

William Beaumont Hospital, Royal Oak, Michigan

Gerald C. Timmis, M.D., Renato Ramos, M.D., V. Gangadharan, M.D., Cindy Tollis, R.N., BSN

University of Vermont Core Hematology Laboratory, Burlington, Vermont

David C. Stump, M.D., Desire Collen, M.D., Ph.D., Dagnija Thornton, B.S., Elizabeth Macy, B.S., Edwin Bovill

St. Vincent's Hospital, Indianapolis, Indiana

Donald Rothbaum, M.D., Cass A. Pinkerton, M.D.

Baptist Memorial Hospital, Memphis, Tennessee

Joseph K. Samaha, M.D., William H. Flanagan, M.D., Bruce Wilson, M.D., Frank McGrew, M.D., Beate Griffin, R.N., Veronica Condon, R.N., Betty Ehemann, R.N., Leighanni White, R.N., Marc Crupie,

M.D., William Falvey, M.D., Fenwick Chappell, M.D., Linda Yates, M.D., James Hannifin, M.D., Marsha Dean, R.N., Carolyn Maroney, R.N., Barbara Wells, R.N. *Collaborating Centers*

Baptist Memorial Hospital-Tipton, Covington, Tennessee: Jesse Cannon, M.D., George Chambers, M.D., Sam Broffitt, M.D., Barrett Matthews, M.D., John Douglas Clark, M.D., Edward Ritch Davis, M.D.

Baptist Memorial Hospital-Forrest City, Forrest City, Arkansas: Frank Schwartz, M.D.

Baptist Memorial Hospital-Lauderdale, Ripley, Tennessee: Joe Hunt, M.D., Arden J. Butler, M.D., William H. Tucker, M.D., B.G. Robbins, M.D., S.M. Fann, M.D.

Baptist Memorial Hospital-Union City, Union City, Tennessee: Halbert Dodd II, M.D., R. Paul Hill, M.D., Laurence Jones, M.D.

Greenwood Leflore Hospital, Greenwood, Mississippi: Jeff Moses, M.D., Timothy Reynolds, M.D.

Missouri Delta Medical Center, Sikeston, Missouri: David Pfefferkorn, M.D., Michael Chouinard, M.D., Jennifer R. Swiney, M.D., William C. Shell, M.D., Jim Heath, M.D., Michael E. Critchlow, M.D., Brad J. Angelos, M.D.

Northwest Mississippi Regional Medical Center, Clarksdale, Mississippi: Timothy H. Lamb, D.O., Travis Wayne Yates, D.O., Andrea Lee Smith, M.D., G.D. Berryhill Jr., M.D., William Bobo, M.D.

Union County General Hospital, New Albany, Mississippi: Thomas F. Barkley, M.D., Thomas A. Shands, M.D.

Lancaster General Hospital, Lancaster, Pennsylvania

Seth J. Worley, M.D., J.H. Gault, M.D., R.D. Gentzler, M.D., I.D. Smith, M.D., J.P. Slovak, M.D., E.W. Supple, M.D., Sherry Lane, R.N., Deborah Leed, R.N., Deborah Ramsey, R.N.

LDS Hospital, Salt Lake City, Utah

Jeffrey L. Anderson, M.D., Labros Karagounis, M.D., Steve Ipsen, R.N., Fidela

Moreno, M.D., Hiram Marshall, M.D. *Collaborating Centers*

St. Mark's Hospital, Salt Lake City, Utah and Cottonwood Hospital, Murray, Utah: J. Joseph Perry, M.D., Keith L. Ritchie, M.D., David C. Boorman, M.D.

Utah Valley Regional Medical Center, Provo, Utah: Charles F. Dahl, M.D., John K. Frischknecht, M.D., Ronald W. Asay, M.D., Douglas R. Smith, M.D.

St. Louis University Medical Center, St. Louis, Missouri

Michel Vandormael, M.D., Frank V. Aguirre, M.D., Bernard Chaitman, M.D., Ubeydullah Deligonul, M.D., Harold Kennedy, M.D., Morton Kern, M.D., Arthur Labovitz, M.D., Leslie Miller, M.D., Larry Samuels, M.D., Robert Weins, M.D., Terri Thornton, R.N., Marti Major, R.N., Lawrence Lewis, M.D., Robert Mecker, M.D., Brent Ruoff, M.D., Trina Stonner, R.N. *Collaborating Centers*

St. John's Mercy Medical Center, St. Louis, Missouri: William Hamilton, M.D., Louis Deane, M.D., Louis Stickley, M.D., Robert Ferrara, M.D., John Lindeman, M.D.

St. Joseph Hospital, Kirkwood, Missouri: James Dwyer, M.D., Paul Gibson, M.D., Duck Sung Chun, M.D.

University of Kentucky Medical Center, Lexington, Kentucky

John Gurley, M.D., Steven Nissen, M.D., David Boothe, M.D., Marcelo Branco, M.D., Denny Gash, M.D., Edward Harlamert, M.D., Anthony DeMaria, M.D., Kim Bennett, R.N., Barbara Cutshaw, R.N. *Collaborating Center*

Middle Kentucky River Medical Center, Jackson, Kentucky: Thomas Benzoni, D.O.

Boston University Medical Center, Boston, Massachussetts

Nicholas A. Ruocco Jr., M.D., John Brush, M.D., David Faxon, M.D., Gary Garber, M.D., Alice Jacobs, M.D., Phillip Podrid, M.D., James Rothendler, M.D., Thomas Ryan, M.D., Beth Hankin, R.N.

St. Patrick Hospital, Missoula, Montana

A.A. Gabster, M.D., C.C. Goren, M.D., L.W. Johnson, M.D., J.F. Knapp, M.D., G.H. Reed, M.D., J.R. Stone, M.D., W.S. Wilson, M.D., Dale Mayer, R.N.

Brooke Army Medical Center, Fort Sam Houston, Texas

Larry Pupa, M.D., Steven Bailey, M.D., Mark Moody, M.D., William Condos, M.D., James Gilman, M.D.

Baylor College of Medicine, Houston, Texas

Neal S. Kleiman, M.D., Pirzada Majid, M.D., Judith Mickelson, M.D., Craig M. Pratt, M.D., Albert Raizner, M.D., Dale Rose, B.S., Kathleen Trainor, R.N.

Cleveland Clinic Foundation, Cleveland, Ohio

Kelly Brezina, R.N.

Geisinger Medical Center, Danville, Pennsylvania

James Blankenship, M.D., N. Patrick Madigan, M.D.

St. Francis Hospital, Beech Grove, Indiana

Mark D. Cohen, M.D., Horace Hickman, M.D., Paula Cross, R.N.

Mercy Hospital, Des Moines, Iowa

Mark Tannenbaum, M.D., Yvette Devine, R.N.

University of Louisville, Louisville, Kentucky

J. David Talley, M.D., Abraham Joseph, M.D., Charles R. Prince, M.D., ZoeAnn Yussman, R.N., Frank Martin, M.D., Brenda Talley, R.N.

Rochester General Hospital, Rochester, New York

Gerald Gacioch, M.D., Valerie Chiodo, R.N.

Address for reprints: Gregory W. Barsness, M.D., Duke University Medical Center, Durham, NC 27708. Fax: (919) 286-4599.

References

1. Anderson JL, Marshall HW, Bray BE, et al. A randomized trial of intracoronary streptokinase in the treatment of acute myocardial infarction. N Engl J Med 1983;308:1312-1318.
2. Kennedy JW, Ritchie JL, Davis KB, et al. Western Washington randomized trial of intracoronary streptokinase in acute myocardial infarction. N Engl J Med 1983;309:1477-1482.
3. Gruppo Italiano per lo Studio della Streptochinasi nell'lnfarto Miocardico (GISSI): Effectiveness of intravenous thrombolytic treatment in acute myocardial infarction. Lancet 1986;I:397-401.
4. Chandler AB, Chapman I, Erhardt LR, et al. Coronary thrombosis in myocardial infarction: Report of a workshop on the role of coronary thrombosis in the pathogenesis of acute myocardial infarction. Am J Cardiol 1974;34:823-833.
5. DeWood MA, Spores J, Notske R, et al. Prevalence of total coronary occlusion during the early hours of transmural myocardial infarction. N Engl J Med 1980;303:897-902.
6. Rude RE, Muller JE, Braunwald E. Efforts to limit the size of myocardial infarcts. Ann Intern Med 1981; 95:736-761.
7. Sobel BE, Bresnahan GF, Shell WE, et al. Estimation of infarct size in man and its relation to prognosis. Circulation 1972;46:640-648
8. Topol EJ, Morris DC, Smalling RW, et al. A multicenter, randomized, placebo-controlled trial of a new form of intravenous recombinant tissue-type plasminogen activator (activase) in acute myocardial infarction. JACC 1987;9:1205-1213.
9. Verstraete M, Bernard R, Bory M, et al. Randomised trial of intravenous recombinant tissue-type plasminogen activator versus intravenous streptokinase in acute myocardial infarction. Lancet 1985;1:842-847.
10. Collen D, Topol EJ, Tiefenbrunn AJ, et al. Coronary thrombolysis with recombinant human tissue-type plasminogen activator: A prospective, randomized, placebo-controlled trial. Circulation 1984;70:1012-1017.
11. Yusuf S, Collins R, Peto R, et al. Intravenous and intracoronary fibrinolytic therapy in acute myocardial infarction: Overview of results on mortality, reinfarction and side-effects from 33 randomised controlled trials. Eur Heart J 1985;6:556-585.
12. The Multicenter Postinfarction Research Group. Risk stratification and survival after myocardial infarction. N Engl J Med 1983;309:331-336.
13. Serruys PW, Simoons ML, Suryapranata H, et al. for the Working Group on Thrombolytic Therapy in Acute Myocardial Infarction of the Netherlands Interuniversity Cardiology Institute. Preservation of global and regional left ventricular function after early thrombolysis in acute myocardial infarction. JACC 1986;7:729-742.
14. Topol EJ, Califf RM, George BS, et al. A randomized trial of immediate versus delayed elective angioplasty after intravenous tissue plasminogen activator in acute myocardial infarction. N Engl J Med 1987;317:581-588.
15. Topol EJ, Califf RM, Kereiakes DJ, et al. Thrombolysis and Angioplasty in Myocardial Infarction (TAMI) trial. JACC 1987;10:65B-74B.
16. Ellis SG, Lincoff AM, George BS, et al. Randomized evaluation of coronary angioplasty for early TIMI 2 flow after thrombolytic therapy for the treatment of acute myocardial infarction: A new look at an old study. The Thrombolysis and Angioplasty in Myocardial Infarction (TAMI) Study Group. Coron Art Dis 1994;5:611-615.
17. Topol EJ, George BS, Kereiakes DJ, et al. Comparison of two dose regimens of intravenous tissue plasminogen activator for acute myocardial infarction. Am J Cardiol 1988; 61:723-728.
18. Stump DC, Califf RM, Topol EJ, et al. Pharmacodynamics of thrombolysis with recombinant tissue-type plasminogen activator. Correlation with characteristics of and clinical outcomes in patients with acute myocardial infarction. The TAMI Study Group. Circulation 1989;80:1222-1230.
19. Mueller HS, Rao AK, Forman SA,

TIMI Investigators. Thrombolysis in myocardial infarction (TIMI): Comparative studies of coronary reperfusion and systemic fibrinogenolysis with two forms of recombinant tissue-type plasminogen activator. JACC 1987;10:479-490.

20. Topol EJ, Califf RM, George BS, et al. Insights derived from the thrombolysis and angioplasty in myocardial infarction (TAMI) trials. JACC 1988; 12:24A-31A.

21. Califf RM Topol EJ, George BS, et al. Characteristics and outcome of patients in whom reperfusion with intravenous tissue-type plasminogen activator fails: Results of the Thrombolysis and Angioplasty in Myocardial Infarction (TAMI) 1 trial. Circulation 1988;77:1090-1099.

22. Califf RM, O'Neil W, Stack RS, et al. Failure of simple clinical measurements to predict perfusion status after intravenous thrombolysis. Ann Intern Med 1988;108:658-662.

23. Collen D, Stassen J, Stump DC, et al. Synergism of thrombolytic agents in vivo. Circulation 1986;74:838-842.

24. Collen D, Stump DC, Van de Werf F. Coronary thrombolysis in patients with acute myocardial infarction by intravenous infusion of synergic thrombolytic agents. Am Heart J 1986;112:1083-1084.

25. Topol EJ, Califf RM, George BS, et al. Coronary arterial thrombolysis with combined infusion of recombinant tissue-type plasminogen activator and UK in patients with acute myocardial infarction. Circulation 1988; 77:1100-1107.

26. Cercek B, Lew AS, Hod H, et al. Enhancement of thrombolysis with issue-type plasminogen activator by pretreatment with heparin. Circulation 1986;74:583-587.

27. Andrade-Gordon P, Strickland S. Interaction of heparin with plasminogen activators and plasminogen: Effects on the activation of plasminogen. Biochemistry 1986;25:4033-4040.

28. Eisenberg PR, Sherman L, Rich M, et al. Importance of continued activation of thrombin reflected by fibrinopeptide A to the efficacy of thrombolysis. JACC 1986;7:1255-1262.

29. Topol EJ, George BS, Kereiakes DJ, et al., and the TAMI Study Group. A randomized controlled trial of intravenous tissue plasminogen activator and early intravenous heparin in acute myocardial infarction. Circulation 1989;79:281-286.

30. Chiariello M, Golino P, Cappelli-Bigazzi M, et al. Reduction in infarct size by the prostacyclin analogue iloprost (ZK 36374) after experimental coronary artery occlusion-reperfusion. Am Heart J 1988;115:499-504.

31. Smith EF, Gallenkamper W, Beckmann R, et al. Early and late administration of a PGI2-analogue, ZK 36 374 (iloprost): Effects on myocardial preservation, collateral blood flow and infarct size. Cardiovasc Res 1984;18:163-173.

32. Melin JA, Becker LC. Salvage of ischemic myocardium by prostacyclin during experimental myocardial infarction. JACC 1983;2:279-286.

33. Thiemermann C, Steinhagen-Thiessen E, Schror K. Inhibition of oxygen-centered free radical formation by the stable prostacyclin-mimetic iloprost (ZK 36 374) in acute myocardial ischemia (letter). J Cardiovasc Pharmacol 1984;6:365-366.

34. Simpson PJ, Mickelson J, Fantone JC, et al. Iloprost inhibits neutrophil function in vitro and in vivo and limits experimental infarct size in canine heart. Circ Res 1987;60:666-673.

35. Schumacher WA, Lee EC, Lucchesi BR. Augmentation of streptokinase-induced thrombolysis by heparin and prostacyclin. J Cardiovasc Pharmacol 1985;7:739-746.

36. Topol EJ, Ellis SG, Califf RM, et al. Combined tissue-type plasminogen activator and prostacyclin therapy for acute myocardial infarction. Thrombolysis and Angioplasty in Myocardial Infarction (TAMI) 4 Study Group. JACC 1989;14:877-884.

37. Kerins DM, Shuh M, Kunitada S, et al. A prostacyclin analog impairs the response to tissue-type plasminogen activator during coronary thrombolysis: Evidence for a pharmacokinetic interaction. J Pharmacol Exp Ther 1991;257:487-492.

38. Kerins DM, Roy L, Kunitada S, et al. Phamacokinetics of tissue-type plasminogen activator during acute myocardial infarction in men. Effect of a prostacyclin analogue. Circulation 1992;85:526-532.

39. A European Collaborative Study.

Controlled trial of urokinase in myocardial infarction. Lancet 1975;624.

40. Brochier M, Raynaud R, Planiol T, et al. Le traitement par l'urokinase des infarctus du myocarde et syndromes de menace: Étude randomisée de 120 cas. Arch Mal Coeur 1975; 68:563-569.

41. Gormsen J, Tidstrom B, Feddersen C, et al. Biochemical evaluation of low dose of urokinase in acute myocardial infarction. Acta Med Scand 1973;194:191-198.

42. Mathey DG, Schofer J, Sheehan FH, et al. Intravenous urokinase in acute myocardial infarction. Am J Cardiol 1985;55:878-882.

43. Neuhaus KL, Tebbe U, Gottwik M, et al. Intravenous recombinant tissue plasminogen activator (rt-PA) and urokinase in acute myocardial infarction: Results of the German Activator Urokinase Study (GAUS). JACC 1988;12:581-587.

44. Wall TC, Phillips HR, Stack RS, et al. Results of high dose intravenous urokinase for acute myocardial infarction. Am J Cardiol 1990;65:124-131.

45. O'Connor CM, Mark DB, Hinohara T, et al. Rescue coronary angioplasty after failure on intravenous streptokinase in acute myocardial: In-hospital and long-term outcomes. J Invas Cardiol 1989;1:85-95.

46. Stack RS, O'Connor CM, Mark DB, et al. Coronary perfusion during acute myocardial infarction with a combined therapy of coronary angioplasty and high-dose intravenous streptokinase. Circulation 1988;1:151-161.

47. Califf RM, Topol EJ, Stack RS, et al. Evaluation of combination thrombolytic therapy and timing of cardiac catheterization in acute myocardial infarction. Circulation 1991;83:1543-1556.

48. Topol EJ, Califf RM, Vandormael M, et al. A randomized trial of late reperfusion therapy for acute myocardial infarction. Circulation 1992; 85:2090-2099.

49. Neuhaus KL, Feuerer W, Jeep-Tebbe S, et al. Improved thrombolysis with a modified dose regimen of recombinant tissue-type plasminogen activator. JACC 1989;14:1566-1569.

50. Carney RJ, Murphy GA, Brandt TR, et al. for The RAAMI Study Investigators. Randomized angiographic trial of recombinant tissue-type plasminogen activator (al-

teplase) in myocardial infarction. JACC 1992;20:17-23.

51. Wall TC, Califf RM, George BS, et al. Accelerated plasminogen activator dose regimens for coronary thrombolysis. JACC 1992;19:482-489.

52. Neuhaus K, VonEssen R, Tebbe U, et al. Improved thrombolysis in acute myocardial infarction with front-loaded administration of alteplase: Results of the rt-PA-APSAC patency study (TAPS). JACC 1992;19:886-891.

53. The GUSTO Investigators. An international randomized trial comparing four thrombolytic strategies for acute myocardial infarction. N Engl J Med 1993;329:673-682.

54. Ohman EM, Califf RM, Topol EJ, et al. Consequences of reocclusion after successful reperfusion therapy in acute myocardial infarction. TAMI Study Group. Circulation 1990; 82:781-791.

55. ISIS-2 (Second International Study of Infarct Survival) Collaborative Group: Randomised trial of intravenous streptokinase, oral aspirin, both, or neither among 17, 187 cases of suspected acute myocardial infarction. Lancet 1988;II:349-360.

56. Roux S, Christeller S, Ludin E. Effects of aspirin on coronary reocclusion and recurrent ischemia after thrombolysis: A meta-analysis. JACC 1992;19:671-677.

57. Yasuda T, Gold HK, Leinbach RC, et al. Kistrin, a polypeptide platelet GPIIb/IIIa receptor antagonist, enhances and sustains coronary arterial thrombolysis with recombinant tissue-type plasminogen activator in a canine preparation. Circulation 1991; 83:1038-1047.

58. Yasuda T, Gold HK, Yaoita H, et al. Comparative effects of aspirin, a synthetic thrombin inhibitor and a monoclonal antiplatelet glycoprotein IIb/IIIa antibody on coronary artery reperfusion, reocclusion and bleeding with recombinant tissue-type plasminogen activator in a canine preparation. JACC 1990;16:714-722.

59. Yasuda T, Gold HK, Leinbach RC, et al. Lysis of plasminogen activator-resistant platelet-rich coronary artery thrombus with combined bolus injection of recombinant tissue-type plasminogen activator and antiplatelet GPIIb/IIIa antibody. JACC 1990; 16:1728-1735.

60. Kleiman NS, Ohman EM, Califf RM, et al. Profound inhibition of platelet aggregation with monoclonal antibody 7E3 Fab after thrombolytic therapy: Results of the thrombolysis and angioplasty in myocardial infarction (TAMI) 8 pilot study. JACC 1993;22:381-389.

61. Gold HK, Coller BS, Yasuda T, et al. Rapid and sustained coronary artery recanalization with combined bolus injection of recombinant tissue-type plasminogen activator and monoclonal antiplatelet GPIIb/IIIa antibody in a canine preparation. Circulation 1988;3:670-677.

62. Forman MB, Bingham S, Kopelman HA, et al. Reduction of infarct size with intracoronary perfluorochemical in a canine preparation of reperfusion. Circulation 1985;71:1060-1068.

63. Nunn GR, Dance G, Peters J, et al. Effect of fluorocarbon exchange transfusion on myocardial infarction size in dogs. Am J Cardiol 1983; 52:203-204.

64. Forman MB, Perry JM, Wilson BH, et al. Demonstration of myocardial reperfusion injury in humans: Results of a pilot study utilizing acute coronary angioplasty with perfluorochemical in anterior myocardial infarction. JACC 1991;18:911-918.

65. Wall TC, Califf RM, Blankenship J, et al., TAMI 9 Research Group. Intravenous fluosol in the treatment of acute myocardial infarction. Results of the thrombolysis and angioplasty in myocardial infarction 9 trial. Circulation 1994;90:114-120.

66. Forman MB, Ingram DA, Murray JJ. Role of perfluorochemical emulsions in the treatment of myocardial reperfusion injury. Am Heart J 1992; 124:1347-1357.

67. Schaer GL, Hursey TL, Abrahams SL, et al. Reduction in reperfusion-induced myocardial necrosis in dogs by RheothRx injection (Poloxamer 188 N.F.), a hemorheological agent that alters neutrophil function. Circulation 1994;90:2964-2975.

68. Carr AME Jr., Powers PL, Jones MR. Effects of poloxamer 188 on the assembly, structure and dissolution of fibrin clots. Thromb Haemostas 1991;66:565-568.

69. Justicz AG, Farnsworth WV, Soberman MS, et al. Reduction of myocardial infarct size by poloxamer 188 and mannitol in a canine model. Am Heart J 1991;122:671-680.

70. Kolodgie FD, Farb A, Carlson GC, et al. Hyperoxic reperfusion is required to reduce infarct size after intravenous therapy with perfluorochemical (Fluosol-DA 20%) or its detergent component (Poloxamer 188) in a poorly collateralized animal model (Absence of a role of polymorphonuclear leukocytes). JACC 1994; 24:1098-1108.

71. Bates ER, Califf RM, Stack RS, et al. Thrombolysis and Angioplasty in Myocardial Infarction (TAMI-1) trial: Influence of infarct location on arterial patency, left ventricular function and mortality. JACC 1989;13:12-18.

72. McNeer JF, Wagner GS, Ginsburg PB, et al. Hospital discharge one week after acute myocardial infarction. N Engl J Med 1978;298:229-232.

73. Califf RM, Topol EJ, George BS, et al. One-year outcome after therapy with tissue plasminogen activator: Report from the Thrombolysis and Angioplasty in Myocardial Infarction trial. Am Heart J 1990;119:777-785.

74. Ohman EM, Topol EJ, Califf RM, et al. Thrombolysis Angioplasty in Myocardial Infarction Study Group: An analysis of the cause of early mortality after administration of thrombolytic therapy. Coron Art Dis 1993; 4:957-964.

75. Muller DW, Topol EJ, George BS, et al. Two-year outcome after angiographically documented myocardial reperfusion for acute coronary artery occlusion. Thrombolysis and Angioplasty Study Group. Am J Cardiol 1990;66:796-801.

76. Chapman GD, Ohman EM, Topol EJ, et al. Minimizing the risk of inappropriately administering thrombolytic therapy: Results from the thrombolysis and angioplasty in myocardial infarction (TAMI) Study Group. Am J Cardiol 1993;71:783-787.

77. Lee KL, Sigmon KN, Topol EJ, et al., and the TAMI Study Group. The utility of easily-obtained noninvasive clinical data for predicting survival following thrombolytic therapy. JACC 1992;19:42A.

78. Lee KL, Woodlief LH, Topol EJ, et al. Predictors of 30-day mortality in the era of reperfusion for acute myocar-

dial infarction, results from an international trial of 41,021 patients. Circulation 1995;91:1659-1668.

79. Lee KL, Sigmon KN, Califf RM, et al., and the TAMI Study Group. How much prognostic information does catheterization after thrombolytic therapy add to noninvasive clinical factors. JACC 1992;19(Suppl A):80A.

80. Kereiakes DJ, Topol EJ, George BS, et al. Myocardial infarction with minimal coronary atherosclerosis in the era of thrombolytic reperfusion. The Thrombolysis and Angioplasty in Myocardial Infarction (TAMI) Study Group. JACC 1991;17:304-312.

81. Mark DB, Sigmon K, Topol EJ, et al. Identification of acute myocardial infarction patients suitable for early hospital discharge after aggressive interventional therapy. Results from the Thrombolysis and Angioplasty in Acute Myocardial Infarction Registry. Circulation 1991;83:1186-1193.

82. Puletti M, Sunseri L, Curione M, et al. Acute myocardial infarction: Sex-related differences in prognosis. Am Heart J 1984;108:63.

83. Kannel WB, Sorlie P, McNamara PM. Prognosis after initial myocardial infarction: The Framingham Study. Am J Cardiol 1979;44:53.

84. Greenland P, Reicher-Reiss H, Goldbourt U, et al., and the Israeli SPRINT Investigators. In-hospital and 1-year mortality in 1,524 women after myocardial infarction. Comparison with 4,315 men. Circulation 1991;83:484-491.

85. Wenger NK. Coronary disease in women. Ann Rev Med 1985;36:285-294.

86. Tofler GH, Stone PH, Muller JE, et al. and the MILIS Study Group. Effects of gender and race on prognosis after myocardial infarction: Adverse prognosis for women, particularly black women. JACC 1987; 9:473-482.

87. Lincoff AM, Califf RM, Ellis SG, et al., for the Thrombolysis and Angioplasty in Myocardial Infarction Study Group. Thrombolytic therapy for women with myocardial infarction: Is there a gender gap? JACC 1993;22:1780-1787.

88. Granger CB, Califf RM, Young S, et al. Outcome of patients with diabetes mellitus and acute myocardial infarction treated with thrombolytic agents. The Thrombolysis and Angioplasty in Myocardial Infarction (TAMI) Study Group. JACC 1993; 21:920-925.

89. Muller DW, Topol EJ, Califf RM, et al. Relationship between antecedent angina pectoris and short-term prognosis after thrombolytic therapy for acute myocardial infarction. Thrombolysis and Angioplasty in Myocardial Infarction (TAMI) Study Group. Am Heart J 1990;119:224-231.

90. AIMS Trial Study Group. Effect of intravenous APSAC on mortality after acute myocardial infarction: Preliminary report of a placebo-controlled clinical trial. Lancet 1988;1:545-549.

91. GISSI-2. A factorial randomised trial of alteplase versus streptokinase and heparin versus no heparin among 12 490 patients with acute myocardial infarction. Lancet 1990;336:65-71.

92. The TIMI Study Group. Comparison of invasive and conservative strategies after treatment with intravenous tissue plasminogen activator in acute myocardial infarction. Results of the Thrombolysis in Myocardial Infarction (TIMI) Phase II Trial. N Engl Med 1989;320:618-627.

93. Grines CL, Topol EJ, O'Neill WW, et al. Effect of cigarette smoking on outcome after thrombolytic therapy for myocardial infarction. Circulation 1995;91:298-303.

94. Wall TC, Califf RM, Harrelson-Woodlief L, et al. Usefulness of a pericardial friction rub after thrombolytic therapy during acute myocardial infarction in predicting amount of myocardial damage. The TAMI Study Group. Am J Cardiol 1990; 66:1418-1421.

95. Belkin RN, Mark DB, Aronson L, et al. Pericardial effusion after intravenous recombinant tissue-type plasminogen activator for acute myocardial infarction. Am J Cardiol 1991; 67:496-500.

96. Bates ER, Clemmensen PM, Califf RM, et al. Precordial ST segment depression predicts a worse prognosis in inferior infarction despite reperfusion therapy. The Thrombolysis and Angioplasty in Myocardial Infarction (TAMI) Study Group. JACC 1990;16; 1538-1544.

97. Clemmensen P, Bates ER, Califf RM, et al., and the TAMI Study Group.

Complete atrioventricular block complicating inferior wall acute myocardial infarction treated with reperfusion therapy. Am J Cardiol 1991; 67:225-230.

98. Grines CL, Topol EJ, Califf RM, et al. Prognostic implications and predictors of enhanced regional wall motion of the noninfarct zone after thrombolysis and angioplasty therapy of acute myocardial infarction. The TAMI Study Groups. Circulation 1989;80:245-253.

99. Harrison JK, Califf RM, Woodlief LH, et al., and the TAMI Study Group. Systolic left ventricular function after reperfusion therapy for acute myocardial infarction: An analysis of determinants of improvement. Circulation 1993;87:1531-1541.

100. Harrison JK, Skelton TN, Davidson CJ, et al. Regional and global left ventricular function evaluated acutely, at 7 days, and at 6 months following thrombolytic therapy. Circulation 1989;80(Suppl II):II-313.

101. Califf RM, Harrelson-Woodlief L, Topol EJ. Left ventricular ejection fraction may not be useful as an end point of thrombolytic therapy comparative trials. Circulation 1990; 82:1847-1853.

102. Granger CB, White HD, Bates ER, et al. A pooled analysis of coronary arterial patency and left ventricular function after intravenous thrombolysis for acute myocardial infarction. Am J Cardiol 1994;74:1220-1228.

103. Lee KL, Sigmon K, George BS, et al., and the TAMI Study Group. Early and complete reperfusion-a key predictor of survival after thrombolytic therapy. Circulation 1988;78(Suppl II)II-501.

104. Lincoff MA, Topol EJ, Califf RM, et al., for the Thrombolysis and Angioplasty in Myocardial Infarction Study Group. Significance of a coronary artery with Thrombolysis In Myocardial Infarction grade 2 flow "patency" (Outcome in the Thrombolysis and Angioplasty in Myocardial Infarction trials). Am J Cardiol 1995;75:871-876 .

105. Krucoff MW, Croll MA, Pope JE, et al. Heuristic and logistic principles of ST-segment interpretation in the time domain. Evolution in the context of the TAMI 7 trial design. J Electrocardiol 1990;23(Suppl):6-10.

106. Krucoff MW, Croll MA, Pope JE, et al. Continuously updated 12-lead ST-segment recovery analysis for myocardial infarct artery patency assessment and its correlation with multiple simultaneous early angiographic observations. Am J Cardiol 1993;71(2):145-151.

107. Krucoff MW, Croll MA, Pope JE, et al., and the TAMI 7 Study Group. Continuous 12-lead ST-segment recovery analysis in the TAMI 7 study. Performance of a noninvasive method for real-time detection of failed myocardial reperfusion. Circulation 1993;88:437-446.

108. Veldkamp RF, Green CL, Wilkins ML, et al., for the Thrombolysis and Angioplasty in Myocardial Infarction (TAMI) 7 Study Group. Comparison of continuous ST-segment recovery analysis with methods using static electrocardiograms for noninvasive patency assessment during acute myocardial infarction. Am J Cardiol 1994;73:1069-1074.

109. Ohman EM, Christenson RH, Califf RM, et al., and the TAMI 7 Study Group. Noninvasive detection of reperfusion after thrombolysis based on serum creatine kinase MB changes and clinical variables. Am Heart J 1993;126:819-826.

110. Califf RM, Topol EJ, Ohman EM, et al. Isolated recurrent ischemia after thrombolytic therapy is a frequent, important and expensive adverse clinical outcome. Am J Cardiol 1992; 19:301A .

111. Ellis SG, Topol EJ, George BS, et al. Recurrent ischemia without warning. Analysis of risk factors for in-hospital ischemic events following successful thrombolysis with intravenous tissue plasminogen activator. Circulation 1989;80:1159-1165.

112. Wall TC, Mark DB, Califf RM, et al. Prediction of early recurrent myocardial ischemia and coronary reocclusion after successful thrombolysis: A qualitative and quantitative angiographic study. Am J Cardiol 1989; 63:423-428.

113. Muller DW, Topol EJ, Ellis SG, et al. Determinants of the need for early acute intervention in patients treated conservatively after thrombolytic therapy for acute myocardial infarction. JACC 1991;18:1594-1601.

114. Stack RS, Califf RM, Hinohara T, et al. Survival and cardiac event rates in the first year after emergency coronary angioplasty for acute myocardial infarction. JACC 1988;11:1141-1149.

115. Abbottsmith CW, Topol EJ, George BS, et al. Fate of patients with acute myocardial infarction with patency of the infarct-related vessel achieved with successful thrombolysis versus rescue angioplasty. JACC 1990; 16:770-778.

116. George BS, Candela RJ, Topol EJ, et al. Brachial approach to emergency cardiac catheterization during thrombolytic therapy for acute myocardial infarction. TAMI Study Group. Cath Cardiovasc Diagn 1990; 20:221-226.

117. Kereiakes DJ, Califf RM, George BS, et al. Coronary bypass surgery improves global and regional left ventricular function following thrombolytic therapy for acute myocardial infarction. TAMI Study Group. Am Heart J 1991;122:390-399.

118. Kereiakes DJ, Topol EJ, George BS, et al. Favorable early and long-term prognosis following coronary bypass surgery therapy for myocardial infarction: Results of a multicenter trial. TAMI Study Group. Am Heart J 1989;118:199-207.

119. Kereiakes DJ, Topol EJ, George BS, et al. Emergency coronary artery bypass surgery preserves global and regional left ventricular function after intravenous tissue plasminogen activator therapy for acute myocardial infarction. JACC 1988;11:899-907.

120. Ohman EM, Califf RM, George BS, et al. The use of intraaortic balloon pumping as an adjunct to reperfusion therapy in acute myocardial infarction. The Thrombolysis and Angioplasty in Myocardial Infarction (TAMI) Study Group. Am Heart J 1991;121:895-901.

121. Ohman EM, Califf RM, Topol EJ, et al., the TAMI Study Group. Aortic counterpulsation with thrombolysis for myocardial infarction: Salutary effect on reocclusion on the infarct related artery. JACC 1992;19(Suppl A):381A.

122. Sane DC, Stump DC, Topol EJ, et al. Correlation between baseline plasminogen activator inhibitor levels and clinical outcome during therapy with tissue plasminogen activator for acute myocardial infarction. Thromb Haemostas 1991;65:275-279.

123. Califf RM, Topol EJ, George BS, et al., the TAMI Study Group.

Hemorrhagic complications associated with the use of intravenous tissue plasminogen activator in treatment of acute myocardial infarction. Am J Med 1988;85:353-359.

124. Wall TC, Califf RM, Ellis SG, et al., for the TAMI Study Group. Lack of impact of early catheterization and fibrin specificity on bleeding complications after thrombolytic therapy. JACC 1993;21:597-603.

125. Popma JJ, Califf RM, Ellis SG, et al. Mechanisms of benefit of combination thrombolytic therapy for acute myocardial infarct: A quantitative angiographic and hematologic study. JACC 1992;20:1305-1312.

126. Harrington RA, Sane DC, Califf RM, et al., for the Thrombolysis and Angioplasty in Myocardial Infarction Study Group. Clinical importance of thrombocytopenia occurring in the hospital phase after administration of thrombolytic therapy for acute myocardial infarction. JACC 1994; 23:891-898.

127. Bernardi MM, Califf RM, Kleiman N, et al., the TAMI Study Group. Lack of usefulness of prolonged bleeding times in predicting hemorrhagic events in patients receiving the 7E3 glycoprotein IIb/IIIa platelet antibody. Am J Cardiol 1993;72:1121-1125.

128. O'Connor CM, Califf RM, Massey EW, et al. Stroke and acute myocardial infarction in the thrombolytic era: Clinical correlates and long-term prognosis. JACC 1990;16:533-540.

129. Tenaglia AN, Califf RM, Candela RJ, et al. Thrombolytic therapy in patients requiring cardiopulmonary resuscitation. Am J Cardiol 1991; 68:1015-1019.

130. Bellinger RL, Califf RM, Mark DB, et al. Helicopter transport of patients during acute myocardial infarction. Am J Cardiol 1988;61:718-722.

131. Mark DB, Hlatky MA, O'Connor CM, et al. Administration of thrombolytic therapy in the community hospital: Established principles and unresolved issues. JACC 1988;12:32A-43A.

132. Wall TC, Strickland J, Masoud J, et al. Thrombolytic therapy on the homefront. Intravenous urokinase in community hos5itals. NC Med J 1989;50:363-366.

Chapter 10

The TEAM Studies:
A Review

Jeffrey L. Anderson, M.D., FACC, and Sanjeev Trehan, M.D.

From the Division of Cardiology, University of Utah, Salt Lake City, Utah

Introduction

The 1980s saw the development of thrombolytic therapy, growing from experimental application to established therapy for acute myocardial infarction (AMI).[1-3] Several intermediate to large scale studies have confirmed the central role of thrombolysis in restoring blood flow in the obstructed coronary artery, reducing infarct size, preserving left ventricular (LV) function, and improving survival.[4-15] The evaluation of new thrombolytic regimens,[16-20] antithrombotic[10,21-24] and other adjunctive therapies,[25,26] strategies for earlier treatment,[27,28] and selection and modification of therapeutic regimens based on individual patient characteristics[29,30] have been some of the recent hallmark advances in management of the acute coronary syndromes.

The Thrombolytic Trials of Eminase for Acute Myocardial Infarction

Among these new studies, the Thrombolytic Trials of Eminase (anistreplase, or anisoylated plasminogen streptokinase activator complex, APSAC) for Acute Myocardial Infarction (TEAM) trials consisted of three pivotal multicenter studies

in the United States and Canada that began in 1985 with recruitment for TEAM-1 and concluded in 1992 with publication of the TEAM-3 study.[31-33] These trials, representing the U.S. evaluation program of anistreplase, focused on reperfusion, patency and reocclusion, and safety and clinical outcome comparisons with approved thrombolytic regimens (streptokinase and alteplase) (Table 1). TEAM-1 compared the efficacy of anistreplase with intracoronary streptokinase,[31] TEAM-2 compared anistreplase with intravenous streptokinase,[32] and TEAM-3 evaluated anistreplase against intravenous tissue plasminogen activator complex (tPA), given as alteplase.[33]

The Open Artery Hypothesis and the TEAM Studies

Theoretical considerations and clinical observations have suggested that achieving a patent coronary artery is of great therapeutic relevance to AMI treatment strategies.[3,34] The benefits of thrombolytic therapy appear to be substantially accounted for by early reestablishment and subsequent maintenance of unimpeded coronary blood flow.[35] Early and maintained vessel patency enables both salvage of ischemic,

Table 1.

Multicenter Thrombolytic Trials of Eminase (APSAC) in Acute Myocardial Infarction (TEAM)

Study (Ref.)	Study Period	Comparison	Number Patients	End Points
TEAM-1 (31)	1985–1986	APSAC vs IC SK	325	Early reperfusion
TEAM-2 (32)	1987–1988	APSAC vs IV SK	370	Early patency
TEAM-3 (33)	1989–1990	APSAC vs tPA	240	LV function
Late patency				

APSAC = anistreplase, eminase; SK = streptokinase; IC = intracoronary; IV = intravenous; tPA = tissue plasminogen activator; LV = left ventricular.

jeopardized but viable myocardium, and improved healing in the infarcted zone, reducing infarct expansion, improving scar formation, and reducing risk of subsequent aneurysm.[3] Further, there is evidence that reperfusion improves electrophysiological substrate, thereby reducing the risk of subsequent ventricular tachyarrhythmias.[3] By establishing a conduit for collateral circulation to other areas with compromised blood flow, it also acts to reduce the risk of subsequent infarction. Given the central role of (re)perfusion to the benefits of thrombolysis, it was the goal of the TEAM studies to evaluate coronary artery reperfusion and patency effects of anistreplase, and compare these with those of other, established regimens. Evaluation of the frequency and time course of initial reperfusion and the contrasting late dynamics of delayed reperfusion and reocclusion was also of interest. Finally, although not of sufficient size to evaluate comparative mortality benefits, the TEAM studies assessed composite clinical events and patient safety (e.g., bleeding).

Properties of Anistreplase and Rationale for its Development

Even before its extensive therapeutic evaluation in AMI, streptokinase was recognized as possessing properties that were not ideal for a thrombolytic. In order to improve on the pharmacological profile of streptokinase, anistreplase was custom-designed and synthesized by chemists at Beecham Laboratories in the United Kingdom in about 1980.[36] After laboratory testing showed promise, clinical trials were begun.

Anistreplase is a 1:1 molar complex of streptokinase and modified (lys) plasminogen that was specifically developed to provide greater fibrin affinity and greater fibrinolytic efficacy, a longer plasma half-life (90–105 min), and greater ease of administration (≤ 5 min injection) than are provided by streptokinase.[37,38] Anistreplase is inactive when injected (its active site is protected by an anisoyl group), but when administered it rapidly circulates, finds and binds to fibrin, and is progressively activated by a simple hydrolysis (deacylation) reaction. Anistreplase was believed to represent a significant advance in drug design for therapeutic thrombolysis based on these features. A schematic representation of the molecular configuration of anistreplase is presented in Figure 1.

Early Investigations with APSAC

An early clinical investigation of anistreplase by Marder and colleagues[39] assessed the effects of different doses of intravenously administered drugs on reperfusion and hematological factors in a limited number of patients with AMI. Outcome was measured as reperfusion efficacy of anistreplase in all patients, as well as in patients who were considered "thrombolysis

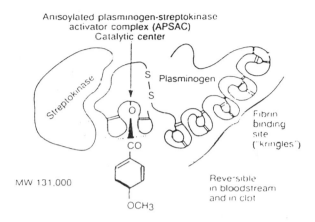

Figure 1. Structure of anistreplase (APSAC).

susceptible" as determined by their ability to show reperfusion of the infarct-related coronary artery by administration of either intravenous (IV) anistreplase or intracoronary (IC) streptokinase (in those who had failed anistreplase). Anistreplase doses of 5, 15, and 30 units (1 U = approximately 1 mg) were administered to 36 patients; the number of patients reperfusing at each of these doses was determined to be 3 (21%) of 14, 3 (42%) of 7, and 9 (60%) of 15, respectively. Reperfusion rates given as a percent of "thrombolysis susceptible" patients were 23%, 43%, and 82%, respectively, as established by subsequent delivery of IC streptokinase in anistreplase resistant cases. Little systemic lytic effect was observed with the 5-U dose, but at doses of ≥ 10 U, progressive reductions in circulating fibrinogen and plasminogen were noted with substantial reductions occurring at the "optimal" reperfusion dose of 30 U.

Early evaluations of anistreplase in Europe also suggested its benefit relative to treatment with nonthrombolytic regimens.[40] Timmis et al.[41] randomized patients with AMI and coronary occlusion, demonstrated by angiography, to receive anistreplase (30 U) or a placebo. Reperfusion within 90 minutes was observed in 56% of patients treated with anistreplase in contrast to only 8% of those treated with placebo.

Based on this early and promising experience, the U.S. clinical trials program for anistreplase was formulated.

TEAM 1

The primary aim of the TEAM-1 trial was to evaluate the reperfusion efficacy, safety, and tolerance of IV anistreplase in patients with AMI and to compare this result with that for the then standard thrombolytic regimen of IC streptokinase given as approved by the U.S. Food and Drug Administration (FDA).[31] The study was designed to evaluate and compare the two methods of applying thrombolytic therapy more than the two agents as such.

Recruitment

Twenty-three U.S. and Canadian centers participated in the study, and 329 patients with AMI were screened and signed consent. Of these, 258 qualified for enrollment by demonstrating coronary occlusion (TIMI flow grade 0 or I[42]) at cardiac catheterization and were randomized to a treatment arm at the time of angiography. Of these, 240 patients fulfilling all angiographic and ECG criteria and actually receiving the assigned study drug regimen were the basis for the study analysis. (Excluded patients were equally divided between groups, and their inclusion in an intention-to-treat approach did not change the conclusions.)

Inclusion Criteria and Treatment Regimens

Qualifying patients had to be < 75 years of age and to have presented within 6 hours of onset of chest pain with> 0.1–0.2 mV (1–2 mm) ECG ST elevation and to show acute coronary occlusion (TIMI grade 0 or I) at acute angiography.[42] These patients then underwent blinded randomization to open label treatment with either IV anistreplase (30 U over 2–4 min) or IC streptokinase (20,000 U as a bolus followed by 2,000 U/min as an infusion for 60 min). Heparin was subsequently given to both groups beginning at 2–6 hours (mean 4.1) after streptokinase or 4–8 hours (mean 6.1) after anistreplase therapy and adjusted to maintain partial thromboplastin time (PTT) at twice normal levels.

Angiographic Evaluation of Reperfusion and Reocclusion

Serial angiographic evaluations of reperfusion were made over 90 minutes, and success was defined as the advancement of grade 0 or I TIMI flow to grade II or III flow at 60 minutes for IC therapy or at 90 minutes for IV therapy. (Angiographic recanalization, the end point in TEAM-1, is a more rigorous evaluation of drug effect on reperfusion than patency because it requires a pretherapy angiogram as well as a posttherapy study, and the pretherapy study must show occlusion [15%–20% of AMI patients will show spontaneous patency at the initial study[14]]).

In TEAM-1, the observed rates of reperfusion were 59 (51%) of 115 for the IV (anistreplase) strategy and 67 (60%) of 111 for the IC (streptokinase) strategy. The reperfusion rate for IV anistreplase was identical to that of IC streptokinase (60%) if treatment was begun within 4 hours of onset of symptoms (Fig. 2). If treatment was begun later than 4 hours, IV therapy was less successful, with only 33% reperfusion at 90 minutes (but this was comparable to or better than the 24% reperfusion rate for treatment beginning after 4 hours with IV streptokinase determined in the TEAM-1 study.[42] These observations are consistent with the traditional perception that fresher, less compact, and "cross-linked" fibrin clots are more susceptible to thrombolysis with streptokinase and related fibrinolytic.

The success of reperfusion was also dependent upon the initial flow grade. For IC streptokinase, the success rate increased from 54% for grade 0 to 78% for grade I flow (P < 0.03); similarly for IV anistreplase, reperfusion was 45% for grade 0 and 77% for grade I arteries (P < 0.002). Hence, even a "trickle" of flow about the obstructing thrombus greatly enhances the chances of subsequent reperfusion success. The location of the infarct related artery did not

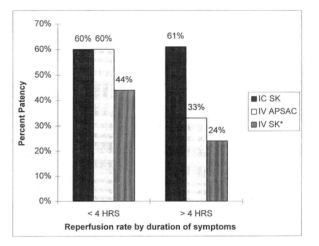

Figure 2. Reperfusion results for IV anistreplase and IC streptokinase in TEAM-1, and comparison with TIMI-1.

substantially affect reperfusion success, although there was a trend favoring reperfusion in the left anterior descending coronary artery.

To evaluate continued artery patency and reocclusion, angiography was repeated after 24 hours in all patients with initial reperfusion who did not undergo additional interventions. Reocclusion rates at 24 hours were low: three of the patients receiving IV anistreplase and one patient receiving IC streptokinase.

Hemodynamic, Hematological, and Clinical Observations

IV anistreplase was generally well tolerated, although a variable, transient decrease in blood pressure was observed, with a median average decline of 10 mmHg at 3 minutes. The 30-U dose of anistreplase caused substantial systemic lytic effects, reducing plasma fibrinogen levels to 32% of pretreatment values at 90 minutes, with a gradual return to normal by 48 hours. The bleeding risks after anistreplase appeared to be similar to those expected for equivalent doses (i.e., ca 1.1 MU) of streptokinase. No intracranial hemorrhages occurred in either group. Significant hemorrhage, defined as a drop in hematocrit of $> 10\%$ points within 24 hours of treatment, was observed in 21 of 113 in the IV anistreplase group versus 15 of 103 in the IC streptokinase group.

TEAM-1 was not designed as a mortality trial, but the low in-hospital death rates observed were reassuring (anistreplase 4%, streptokinase 8%).

Other Studies Comparing IV APSAC and IC Streptokinase

The findings of the TEAM-1 study were similar to those of other reperfusion studies of similar design that included comparisons with IC streptokinase. Most notable of these studies was a concurrent Dutch multicenter study[43] that also compared the reperfusion efficacy of IV anistreplase (30 U over 5 min) with IC streptokinase (mean 275,000 U over 60 min). In the Dutch study, patients with AMI presented within 4 hours of symptom onset, and reperfusion was achieved in 23 (65%) of 26 patients treated with anistreplase compared to 25 (67%) of 37 of those treated with IC streptokinase. The TEAM-1 study (60% reperfusion success) and the Dutch study (65% reperfusion success) results thus were similar for the subgroups treated within 4 hours of onset of symptoms. The mean times to achieve reperfusion following IV anistreplase therapy also were comparable in the U.S. (average, 43 min) and the Dutch (46 min) studies.

Summary of TEAM-1

In summary, for AMI patients selected for angiographic coronary occlusion (i.e., representing about 80% of those with ST elevation[14]), anistreplase, given in a convenient, IV bolus form, was shown to be effective in restoring reperfusion within 90 minutes in 60%–65% of patients treated within 4 hours, a percentage equivalent to that of IC streptokinase, the approved "gold standard" at the time of study initiation. Time to reperfusion averaged 45 minutes. Tolerance was good. These reperfusion results provided a promising basis for the further evaluation of the IV strategy of administering anistreplase for early therapy of patients with AMI.

TEAM-2

The Second Thrombolytic Trial of Eminase in AMI, TEAM-2,[32] aimed to determine the therapeutic effects of anistreplase on patency assessed qualitatively and quantitatively early after MI and compare these patency results with a standard thrombolytic regimen of IV streptokinase and to determine absolute and relative reocclusion rates within 1–2 days of therapy. With FDA approval of the IV route for streptokinase, and given its greater ease of use than IC delivery and its rapid acceptance into clinical practice, it was appropriate that the second thrombolytic trial was planned to directly compare IV administration of anistreplase to streptokinase.

TEAM-2 Entry Criteria and Enrollment

TEAM-2 enrolled 370 patients with AMI, age < 75 years, and with symptoms lasting > 30 minutes but < 4 hours, and with ST segment elevation of 0.1 mV or more in one or more limb leads or 0.2 mV or more in one or more precordial leads, suggestive of ischemic injury associated with pain not relieved by sublingual or IV nitroglycerin.

Exclusion

Patients with contraindications to thrombolytic therapy and with ongoing cardiogenic shock on vasopressors or intraaortic balloon pump, or with a history of coronary artery bypass surgery or balloon angioplasty within the last 1 month were excluded from the study. Qualifying patients were randomized in a double-blind fashion to receive either 30 U of IV anistreplase over 2–4 minutes or 1.5 million IU of streptokinase over 60 minutes. Early coronary patency rates were determined angio-

graphically at 90–240 minutes (median, 2.1 hours) and late patency rates were assessed after 1 day (18–48 hours, mean 28 hours). All patients received adjunctive antithrombotic therapy with IV heparin, which was titrated to maintain effective anticoagulation, defined as a PTT 1.5–2.5 times the upper normal limit.

Early Patency Results

The two groups were evenly matched, though there was a significant excess of women in the anistreplase group (P = 0.05). The early angiographic patency results were comparable in the two groups: 72% (anistreplase) and 73% (streptokinase). However, TIMI-III flow (complete reperfusion; now known to be associated with optimal outcome[44]) tended to be higher with anistreplase (60%) than with streptokinase (53%) (Fig. 3). Thus, among patients with patent arteries as defined by TIMI II or III flow at early angiography, 82% showed TIMI-III flow with anistreplase versus 72% with streptokinase (P = 0.03).

When analyzed by coronary artery, there was a marginally greater patency success among patients with right coronary occlusion, 79% versus 66% for the left anterior descending artery, in contrast to the trend observed in TEAM-1.[31] The reasons for these differing trends is unclear and may be due to differences in biological responses

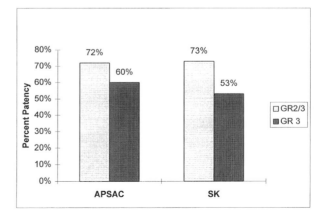

Figure 3. Patency results for IV anistreplase and IV streptokinase in TEAM-2.

by coronary artery, to study design differences, or to chance. Taken together, TEAM-1/2 would suggest approximately equivalent patency effects of anistreplase or streptokinase on the two major infarct related coronary arteries.

Delayed Patency and Reocclusion

One hundred and ninety patients with initially patent arteries without interventions were restudied angiographically after 1 day (18–48 hours, mean 28 hours). Only 1 of the 96 anistreplase and 2 of the 94 streptokinase-treated patients had reoccluded. Among the 98%–99% of restudied patients with continued patency, TIMI-III perfusion was present in 93% of the anistreplase and 91% of the streptokinase group (the rest, 7%–9%, had grade II perfusion). Thus, the risk of unanticipated reocclusion was very low with these regimens, whereas a progressive increase in perfusion grade (percent TIMI-III flow) was common during the first day after therapy.

Hemodynamic and Hematological Results

The hemodynamic and laboratory evaluations in the two treatment groups suggested comparability. The incidence of hypotension was not significantly greater with anistreplase than streptokinase, despite rapid injection. The observed changes in hemoglobin, fibrinogen, and plasminogen after both therapies were comparable and of an expected degree based upon previous studies. Fibrinogen fell to an average of 24% of baseline after anistreplase and to 21% of baseline after streptokinase (P = 0.05). Plasminogen fell to 18% and 14% of baseline in the two treatment groups, respectively. The reduction in hematocrit and hemoglobin levels after anistreplase and streptokinase therapy were similar at 24 hours and 3 days, as were the nadir values. Stroke occurred in 3 patients (1.6%) in the streptokinase group and 1 (0.5%, P = 0.32) in the anistreplase group.

Enzymatic Confirmation and Sizing of MI

Enzymatic confirmation of MI as defined by an elevation of creatinine kinase (CK) to 1.5 times or more of the upper limits of normal during serial testing was present in 97% of the anistreplase-treated patients and 96% of the streptokinase-treated patients. However, the elevations were present in the initial sample at study entry in only 9% and 11%, respectively, confirming the early acquisition of patients. Karagounis et al.[45] reported on the effects of thrombolytic therapy on the infarct size in TEAM-2 as assessed by enzymatic (CK, CK-MB, LDH, and LDH-1) and ECG determinations. A trend toward lower peak enzymes was noted for each of the four enzymes in the anistreplase group compared to the streptokinase group, with reductions averaging 6%–16%. Differences approached significance for LDH (P < 0.07) and achieved significance for LDH-1 (P = 0.035). Moreover, a significant difference was observed for all four cardiac enzymes in time-activity kinetics for patients with, versus patients without, early coronary patency. Regardless of thrombolytic agent, enzyme levels were lower (P ≤ 0.05) and the shape of the curves differed favorably in patients with patent arteries (P ≤ 0.0005).

ECG Markers of Outcome by Therapy and Patency

There was no significant difference in the ECG indices of myocardial injury or infarction between the two treatment groups with the exception of the loss of R wave amplitude, and this was attributed to differences in baseline values. In contrast, there was a significant reduction in the summed Q wave amplitude overall and at discharge when results were compared by patency outcomes (P = 0.04).

Summary of TEAM-2

In summary, there was a general comparability in patency, clinical, ECG, and enzymatic evolution of AMI with anistreplase and streptokinase (grade III patency and enzyme peaks favored anistreplase). Also, there were significant reductions in the extent of infarction with the achievement of early patency by either therapy.

TIMI Grade Patency and Outcome: Is Grade II Optimal?

While the primary mechanism by which thrombolytic therapy reduces mortality is believed to be the restoration of patency of the infarct related artery, it only recently has been realized that not just the presence of patency, but also the degree of perfusion may play an important role in the reduction in mortality and morbidity that accompanies thrombolysis. Traditionally, the TIMI scale has been utilized for assessment of patency success, based on a logical but arbitrary classification. TIMI grades 0 (totally occluded artery) and I (minimally perfused) have been considered to represent reperfusion failures, whereas TIMI grades II (partially perfused) and III (fully perfused) have been considered to be patency successes.[42]

Analysis of the TEAM-2 data first suggested that TIMI grade II flow leads to suboptimal results (i.e., closer to those of occluded [grades 0/I] than fully perfused [grade III] coronary arteries).[46] In TEAM-2, patients with TIMI grade II perfusion had enzymatic peaks and times to peak activity, and also ECG evolution of summed ST segments, Q waves and R waves that were not significantly different from those of patients with grade 0 or I flow. In contrast, patients with grade III perfusion had significantly lower enzyme peaks (for 3 of the 4 enzymes, $P < 0.005$–0.0003) (Table 2) and shorter times to peak activity (also for 3 of the 4 enzymes, $P < 0.03$–0.002) than other patients.

For ECG indices, summed ST elevations resolved more quickly and completely in the grade III patency group ($P = 0.008$), but not with grade II; Q wave development was blunted ($P = 0.001$) and R

wave amplitude was better preserved ($P = 0.01$), but only in the grade III patients; final Selvester QRS infarct score was least in the grade III group ($P = 0.03$) (Table 2).

On the basis of these results, it was first proposed that while establishment of TIMI grade II flow results in some perfusion of the infarcted coronary artery bed, perfusion is inadequate to meet the metabolic demands of the jeopardized myocardium, falling below a critical threshold sufficient to relieve myocardial ischemia. It was recognized, however, that not only persistent epicardial coronary artery occlusion, but also arteriolar/capillary flow insufficiency (no-reflow phenomenon) due to extensive tissue damage might contribute to grade II flow in some cases (i.e., TIMI-II might be a consequence, not a cause of, a poor outcome). Nonetheless, overall analysis of the data from TEAM-2 and several subsequent trials[35,44,47–51] suggest that TIMI perfusion grade II is usually a consequence of inadequate thrombolysis and behaves more like a mostly occluded than a well-perfused artery, contrary to previous assumptions. Thus, achievement of grade II flow is not optimal for myocardial salvage and the goal of reperfusion should be to quickly achieve and maintain grade III perfusion.

Observations from TEAM-2 on Myocardial Electrical Stability and Perfusion: QT Dispersion

The TEAM-2 study also provided indirect evidence of the benefit of thrombolytic therapy on the risk for ventricular arrhythmia.[52] Electrocardiographic QT interval is a measure of regional ventricular repolarization time. The maximum interregional (interlead) difference in QT interval, designated QT dispersion or QTd, has been proposed as a measure of heterogeneity of ventricular recovery, and consequently, of arrhythmia vulnerability.[53] Moreno et al.[52] demonstrated that QTd (maximum minus minimum QT interval) on the standard 12-lead ECG was markedly reduced in patients achieving successful thrombolysis

Table 2.

Enzyme Peaks and QRS Scores by Therapy and Patency in TEAM-2 (Refs. 32, 45, 46)

A. Enzyme Peaks (IU/L), Mean

	APSAC	SK	P Value	Grade 0	Grade I	Grade II	Grade III	P Value	P Value (Gr III vs < Gr III)
CK	2438	2761	0.13	3129	2954	2931	2292	0.01	0.002
CK-MB	265	282	0.53	349	303	273	247	0.06	—
LDH	619	699	0.07	826	655	742	570	0.0001	0.0003
LDH-1	279	332	0.04	443	338	362	256	0.004	0.005

B. QRS Score at Discharge (after Selvester—see refs. 45, 46)

APSAC	SK	P Value	Grade 0	Grade I	Grade II	Grade III	P Value	P Value
5.57 ± 0.31	5.50 ± 0.38	NS	6.9 ± 0.7	$5.7 + 0.8$	5.4 ± 0.6	5.0 ± 0.3	0.03	0.0001

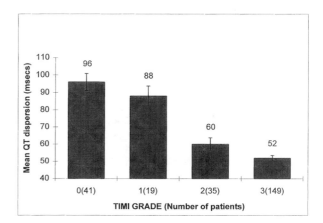

Figure 4. Convalescent QT dispersion grouped by early coronary patency grade in TEAM-2.

compared with those with persistently occluded coronary arteries in TEAM-2 (Fig. 4). QTd was progressively reduced with increasing grades of perfusion, with maximum benefit (minimum QTd, near the normal range) in those achieving TIMI grade III flow. Moreover, the association of QTd with patency was independent of other patient characteristics.

Thus, achieving patency of the infarct related artery appears to reduce the degree to which an abnormal electrophysiological milieu develops following AMI and may be an explanation for the low rates of total and sudden death observed after successful thrombolysis. The clinical consequence of the effect of patency on QTd should be evaluated in other studies because sufficient long-term clinical outcome data to directly do this were not available in TEAM-2.

TEAM-2 and the Smoker's Paradox

A smoker's paradox has been described such that patients who smoke and sustain an AMI paradoxically show improved short-term prognosis when compared with nonsmokers.[54] Gomez et al.[55] investigated the smoker's paradox and its angiographic correlates within the TEAM-2 database with interesting findings. Smokers tended to be younger (mean age of 53 vs 59 years) and were more likely to be men (80% vs 73%), normotensive (74% vs 58%), and have an inferior infarction (66% vs 51%) than nonsmokers. After correcting for the imbalances in baseline and angiographic variables, multivariate logistic regression analysis still identified smoking as an independent predictor for achieving grade III flow, with an odds ratio of 1.8 (P = 0.01). These findings suggested the hypothesis that, in addition to identifying younger patients generally more likely to have a good treatment response and a favorable outcome, smoking may be associated with more active thrombogenic mechanisms, leading to a greater thrombus component of the coronary occlusion and making it more susceptible to lytic therapy.

TEAM-3

The TEAM-3 study was designed to be a controlled, multicenter trial of intermediate size comparing the two second-generation thrombolytic regimens, anistreplase and standard dose tPA (alteplase), in patients with AMI.[33] The specific objectives of TEAM-3 were: (1) to compare left ventricular ejection fraction (LVEF) at rest and during exercise by treatment before hospital discharge and at 30 days; (2) to compare clinical morbidity after anistreplase and tPA therapy and the need for mechanical interventions; and (3) to assess patency of the coronary arteries at 1 day.

Study Design

The study was designed as a double-blind, double-dummy comparison of anistreplase, given over 2–5 minutes, and tPA, given over 3 hours (standard dosing regimen), in patients with documented AMI who could be treated within 4 hours of symptom onset. The inclusion and exclusion criteria were otherwise similar to those of the earlier TEAM-2.[32] With both therapies, heparin was administered, beginning 2 hours after the start of thrombolytic therapy, with an IV bolus of 5,000 U followed by an infusion of 1,000 U/hour. The heparin dose was adjusted to maintain an activated PTT 1.5–2.5 times the upper limit of normal and heparin was continued for at least 48 hours. Aspirin was also given to all patients, immediately on study entry in a dose of 160 mg and daily thereafter in a 160–320 mg dose for at least the 1-month duration of the study. The administration of beta blockers and calcium antagonists was not specified by the protocol, but left to the discretion of individual study investigators.

Coronary angiography was undertaken at 1 day (18–48 hours) after the start of thrombolytic therapy to assess plateau coronary patency rate in the absence of intervening interventions. ("Plateau," or maximum coronary patency rate, is the net result of early and delayed achievement of patency minus coronary reocclusion, is achieved within 1 day, and was believed to be important and complementary to the assessment of 90-minute patency, determined in TEAM-2). Again, angiographic perfusion in an infarct related artery was graded according to the TIMI classification by a blinded investigator at the TEAM core angiographic laboratory. The guidelines for mechanical intervention suggested that elective angioplasty not be performed before the angiographic study at 1 day and then only for persistently occluded (grades 0 or I) arteries, if clinically indicated. Allowance for emergent angiography, angioplasty, and bypass surgery was made for patients who developed cardiogenic shock or early hemodynamic failure and patients who developed recurrent, medically unresponsive pain accompanied by ischemic ECG changes.

Rest radionuclide ventriculography was first performed as soon as possible after administration of thrombolytics, within a maximum of 4 hours, to provide an early posttherapy result. Convalescent radionuclide ventriculography (the primary end point) was performed 7–10 days after dosing or at the time of hospital discharge (whichever came first) and again at 1 month. In addition to the rest studies, exercise was performed at the 7- to 10-day and the 1-month assessments to determine exercise LVEF.

Patient Acquisition and Rest LV Function Results

A total of 325 patients were enrolled in the study: 161 were randomized to receive anistreplase and 164 to receive tPA. The two groups were comparable in their pretreatment medical history, age, gender, time to therapy, entry hemodynamics, and the location of the infarct, except for the slightly greater frequency of diabetes in the anistreplase compared to the tPA group (21% vs 12%, P = 0.03).

Resting LVEF, measured predischarge, averaged 51.3% in the anistreplase group and 54.2% in the tPA group (P = 0.038)(Fig. 5). At 1 month, EF averaged 50.2% in the anistreplase group versus 54.8% in the tPA group (P = 0.002) (Fig. 5). In neither group was there a large proportion of patients with substantially depressed EFs at 1 month; only 5% of the patients in each group had severe LV dysfunction (EF < 0.30). These differences in global EF were accompanied and explained by parallel differences in systolic volumes and infarct-zone EFs. In contrast to the differences observed in the convalescent studies, EFs were similar by therapy in the early posttreatment baseline study (at a median of 2.9 hours).

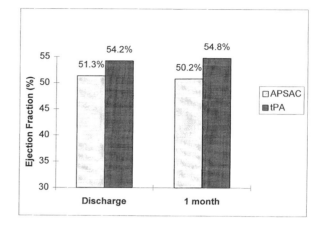

Figure 5. Convalescent LVEF by therapy (anistreplase vs tPA) in TEAM-3.

Exercise EF

Little further difference over the rest results was elicited by exercise. EF increase at submaximal exercise at predischarge testing tended to be greater for tPA (P = 0.052). However, maximal exercise at 1 month elicited a similar augmentation in EF after APSAC (+ 4.3% points) and tPA (+ 4.6% points) therapies and exercise times were comparable.

Clinical Events

The occurrence of major clinical events was generally comparable in the two groups and within the range anticipated for these thrombolytic therapies. The 1-month mortality was 6% in the anistreplase group and 8% in the tPA group; stroke rates were 2% and 1%, and reinfarction rates 2% and 4%, respectively. There was no significant difference in heart failure, recurrent ischemia, ventricular tachycardia, or fibrillation incidence. Bleeding episodes occurred more frequently in the anistreplase than the tPA group (28% vs 17% transfused, P = 0.01). Overall clinical outcomes were compared with a combined morbidity index using an ordinal logistic regression approach. Results showed an equivalent outcome for the two treatments, with an odds ratio of all adverse outcomes for anistreplase versus tPA-treated patients of 1.05

(95% confidence intervals 0.74–1.5, P = 0.82).

One-Day Coronary Patency Rates

Coronary angiography at 1 day (median, 26 hours) revealed comparable distributions of TIMI perfusion grades II and III in both treatment groups. The total coronary artery patency rate (TIMI II + III) was high after both anistreplase (89%) and tPA (86%) (P = 0.37). The success of patency also was not significantly different by infarct related artery or by anterior versus inferior infarct location. Consistent with the similar patency outcomes, there was no difference in the frequency of mechanical interventions following therapy with anistreplase and tPA.

Hematological Effects

As expected, the hematological effects of anistreplase were more pronounced than tPA, with greater decreases in fibrinogen and plasminogen (28% vs 65% of baseline for fibrinogen and 22% vs 58% of baseline for plasminogen for anistreplase and tPA, respectively).

Summary of TEAM-3

The TEAM-3 study compared standard regimens of anistreplase and tPA and the primary end point of resting EF measured at discharge and at 1 month favored tPA, with the small difference (2%–4% points) associated with parallel differences in infarct zone function and systolic volumes. However, the convalescent EF was excellent in both groups and exercise performance was comparable. Differences in EF could not be ascribed to differences in 1-day patency, which were comparably high in both groups, but perhaps reflect a difference in very early (60–90 min) patency, which was not assessed in TEAM-3. Clinical outcomes as assessed by a morbidity index were comparable and favorable in both groups.

Subsequent comparisons of anistreplase with tPA have used an accelerated dosing regimen for alteplase and have reported early patency and subsequent functional and clinical advantages for tPA.[56,57]

TIMI Flow Grade and LV Function in TEAM-3: Only Grade III is Optimal

The TEAM-3 study allowed an evaluation of the association of 1-day coronary patency with convalescent LV function. TIMI perfusion grade III flow was found to be associated with better EF outcome irrespective of the thrombolytic agent used.[47] In contrast, the outcomes for EF, enzyme peaks, ECG markers, and morbidity index associated with grade II perfusion were

worse, and did not differ significantly from grades 0 and I perfusion groups. TIMI perfusion grade III patients, when compared with grade 0, I, or II patients, showed a much improved global EF at 1 week (54% vs 49%, P = 0.006) and 1 month (54% vs 49%, P = 0.01) (Fig. 6). Similarly, infarct zone EF was greater at 1 week, 41% versus 32%; and at 1 month, 42% versus 32% (P = 0.03), in patients achieving grade III patency (Fig. 6). As in TEAM-2, smaller enzyme peaks (significant for LDH) and shorter times to peak (significant for all four enzymes) were observed in association with TIMI-III flow. Also, infarct size was smaller by ECG criteria, as evidenced by a smaller QRS score at discharge and at 1 month in patients with TIMI-3 flow. The power of clinical end point comparisons was limited by the relatively small number of events, but a trend toward a lower morbidity index was also observed.

Implications of TEAM-3 Patency Substudy

The implication of this patency together with the TEAM-2 substudy is that grade II perfusion is not associated with optimal myocardial salvage (assessed by ventriculographic, enzymatic, and ECG criteria) and clinical outcome, and therefore, TIMI grade III perfusion should be considered the best measure for success of throm-

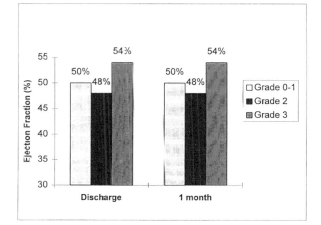

Figure 6. Convalescent LVEF by 1-day coronary patency grade in TEAM-3.

bolytic therapy and the goal for reperfusion therapies. These seminal observations have now been confirmed and extended to mortality differences among perfusion grades by studies from the U.S. and Europe, placing the patent coronary artery hypothesis on firm ground.[44–51]

Anistreplase and tPA Dosing and Patient Weight

Generally, thrombolytics have been given in fixed doses, with little regard for patient weight (except for a reduction in dose of tPA with body weight < 60 kg for safety reasons). The question of whether very large patients are optimally treated with standard drug doses also was raised in the rt-PA-APSAC Patency Study (TAPS).[56,57] We looked at the question of body weight and patency outcome in the TEAM-3 database.[58] In anistreplase-treated patients, coronary patency rates at 1 day were found to be similar in those in the upper quintile of weight (> 94 kg) and in low- to normal-weight patients (86% vs 90%, respectively, for grades II or III; 82% vs 74% for grade III). In contrast, for tPA-treated patients, heavy patients showed lower 1-day patency rates compared to lighter patients (74% vs 89% for grade II or III [P = 0.02], 59% vs 77% for grade III [P = 0.03]).

The results differ from TAPS, in which early (90-min) patency rates were unaffected by weight with tPA therapy, but reduced in heavy patients with anistreplase.[56] The two studies are consistent if it is assumed that tPA (accelerated dosing) achieves optimal early patency rates, even in heavy patients, whereas 90 minutes is too early for anistreplase to achieve its optimal patency rate in the obese, which occurs later; in contrast, heavy patients treated with tPA lose patency advantage over the first day (perhaps because of less adequate heparinization as well as tPA use for thrombolysis). These observations suggest that optimization of thrombolytic therapy by body weight is a fertile area for further investigation.

Effects of Thrombolysis on Measures of Myocardial Electrical Stability in TEAM-3

The hypothesis, generated in TEAM-2, that increased dispersion of ventricular repolarization (measured as QTd) associated with coronary occlusion may be reversed with reperfusion,[52] was prospectively tested in TEAM-3.[59] The results verified that patency grade is inversely related to QT dispersion. Furthermore, TIMI grade was the most significant multivariate associate, followed by reinfarction status and LVEF. The consequences of these differences for long-term arrhythmic events should be assessed in additional studies.

Low amplitude, high frequency signals in the terminal portion of the QRS complex ("late potentials") are believed to correspond to fragmented activation of ventricular tissue and inhomogeneous conduction within diseased myocardium and are also associated with the risk of tachyarrhythmias and sudden death.[60,61] We tested the ability of thrombolytic related achievement of early patency to reduce ECG late potential after AMI.[62] Although not a formal TEAM substudy, the trial included many patients in the TEAM-2 and TEAM-3 studies entered at our center. Among 101 well-characterized patients, a highly significant difference in the incidence of late potentials was found comparing those achieving patency (TIMI II or III) to those remaining occluded (TIMI 0 or I), 18% versus 50%, respectively, P = 0.006. The odds ratio for developing a late potential was 0.39 for thrombolysis versus no thrombolysis and 0.22 for patency versus no patency (both P < 0.05). Furthermore, late potentials tended to occur less often after early than late patency. The reduction of late potentials by thrombolytic related perfusion may be an additional important mechanism of benefit in stabilizing myocardial electrical function and reducing future arrhythmic events.

Conclusion

The U.S./Canadian TEAM trials program contributed importantly in evaluating a new thrombolytic (anistreplase) and comparing it with other agents (streptokinase, tPA). Anistreplase was found to achieve thrombolysis with nearly equivalent efficacy to IC streptokinase if administered early after MI and was comparable to or better (and more convenient) than IV streptokinase. Although markers of ventricular function and infarct size suggested comparable or somewhat better results with standard regimen tPA, coronary patency at 1 day was identical.

The TEAM studies also played a pivotal role in addressing more general questions surrounding thrombolysis, including IV versus IC therapy strategies, outcomes by TIMI patency grade, the smoker's paradox, thrombolytic efficacy by patient weight, and the influence of reperfusion on myocardial electrical stability. As such, they contributed together with many other efforts world-wide in a veritable revolution in AMI therapy, to the good of patients.

References

1. Laffel GL, Braunwald E. Thrombolytic therapy: A new strategy for the treatment of acute myocardial infarction. N Engl J Med 1984;311:710,770.
2. Marder VJ, Sherry S. Thrombolytic therapy: Current status. N Engl J Med 1988;318:1512-1520,1585-1594
3. Gersh BJ, Anderson JL. Thrombolysis and myocardial salvage. Results of clinical trials and the animal paradigm-paradoxic or predictable? Circulation 1993;88:296-306
4. ISAM (Intravenous Streptokinase in Acute Myocardial Infarction) Study Group. A prospective trial of intravenous streptokinase in acute myocardial infarction (ISAM): Mortality, morbidity, and infarct size at 21 days. N Engl J Med 1986;314:1465-1471.
5. White HD, Norris RM, Brown MA, et al. Effect of intravenous streptokinase on left ventricular function and early survival after acute myocardial infarction. N Engl J Med 1987;317:850-855.
6. Guerci AD, Gerstenblith G, Brinker JA, et al. A randomized, placebo-controlled, double-blind trial of intravenous tissue plasminogen activator for acute myocardial infarction with subsequent randomization to elective coronary angioplasty. N Engl J Med 1987;317:1613-1618.
7. O'Rourke M, Baron D, Keogh A, et al. Limitation of myocardial infarction by early infusion of recombinant tissue-type plasminogen activator. Circulation 1988;77:1311-1315.
8. Bassand J-P, Machecourt J, Cassagnes J, et al., for the APSIM Study Investigators. Multicenter trial of intravenous anisoylated plasminogen streptokinase activator complex (APSAC) in acute myocardial infarction: Effects on infarct size and left ventricular function. JACC 1989; 13:988-997.
9. Gruppo Italiano per lo Studio della Streptochinasi nell' Infarcto Miocardico (GISSI). Effectiveness of intravenous thrombolytic treatment in acute myocardial infarction. Lancet 1986;i:397-401.
10. ISIS-2 Collaborative Group. Randomized trial of intravenous streptokinase. Oral aspirin, both, or neither among 17,187 cases of suspected acute myocardial infarction: ISIS-2. Lancet 1988;ii:349-360.
11. Wilcox RG, Lippe GV, Olsson DB, et al. Trial of tissue plasminogen activator for mortality reduction for acute myocardial infarction: Anglo-Scandinavian study of early thrombolytic therapy (ASSET). Lancet 1988;ii:525-530.
12. AIMS Trial Study Group. Long-term effects of intravenous anistreplase in acute myocardial infarction: Final report of the AIMS study. Lancet 1990; 335:427-431.
13. Braunwald E. Myocardial reperfusion limitation of infarct size, reduction of left ventricular dysfunction, and improved survival. Should the paradigm be expanded? Circulation 1989; 79:441-444.
14. Granger CB, Califf RM, Topol EJ. Thrombolytic therapy for acute my-

ocardial infarction. A review. Drugs 1992;44:293.

15. Fibrinolytic Therapy Trialists' (FTT) Collaborative Group. Indications for fibrinolytic therapy in suspected acute myocardial infarction: Collaborative overview of early mortality and major morbidity results from all randomised trials of more than 1000 patients. Lancet 1994;343:311-322.

16. PRIMI Trial Study Group. Randomized double-blind trial of recombinant pro-urokinase against streptokinase in acute myocardial infarction. Lancet 1989;i:863-868.

17. Neuhaus K-L, von Essen R, Tebbe U, et al. Improved thrombolysis in acute myocardial infarction with front-loaded administration of alteplase: Results of the rt-PA-APSAC Patency Study (TAPS). JACC 1992;19:885.

18. The INJECT Study Group. A randomized, double blind comparison of reteplase, 10 + 10 MU double bolus administration, with streptokinase in patients with acute myocardial infarction (INJECT). Lancet 1995;346:329-336.

19. Vanderschueren S. Barrios L, Kerdsinchai P, et al., for the STAR Trial Group. A randomized trial of recombinant staphylokinase versus alteplase for coronary artery patency in acute myocardial infarction. Circulation 1995;92:2044-2049.

20. Cannon CP, McCabe CH, Ghali M, et al., and the TIMI 10A Investigators. TNK-tissue plasminogen activator in acute myocardial infarction: Results of the Thrombolysis in Myocardial Infarction (TIMI) 10A dose-ranging trial. Circulation 1996 (In press).

21. ISIS-3 Collaborative Group. ISIS-3: A randomised comparison of streptokinase vs tissue plasminogen activator vs anistreplase and of aspirin plus heparin vs aspirin alone among 41,299 cases of suspected acute myocardial infarction. Lancet 1992;339:753.

22. The International Study Group. In-hospital mortality and clinical course of 20,891 patients with suspected acute myocardial infarction randomised between alteplase and streptokinase with or without heparin. Lancet 1990;336:71-75.

23. Cannon CP, McCabe CH, Henry TD, et al., for the TIMI 5 Investigators. A pilot trial of recombinant desulfato-

hirudin compared to heparin in conjunction with tissue plasminogen activator and aspirin for acute myocardial infarction: Results of the Thrombolysis in Myocardial Infarction (TIMI) 5 Trial. JACC 1994;23:993-1003.

24. The EPIC Investigators. Use of a monoclonal antibody directed against the platelet glycoprotein IIb/IIIa receptor in high-risk coronary angioplasty. N Engl J Med 1994;330:956-961.

25. The GISSI-3 Investigators. Effects of lisinopril and transdermal glyceryl trinitrate singly and together on 6-week mortality and ventricular function after acute myocardial infarction: The Gruppo Italiano per lo Studio della Sopravvivenza nell'infarcto Miocardico (GISSI)-Study. Lancet 1994;343:1115-1122.

26. ISIS-4 Collaborative Group. ISIS-4: A randomized factorial trial assessing early oral captopril, oral mononitrate, and intravenous magnesium sulphate in 58,050 patients with suspected acute myocardial infarction. Lancet 1995;345:669-685.

27. The European Myocardial Infarction Project Group (EMIP). Prehospital thrombolytic therapy in patients with suspected acute myocardial infarction. N Engl J Med 1993;329:383.

28. Weaver WD, Cerqueira M, Hallstrom AP, et al., for the MITI Study Group. Prehospital-initiated vs hospital-initiated thrombolytic therapy. The Myocardial Infarction Triage and Intervention (MITI) Trial. JAMA 1993;270:1211-1216.

29. Fuster V. Coronary thrombolysis-a perspective for the practicing physician. N Engl J Med 1993;329:723-725.

30. Simoons ML, Arnold AE. Tailored thrombolytic therapy. A perspective. Circulation 1993;88:2556-2564.

31. Anderson JL, Rothbard RL, Hackworthy RA, et al., for the APSAC Multicenter Investigators. Multicenter reperfusion trial of intravenous anisoylated plasminogen streptokinase activator complex (APSAC) in acute myocardial infarction: Controlled comparison with intracoronary streptokinase. JACC 1988;11:1153-1163.

32. Anderson JL, Sorensen SG, Moreno FL, et al., and the TEAM-2 Investigators. Multicenter patency trial of intravenous anistreplase com-

pared with streptokinase in acute myocardial infarction. Circulation 1991; 83:126-140.

33. Anderson JL, Becker LC, Sorensen SG, et al., for the TEAM-3 Investigators. Anistreplase versus alteplase in acute myocardial infarction: Comparative effects on left ventricular function, morbidity, and 1 day patency. JACC 1992;20:753-766.

34. Braunwald E. The open-artery theory is alive and well again. N Engl J Med 1993;329:1650-1652

35. Simes RJ, Topol DJ, Holmes DR, et al., for the GUSTO-1 Investigators. Link between the angiographic substudy and mortality outcomes in a large randomized trial of myocardial reperfusion. Circulation 1995; 91:1923-1928.

36. Smith RAG, Dupe RJ, English PD, et al. Fibrinolysis with acyl-enzymes: a new approach to thrombolytic therapy. Nature 1981;290:505-508.

37. Anderson JL, Boissel J-P, Chamberlain DA (eds.): Symposium on anisoylated plasminogen streptokinase activator complex APSAC. Drugs 1987;33(Suppl 3).

38. Anderson JL, Califf RA. Anisoylated plasminogen streptokinase activator complex (APSAC) in cardiovascular therapy. In: Messerli F, ed. Drugs for the Heart and Circulation. 2nd edition. Philadelphia, PA: WB Saunders, 1996, pp. 1553-1566.

39. Marder VJ, Rothbard RL, Fitzpatrick PG, et al. Rapid lysis of coronary artery thrombi with anisoylated plasminogen-streptokinase activator complex: Treatment by bolus intravenous injection. Ann Intern Med 1986; 104:304-310.

40. Johnson ES, Cregeen RJ. Anisoylated plasminogen streptokinase activator complex in perspective: an interim report of efficacy and safety. Drugs 1987; 33(Suppl 13):298-311.

41. Timmis AD, Griffin B, Crick J, et al. Anisoylated plasminogen streptokinase activator complex in acute myocardial infarction: A placebo-controlled arteriographic coronary recanalization study. JACC 1987; 10:205-210.

42. Chesebro JH, Knatterud G, Roberts R, et al. Thrombolysis in myocardial infarction (TIMI) trial phase I: A comparison between intravenous plasminogen activator and intravenous streptokinase. Circulation 1987; 76:142-154.

43. Bonnier HJRM, Visser RF, Klomps HC, et al., and the Dutch Invasive Reperfusion Study Group. Comparison of intravenous anisoylated plasminogen streptokinase activator complex and intracoronary streptokinase in acute myocardial infarction. Am J Cardiol 1988;62:25-30.

44. Anderson JL, Karagounis LA, Califf RA. Metaanalysis of 5 reported studies on the relation of early coronary patency grades with mortality and outcomes after acute myocardial infarction. Am J Cardiol 1996;78:1-8.

45. Karagounis L, Ipsen S, Moreno F, et al., and the TEAM-2 Investigators. Effects of early thrombolytic therapy on enzymatic and electrocardiographic infarct size: results of a randomized, blinded study of anistreplase versus streptokinase in acute myocardial infarction. Am J Cardiol 1991;68:848-856.

46. Karagounis L, Sorensen SG, Menlove RL, et al., for the TEAM-2 Investigators. Does Thrombolysis In Myocardial Infarction (TIMI) perfusion grade 2 represent a mostly patent artery or a mostly occluded artery? Enzymatic and electrocardiographic evidence from the TEAM-2 study. JACC 1992;19:1-10.

47. Anderson JL, Karagounis LA, Becker LC, et al., for the TEAM-3 Investigators. TIMI perfusion grade 3 but not grade 2 results in improved outcome after thrombolysis for myocardial infarction. Circulation 1993; 87:1829-1839.

48. Vogt A, von Essen R, Tebbe U, et al. Impact of early perfusion status of the infarct-related artery on short term mortality after thrombolysis for acute myocardial infarction: Retrospective analysis of four German multicenter studies. JACC 1993;21:1391-1395.

49. Simes RJ, Topol DJ, Holmes DR, et al., for the GUSTO-1 Investigators. Link between the angiographic substudy and mortality outcomes in a large randomized trial of myocardial reperfusion. Circulation 1995; 91:1923-1928.

50. Lincoff AM, Topol EJ, Califf RM, et al., for the TAMI Study Group. Significance of a coronary artery with

thrombolysis in myocardial infarction grade 2 flow "patency" outcome in the Thrombolysis and Angioplasty in Myocardial Infarction Trials). Am J Cardiol 1995;75:871-876.

51. Zahger D, Karagounis LA, Cercek B, et al., for the TEAM Investigators. Incomplete recanalization as an important determinant of thrombolysis in myocardial infarction (TIMI) grade 2 flow after thrombolytic therapy for acute myocardial infarction. Am J Cardiol 1995;76:749-752.

52. Moreno FM, Villanueva MA, Karagounis LA, et al., for the TEAM-2 Study Investigators. Reduction in QT interval dispersion by successful thrombolytic therapy in acute myocardial infarction. Circulation 1994; 90:94-100.

53. Statters DJ, Malik M, Ward DE, et al. QT dispersion: Problems of methodology and clinical significance. J Cardiovasc Electrophysiol 1994;5:672-685.

54. Mueller HS, Cohen LS, Braunwald E, et al., for the TIMI investigators. Predictors of early morbidity and mortality after thrombolytic therapy of acute myocardial infarction. Circulation 1992;85:1254-1264.

55. Gomez MA, Karagounis LA, Allen A, et al., for the TEAM-2 Investigators. Effect of cigarette smoking on coronary patency after thrombolytic therapy for myocardial infarction. Am J Cardiol 1993;72:373-378.

56. Neuhaus K-L, von Essen R, Tebbe U, et al. Improved thrombolysis in acute myocardial infarction with front-loaded administration of alteplase: Results of the rt-PA-APSAC Patency Study (TAPS). JACC 1992;19:885.

57. Cannon CP, McCabe CH, Diver DJ, et al., and the TIMI 4 Investigators. Comparison of front-loaded tissue-type plasminogen activator, anistreplase and combination thrombolytic therapy for acute myocardial infarction: Results of the thrombolysis in myocardial infarction (TIMI) 4 trial. JACC 1994;24:1602-1610.

58. Karagounis LA, Anderson JL, Sorensen SG, et al., for the TEAM-3 Investigators. Relation of reperfusion success with anistreplase or alteplase in acute myocardial infarction to body weight. Am J Cardiol 1994;73:16-22.

59. Karagounis LA, Moreno FM, Sorensen SG, et al., for the TEAM-3 Investigators. Multivariate determinants of QT dispersion in patients with acute myocardial infarction: Primary patency status of the infarct-related artery. Circulation 1994;90:I-662.

60. Cain ME, Anderson JL, Arnsdorf MF, et al., for the American College of Cardiology. Signal-averaged electrocardiography expert consensus document. JACC 1996;27:238-249.

61. El-Sherif N, Denes P, Katz R, et al., for the CAST/SAECG Substudy Investigators. Definition of the best prediction criteria of the time domain signal-averaged electrocardiogram for serious arrhythmic events in the postinfarction period. JACC 1995; 25:908-914.

62. Moreno FM, Karagounis L, Marshall H, et al. Thrombolysis-related early patency reduces ECG late potential after myocardial infarction. Am Heart J 1992;124:557-564.

Address for reprints: Jeffrey L. Anderson, M.D., FACC, Chief, Division of Cardiology, LDS Hospital, 8th Ave. and C St., Salt Lake City, UT 84123. Fax: (801) 321-5087.

Chapter 11

The GUSTO Trials

Christopher B. Granger, M.D.
and Robert M. Califf, M.D.

From the Duke University Medical Center, Durham, North Carolina

Genesis of the GUSTO Trials

The Global Utilization of Streptokinase and Tissue Plasminogen Activator (alteplase) for Occluded Coronary Arteries (GUSTO) trial organization was envisioned by its leaders as an international group specializing in acute care cardiology and clinical trials methods, and executed by a worldwide network of dedicated clinical investigators. The organization relied on the broad experience of its Steering Committee members, including representatives from the Thrombolysis and Angioplasty in Myocardial Infarction (TAMI) trial and other North American trials, the Gruppo Italiano per lo Studio della Streptochinasi nell'Infarto Miocardico (GISSI)/International Trial, and the International Study of Infarct Survival (ISIS) trial. The trial methods were a modification of the large, simple trial approach popularized by the leaders of the ISIS trials. Relatively small amounts of the most important data were colleted from a large number of patients to ensure adequate ability to determine the effect of therapy on mortality itself, rather than on surrogate endpoints. The simple trial approach was blended with moderate levels of data monitoring and on-site investigator training, collection of additional data to address important secondary issues, and incorporation of selected ancillary studies to provide a mechanistic understanding of the treatment effect and other important clinical topics.

The underlying theme of the original GUSTO trial, a principle that would serve as a common thread throughout the series of trials, was that rapid and stable reperfusion in acute myocardial infarction is important for improved survival. The trial included enough patients to detect the smallest difference in mortality considered to be clinically important (a 14% relative or 1% absolute difference in mortality) and enough patients in an angiographic substudy to determine coronary artery patency and reocclusion rates.

Strict guidelines were developed and published[1] to address the political and economic considerations related to the development of thrombolytic agents, avoid conflicts of interest, and maintain independence from the sponsors. Moreover, compared with previous large thrombolytic trials, greater effort was made in GUSTO-I to ensure data quality and to collect key information to address ancillary issues of major clinical importance. Medical records were reviewed for 10% of all patients enrolled and for 100% of patients who suffered a stroke. These records underwent thorough, detailed adjudication. Serious adverse event reporting (beyond those collected on the standard case report form) was limited to serious, unexpected adverse events. The simpler adverse event reporting used in the GUSTO-I trial is now standard in large thrombolysis trials of agents that have been given to at least 1,000 patients in Phase II.

The experience of GUSTO-I provided the enthusiasm, excitement, and momentum for the investigators to continue a series of large trials that test many areas of reperfusion therapy, including several thrombolytic agents, direct angioplasty, and novel antithrombin and antiplatelet agents. By including over 600 centers in the United States and over 3,000 worldwide, the GUSTO trials would enable tens of thousands of participating physicians and nurses to contribute to, and benefit from, a series of large trials that could result in major advances in the treatment of acute coronary syndromes.

The GUSTO trials have provided some of the world's largest quality-controlled databases of patients with acute coronary syndromes, databases that contained selected, comprehensive, verified information using common definitions. These databases, combined with a group of investigators who had the energy, dedication, and capacity to address important clinical questions, have resulted in a comprehensive reassessment of acute coronary syndromes.

The most important legacy of the GUSTO trials may have been the establishment of an international group of leaders in clinical trials and a worldwide network of investigators to conduct clinical trials. This group of investigators would extend and mature the concept that clinical research can be incorporated into routine clinical practice worldwide to test new therapies rapidly and accurately and thus improve patient care.[2]

GUSTO-I

The concept that earlier, more complete infarct related coronary artery patency results in better left ventricular function and better survival was challenged by the results of GISSI-2[3] and ISIS-3.[4] These trials found that alteplase, which was known to produce more complete early patency than streptokinase,[5] did not produce better survival. One of the most strongly argued explanations for the lack of survival difference was that intravenous heparin, which was thought to be necessary with alteplase treatment to avoid increased reocclusion, was not used in these trials. This might have negated alteplase's early advantage. A group of angiographic studies fueled this hypothesis; they found that without intravenous heparin, high rates of reocclusion were common after alteplase treatment.[6,7] At the same time, other investigations showed that alteplase given in an accelerated fashion resulted in even better early patency without an apparent increase in bleeding.[8–10] Still other studies showed that the combination of alteplase and a nonfibrin-specific thrombolytic agent resulted in low rates of reocclusion.[11,12]

These findings led to the conception of the GUSTO-I trial, which was designed to test the hypothesis that rapid and durable infarct-artery patency correlates with survival (Fig. 1).[13] There were two control arms reflecting the different approaches to the use of heparin with thrombolytic agents around the world. The first, the standard regimen in much of the world, was streptokinase with subcutaneous heparin (12,500 U subcutaneously twice daily beginning 4 hours after initiation of streptokinase) that was used in the GISSI-2 and ISIS-3 trials. The second, streptokinase with intravenous heparin was the standard United States approach and was included so as not to disad-

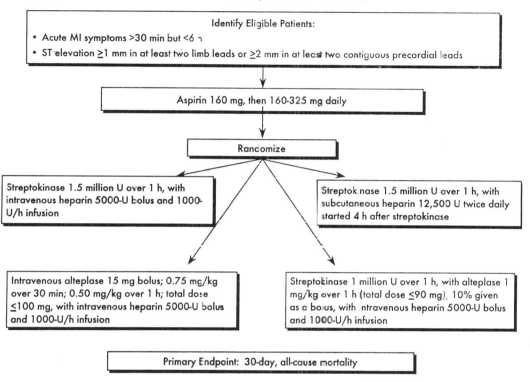

Figure 1. The design of the GUSTO-I trial. MI = myocardial infarction.

vantage streptokinase should intravenous heparin be an important component of its benefit. The experimental arms both included intravenous heparin used to attempt to reduce the incidence of early reocclusion. The first was an accelerated dose (or "front-loaded") of alteplase that was given as a 15-mg bolus, followed by 0.75 mg/kg over 30 minutes (50 mg maximum), and then 0.5 mg/kg over 60 minutes (35 mg maximum), or an overall total of up to 100 mg of alteplase over 90 minutes. This arm was intended to test the effect of more rapid coronary reperfusion on survival. The second was a combination of alteplase (1 mg/kg over 60 minutes, up to 90 mg, with 10% of the dose given as a bolus) and streptokinase (1 MU over 60 minutes) That was intended to test the importance of sustained reperfusion.

The analysis plan called for the two streptokinase arms to be combined should there be no appreciable difference between the two arms. This allowed for a more robust comparison with the experimental arms. Because it was recognized that the two experimental arms were likely to result in a higher risk of intracranial hemorrhage, a secondary endpoint considered survival benefit and stroke risk by combining death and disabling stroke into a single measure called "net clinical benefit."

Because the importance of earlier reperfusion was expected to be more evident in patients presenting earlier symptom onset, only patients who presented within 6 hours of symptom onset were eligible (Table 1). In an attempt to maximize the relevance of the trial results to general practice, exclusion criteria were kept to a minimum.

Patients were enrolled from December 27, 1990 to February 22, 1993. The primary results were presented only 9.5 weeks later,

Table 1

The GUSTO Trials

Trial	Patients	Countries	Hospitals	Patient Population	Enrollment Period	Experimental Treatment(s)
GUSTO-I[13]	41,021	15	1,081	ST elevation MI, symptoms < 6 hours	12/90–2/93	Accelerated alteplase; alteplase-streptokinase combined
GUSTO-IIa[32]	2,564	12	275	Acute coronary syndromes, symptoms < 12 hours	9/93–4/94	Hirudin
GUSTO-IIb[33]	12,142	13	373	Acute coronary syndromes, symptoms < 12 hours	4/94–2/95	Hirudin
GUSTO-III[51]	15,059	20	807	ST elevation MI, symptoms < 6 hours	10/95–1/97	Reteplase

MI: myocardial infarction.

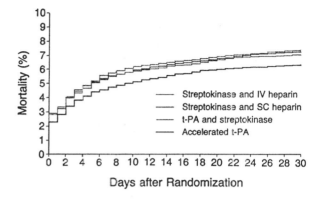

Figure 2. Thirty-day mortality in the four treatment arms of the GUSTO-I trial. IV = intravenous; SC = subcutaneous; tPA = alteplase. (Reprinted from The GUSTO Investigators[13] with permission.)

with 30-day mortality data that were > 99% complete on 41,021 patients from 1,081 hospitals in 15 countries on 5 continents. This accomplishment resulted from the hard work of the investigators and other study personnel and the efficient systems for collection and processing of large amounts of data.

The principal finding of GUSTO-I was that compared with streptokinase, accelerated alteplase resulted in a 1% absolute, or 14% relative, reduction in 30-day mortality (Fig. 2).[13] This reduction was highly significant, whether compared with the streptokinase arms combined (P = 0.001) or separately (P = 0.009 for subcutaneous heparin, P = 0.003 for intravenous heparin). Moreover, the 1% survival advantage with alteplase persisted at 1 year.[14]

The second experimental arm, the combination of streptokinase and alteplase, was not better than streptokinase alone and was marginally worse (P = 0.04) than accelerated alteplase. Somewhat surprisingly, the use of full dose intravenous heparin was not better than the use of delayed subcutaneous heparin with streptokinase. In fact, there was a nonsignificant increase in mortality with intravenous (7.4%) versus subcutaneous (7.2%) heparin, although the rates were identical at 1 year.[14]

Because of the importance of understanding the effect of the new treatment strategies on stroke, a great deal of care was taken in its accurate determination and classification. An expert, blinded committee reviewed the medical records of every

case of suspected stroke. Over 93% of all stroke pathology was documented by brain imaging or autopsy ensuring that precise rates of actual, rather than suspected, intracranial hemorrhage and other stroke were ascertained. Perhaps most important, data were collected from investigators on the degree of disability after stroke. This information was found to be highly accurate when compared with direct telephone interviews of patients with stroke in North America.[15]

As had been expected based on earlier trials,[3,4] accelerated alteplase was associated with an increase of two primary intracranial hemorrhages per 1,000 patients treated compared with streptokinase (0.72% vs 0.52%, P = 0.03).[13] The incidence of "net clinical outcome" (death or nonfatal, disabling stroke) was significantly lower with accelerated alteplase than with streptokinase (6.9% vs 7.8%, P = 0.006).

On average, accelerated alteplase reduced mortality by 1%, which was economically attractive by United States standards at an average of $33,000 per year of life saved.[16] However, there has been substantial interest in and speculation about which patients had the greatest benefit and which patients had no benefit or a greater risk with alteplase and might therefore receive the less expensive drug, streptokinase.[17,18] In fact, the relative reduction in death with accelerated alteplase was similar across patients subgrouped by age, infarct location, time from symptom onset, blood pressure, heart rate, Killip class, or prior infarction.

The absolute benefit, therefore, is best estimated by determining the absolute risk, and a simple nomogram has been developed to do this in clinical practice.[19]

Angiographic Substudy.

An integral part of the GUSTO-I trial was a 2,431-patient angiographic substudy.[20] This substudy was designed to determine the patency profiles, reocclusion rates, and left ventricular function measures of the four treatment strategies to serve as a mechanistic underpinning of the overall trial. The major findings were that infarct-artery patency was greater at 90 minutes with accelerated alteplase, and reocclusion rates were low in all treatment groups. Accelerated alteplase resulted in an 81% incidence of thrombolysis in myocardial infarction (TIMI) grade II or III flow at 90 minutes, compared with an incidence of 54% to 60% for streptokinase. Although the incidence of TIMI grade III flow was highest with accelerated alteplase, it was present in only 54% of patients, leaving substantial room for improvement and creating an objective for future trials.

The substudy has provided a database to address a wide variety of issues in acute myocardial infarction. It confirmed earlier studies that had found better survival with a higher TIMI flow grade,[21,22] even after adjustment for other patient characteristics (Fig. 3).[23] TIMI flow grade also was found to be an independent predictor of long-term survival, along with younger age, higher left ventricular ejection fraction, and the absence of diabetes.[24] Better measures of left ventricular function and smaller left ventricular volumes generally were found with accelerated alteplase, and they were associated with better survival.[20,25]

Given the underlying hypothesis of GUSTO-I that accelerated alteplase would result in better early patency (which would result in better survival), and that both better patency and survival were observed, the question arises: can the better survival be completely explained by the better patency? This question was addressed in an analysis using simple regression models for the relationships between thrombolytic strategy and patency, and between patency and survival, to see if those relationships completely explained the relationship between thrombolytic strategy and survival.[23] In fact, the better survival with accelerated alteplase was almost completely explained by the better early patency (Fig. 4). This linkage of early patency and survival was perhaps the most important message from the GUSTO-I trial, and it provided a compelling basis to continue to develop therapies that can establish earlier and more complete reperfusion.

GUSTO-II

If GUSTO-I addressed the "open-artery hypothesis," that is, that early and sustained reperfusion is important, GUSTO-II (Global Use of Strategies To Open Occluded Arteries in Acute Coronary Syndromes) was intended to test the "thrombin hypothesis": more effective inhibition of thrombin will help improve patient outcome in acute coronary syndrome.

Figure 3. Relation between Thrombolysis In Myocardial Infarction (TIMI) flow grade and 30-day mortality after thrombolysis in the GUSTO-I trial, before and after adjustment for sex, age, previous infarction, infarct location, height, systolic blood pressure, and heart rate. (Reprinted from Simes et al.[23] with permission.)

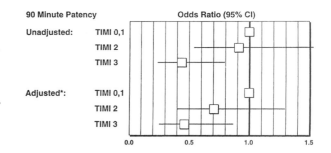

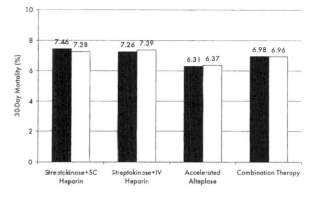

Figure 4. Predicted (black bars) versus observed (white bars) 30-day mortality in the GUSTO-I trial, on the basis of TIMI flow grade at 90 minutes. Mortality was predicted using 1,210 patients randomized to undergo angiography at 90 minutes; observed mortality refers to the other 39,811 patients in GUSTO-I. SC = subcutaneous; IV = intravenous. (Reprinted from Simes et al.[23] with permission.)

One of the lessons from GUSTO-I was that intravenous heparin has major limitations when used with thrombolytics. There was no advantage of intravenous compared with subcutaneous heparin with streptokinase, and there were more complications (without more benefit) with higher levels of heparin anticoagulation.[26] In fact, the lowest mortality and bleeding rates were associated with an activated partial thromboplastin time (aPTT) in the 50- to 75-second range (Fig. 5), and higher aPTTs did not confer lower rates of reinfarction. Moreover, a coagulation marker substudy found that heparin was ineffective at suppressing thrombin generation and activity.[27]

As GUSTO-I was being completed, a more potent class of antithrombin agents was being tested in pilot studies. The prototype was hirudin, a direct thrombin inhibitor derived from leech saliva. Hirudin seemed to overcome all the major disadvantages of heparin; it does not require antithrombin-III as a cofactor, it is small enough to effectively inhibit clot-bound thrombin, it is not neutralized by circulating proteins such as platelet factor 4, it does not cause immune reactions such as heparin-induced thrombocytopenia, and it has a more predictable anticoagulant effect. Pilot studies in both unstable angina[28] and ST-segment elevation acute infarction[29] were promising, showing better early patency with hirudin than with heparin and strong tendencies toward reduced event

rates. Because these studies were small and studied relatively young, healthy patients, the risk of toxicity, especially with the higher doses, may have been underestimated.

Simultaneously with two other large trials, TIMI-9a[30] and the r-Hirudin for Improvement of Thrombolysis (HIT-III) trial,[31] the GUSTO group began a large trial of hirudin versus heparin across the spectrum of acute coronary syndromes.[32] The GUSTO and TIMI groups decided to use the same dose of hirudin in their trials. Because aPTTs had been found to be reduced in heavier patients, a modestly higher dose of intravenous heparin was used in heavier patients in the control arm. All three of these trials had to be stopped early because of unacceptably high rates of intracranial hemorrhage with hirudin, especially in conjunction with thrombolytic therapy (Table 2).[30–32] Moreover, even the patients treated with the modestly higher dose of heparin, which was associated with a median 5-second higher aPTT at 24 hours, had a twofold increase in the risk of intracranial hemorrhage. The increased risk appeared to be related to greater anitcoagulation and was not explained by a change to a higher risk patient population. In fact, a reduction in the rate of intracranial hemorrhage (to that expected from earlier trials) with reduced doses of hirudin and heparin in GUSTO-IIb[33] and TIMI-9b[34] provided fundamental support to the conclusion that lower levels of anticoagulation after throm-

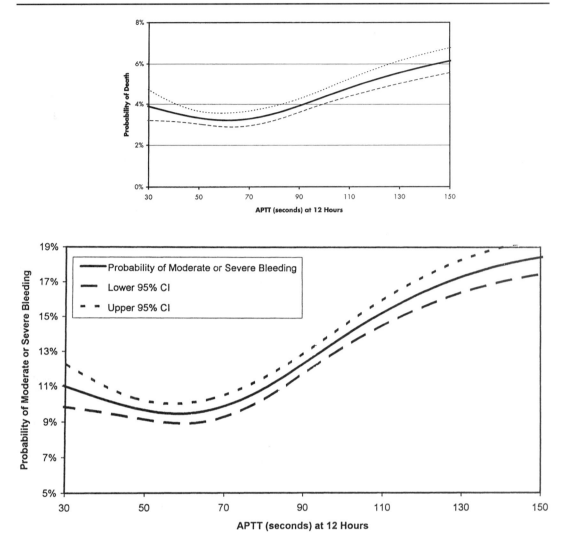

Figure 5. Mortality at 30 days (A) and in-hospital bleeding (B) rates by activated thromboplastin time (aPTT) in the GUSTO-I trial. (Reprinted from Granger et al.26. with permission.)

bolysis should be the goal in patient care.

GUSTO-IIa and TIMI-9A were resumed as GUSTO-IIb and TIMI-9b with lower doses of hirudin and heparin. The principle finding of GUSTO-IIb was a small reduction in death or myocardial (re)infarction at 30 days that fell just short of statistical significance (Fig. 6).[33] The point estimate was a prevention of 2 deaths and 9 nonfatal (re)infarctions per 1,000 patients treated. There was clear evidence of a treatment effect during study drug administration; at 24 and 48 hours, there were highly significant (P = 0.001) reductions in death or (re)infarction. Although there was no increase in death or myocardial infarction in the hirudin group for the remainder of the 30 days, there was likewise no further benefit. The treatment effect appeared to be similar across major patient subgroups, including patients with or without ST-segment elevation at baseline. With the GUSTO-IIb and TIMI-9b trial results were combined,[35] myocardial (re)infarction was significantly reduced with hirudin, but not the composite of death or (re)infarction at 30 days.

Table 2

Rates of Intracranial Hemorrhage in Randomized Trials of Heparin versus Hirudin with Thrombolytic Therapy Compared with the GUSTO-I Trial

	Thrombolysis + Hirudin	Thrombolysis + Heparin	GUSTO-I Thrombolysis + Heparin
GUSTO-IIa[32]	13/677 (1.9%)	8/660 (1.2%)	—
TIMI-9A[30]	6/345 (1.7%)	7/368 (1.9%)	—
HIT-III[31]	5/148 (3.4%)	0/154 (0%)	—
Combined (%, 95% CI)	24/1,170 (2.1%, 1.2%–2.9%)	15/1,182 (1.3%, 0.6%–1.9%)	268/41,021 (0.65%, 0.53–0.73%)

CI = confidence interval.

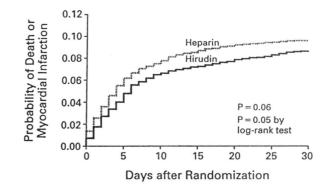

Figure 6. Mortality or (re)nonfatal infarction at 30 days in patients receiving heparin or hirudin in the GUSTO-IIb trial. (Reprinted from The GUSTO-IIb Investigators[33] with permission.)

The overall impression that hirudin is more effective than heparin was further supported by the 6-month follow-up results, at which time hirudin did confer a significant reduction in death or (re)infarction (12.3% vs 13.6%, P = 0.039).[36]

One subgroup of special interest and relevance to future studies of the GUSTO group was patients treated with streptokinase. In this population, hirudin had a marked benefit compared with hirudin.[37] At 6 months, among patients treated with streptokinase, there was a 38% relative and 7.3% absolute reduction in death and myocardial infarction with hirudin.[36] These data, combined with studies showing better early coronary artery patency with streptokinase and hirulog,[38] raise the possibility that direct thrombin inhibitors may be more important with streptokinase. This is being tested directly in the 17,000-patient HERO-2 trial of hirulog versus heparin combined with streptokinase, which is being conducted within the GUSTO investigator network.

Direct Angioplasty Substudy.

A series of small studies, highlighted by three published in 1993,[39-41] have compared primary angioplasty with thrombolysis for acute myocardial infarction and found a large, statistically significant reduction in mortality. A systematic overview confirmed a substantial reduction in death, reinfarction, and stroke with primary an-

gioplasty.[42] These earlier studies were generally conducted by primary angioplasty enthusiasts in high volume centers with small sample sizes, leading to uncertainty as to the reliability and relevance of the results in guiding mainstream clinical practice.[43]

The GUSTO-IIb direct angioplasty substudy was designed to compare direct angioplasty with thrombolysis in a more relevant way for most cardiologists by addressing each of the limitations of previous studies. The trial used accelerated alteplase (the best available thrombolytic regimen), a larger group of highly experienced investigators (but who were more representative of the overall population of cardiologists performing primary angioplasty), and a larger sample size (allowing a more accurate estimate of treatment effects).[44]

The major finding of the substudy was a statistically significant, modest reduction in the primary endpoint of death, reinfarction, or disabling stroke at 30 days, with a 13.7% incidence in the alteplase group compared with 9.6% in the angioplasty group (P = 0.033 (Fig. 7). By 6 months, the absolute benefit had been reduced to just over half of that at 30 days with rates of 15.9% and 13.3%, and an advantage of primary angioplasty that was no longer significant (P = 0.23).[45]

Compared with previous studies, which generally did not use rigorous, independent methods to review angiographic results, the acute angiographic success was

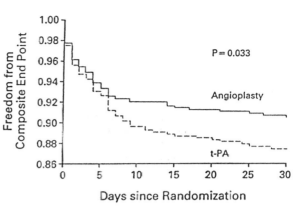

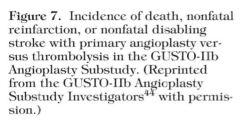

Figure 7. Incidence of death, nonfatal reinfarction, or nonfatal disabling stroke with primary angioplasty versus thrombolysis in the GUSTO-IIb Angioplasty Substudy. (Reprinted from the GUSTO-IIb Angioplasty Substudy Investigators[44] with permission.)

lower in the substudy. The core laboratory and the investigators reported TIMI grade III flow rates of 73% and 85%, respectively.[44] The median time from randomization to angioplasty balloon inflation was 1.3 hours.

The modest early advantage of primary angioplasty supports its use as an excellent alternative to thrombolysis in experienced hands and is consistent with the concept of earlier reperfusion resulting in better outcomes. However, the magnitude of the benefit was less than found in previous studies. Of interest, patients who presented later after symptom onset tended to have more treatment advantages with direct angioplasty,[46] although this finding could reflect the play of chance. Markers of high risk, such as advanced age, anterior infarction, or tachycardia, did not identify patients who derived a greater benefit from direct angioplasty.

GUSTO-III

The GUSTO-III (Global Use of Strategies to Open Occluded Coronary Arteries) trial marked a return to the study of thrombolytic agents, namely reteplase, a deletion mutant of tissue plasminogen activator (tPA). The removal of the finger, epidermal growth factor, and kringle-1 regions of native tPA gives the molecule a longer half-life, allowing double-bolus administration, and causes less fibrinogen depletion.

Angiographic studies of reteplase found higher early rates of TIMI grade III flow in the infarct related artery compared with streptokinase, a 3-hour infusion of alteplase,[47] or accelerated alteplase.[48] Based on these studies, expectations were that the more complete restoration of early coronary flow with reteplase would translate into better survival.

The International Joint Efficacy Comparison of Thrombolytics (INJECT) trial compared reteplase with streptokinase in a 6,000-patient trial designed to show that reteplase was at least as good as streptokinase for patient survival.[49] The point estimate was 0.5% better survival with reteplase at 30 days. The 95% confidence interval excluded the possibility that patients randomized to reteplase had > 1% higher mortality than streptokinase. At 6 months, the survival advantage of reteplase was close to 1%.[50]

In the GUSTO-III trial, 15,059 patients within 6 hours of symptom onset of acute myocardial infarction and with ST-segment elevation were randomized in a 2:1 ratio to reteplase (2 boluses of 10 MU each, 30 minutes apart) or to accelerated alteplase. The mortality rates at 30 days were 7.47% for reteplase and 7.24% for accelerated alteplase, for an absolute difference of 0.23%.[51] The 95% confidence interval of the difference included a 1.1% higher mortality with reteplase and a 0.66% higher mortality with alteplase. The net clinical effect (composite and death or nonfatal, disabling stroke) was 7.89% with reteplase and 7.91% with alteplase. In both treatment groups the primary intracranial hemorrhage rates were similar and higher than in previous trials.

The reason that the better patency observed in the angiographic trials did not translate into better survival in GUSTO-III is not known. Review of the Reteplase versus Alteplase Potency Investigation During myocardial infarction (RAPID-2) study shows that in a subset of patients with early (30-minute) angiography, reteplase was associated with TIMI grade III flow in 39% of patients versus 27% for alteplase.[48] Other possible explanations include overestimation of the patency advantage of reteplase, a higher reocclusion rate with reteplase (not evaluated in RAPID 2), an underestimate of survival with reteplase in GUSTO-III, or simply the play of chance.

Perhaps the most important outcome of GUSTO-III was the resulting focus on the issue of therapeutic equivalence. The GUSTO-III Steering Committee believed that the results did not show equivalence between reteplase and accelerated alteplase, because the 95% confidence interval included the possibility that reteplase was > 1% worse than alteplase. Because the 1% advantage of alteplase in GUSTO-I was widely interpreted and applied as being clinically relevant, exclusion of a 1% worse

survival with a new therapy should be a requisite for declaring clinical equivalence. The findings of similar rates of the composite of death and stroke with reteplase versus alteplase and of better patency with reteplase in the angiographic studies support the interpretation that the treatments are similar. Many hospitals and practitioners have switched from alteplase to reteplase in clinical care.

Predictive Models of Major Clinical Outcomes

The GUSTO trials provide a unique, powerful database because of the large population for whom common nomenclature has been used to describe baseline characteristics and clinical outcomes. By using sophisticated statistical methods to describe and validate complex multivariable relationships, robust models to estimate the risk of clinical outcomes have been derived from these databases.[15,25,52–66] Selected predictive models are listed in Table 3.

Mortality.

In the GUSTO-I population,[52] and validated in GUSTO-IIb,[53] multivariable analysis identified age as the most important factor influencing 30-day mortality with rates from 1.1% in the youngest decile (< 45

Table 3
Selected Predictive Models from the GUSTO Trial Databases

Model	Events (n)	C-index*	Most Important Predictor
30-day mortality[52]	2,851	0.84	Age
Intracranial hemorrhage[15]	268	0.77	Age
Death after intracranial hemorrhage[62]	105	0.93	Glasgow coma scale score
Nonhemorrhagic stroke[69]	247		Age
Death after cardiogenic shock[61]	1,647		Age
Moderate or severe bleeding[58]	5,154	0.83	Age

*The C-index provides a measure of the ability of a model to discriminate risk, with 0.50 being equal to chance (no discriminative power) and 1.0 being perfect discrimination.

Table 4

Independent, Significant Baseline Predictors of 30-day Mortality in the GUSTO-I Trial

Variable	Adjusted χ^2*
Advanced age	717
Lower systolic blood pressure (mmHg)	550
Worse Killip Class	350 (3 df)
Increased heart rate	275 (2 df)
Anterior location of infarction	143 (2 df)
Previous infarction	64
Age-by-Killip Class interaction	29
Shorter height	31 (4 df)
Longer time to treatment	23
Diabetes	21
Reduced weight	16
Nonsmoking status	22 (2 df)
Use of streptokinase	15 (3 df)
Previous bypass surgery	16
Hypertension	14
Prior cerebrovascular disease	10

*Indicates relative prognostic importance of each variable after adjusting for all other factors listed. df = degrees of freedom. (Reprinted from Lee et al.[52] with permission.)

years of age) to 20.5% for patients over age 75. The other most important factors, in order of importance, were lower systolic blood pressure, higher Killip class, elevated heart rate, and anterior infarct location. Together, these five variables contained 90% of the prognostic information derived from baseline characteristics. The entire list of independent risk factors for mortality is seen in Table 4.[52] From this model, a simple nomogram to estimate the risk of death in individual patients was developed,[19] as well as a second nomogram that also incorporates variables from the presenting electrocardiogram.[56] The most important independent prognostic variables from the electrocardiogram were the total amount of ST-segment deviations and the QRS durations.

A humbling observation to practitioners is that modifiable factors associated with better outcome–shorter time to treatment, treatment in the United States health care system with more revascularization, and use of accelerated alteplase–are minor determinants of outcome compared with baseline factors that cannot be changed. This observation explains why comparison outcomes by treatment across different studies, especially without careful adjustment for differences in risk, is often misleading.

Intracranial Hemorrhage.

The incidence of intracranial hemorrhage among patients with ST-segment elevation treated with thrombolytic therapy was 0.65% in GUSTO-I, 1.6% in GUSTO-IIa (with high dose hirudin and higher dose heparin), 0.6% in GUSTO-IIb, and 0.90% in GUSTO-III. The higher rate of intracranial hemorrhage in GUSTO-III was only partly explained by advanced age and may have been due in part to more thorough ascertainment. The median time intracranial hemorrhage in GUSTO-I was 10 hours after initiation of accelerated alteplase and 60% of patients died. Only 13% recovered with mild or no deficits.[15]

The most comprehensive previous analysis of predictors of intracranial hemorrhage after thrombolytic therapy, based on 150 patients with intracranial hemorrhage and 294 matched controls, found that advanced age, lower body weight, higher blood pressure, and use of alteplase correlate with a higher risk of intracranial hemorrhage with thrombolysis.[67] Among the 268 patients with intracranial hemorrhage in GUSTO-I (more patients than in all previous studies of imaging documented intracranial hemorrhage combined), age was the most important predictor, followed by lower body weight and previous cerebrovascular disease (Table 5).[15] Less powerful but still significant risk factors were higher diastolic or systolic blood pressure, history of hypertension, and randomization to either the combination alteplase-streptokinase strategy or to accelerated alteplase. A significant interaction between hypertension and age suggested that a history of hypertension is a less important risk factor in older patients. Even with this large

database to generate a predictive model, however, the ability to discriminate between high and low risk for intracranial hemorrhage was relatively poor (C-index = 0.54).

Detailed review of brain images from patients suffering intracranial hemorrhage in GUSTO-I revealed a heterogeneous set of findings, with larger volumes in the elderly, more subdural hematomas after head trauma or syncope, and deeper hemorrhages in patients with a history of hypertension.[68]

The ability to predict the likelihood of death after intracranial hemorrhage may help in counseling patients and families and in guiding aggressiveness of care. Analysis of the GUSTO-I data found three expected predictors and one unexpected predictor of mortality.[62] The most important predictor was the Glasgow coma scale score on the initial exam after intracranial hemorrhage. A larger total volume of intracranial hemorrhage (based on computed tomography or magnetic resonance imaging) and advanced age also were independent predictors. The unexpected independent predictor was earlier stroke onset after thrombolytic therapy. A simple nomogram has been developed that can be used in clin-

Table 5

Independent Predictors of Intracranial Hemorrhage After
Thrombolysis in the GUSTO-I Trial

Variable	Adjusted χ^2*
Older age	65
Lower weight	35
Prior cerebrovascular disease	20
Higher diastolic blood pressure	14
Combination alteplase-streptokinase therapy	14
Hypertension	7
Hypertension-by-age interaction	6
Accelerated alteplase therapy	4
Higher systolic blood pressure	4

*Indicates relative prognostic importance of each variable after adjusting for all other factors listed. (Adapted from Gore et al.[15] with permission.)

Table 6

Independent Predictors of Moderate or Severe Bleeding
(Noncerebral) After Thrombolysis in GUSTO-I, Excluding the Use
of Procedures

Variable	Adjusted χ^{2}*
Advanced age	147
Reduced weight	72
Female sex	30
Streptokinase with intravenous heparin	20
African ancestry	20
Increased heart rate	12

*Indicates the relative prognostic importance of each variable after adjusting
for all other factors listed. (Adapted from Berkowitz et al.[58] with permission.)

ical practice.[62] This model provides highly accurate discrimination of the likelihood of death (C-index = 0.93).

Nonhemorrhagic Stroke.

Ischemic stroke without hemorrhage occurred in 0.6% of the GUSTO-I population. In that group, 17% of patients died, and 38% had mild or no deficit.[69] The statistically significant independent predictors of nonhemorrhagic stroke were advanced age (> 50% increased risk per 10 additional years of age), increased heart rate, history of stroke or transient ischemic attack, diabetes, prior angina, and history of hypertension. A simple nomogram that can be used in clinical care has been published.[69]

Moderate or Severe Bleeding. In the GUSTO-I database, 12.6% of patients had either moderate (requiring transfusion) or severe (hemodynamically significant) bleeding.[58] This database contained nearly 100 times the number of events compared with the two previous studies of predictors of bleeding after thrombolysis.[70,71] The most important predictor of bleeding was coronary artery bypass surgery; 50% of patients undergoing coronary artery bypass surgery had transfusions for blood loss. Coronary angiography and angioplasty also were significant predictors. Excluding

procedures, the most important predictor was advanced age, such that there was a 40% increased risk of bleeding with each additional 10 years of age (Table 6). The next most important independent factor was lighter body weight, followed by female sex, thrombolytic assignment, and African ancestry. The greater likelihood of bleeding in patients of African ancestry after adjusting for all other risk factors is intriguing, and it may relate to the greater sensitivity of African-Americans to the fibrinolytic alteplase as noted in the TAMI trials.[72]

Patient Characteristics. The GUSTO databases have provided an opportunity to describe various baseline patient characteristics, related conditions, and related outcomes.

Age.

Patient age in GUSTO-I spanned a remarkable range, from 19 to 110 years.[73] Older patients had similar early infarct-artery patency, but worse regional left ventricular function and higher left ventricular volumes than younger patients.[74] Age was the most important independent predictor of most major adverse outcomes after thrombolysis, including mortality, with the risk of death increasing in more of an expo-

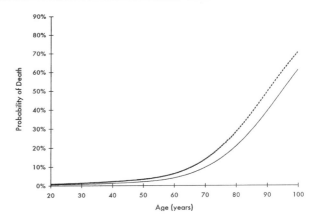

Figure 8. Mortality at 30 days (solid line) and at 1 year (dashed line) in the GUSTO-I trial as a function of age. (Reprinted from White et al.[75] with permission.)

nential than linear fashion beyond age 60 (Fig. 8).[75] However, older patients also have at least as large an absolute survival benefit from thrombolysis as do younger patients.[76] In GUSTO-I, all but the oldest patients (> 85 years) had lower mortality and lower death or disabling stroke when treated with accelerated alteplase.

Sex. In GUSTO-I, typical of thrombolytic trials, 25% of the population was female. In the non–ST-elevation cohort of GUSTO-IIb, women made up a greater proportion (33%) of the population. Women on average were older than men (by 7 years in GUSTO-I), took 18 minutes longer to arrive at the hospital, and had a longer hospital delay until thrombolytic therapy was begun.[77] Cigarette smoking, after adjusting for age, was more common in women, in and outside the United States. Nearly all complications were more common in women, including shock, congestive heart failure, bleeding, stroke, and reinfarction. Revascularization rates were similar between the sexes. Although the unadjusted 30-day mortality rate was twice as high in women as in men (11.3% vs 5.5%), after adjustment for age and other baseline differences, mortality was only slightly higher at 30 days (P = 0.04)[77] and was not different from 30 days to 1 year.[78]

Smoking. Cigarette smoking provides a good illustration of the hazards of making clinical decisions on the basis of univariable, observational analyses. In GUSTO-I, similar to previous trials, cigarette smokers had much lower 30-day mortality than nonsmokers (4.0% vs 10.3%, P < 0.001).[79] However, this appears to be explained by the findings that cigarette smokers have infarctions much earlier (mean = 11 years), are more often men, and have better left ventricular function and less reocclusion than do nonsmokers. Current cigarette smokers composed a large proportion of the overall study population (42%), whereas only 29% had never smoked.

Menstruation. Considerable confusion has existed about the advisability of treating a menstruating woman with thrombolytic therapy due to the uncertain effects of this therapy on menstrual flow and the risk of serious hemorrhage. An advantage of the unrestricted enrollment criteria in GUSTO-I is the opportunity to examine groups of patients who might have been excluded from other trials and, in fact, may commonly be excluded from receiving thrombolytic therapy in routine practice. In GUSTO-I, we collected information on 12 menstruating women treated with thrombolysis.[80] Although three patients did receive transfusions for bleeding, and in two of these it was for increased vaginal bleeding, none had severe bleeding and none died. This experience suggests that the life-saving benefit of thrombolysis should generally not be withheld because of menstruation.

Hypertension. A history of hypertension and an elevated blood pressure on admission were associated in GUSTO-I with a higher risk of bleeding, including intracranial hemorrhage. History of hypertension also was an independent predictor of increased risk of death, but elevated blood pressure on admission was not; in fact, it identified a relatively low risk population for death.[81] Combined with a substantially increased risk of intracranial hemorrhage in patients with a very elevated blood pressure on presentation, this suggests that for some patients with an otherwise low risk of death (no prior infarction, Killip class 1), the balance could favor withholding thrombolytic therapy, especially if direct angioplasty is available. When a thrombolytic agent is used in patients presenting with very high blood pressure, in spite of some suggestions to the contrary,[18] data from GUSTO-I suggest that accelerated alteplase results in a lower likelihood of death or disabling stroke than does streptokinase.[81]

Diabetes. In the GUSTO-I Angiographic Substudy, patients with and without diabetes were found to have similar coronary patency rates after thrombolysis.[82] In spite of this, 30-day mortality was higher among patients with diabetes, with higher mortality for diabetic patients treated with insulin (12.5%) than in other diabetic (9.7%) and nondiabetic (6.2%) patients ($P < 0.001$).[83] Patients with diabetes had higher risk baseline clinical and angiographic characteristics, including being older and more often female, having a longer time to thrombolysis, and more often having anterior location and more extensive coronary artery disease. In spite of similar overall left ventricular function, congestive heart failure was more common among patients with diabetes (22% vs 15%), which may relate to the reduced hyperkinesis in the noninfarct zone.[82] After adjustment for differences in clinical and angiographic baseline characteristics, diabetes remained an independent risk factor for 30-day and 1-year mortality. In spite of a theoretical concern over ocular bleeding due to diabetic retinopathy, review of the experience in GUSTO-I shows that risk of ocular hemorrhage is exceedingly low, estimated to be $< 0.05\%$.[84] Thus diabetic retinopathy should not be a contraindication to thrombolysis.

Time to treatment. The GUSTO-I trial provides data that strongly support the importance of rapid treatment with thrombolytic therapy. The overall results showed that treatment that most rapidly restored perfusion resulted in better survival. After adjustment for other variables, time to treatment was a significant predictor of mortality, with each hour of additional delay being associated with roughly a 0.5% increase in 30-day mortality.[52] Unfortunately, $< 3\%$ of the overall population actually received thrombolytic therapy in the "golden hour" after symptom onset.[85] Moreover the data from GUSTO-I show that higher risk patients, who would have the most to gain from earlier treatment, tended to have the longest delays, from symptom onset to hospital arrival and from hospital arrival until initiation of thrombolytic therapy.[85] These patients include the elderly, women, and patients with diabetes or a history of hypertension.

Electrocardiographic variables. A core laboratory review of tens of thousands of electrocardiograms (ECGs) in the GUSTO trials has allowed careful evaluation of the relationship of the presenting ECG and outcome. A wide variety of ECG characteristics are associated with increased mortality, including higher heart rate, rhythm other than sinus, bundle branch block,[86] hemiblock, longer QRS duration, anterior infarction, and greater ST elevation or depression.[56] Precordial ST-segment depression added substantially to risk of death among patients with inferior infarction.[87] Higher T wave amplitude that was associated with shorter time since symptom onset was independently associated with a lower risk of death.[88]

About 20% of patients who did not develop Q waves by the predischarge ECG had an excellent 30-day and 1-year survival, as well as fewer nonfatal complications.[89] Analysis of non-Q wave myocardial infarction in the angiographic substudy population showed that the better clinical course was associated with better early patency and better left ventricular function.[90]

Atrial fibrillation.

In GUSTO I, atrial fibrillation was noted in 2.5% of patients on the admission ECG and in 7.9% of patients after enrollment.[91] Atrial fibrillation was related to advanced age, higher cardiac enzyme levels, more heart failure, and faster heart rate, more extensive coronary artery disease, and a lower early TIMI flow grade. Stroke, especially ischemic (1.8% vs 0.5%), and mortality (14.3% vs 6.2%) were increased in patients with atrial fibrillation. After adjusting for other factors, atrial fibrillation was associated with a 30% increased risk of death.

Prior cardiac procedures. Prior bypass surgery was an independent predictor of 30-day mortality.[52] The point estimate of the absolute survival advantage of accelerated alteplase compared with streptokinase in this patient subset was greater than in most subsets, at 2.7%. Patients with prior angioplasty had a lower risk of 30-day mortality, most of which could be explained by more favorable baseline characteristics (such as being younger and having a shorter time to thrombolysis).[92]

Prior infarction. Patient with prior myocardial infarction had a higher overall risk of death despite similar rates of early coronary patency, and they had a similar relative treatment effect with accelerated alteplase compared with the rest of the population.[93] Although presentation to the hospital was somewhat faster, treatment after arrival to the hospital was delayed.

Cardiogenic shock. Shock was present at enrollment in 1% of patients and developed later in 6.5% of patients.[60] In spite of advances in treatment of acute myocardial infarction mortality remained high. Within 30 days of presentation, 57% of patients presenting with shock and 55% of patients developing shock died. Similar to the lower mortality of patients in shock treated with

streptokinase in the International Study Group,[94] mortality tended to be lower (P = 0.06) with streptokinase than with accelerated alteplase in GUSTO-I in patients presenting with shock. In GUSTO-III, patients in shock treated with reteplase tended to have lower mortality than those given alteplase. These results in aggregate raise the possibility that a less fibrin-specific agent may be advantageous in shock, where delivery of the thrombolytic agent to the clot may be impaired due to generalized hypoperfusion.

Two analyses from the GUSTO-I database support the concept that the aggressive use of revascularization and other interventions may improve outcome in patients with shock. Patients with shock who underwent early catheterization and revascularization had a better 30-day survival, even after adjusting for baseline differences and attempting to account for other factors (such as timing of death) that could have confounded the analysis.[95] Perhaps more convincing, patients in cardiogenic shock treated in the United States had significantly lower (P < 0.001) adjusted 30-day (50% vs 66%) and 1-year (56% vs 70%) mortality than did patients outside the United States. This better outcome was accompanied by a substantially higher use of catheterization, angioplasty, bypass surgery, and use of Swan-Ganz catheters and intra-aortic balloon pumping in the United States[96] Although this could theoretically be explained in part by physicians in the United States more readily identifying shock and therefore defining a less-sick population, the consistent findings of the association of better outcome with more aggressive intervention support this approach.

Nonrandomized Treatment Comparisons.

Data collection for the use of adjunctive therapies (other than the primary randomized comparison) and patient outcomes has allowed comparisons of their effects. These analyses are confounded by at least three factors that limit our ability to determine treatment effects; thus these analyses should be used primarily for hypothesis generation. The first factor, and the one that can be moderately well controlled, is the difference in characteristics collected at randomization, such as age. As described above, mortality models can adjust for much of the differences in the likelihood of death based on these characteristics. The second confounder is that of interval events, such as reinfarction or congestive heart failure, that occur after randomization. Because details of these events were not collected, their effects cannot adequately be accounted for. The third confounder is that of timing of the adjunctive treatment. Because the patient must survive long enough to begin the use of a given adjunctive treatment, there is an inherent tendency to relate better survival with its use, even if the treatment does not improve survival.

Beta blockers.

Because the GUSTO-I protocol recommended the use of intravenous followed by oral atenolol for all eligible patients, 75% of patients received this beta blocker in some form and 44% received intravenous drugs. After attempts to adjust for all confound factors, atenolol use was associated with better survival.[97] However, when use of intravenous followed by oral beta blocker was compared with the use of oral beta blocker alone (generally started on day 1 or 2), survival appeared to be no worse with forgoing the use of an acute intravenous beta blocker.

Lidocaine. During GUSTO-I enrollment, the use of prophylactic lidocaine was still common practice in the United States, where 25% of patients received it. In contrast to prior meta-analyses that suggested harm from prophylactic lidocaine in the prethrombolytic era, the GUSTO-I and -II

data suggest that lidocaine is associated with no worse mortality, and lower rates of ventricular arrhythmias.[98]

Bypass surgery. Nearly 9% of patients in GUSTO-I underwent coronary artery bypass surgery during the initial hospitalization. Because more patients assigned accelerated alteplase than streptokinase underwent bypass, there was speculation that the better survival with alteplase could have been related to benefits from surgery.[17] However, nearly half of the survival advantage of alteplase was evident by the end of the first 24 hours[99] before bypass would be electively performed. In addition, the 15% relative reduction in mortality with alteplase was present by the end of the first week when bypass rates were similar across treatment arms. Compared with patients not undergoing bypass, with adjustment for differences in baseline characteristics and time of surgery examined as a time dependent covariate in a Cox survival model, bypass was associated with higher 30-day (risk ratio 1.87, $P < 0.001$) and 1-year mortality (risk ratio 1.21).[100] These data are consistent with previous studies that show an increased risk of death for the first year after bypass followed by a long-term net benefit for patients with multivessel disease.

Other Substudies.

The GUSTO-I study was notable for the consistency in the findings that accelerated alteplase resulted in greater early patency, better left ventricular function, fewer clinical events related to infarct size (such as heart failure, shock, and even arrhythmias), and better survival. Also consistent with these findings was a substudy performed in Europe using quantitative cardiac enzyme release kinetics to measure infarct size.[101]

One substudy that failed to support the overall GUSTO results used continuous monitoring of the ST segment to assess the speed and stability of reperfusion.[65]

Despite data showing that rapid resolution of ST elevation correlates with angiographic reperfusion[102] and predicts improved clinical outcomes,[103] accelerated alteplase was not associated with significantly faster resolution of ST elevation in this 1,067-patient study. The failure of continuous ST-segment monitoring to discriminate between thrombolytic regimens that produce different early patency rates may relate to technical difficulties in applying the monitors and collecting data.

The data from the ST-segment monitoring substudy were used to show that recurrence of ST segment shift of ≥ 0.1 mV occurring in 33% of patients was an independent predictor of 30-day (P = 0.0001) and 1-year (P = 0.008) mortality.[104] Clinical evidence of recurrent ischemia, as collected in the overall GUSTO-I population, also related to worse prognosis. Among the 20% of patients who had recurrent ischemia, mortality was higher in the presence of ST-segment changes and substantially higher when accompanied by hemodynamic changes.[105]

In GUSTO-IIa, the prognostic value of troponin-T was shown in a substudy including 855 patients with acute coronary syndromes in 96 North American hospitals.[54] Thirty-six percent of patients had a positive troponin T value (> 0.1 ng/mL) at presentation; their 30-day mortality was significantly higher (11.8%) than that of patients with a negative value (3.9%). In a multivariable model, troponin T was a more important predictor than creatine kinase-MB or ST-segment changes on the baseline ECG.

International and Regional Geographic Differences.

Marked regional and international heterogeneity in medical care has provided the opportunity to examine important regional differences in medical care and in outcomes in the GUSTO trials. As expected, high technological procedures were used more commonly in the United States than in other areas of the world. Patients in the United States were more likely to undergo angiography, angioplasty, bypass surgery, and right heart catheterization. These differences were associated with a measurable, but small, improvement in survival, with a 6.8% 30-day mortality in the United States versus 7.2% elsewhere (P = 0.047).[52]

A prospective substudy comparing medical care, resource use, quality of life, and outcomes in the United States and Canada was performed using a randomly selected population.[16] Patients in the United States had twice as many procedures, more specialty care, and shorter hospital stays. Canadian patients had more primary care physician follow-up visits. Measures of quality of life were significantly better for patients in the United States, especially less limiting angina. Again, there was a small but measurable survival advantage for patients from the United States.

Important differences in medical care were also measured within different regions of the United States.[106] In the Northeast, patients were much more likely to be treated according to published guidelines based on the results of randomized clinical trials, and they were much less likely to undergo angiography and revascularization. The use of angiography was generally related to its availability, except for the Northeast, where the use was less than expected based on availability.

To better understand what determines whether catheterization and revascularization will be performed in the United States, a model was developed to determine which factors lead to their use.[59] In spite of national guidelines and randomized trial data indicating that recurrent ischemia and left ventricular dysfunction should be the major criteria for revascularization,[107] the predominant factor was age, with 76% of patients under age 73 undergoing angiography versus 53% of patients over age 73. The second most important factor was whether the hospital had catheterization facilities, and the third most important factor was recurrent ischemia. Unfortunately, patients with most to gain from an aggressive approach, those in cardiogenic shock, had a lower rate of catheterization than did patients who were hemodynamically stable.

Cost-effectiveness.

A critical piece of the GUSTO-I trial was the cost-effectiveness analysis, which enabled physicians, health care systems, or societies to determine whether the substantially higher cost of alteplase was worthwhile relative to other resource demands in medical care.[108] Detailed resource use and hospital cost data were collected from randomly selected patients in the United States. At 1 year, patients treated with alteplase had higher costs and higher survival (by 1.1 %) than patients treated with streptokinase. On the basis of projected average life expectancy of 14 years based on database information after acute myocardial infarction, the incremental cost per year of life saved was $32,678. This estimate was sensitive to changes in life expectancy, but it was relatively insensitive to changes in costs of disabling stroke. The cost is quite favorable compared with benchmarks of what society considers to be cost-effective, such as hemodialysis that costs about $50,000 per year to keep a patient alive. By explicitly measuring cost-effectiveness, the GUSTO-I trial set a standard against which other incrementally beneficial therapies in acute coronary syndromes will be compared.

The GUSTO-IIb direct angioplasty substudy also included a prospective cost-effectiveness analysis. At 6 months, the costs of alteplase and of primary angioplasty were very similar.[109]

The Future

The original GUSTO organization, which has now adopted the name VIGOUR (Virtual Coordinating Center for Global Collaborative Cardiovascular Research), is currently involved in several large trials of acute coronary syndromes. The GUSTO-IV trial (preceded by its pilot trial, SPEED) will evaluate abciximab in acute coronary syndromes, SYMPHONY (sibrafiban versus aspirin to yield maximum protection from ischemic heart events post acute coronary syndromes) is studying the oral platelet glycoprotein IIb/IIIa receptor antagonist sibrafiban in acute coronary syndromes without ST elevation, ASSENT-2 (Assessment of the Safety and Efficacy of a New Thrombolytic agent) is comparing the novel thrombolytic agent TNK-tPA to accelerated alteplase, and HERO-2 is comparing hirulog versus heparin in addition to streptokinase for acute myocardial infarction.

We are in an era during which the number of promising therapeutic agents is growing exponentially based on molecular engineering and an enhanced understanding of the genetic basis of disease. Rapidly determining which of these potential therapies will most improve patient care is going to require increasingly efficient and effective approaches. The GUSTO organization has shown that an alliance between industry and practitioners, organized by a group of representative leaders in cardiology and clinical trials, can achieve this goal while providing added insight into major issues concerning the treatment of the disease being studied.

References

1. Topol EJ, Armstrong P, Van de Werf F, et al. Confronting the issues of patient safety and investigator conflict of interest in an international clinical trial of myocardial infarction. JACC 1992;19: 1123-1128.
2. Topol EJ, Califf RM, Van de Werf F, et al. Perspectives on large scale cardiovascular clinical trials for the new millennium. Circulation 1997;95:1072-1082.
3. Gruppo Italiano per lo Studio della Sopravvivenza nell'Infarto Miocardico. GISSI-2: A factorial randomised trial of alteplase versus streptokinase and heparin versus no heparin among 12 490 patients with acute myocardial infarction. Lancet 1990;336:65-71.
4. Third International Study of Infarct Survival Study Group. ISIS-3: A randomised comparison of streptokinase vs tissue plasminogen activator vs anistreplase and of aspirin plus heparin vs aspirin alone among 41 299 cases of suspected acute myocardial infarction. Lancet 1992;339:753-770.
5. Granger CB, Califf RM, Topol EJ. Thrombolytic therapy for acute myocardial infarction. A review. Drugs 1992; 44:293-325.
6. Hsia J, Hamilton WP, Kleiman N, et al. A comparison between heparin and low-dose aspirin as adjunctive therapy with tissue plasminogen activator for acute myocardial infarction. N Engl J Med 1990;323:1433-1437.
7. Bleich SD, Nichols TC, Schumacher RR, et al. Effect of heparin on coronary arterial patency after thrombolysis with tissue plasminogen activator in acute myocardial infarction. Am J Cardiol 1990;66:1412-1417.
8. Neuhaus KL, Feuerer W, Jeep-Tebbe S, et al. Improved thrombolysis with a modified dose regimen of recombinant tissue-type plasminogen activator. JACC 1989;14: 1566-1569.
9. Neuhaus KL, von Essen R, Tebbe U, et al. Improved thrombolysis in acute myocardial infarction with front-loaded administration of alteplase: Results of the rtPA-APSAC patency study (TAPS). JACC 1992;19:885-891.
10. Carney RJ, Murphy GA, Brandt TR, et al. Randomized angiographic trial of recombinant tissue-type plasminogen activator (alteplase) in myocardial infarction. RAAMI Study Investigators. JACC 1992;20:17-23.
11. Califf RM, Topol EJ, Stack RS, et al. Evaluation of combination thrombolytic therapy and timing of cardiac catheterization in acute myocardial infarction. Results of thrombolysis and angioplasty in myocardial infarction-phase 5 randomized trial. TAMI Study Group. Circulation 1991; 83:1543-1556.
12. Grines CL, Nissen SE, Booth DC, et al. A prospective, randomized trial comparing combination half-dose tissue-type plasminogen activator and streptokinase with full-dose tissue-type plasminogen activator. Kentucky Acute Myocardial Infarction Trial (KAMIT) Group. Circulation 1991; 84: 540-549.
13. The GUSTO Investigators. An international randomized trial comparing four thrombolytic strategies for acute myocardial infarction. N Engl J Med 1993;329:673-682.
14. Califf RM, White HD, Van de Werf F, et al. One-year results from the Global Utilization of Streptokinase and TPA for Occluded Coronary Arteries (GUSTO-I) Trial. Circulation 1996;94: 1233-1238.
15. Gore JM, Granger CB, Sloan MA, et al. Stroke after thrombolysis: Mortality and functional outcomes in the GUSTO-I trial. Circulation 1995;92: 2811-2818.
16. Mark DB, Naylor CD, Hlatky MA, et al. Use of medical resources and quality of life after acute myocardial infarction in Canada and the United States. N Engl J Med 1994; 331:1130-1135.
17. Ridker PM, O'Donnell C, Marder VJ, et al. Large-scale trials of thrombolytic therapy for acute myocardial infarction: GISSI-2, ISIS-3, and GUSTO1. Ann Intern Med 1993; 119:530-532.
18. Sleight P. Thrombolysis after GUSTO: A European perspective. J Myocard Ischemia 1993;5:25-30.
19. Califf RM, Woodlief LH, Harrell FE Jr, et al. Selection of thrombolytic therapy for individual patients: Development of a clinical model. Am Heart J 1997;133:630-639.
20. The GUSTO Angiographic Investigators. The effects of tissue plasminogen activator, streptokinase, or both

on coronary-artery patency, ventricular function, and survival after acute myocardial infarction. N Engl J Med 1993;329: 1615-1622.

21. Karagounis L, Sorensen SG, Merlove RL, et al., for the TEAM-2 Investigators. Does Thrombolysis In Myocardial Infarction (TIMI) perfusion grade II represent a mostly patent artery or a mostly occluded artery? Enzymatic and electrocardiographic evidence from the TEAM-2 study. JACC 1992;19:1-10.

22. Vogt A, von Essen R, Tebbe U, et al. Impact of early perfusion status of the infarct-related artery on short-term mortality after thrombolysis for acute myocardial infarction: Retrospective analysis of four German multicenter studies. JACC 1993;21:1391-1395.

23. Simes RJ, Topol EJ, Holmes DRJ, et al. Link between the angiographic substudy and mortality outcomes in a large randomized trial of myocardial reperfusion: Importance of early and complete infarct artery reperfusion. Circulation 1995;91:1923-1928.

24. Ross AM, Coyne KS, Moreyra E, et al. Extended mortality benefit of early postinfarction reperfusion. Circulation 1998;97:1549-1556.

25. Migrino RQ, Young JB, Ellis SG, et al. End-systolic volume index at 90 to 180 minutes into reperfusion therapy for acute myocardial infarction is a strong predictor of early and late mortality. Circulation 1997;96:116-121.

26. Granger CB, Hirsh J, Califf RM, et al. Activated partial thromboplastin time and outcome after thrombolytic therapy for acute myocardial infarction: Results from the GUSTO-I trial. Circulation 1996;93:870-878.

27. Granger CB, Becker R, Tracy RP, et al. Thrombin generation, inhibition and clinical outcomes in patients with acute myocardial infarction treated with thrombolytic therapy and heparin: Results from the GUSTO-I trial. JACC 1998; 31:497-505.

28. Topol EJ, Fuster V, Harrington RA, et al. Recombinant hirudin for unstable angina pectoris: A multicenter, randomized angiographic trial. Circulation 1994;89:1557-1566.

29. Cannon CP, McCabe CH, Henry TD, et al. A pilot trial of recombinant desulfatohirudin compared with heparin in conjunction with tissue-type plasminogen activator and aspirin for acute myocardial infarction: Results of the Thrombolysis In Myocardial Infarction (TIMI) 5 trial. JACC 1994;23: 993-1003.

30. Antman EM, for the TIMI 9A Investigators. Hirudin in acute myocardial infarction: Safety report from the Thrombolysis and thrombin inhibition In Myocardial Infarction (TIMI) 9A trial. Circulation 1994;90:1624-1630.

31. Neuhaus KL, vonEssen R, Tebbe U, et al. Safety observations from the pilot phase of the randomized r-Hirudin for Improvement of Thrombolysis (HIT-111) study: A study of the Arbeitsgemeinschaft Leitender Kardiologischer Krankenhausarzte (ALKK). Circulation 1994;90:1638-1642.

32. The Global Use of Strategies to Open Occluded Coronary Arteries (GUSTO) IIa Investigators. Randomized trial of intravenous heparin versus recombinant hirudin for acute coronary syndromes. Circulation 1994;90:1631-1637.

33. The Global Use of Strategies to Open Occluded Coronary Arteries (GUSTO) IIb Investigators. A comparison of recombinant hirudin with heparin for the treatment of acute coronary syndromes. N Engl J Med 1996;335:775-782.

34. Antman EM. Hirudin in acute myocardial infarction. Thrombolysis and thrombin inhibition in myocardial infarction (TIMI) 9B trial. Circulation 1996;94:911-921.

35. Simes RJ, Granger CB, Antman EM, et al. Impact of hirudin versus heparin on mortality and (re)infarction in patients with acute coronary syndromes: A prospective meta-analysis of the GUSTO-IIb and TIMI 9b trials. (abstract) Circulation 1996;94:1-430.

36. Granger CB, Van de Werf F, Armstrong PW, et al. Hirudin reduces death and myocardial (re)infarction at 6-months: Follow-up results of the GUSTO-IIb trial. (abstract) JACC 1998;31:79A.

37. Metz BK, Granger CB, White HD, et al. Streptokinase and hirudin reduces death and reinfarction in acute myocardial infarction compared with streptokinase and heparin: Results from Gusto IIb. (abstract) Circulation 1996;94(Suppl 1):I430.

38. White HD, Aylward PE, Frey MJ, et al.

Randomized, double-blind comparison of hirulog versus heparin in patients receiving streptokinase and aspirin for acute myocardial infarction (HERO). Circulation 1997;96:2155-2161.

39. Grines CL, Browne KF, Marco J, et al. A comparison of immediate angioplasty with thrombolytic therapy for acute myocardial infarction. The Primary Angioplasty in Myocardial Infarction Study Group. N Engl J Med 1993;328:673-679.

40. Zijlstra F, de Boer MJ, Hoorntje JC, et al. A comparison of immediate coronary angioplasty with intravenous streptokinase in acute myocardial infarction. N Engl J Med 1993;328:680-684.

41. Gibbons RJ, Holmes DR, Reeder GS, et al. Immediate angioplasty compared with the administration of a thrombolytic agent followed by conservative treatment for myocardial infarction. The Mayo Coronary Care Unit and Catheterization Laboratory Groups. N Engl J Med 1993;328:685-691.

42. Weaver WD, Simes RJ, Betriu A, et al. Comparison of primary coronary angioplasty and intravenous thrombolytic therapy for acute myocardial infarction-A quantitative review. JAMA 1997;278:2093-2098.

43. Jollis JG, Peterson ED, Nelson CL, et al. Relationship between physician and hospital coronary angioplasty volume and outcome in elderly patients. Circulation 1997;95: 2485-2491.

44. The Global Use of Strategies to Open Occluded Coronary Arteries in Acute Coronary Syndromes (GUSTO IIb) Angioplasty Substudy Investigators. A clinical trial comparing primary coronary angioplasty with tissue plasminogen activator for acute myocardial infarction [erratum published N Engl J Med 1997;337:287]. N Engl J Med 1997;336:1621-1628.

45. Granger CB, Betriu A, Phillips HR, et al. Nearly half of early benefit of direct angioplasty lost in longer-term follow-up: 6-month results from the GUSTO-IIb direct angioplasty substudy. (abstract) Circulation 1997;96:I-205.

46. Granger CB, Phillips HR, Betriu A, et al. Direct angioplasty may be less advantageous in patients presenting early after symptom onset: Results from GUSTO IIb. (abstract) JACC 1997;29(Suppl A):366A.

47. Smalling RW, Bode C, Kalbfleisch J, et al. More rapid, complete, and stable coronary thrombolysis with bolus administration of reteplase compared with alteplase infusion in acute myocardial infarction. Circulation 1995; 91:2725-2732.

48. Bode C, Smalling RW, Berg G, et al. Randomized comparison of coronary thrombolysis achieved with double-bolus reteplase (recombinant plasminogen activator) and front-loaded, accelerated alteplase (recombinant tissue plasminogen activator) in patients with acute myocardial infarction. Circulation 1996;94:891-898.

49. International Joint Efficacy Comparison of Thrombolytics. Randomised, double-blind comparison of reteplase double-bolus administration with streptokinase in acute myocardial infarction (INJECT): Trial to investigate equivalence. Lancet 1995;346:329-336.

50. Wilcox RG. Clinical trials in thrombolytic therapy: What do they tell us? INJECT 6-month outcomes data. Am J Cardiol 1996;78(Suppl 12A):20-23.

51. The Global Use of Strategies to Open Occluded Coronary Arteries (GUSTO 111) Investigators. A comparison of reteplase with alteplase for acute myocardial infarction. N Engl J Med 1997;337:1118-1123.

52. Lee KL, Woodlief LH, Topol EJ, et al. Predictors of 30-day mortality in the era of reperfusion for acute myocardial infarction: Results from an international trial of 41,021 patients. Circulation 1995;91:1659-1668.

53. Woodlief LH, Lee KL, Califf RM, for the GUSTO IIa Investigators. Validation of a mortality model in 1384 patients with acute myocardial infarction. (abstract) Circulation 1995; 92(Suppl I):I-776.

54. Ohman EM, Armstrong PW, Christenson RH, et al. Cardiac troponin T levels for risk stratification in acute myocardial ischemia. N Engl J Med 1996;335:1333-1341.

55. Christenson RH, Duh S-H, Newby LK, et al. Cardiac troponin T and cardiac troponin 1: Relative values in short-term risk stratification of patients with acute coronary syndromes. Clin Chem 1998;44:494-501.

56. Hathaway WR, Peterson ED, Wagner GS, et al. Prognostic significance of the initial electrocardiogram in patients with acute myocardial infarction. JAMA 1998;279: 387-391.

57. Pilote L, Ohman M, Miller DP, et al., GUSTO-I Investigators. Ischemia after thrombolysis is frequent, somewhat predictable, and pre-empted by early angiography. (abstract) JACC 1996;28:249A.

58. Berkowitz SD, Granger CB, Pieper KS, et al. Incidence and predictors of bleeding after contemporary thrombolytic therapy for myocardial infarction. Circulation 1997;95: 2508-2516.

59. Pilote L, Miller DP, Califf RM, et al. Determinants of the use of coronary angiography and revascularization after thrombolysis for acute myocardial infarction. N Engl J Med 1996;335: 1198-1205.

60. Holmes DR Jr, Bates ER, Kleiman NS, et al. Contemporary reperfusion therapy for cardiogenic shock: The GUSTO-I trial experience. JACC 1995; 26:668-674.

61. Holmes DR, Berger PB, Bates E, et al. Predictors of mortality in cardiogenic shock: The GUSTO experience. (abstract) JACC 1995;25:86A.

62. Sloan MA, Sila CA, Mahaffey KW, et al. Prediction of 30-day mortality among patients with thrombolysis-related intracranial hemorrhage. Circulation 1998;(In Press).

63. Tsang TSM, Califf RM, Stebbins AL, et al. Incidence and impact on outcome of streptokinase allergy in the GUSTO-I trial. Am J Cardiol 1997;79: 1232-1235.

64. Klootwijk P, Langer A, Meij S, et al. Non-invasive prediction of reperfusion and coronary artery patency by continuous ST segment monitoring in the GUSTO-I trial. Eur Heart J 1996;17: 689-698.

65. Langer A, Krucoff MW, Klootwijk P, et al. Noninvasive assessment of speed and stability of infarct-related artery reperfusion: Results of the GUSTO ST segment monitoring study. JACC 1995;25:1552-1557.

66. Sgarbossa EB, Pinski SL, Gates K, et al. Predictors of in-hospital bundle branch block reversion after presenting with acute myocardial infarction and bundle branch block. Am J Cardiol 1998;(In Press).

67. Simoons ML, Maggioni AP, Knatterud G, et al. Individual risk assessment for intracranial hemorrhage during thrombolytic therapy. Lancet 1993; 342:1523-1528.

68. Gebel JM, Sila CA, Sloan MA, et al. Thrombolysis-related intracranial hemorrhage radiographic analysis of 244 cases from the GUSTO-I trial with clinical correlation. Stroke 1998;29: 563-569.

69. Mahaffey KW, Granger CB, Sloan MA, et al. Risk factors for in-hospital nonhemorrhagic stroke in patients with acute myocardial infarction treated with thrombolysis. Results from GUSTO-I. Circulation 1998;97:757-764.

70. Califf RM, Topol EJ, George BS, et al. Hemorrhagic complications associated with the use of intravenous tissue plasminogen activator in treatment of acute myocardial infarction. Am J Med 1988;85:353-359.

71. Bovill EG, Terrin ML, Stump DC, et al. Hemorrhagic events during therapy with recombinant tissue-type plasminogen activator, heparin, and aspirin for acute myocardial infarction. Ann Intern Med 1991;115:256-265.

72. Sane DC, Califf RM, Topol EJ, et al. Bleeding during thrombolytic therapy for acute myocardial infarction: Mechanisms and management. Ann Intern Med 1989;111:1010-1022.

73. Katz A, Cohn G, Mashal A, et al. Thrombolytic therapy for acute myocardial infarction in a 110-year old man. Am J Cardiol 1993;71:1122-1123.

74. Lesnefsky EJ, Lundergan CF, Hodgson JM, et al. Increased left ventricular dysfunction in elderly patients despite successful thrombolysis: The GUSTO-I angiographic experience. JACC 1996;28:331-337.

75. White HD, Barbash GI, Califf RM, et al. Age and outcome with contemporary thrombolytic therapy: Results from the GUSTO-I trial. Circulation 1996;94:1826-1833.

76. Fibrinolytic Therapy Trialists' (FTT) Collaborative Group. Indications for fibrinolytic therapy in suspected acute myocardial infarction: Collaborative overview of early mortality and major morbidity results from all randomised trials of more than 1000 patients. Lancet 1994;343:311-322.

77. Weaver WD, White HID, Wilcox RG, et al. Comparisons of characteristics and outcomes among women and men with acute myocardial infarction treated with thrombolytic therapy. JAMA 1996;275:777-782.

78. Moen EK, Asher CR, Miller DIP, et al. Long-term follow-up of gender-specific outcomes after thrombolytic therapy for acute myocardial infarction from the GUSTO-I trial. J Womens Health 1997;6:285-293.

79. Barbash GI, Reiner J, White HID, et al. Evaluation of the paradoxical beneficial, effects of smoking in patients receiving thrombolytic therapy for acute myocardial infarction: Mechanism of the "smoker's paradox" from the GUSTO-I trial, with angiographic insights. JACC 1995;26:1222-1229.

80. Karnash SL, Granger CB, White HD, et al. Treating menstruating women with thrombolytic therapy: Insights from the Global Utilization of Streptokinase and Tissue Plasminogen Activator for Occluded Coronary Arteries (GUSTO-I) trial. JACC 1995;26:1651-1656.

81. Aylward PE, Wilcox RG, Horgan JH, et al. Relation of increased arterial blood pressure to mortality and stroke in the context of contemporary thrombolytic therapy for acute myocardial infarction. Ann Intern Med 1996;125:891-900.

82. Woodfield SL, Lundergan CF, Reiner JS, et al. Angiographic findings and outcome in diabetic patients treated with thrombolytic therapy for acute myocardial infarction: The GUSTO-I experience. JACC 1996;28:1661-1669.

83. Mak KH, Moliterno DJ, Granger CB, et al. Influence of diabetes mellitus on clinical outcome in the thrombolytic era of acute myocardial infarction. JACC 1997;30:171-179.

84. Mahaffey KW, Granger CB, Toth CA, et al. Diabetic retinopathy should not be a contraindication to thrombolytic therapy for acute myocardial infarction: Review of ocular hemorrhage incidence and location in the GUSTO-I trial. JACC 1997;30:1606-1610.

85. Newby LK, Rutsch WR, Califf RM, et al. Time from symptom onset to treatment and outcomes after thrombolytic therapy. JACC 1996;27:1646-1655.

86. Sgarbossa EB, Pinski SL, Topol EJ, et al. Acute myocardial infarction and complete bundle branch block at hospital admission: Clinical characteristics and outcome in the thrombolytic era. JACC 1998;31:105-110.

87. Peterson ED, Hathaway WR, Zabel KM, et al. Prognostic significance of precordial ST depression during inferior myocardial infarction in the thrombolytic era: Results in 16,521 patients. JACC 1996;28:305-312.

88. Hochrein J, Sun F, Pieper KS, et al. Higher T-wave amplitude associated with better prognosis in patients receiving thrombolytic therapy for acute myocardial infarction (a GUSTO-I substudy). Am J Cardiol 1998;81:1078-1084.

89. Barbagelata A, Califf RM, Sgarbossa EB, et al. Thrombolysis and Q wave versus non-Q wave first acute myocardial infarction: A GUSTO-I substudy. JACC 1997;29:770-777.

90. Goodman SG, Langer A, Ross AM, et al. Non-Q-wave versus Q-wave myocardial infarction after thrombolytic therapy. Angiographic and prognostic insights from the global utilization of streptokinase and tissue plasminogen activator for occluded coronary arteries-I angiographic substudy. Circulation 1998;97:444-450.

91. Crenshaw BS, Ward SR, Granger CB, et al. Atrial fibrillation in the setting of acute myocardial infarction: The GUSTO-I experience. JACC 1997;30:406-413.

92. Labinaz M, Sketch MH, Stebbins AL, et al. Thrombolytic therapy for patients with prior percutaneous transluminal coronary angioplasty and subsequent acute myocardial infarction. Am J Cardiol 1996;78:1338-1344.

93. Brieger DB, Mak K-H, White HD, et al. Benefit of early sustained reperfusion in patients with prior myocardial infarction (The GUSTO-I Trial). Am J Cardiol 1998;81:282-287.

94. The International Study Group. In-hospital mortality and clinical course of 20,891 patients with suspected acute myocardial infarction randomised between alteplase and streptokinase with or without heparin. Lancet 1990;336:71-75.

95. Berger PB, Holmes DR Jr., Stebbins AL, et al. Impact of an aggressive invasive catheterization and revascularization strategy on mortality in patients with cardiogenic shock in the Global Utilization of Streptokinase and Tissue Plasminogen Activator for

Occluded Coronary Arteries (GUSTO-I) Trial: An observational study. Circulation 1997;96:122-127.

96. Holmes DR, Califf RM, Van de Werf F, et al. Difference in countries' use of resources and clinical outcome for patients with cardiogenic shock after myocardial infarction: Results from the GUSTO trial. Lancet 1997;349:75-78.

97. Pfisterer M, Cox JL, Granger CB, et al. Atenolol use and clinical outcomes after thrombolysis for acute myocardial infarction: The GUSTO-I experience. JACC 1998;(In Press).

98. Alexander JH, Granger CB, Thompson TD, et al., GUSTO Coordinating Center DN. Prophylactic lidocaine use in GUSTO-I and GUSTO-II: Incidence and outcomes. (abstract) Circulation 1996;94(Suppl I):I-197.

99. Kleiman NS, White HD, Ohman EM, et al. Mortality within 24 hours of thrombolysis for myocardial infarction: The Importance of early reperfusion. Circulation 1994;90: 2658-2665.

100. Tardiff BE, Califf RM, Morris D, et al. Coronary revascularization surgery after myocardial infarction: Impact of bypass surgery on survival after thrombolysis. JACC 1997;29: 240-249.

101. Baardman T, Hermens WT, Lenderink T, et al. Differential effects of tissue plasminogen activator and streptokinase on infarct size and on rate of enzyme release: Influence of early infarct related artery patency: The GUSTO enzyme substudy. Eur Heart J 1996; 17:237-246.

102. Krucoff MW, Croll MA, Pope JE. et al. Continuous 12-lead ST segment recovery analysis in the TAMI 7 Study: Performance of a noninvasive method for real time detection of failed myocardial reperfusion. Circulation 1993;88:437-446.

103. Schroder R, Dissmann R, Bruggemann T, et al. Extent of early ST segment elevation resolution: A simple but strong predictor of outcome in patients with acute myocardial infarction. JACC 1994;24:384-391.

104. Langer A, Krucoff MW, Klootwijk P, et al. Prognostic significance of ST segment shift early after resolution of ST elevation in patients with myocardial infarction treated with thrombolytic therapy: The GUSTO-I ST segment monitoring substudy. JACC 1998;31: 783-789.

105. Betriu A, Califf RM, Bosch X, et al. Recurrent Ischemia after thrombolysis: Importance of associated clinical findings. JACC 1998;31:94-102.

106. Pilote L, Califf RM, Sapp S, et al. Regional variation across the United States in the management of acute myocardial infarction. N Engl J Med 1995;333:565-572.

107. Ryan TJ, Anderson JL, Antman EM, et al. ACC/AHA guidelines for the management of patients with acute myocardial infarction: A report of the American College of Cardiology/American Heart Association Task Force on practice guidelines (Committee on Management of Acute Myocardial Infarction). JACC 1996;28:1328-1428.

108. Mark DB, Hlatky MA, Califf RM, et al. Cost effectiveness of thrombolytic therapy with tissue plasminogen activator as compared with streptokinase for acute myocardial infarction. N Engl J Med 1995;332:1418-1424.

109. Mark DB, Granger CB, Ellis SG, et al. Costs of direct angioplasty versus thrombolysis for acute myocardial infarction: Results from the GUSTO II randomized trial. (abstract) Circulation 1996;94:I-168.

Chapter 12

Prehospital Thrombolysis in Acute Myocardial Infarction Salvages Myocardium

Mervyn S. Gotsman, M.D., F.R.C.P., FACC,* A. Teddy Weiss, MD, FACC,** Yoseph Rozenman, M.D., FACC, Chaim Lotan, M.D., FACC, Doron Zahger, M.D.. and Morris Mosseri, M.D.

From the Department of Cardiology, Hadassah University Hospital, Jerusalem, Israel

Early thrombolysis can be given at home, by a medical intensive care unit ambulance team, in the emergency room, or in the coronary care unit. Thrombolysis should be given very early (< 2 or 4 hours) and reestablish normal or near normal coronary blood flow. Methods of management include home monitoring of high risk patients with a transtelephonic 12-lead monitor ECG, the management of the patient at home by a trained GP, physician, or medical technician controlled intensive care ambulance team, or a rapid "door to needle" time in the emergency room. Each of these systems requires patient and physician reeducation, to make each group aware of the advantages of early and complete revascularization. An alternative fast track can be provided by immediate percutaneous transluminal coronary angioplasty if the hospital can be prewarned by the physician outside. This article reviews the current published literature and also our experience in 760 patients in Jerusalem. Infarct size, complication rate, and long-term prognosis is related to early complete restoration of coronary blood flow. (J Interven Cardiol 1997;10:315-325)

Introduction

The mortality of acute myocardial infarction (MI) has fallen from 32% in 1966 to 14% after the introduction of intensive coronary care units.[1,2] Our present mortality in the coronary intensive care unit is now 10% for all patients, but less than 2% for patients who undergo thrombolysis for acute MI.[3] Similar improvement has been observed in the CAMI study.[4]

Acute MI is a consequence of rupture of an atheromatous plaque with the generation of acute intramural and intraluminal thrombosis. This may have a sudden or intermittent onset, progressing rapidly or slowly to acute occlusion and may be followed by spontaneous stuttering reperfu-

*David and Rose Orzen Professor of Cardiology; **Aaron and Nettie Zuckerman Professor of Cardiology.

sions.[5-10] Myocardial necrosis is a time dependent process starting in the endocardium after 20 minutes of total occlusion and is largely transmural and complete after 2-4 hours.[11] The extent of myocardial damage in necrosis is related to the volume of myocardium at risk (subtending the occluded vessel and modified by a collateral circulation) but is determined mainly by the integral of the reduction in coronary blood flow and its duration.[12] Thus, proximal disease of the left anterior descending artery causes more damage than occlusion of a small marginal branch of the circumflex artery, but therapeutic improvement is achieved best by very early and complete reperfusion of the infarct related vessel.[13]

It has been shown that in acute impending MI, the time delay from the onset of chest pain until initiation of treatment (or reperfusion) and the degree of reperfusion (TIMI Grade 0-II [poor] vs TIMI Grade III [good reperfusion]) determines the outcome, defined as mortality, infarct size, left ventricular remodeling, and long-term prognosis.[14-19]

The GISSI-I, GUSTO-I, EMIP, GREAT, and our own studies have all shown that earlier reperfusion reduces mortality and infarct size.[15-24] The TEAM[25,26] and GUSTO Angiographic and Direct Angioplasty studies[27-31] have shown that more complete reperfusion also reduces infarct size. There are two important goals of reperfusion in acute MI: early reperfusion and complete reperfusion. This paper will deal with current experience of different techniques of early reperfusion and will comment on methods of complete reperfusion.

Delay to Reperfusion Increases Infarct Size

There are four time delays in reperfusion[14,32-35]: (1) the patient delays in calling for medical care; (2) there is a delay in the provision of medical service; (3) there is a delay in the medical diagnosis, triage, and treatment; or (4) there is a delay until the artery is opened by chemical or mechanical

processes. Patient delay depends on the abruptness of the onset of the ischemic event, the patient's appreciation of the initial symptoms (threshold for pain, shortness of breath, vomiting, faintness, or collapse), his awareness that the symptoms are the first events reflecting an impending infarct, his/her willingness to call and submit to medical care, and the availability of emergency diagnostic and thrombolytic services.[3,16,32]

Patient delay can be shortened by an educational program relating to three different patient populations.[36] One population is *healthy patients* who have no major risks. Education can take place in the school, newspaper, radio, and television, but this requires continuous reinforcement in a well population which is at low risk of developing infarction. A second population is *high risk* patients. Those who have risk factors can also receive guidelines, but this increases their apprehension and over-use of services. The third population, patients with *previous infarction*, requires intensive education. In this group, many patients have stable angina pectoris and they need to appreciate the difference between a simple anginal attack, an unstable syndrome, and impending acute MI.[37]

The US Myocardial Infarction Survey has shown that the average patient delay is 4-6 hours.[38] Compare this to our own patient delay for home thrombolysis of 1.4 hours.[3] Patient education was examined in Seattle by the myocardial infarction and triage (MITI) study; there was a reduction in call time after a community education program, but this had only a small influence on shortening delay.[37]

Examination of delay times in the major studies does not reflect overall patient-medical care behavior in the general population: most controlled double-blind studies have limited inclusion criteria to delay times of < 4 hours, and this of course eliminates patients who present late. It does not represent the real-life situation. Nonetheless, a national educational program using television and the national and regional press to emphasize the importance of early diagnosis and that delay in making diagnosis increases infarct size should continue and teach the normal population and "at risk" subjects that early treatment improves outcome.

Delay in Providing a Medical Service: Practical Methods of Delivering Thrombolytic Therapy and Their Delays

Transtelephonic Monitoring.

This provides very rapid access to medical care. In Israel, high risk patients (after an ischemic episode, an infarct, or arrhythmias), carry a transtelephonic ECG monitor. This records a 1-, 3-, or 12-lead ECG that preserves the recording in microcomputer memory until the patient can transmit the recording by telephone to a central station. The station has the patient's background, history, basic ECG, and personal details on file and these are stored in the central computer. The station is serviced by a 24-hour duty trained nurse or emergency medical technician under medical supervision. The station nurse receives the patient's history and his/her transtelephonic ECG. This is compared to the patient's past history and their previously stored, computerized baseline ECG record. The on-duty staff make a provisional diagnosis and decide whether to reassure the patient, or dispatch an ambulance with an attending physician. The physician in the ambulance arrives within minutes, retakes the history, examines the patient, starts ECG rhythm monitoring and records a further 12-lead ECG. Immediate diagnosis and early management, including thrombolysis, can be provided at home until the patient is transferred gently to the duty hospital. The Mobile Intensive Care Unit (MICU) can communicate with the hospital and the patient's physician before transfer. The ECG record can also be transmitted by facsimile to the patient's treating physician or cardiologist.

Communal monitor transmitters can be provided for high risk populations in old age homes, protected housing estates, large businesses, factories, and banks. The duty nurse in the institution has the transtelephonic monitor transmitter and any symptomatic person can use the transmitter to call the central station.

The major drawback is "over call." Many patients are apprehensive and use the service liberally for mild chest discomfort, palpitations, or even other medical problems. The nurse/coordinator dispatches the ambulance whenever there is any doubt about the symptomatology, while the MICU team transfers the patient to the hospital when they are uncertain about diagnosis. The service has an important medico-legal responsibility: it takes legal responsibility for patient care and is liable for misdiagnosis or incorrect management.

The Mobile Intensive Care Unit.

Most major cities have an emergency ambulance system, staffed either by a well-trained medical orderly and sometimes an additional physician (Table 1). This system started in Jerusalem in 1972 and has acquired extensive experience in the management of acute MI and arrhythmias (as well as other major medical emergencies, mass casualties, and car accidents). The mean response time of the Jerusalem ambulance, when available, is 5-10 minutes.[32,33,39,40] The physician and medical orderly, together with an assistant and trained driver, set up intensive care in the patient's home so that the ambulance provides prehospital medical care with all equipment (defibrillators, pacemakers, and monitors) and the appropriate drugs available for diagnosis, resuscitation, and management. The ambulance team has written guidelines for diagnosis and treatment and is trained to manage emergency situations. It is effective in making an early diagnosis of MI, managing

Table 1

The Mobile Intensive Care Unit

The Medical Intensive Care Unit Ambulance

Physician, driver, and two paramedics
Portable ECG machine
Portable patient ECG monitor
Defibrillator
Facilities for treatment and resuscitation
Radio/telephone contact with central station
Transport system

ECG = electrocardiogram.

life-threatening arrhythmias (ventricular fibrillation, complete heart block, or malignant ventricular arrhythmias) and managing shock-like states and acute pulmonary edema. Patients can be intubated and ventilated if needed. Front-line, emergency home therapy is effective and saves lives. The provision of additional home thrombolytic therapy is quite simple since the physician has been trained in the diagnosis of acute infarction, indications for thrombolytic therapy, and in particular the major contraindications (severe hypotension, a bleeding tendency, a recent operation, pericarditis, or a dissecting aneurysm). The public ambulance system has been so successful in Israel that two major companies have started their own private service to supplement transtelephonic monitoring. Nonetheless, the addition of thrombolysis has two further disadvantages. The ambulance team may be uncertain of the diagnosis of impending MI. Many patients, when seen initially, do not have ST segment elevation. In some patients arterial occlusion has a stuttering onset and the pain may disappear and ST segment and T-waves return to normal. Some patients have continuing pain with minimal T-wave changes while others have T-wave changes only; only one-third have unequivocal transmural ischemia with ST segment elevation. In some instances the pain disappears, the patient is left at home, and the pain reoccurrs a few

hours later. This too is important to recognize, as sudden return of chest pain, ST segment elevation, and extensive MI or ischemia may cause sudden death.

The second element is expense: streptokinase costs $200 per injection and tPA costs $1400.

We have shown that prehospital thrombolysis with an effective MICU shortens time delay of thrombolysis significantly. In a cohort of 760 patients, our delay time for prehospital administration of thrombolysis is 1.4 hours, compared to 2.1 hours for hospital therapy. In patients with first anterior MI, home thrombolysis salvaged 50% of myocardium in risk whereas in-hospital thrombolysis salvaged only 25%.[3]

The EMIP Study was a randomized European study of prehospital thrombolysis: half the patients received thrombolysis at home; the other half received heparin only and were given thrombolytic therapy when they arrived in the hospital (Table 2). In this study 5,469 patients were randomized. There was a 13% reduction in overall mortality (9.7% vs 11.1%, $P = 0.08$) and a 16% reduction in cardiac mortality ($P = 0.049$). Their delay times were longer; the mean delay to prehospital thrombolysis was 130 minutes and to in-hospital thrombolysis was 190 minutes. Unfortunately in both groups, treatment was delayed and most of the myocardial damage had already occurred in each group.[22-23]

The MITI study from Seattle had similar results. In Seattle, the ambulance is staffed by paramedics, and although the ECG is transmitted to the central hospital,

Table 2

Indications of Thrombolytic Therapy in Acute Myocardial Infarction

Criteria for Thrombolysis:

Ischemic chest pain < 4 hours
ST-segment elevation in 2 leads > 2 mm
No response to sublingual vasodilators

medico-legal problems still occur. They found that the best result was achieved by warning the emergency room that the patient was about to arrive: this significantly reduced delay time by 40 minutes.[34]

In Rotterdam the ambulance uses an automatic monitor and the service has accumulated extensive practical experience.[35,41] The short- and long-term results of the REPAIR study (repertusion in acute infarction, Rotterdam) has shown a clear short- and long-term advantage of prehospital lytic therapy. They treated 529 patients in the prehospital setting with high dose IV thrombolytic therapy. Time gained for prehospital therapy was 50 minutes. Hospital mortality was 2%, 1-year mortality 3%, and the cumulative mortality until the end of the fifth year was 8%. The long-term outcome was better than a 16%, 5-year mortality in patients treated with alteplase after arriving at the hospital.

The General Practitioner.

The general practitioner has a longer delay time: he or she may be busy in surgery, be asleep at night, off duty, or may not have adequate training or experience, nor sufficient ECG equipment or adequate therapeutic means at their disposal.

The GREAT study was a randomized, double-blind trial undertaken by general practitioners in the rural Grampian region near Aberdeen.[24,42] They were trained to make an initial diagnosis of impending MI and provide immediate thrombolysis. Half the patients were given APSAC at home and the other half on admission to hospital. Prehospital initiation of thrombolytic therapy saved 1 hour (105 vs 240 minutes) and was associated with the halving of the 3-month mortality (from 15.5% to 8%). Besides the reduction in mortality there were fewer cardiac arrests, fewer Q-wave MIs, and improved left ventricular function. GP training improved the speed of physician response, clinical assessment and diagnosis, relief of pain and anxiety, correc-

tion of autonomic disturbances, and arrhythmias and resuscitation. Telephonic transmission of the ECG by the general practitioner to a regional hospital may be the most effective approach in rural areas where the ambulance service is slow or the local hospital is 1-2 hours away from the patient.

Emergency Room.

This is the current practical method. "Door to needle time" in the emergency room is used as a measure of thrombolytic therapeutic delay, but it ignores the important prehospital delay time.[18,43-46] The NHLBI (National Heart, Lung and Blood Institute) has a major project to reduce this interval to less than 1 hour.[46] Delay is caused by emergency room congestion, lack of training or zealousness of emergency room physicians, and sometimes by the need to call a duty cardiologist. The emergency room physicians need to be trained so that chest pain should be regarded an acute emergency that requires an immediate history, ECG record, recognition of ST segment elevation, and prompt triage. This should include comprehensive inclusion and exclusion criteria protocols. Emergency room physicians can and should provide immediate intravenous thrombolytic therapy.

The delay is reduced if the emergency ambulance technician alerts the emergency staff about the arrival of a patient with impending MI and the hospital staff is immediately available to provide prompt intravenous thrombolytic therapy. Nonetheless, GUSTO I showed the clear relationship between treatment delay and mortality (< 1 hour, 5.6%, and > 4hours, 8.6%).[19]

Intensive Coronary Care Unit Management.

This is too late since the triage delays in the home, emergency room, and ICCU are cumulative and occur in series so that each delay further hinders immediate thrombolysis.[34,43,46-48]

Improving the Rate of Reperfusion and Preventing Reocclusion

Pharmacological thrombolysis induces a biochemical cascade in the coronary artery that has its own finite time delay: reopening may take from 15-60 minutes depending on the drug used.

What drugs and ancillary treatment therefore can improve thrombolysis? TIMI-I showed that tPA improved 90-minute reperfusion when compared to streptokinase (31% vs 62%), but the GUSTO angiographic study showed that after 2.5 hours, the reperfusion rate was similar.[27,49] Front-loaded tPA and rPA are more effective in opening the artery earlier than streptokinase, while staphylokinase and TNK are promising alternatives.[50-52]

Platelet inhibiting drugs are complementary ancillary drugs. Aspirin has been shown to be as effective in improving mortality in acute MI as streptokinase (ISIS-II) and the Tel Aviv study showed that aspirin given at home is associated with improved reperfusion by the time the patient reaches the hospital.[53,54] The platelet IIb/IIIa blocking agents and antibodies are also promising since they prevent reocclusion by platelet-rich thrombi. Abciximax is effective in high risk PTCA patients, and theoretically, can be added to home thrombolysis. Its present disadvantage is cost and probably it does not increase the risk of bleeding.[55,56]

Heparin is an important anticoagulant. The HART study showed that intravenous heparin improves mortality in reperfusion. We have given intravenous heparin from the moment the impending infarct is diagnosed, but there is no doubt that heparin increases the number of bleeding episodes.[54] Hirudin a more effective antithrombin agent, has not been shown to have an advantage over heparin.[57]

Bleeding is a continuing hazard, but home thrombolysis does not induce bleeding before the patient comes to the hospital.[3,58,59]

Reperfusion arrhythmias are common, but can be treated comfortably by an ambulance team that has continuous monitoring, antiarrhythmic therapy, and electrical defibrillation available and at hand.[3,60]

Complete Reperfusion

Our studies with early reperfusion in MI showed a wide variation in ventricular function in patients who received thrombolytic therapy with the same time delay after pain onset. There was a subset of patients in whom thrombolysis was ineffective and the artery remained closed, opened partially, or reoccluded after reperfusion (delayed relief of pain, or return of an elevated ST segment to the isoelectric line, and a larger CK): these subsets had a larger infarct.[61]

The TEAM studies and the angiographic subset of the GUSTO study examined blood flow in the culprit coronary artery at angiography 90 minutes after administration of a thrombolytic drug.[25,27] They used the TIMI grade flow to assess the degree of reperfusion. The study showed that grade III flow was essential to preserve myocardium and that TIMI II flow (reduced flow) was no better than TIMI grades I or 0. It is clear that grades I or II represent incomplete reopening of the artery with decreased myocardial perfusion and flow insufficient to protect and salvage myocardium. There is a clear linear relationship between time to TIMI III flow, myocardial preservation, and mortality (patency to survival ratio). Angiographic studies have also shown that severe residual stenosis or a minimal lumen diameter of < 0.7 millimeters represents significant stenosis with reduction in blood flow incomplete reperfusion, persistent severe ischemia, and ongoing necrosis.[62]

We examined residual stenosis in the infarct related artery 7 days after reperfusion therapy. In a group of patients with anterior MI who received thrombolytic therapy after 2 hours, there was no relationship between the degree of residual stenosis and infarct size: all the infarcts were large, indicating that thrombolysis after 2 hours was insufficient to salvage myocardium. In contrast, in patients who underwent reperfusion in less than 2 hours, infarct size was related to residual stenosis. Patients with < 75% stenosis had a small infarct, those with > 75% stenosis a large infarct, and in the intervening zone there was a linear relationship between infarct size and residual coronary artery narrowing. It is clear therefore that the major determinants of infarct size are early reopening and effective reperfusion.[9,10,63-65]

Home thrombolysis always aims at complete, early coronary reperfusion (TIMI Grade III). Earlier, more complete thrombolysis is possible if the thrombus is fresher (with less Factor XIII and clot retraction), the use of more powerful agents (front-loaded tPA or TNK) or adjuvant therapy with antiplatelet drugs (IIb/IIIa antagonists).

The Hadassah Hospital Experience in Jerusalem

We treated 760 patients with early thrombolytic therapy.[3,56] In this group the mean delay for prehospital thrombolysis was 1.4 ± 8 hours and for hospital treatment 2.1 ± 1 hours (Fig. 1). Mortality was 2.1%. Stroke occurred in 0.4% and major bleeding in 1.6%. Major arrhythmias were common but were all treated successfully (ventricular fibrillation in 7%, accelerated ventricular rhythm or ventricular tachycardia in 25%, atrial fibrillation in 9%, and atrial ventricular block in 7.4%).

Coronary angiography was undertaken 7 days after the acute event. Ventricular function was measured by left ventricular angiography. The extent of left ventricular dysfunction was measured as a "dysfunction index."[13] Smaller infarcts (or more myocardial salvage) were related to the site of arterial obstruction (inferior infarction < anterior infarction, prehospital rather than in-hospital thrombolysis, patients treated in < 2 hours after pain onset, and patients in whom the total duration of pain was < 4 hours) (Figs. 2-4). There was a clear relationship between the duration of pain and infarct size, provided the artery had been opened and Grade III TIMI flow restored. We concluded that time was of the essence. Every minute of delay in applying thrombolytic therapy increased infarct size. The artery had to open as early, and as nearly completely, as possible.[3,10,13,15,19,65]

Reocclusion of the Infarct Related Coronary Artery

The Aachen Group studied patients with impending MI sequentially: immediately after intracoronary thrombolysis, followed by second angiography after 24 hours, and then a third angiogram 1-2 years after the acute event.[66] The initial occlusion rate was 8.5% and the reocclusion rate 13.4%. In our own series of patients studied 3 months after the acute event, 20% of the arteries had reoccluded. This was often silent and occurred in arteries with more

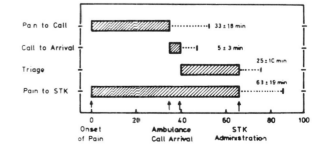

Figure 1. Time delay in the management of prehospital thrombolysis (reproduced with permission from Chest).

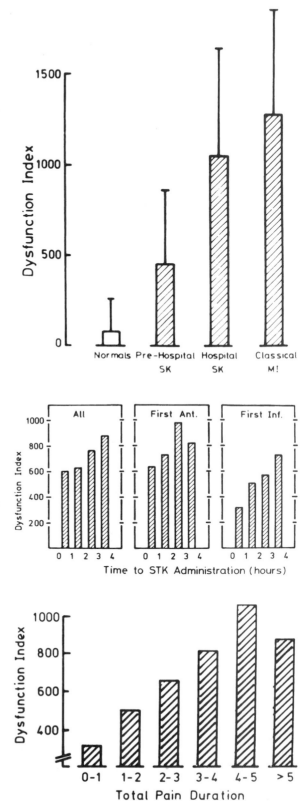

Figure 2. Myocardial dysfunction according to site of administration of thrombolytic therapy. This includes the patients with first anterior myocardial infarction only. The normal dysfunction index is 0 and that of an established anterior infarction 1200. Note how hospital treatment (time delay from onset of pain to treatment 2.1 hours) saves 30% of myocardium at risk, whereas prehospital therapy (mean delay 1.4 hours) saves 66%.

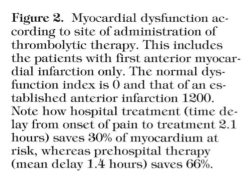

Figure 3. Relationship between time delay to thrombolytic therapy administration and infarct size. The anterior infarct are bigger than inferior infarcts and infarct size increases progressively with time delay. Maximal salvage occurs in the first 2 hours after the onset of pain.

Figure 4. Relationship between total pain duration (hours) and infarct size (dysfunction index). Total pain duration of greater than 4 hours is associated with a large infarct.

severe obstruction.[40] The APRICOT and RAPID I and II angiographic studies showed that in-hospital reocclusion rates range from 2.9-9% depending upon the type of drug given. If thrombolytic therapy is given early and more myocardium preserved, then it is more important to prevent reocclusion.[67,68] The IIb/IIIa antagonists and other antiplatelet drugs should prevent this process.

Arterial patency is best monitored by dynamic continuous ECG recording. Arterial reperfusion is not a sudden event due to prompt dissolution of the clot. There is gradual dissolution, usually with a stuttering course, minor reperfusion and then reocclusion, followed by reperfusion and finally patency. It is essential to monitor blood flow in the infarct related coronary artery and the state of the ischemic myocardium. This can be judged by the degree and extent of ST segment elevation which reflects the status of the myocardial injury or ischemia, although it is not a precise surrogate of TIMI III perfusion. Studies were undertaken by the Aachen Group using a 40-lead anterior chest wall ECG array,[69] but much more simply by Krukoff et al.[70,71] who use a mobile commercial 12-lead ECG package in which ST segment elevation and its return to normal is used as a fingerprint of coronary blood flow and myocardial ischemia. We believe that continuous monitoring of the appropriate ST segments will become everyday practice in addition to continuous arrhythmia monitoring.

The open artery hypothesis implies the early restoration of TIMI Grade III flow; this will restore and preserve myocardial function, improve remodeling, and enhance healing with a better long-term prognosis.[72,73]

Direct Percutaneous Transluminal Coronary Angioplasty (PTCA)

PTCA is an effective alternative to chemical lysis and several studies have shown that mortality, infarct size, reocclu-sion rates, and bleeding complications are reduced. The procedure is invasive and requires a catheterization theater available 24 hours a day with immediate on-call staff and experienced operators: however, the required facilities are not always available in some large hospitals, while others do not have a cardiac interventional unit.[28-31]

In the ideal mileau for direct PTCA, the patient with impending infarction is given aspirin at home and the ECG is transmitted by telephone or radio from the ambulance to a receiving hospital. Triage is then continued during transport to the hospital and the patient is taken directly to an available, vacant catheterization theater staffed by an experienced interventional team. It bypasses the emergency room or ICCU. This should reduce the delay time to under 1 hour. The results of PTCA are excellent, and additional thrombolysis is probably unnecessary: the thrombolytic drugs increase the risk of bleeding and may up-regulate the thrombotic cascade. There is the need for a carefully controlled double-blinded study to compare direct PTCA to prehospital thrombolytic therapy.

Late PTCA After Home Thrombolysis

Salvage PTCA was undertaken in eight of our patients because of prolonged unresponsive pain and persistent ST segment elevation. Two patients had progressive cardiogenic shock. All the patients except one had severe multiple vessel disease.

Elective PTCA after lytic therapy rarely lyses the entire thrombus, nor does it affect the underlying ruptured plaque. Most patients have a critical residual stenosis in the infarct related coronary artery. They underwent coronary angiography 7 days after the acute event and it was found that 70% of patients had > 70% residual stenosis in the infarct related coronary artery. We routinely undertook PTCA, although this is at variance with the results of the TIMI IIb study showing that PTCA altered the long-term prognosis only in patients with residual clinical or exercise induced ischemia.[74] We do not have any long-term comparative data to show that the interventional algorithm altered mortality or improved left ventricular remodeling since there was no control group, but all the patients had a patent artery. When the patients were restudied several years later after they returned with a ruptured plaque in another artery, restenosis of the initial lesion occurred in less than 15%.

Setting Up a Home Thrombolysis Program

Most cities have an emergency ambulance system to deal with major medical crises and mass catastrophes. The ambulance is equipped with an ECG recorder, a continuous ECG monitor, intravenous therapy and resuscitation equipment, defibrillators, and external pacemakers. The paramedic staff are trained to diagnose acute MI and manage arrhythmias such as ventricular fibrillation, complete heart block, cardiogenic shock, and initiate resuscitation (intravenous infusions and intubation). In many cities, particularly in Europe, the service has a trained flying squad emergency physician. This physician can be trained to understand the clinical syndrome of acute MI, interpret the ECG, know when and how to administer thrombolytic therapy, its indications and contraindications, and be aware of its complications. In these circumstances prehospital thrombolytic care is relatively simple.

Where an ambulance physician is unavailable, paramedics can be supplied with an automatic ECG recorder which is capable of interpretating the ECG tracing, and also a transtelephonic or radio device to transmit the ECG to a central station (often the regional hospital) and have available, an interactive medical supervisor to provide instructions about how to manage the patient. Without onsite medical supervision, there remains the medico-legal implications of partially supervised thrombolytic therapy and the possibility of inadvertent administration and its potential complications.

Guidelines for the Management of Patients

Patients with ischemic chest pain for < 4 hours or ST segment elevation in two or more leads of > 2 mm unresponsive to sublingual vasodilators are suitable candidates for thrombolytic therapy.[75] They have impending transmural MI. Contraindications to thrombolytic therapy include acute pericarditis, dissecting aneurysm, severe hypertension (>180/120 mmHg), fluctuating hypo- and hypertension, a history of bleeding (peptic ulcer, stroke, or recent operation during the previous 6 weeks), recent trauma during falling, or major resuscitation. If the patient has clinical or ECG evidence of impending MI and there are no contraindications to lytic therapy, an intravenous line is placed, continuous ST segment and arrhythmia monitoring started and the patient is started with streptokinase, APSAC or front-loaded tPA according to the individual preference. Streptokinase and APSAC can cause allergic manifestations and the patient should be given an initial bolus of 250 cc of intravenous saline, together with half a gram of hydrocortisone. Some centers start heparin immediately with a dose of 500,000 units together with aspirin 500 mg chewed sublingually. Intravenous morphine (3-10 mg) is given to control pain; hypotension, cardiac failure, or pulmonary edema are treated appropriately. The patient is stabilized and can be transferred slowly and gently to the hospital under careful ECG monitoring control, so that any sudden arrhythmias can be managed immediately.

Improving the Availability of Thrombolytic Therapy in Acute MI: The Illusion of Reperfusion

In Israel, 50% of patients receive thrombolytic therapy, but this is much lower in other countries.[76]

Lincoff and Topol have examined the number of patients who receive thrombolysis and the percentage in whom it is successful.[77] They have shown that of subjects who are thrombolyzed, 85% have coronary artery patency at 90 minutes, 75% at 60 minutes, but only 57% have TIMI-Grade III perfusion. Of these, 23% do not have myocardial reperfusion (despite patent coronary arteries), another 34% have intermittent patency, and another 30% of arteries undergo reocclusion, so that only 25% of patients who receive thrombolytic therapy have adequate early reperfusion.

Thus, despite our present theoretical knowledge, extensive clinical experience and the widespread use of thrombolysis effective treatment still has to be brought to more patients with impending MI; it needs to be given earlier and to take advantage of drugs and technologies that can induce TIMI Grade III reperfusion within 2 hours after the onset of chest pain.

Disease

Thrombolysis, and in particular, early and complete restoration of coronary artery patency with good coronary blood flow, has altered the natural history of coronary artery disease. Atheroma accretion is a continuous time dependent process, accelerated by risk factors, but this gradual and inexorable process is punctuated by episodes of acute plaque rupture. The natural history of a patient with coronary artery disease therefore does not follow a progressive linear downhill course, but consists of a series of cliffs or precipices down which the patient falls. Figure 5 shows the progressive nature of the disease and the projected fall in ejection fraction after a first anterior infarct, poor remodeling, after a second inferior infarct, and then further remodeling. Early effective lytic therapy that reopens the coronary artery within 2 hours alters and modulates this process; the improvement or prevention of deterio-

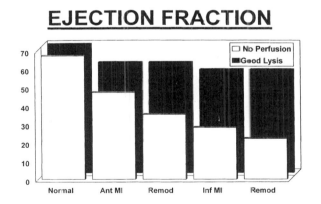

EJECTION FRACTION

Figure 5. Quantum leaps after acute myocardial infarction The theoretical model of "excellent or no reperfusion." In the typical patient with an anterior myocardial infarction and no reperfusion the ejection fraction falls from 66% to 45% and later to 35% due to poor remodeling. After a further inferior infarct, some years later, the ejection fraction falls to 30% and with poor remodeling to 18%. Compare this to the patient who received good early thrombolysis. The final effective ejection fraction after the second infarct was 50%. Effective thrombolysis is important in preserving myocardium and left ventricular function during the first and subsequent infarcts. The final outcome of thrombolysis and its main effect is seen usually after the second or even the third infarct (reproduced with permission from International Journal of Cardiology).

rating ventricular function is shown in Figure 5. Thrombolytic therapy preserves myocardium, improves remodeling and prevents and modifies the electrical instability of the ventricle.

Long-term studies have shown that after the initial improvement in mortality, the survival curves in the thrombolytic and control groups are parallel. Secondary prevention (lipid lowering, management of hypertension, diabetes, and other risk factors) and further prompt thrombolysis in second infarcts is important to modify further the outcome.[78]

Conclusions

Thrombolysis is now routine practice in acute MI.[75] Very early thrombolysis (particularly before hospital admission), complete reopening of the artery, and the prevention of reocclusion both protects and preserves myocardium. Prevention of plaque rupture, patient education, physician training in reperfusion therapy, and the development of new thrombolytic and platelet antagonist drugs will salvage more myocardium, reduce morbidity, and ultimately improve outcome and long-term morbidity and mortality.

References

1. Gotsman MS, Schrire V. Recent myocardial infarction in a teaching hospital: Results without intensive care. S Afr Med J 1967;41:1166-1169.
2. Gotsman MS, Schrire V. Acute myocardial infarction: Results of intensive coronary care. S Afr Med J 1968;42:1223-1230.
3. Rozenman Y, Gotsman MS, Weiss AT, et al. Very early thrombolysis in acute myocardial infarction: A light at the end of the tunnel. Isr J Med Sci 1994;30:99-107.
4. Rouleau JL, Talajic M, Sussex B, et al. Myocardial infarction patients in the 1990s: Their risk factors, stratification and survival in Canada: The Canadian Assessment of Myocardial Infarction (CAMI) Study. J Am Coll Cardiol 1996;27:1119-1127.
5. A report from the Committee on Vascular Lesion of the Council on Arteriosclerosis, American Heart Association. A definition of advanced types of atherosclerotic lesions and a histological classification of atherosclerosis. Circulation 1995;92:1355-1374.
6. Davies MJ, Thomas AC. Plaque fissuring: The cause of acute myocardial infarction, sudden ischaemic death, and crescendo angina. Br Heart J 1985;53:363-373.
7. Falk E. Coronary Thrombosis: Pathogenesis and clinical manifestations. Am J Cardiol 1991;68:288-358.
8. Fuster V. Lewis A. Conner Memorial Lecture. Mechanisms leading to myocardial infarction: Insights from studies of vascular biology. Circulation 1994;90:21-46.
9. Gotsman MS, Rosenheck S, Nassar H, et al. Angiographic findings in the coronary arteries after thrombolysis in acute myocardial infarction. Am J Cardiol 1992;70:715-723.
10. Rozenman Y, Rosenheck S, Nassar H, et al. Acute myocardial infarction: The angiographic picture: New insights into the pathogenesis of myocardial infarction. Int J Cardiol 1995;49:S11-S16.
11. Reimer KA, Lowe JE, Rassmussen MM, et al. The wavefront phenomenon of ischemic cell death: Myocardial infarct size vs. duration of coronary occlusion in dogs. Circulation 1977;56:786-794.
12. Braunwald E, Pfeffer MA. Ventricular enlargement and remodeling following acute myocardial infarction: Mechanisms and management. Am J Cardiol 1991;68:1D-6D.
13. Fine DG, Vinker S, Weiss AT, et al. Influence of vessel involvement and early streptokinase therapy on regional and global left ventricular function in acute myocardial infarction. Herz 1987;12:398-404.
14. Newby LK, Rutsch WR, Califf RM, et al. for the GUSTO-I Investigators. Time from symptom onset to treatment and outcomes after thrombolytic therapy. J Am Coll Cardiol 1996;27:1646-1655.
15. Rozenman Y, Gotsman MS, Weiss AT, et al. Early intravenous thrombolysis in acute myocardial infarction: The Jerusalem experience. Int J Cardiol 1995;49:S21-S28.

16. Gotsman MS, Weiss AT. Immediate reperfusion in acute myocardial infarction. Bibltheca Cardiol 1986;40 30-51.

17. Gotsman MS, Weiss AT, Mosseri M, et al. Prehospital and very early hospital management of acute myocardial infarction by high-dose rapid infusion of streptokinase. In Sleight P, ed. Streptokinase for Acute Myocardial Infarction: Results and Implications of the Major Clinical Studies. Kent England: MCS Consultants, 1989, pp. 25-38.

18. Julian DG. Time as a factor in thrombolytic therapy. Int J Cardiol 1995;49: S17-S19.

19. The GUSTO Investigators. An international randomized trial comparing four thrombolytic strategies for acute myocardial infarction. N Engl J Med 1993; 329:673-682.

20. GISSI. Effectiveness of intravenous thrombolytic treatment in acute myocardial infarction. Lancet 1986;1:397-401.

21. Gotsman MS, Lotan C, Weiss AT, et al. Early and prehospital thrombolytic therapy in acute myocardial infarction. In: Bossaert L, Gotsman MS, eds. Prehospital Thrombolytic Treatment of Acute Myocardial Infarction. Brussels, Belgium: Congress Magazine.

22. The European Myocardial Infarction Project Group. Prehospital thrombolytic therapy in patients with suspected acute myocardial infarction. N Engl J Med 1993;320:383-389.

23. Boissel JP. The European Myocardial Infarction Project: An assessment of prehospital thrombolysis. Int J Cardiol 1995;49:S29-S37.

24. GREAT Group. Feasibility, safety and efficacy of domiciliary thrombolysis by general practitioners: Grampian Region Early Anistreplase Trial. Br Med J 1992;305:548-553.

25. Anderson JL, Karagounis LA, Becker LC, et al. for the TEAM-3 investigators. TIMI perfusion grade 3 but not grade 2 results in improved outcome after thrombolysis for myocardial infarction. Ventriculographic, enzymatic and electrocardiographic evidence from the TEAM-3 study. Circulation 1993;87: 1829-1839.

26. Anderson JL, Karagounis LA, Califf RM. Meta analysis of five reported studies on the relation of early coronary patency grades with mortality and outcomes after acute myocardial infarction. Am J Cardiol 1996;78:1-8.

27. The GUSTO Angiographic Investigators. The effects of tissue plasminogen activator, streptokinase, or both on coronary artery patency, ventricular function, and survival after acute myocardial infarction. N Engl J Med 1993;329:1615-1622.

28. Grines CL, Browne KF, Marco J, et al. A comparison of immediate angioplasty with thrombolytic therapy for acute myocardial infarction. N Engl J Med 1993; 328:673-679.

29. Zijlstra F, deBoer MJ, Hoorntje JCA, et al. A comparison of immediate coronary angioplasty with intravenous streptokinase in acute myocardial infarction. N Engl J Med 1993;328:680-684.

30. Gibbons RJ, Holmes DR, Reeder GS, et al. Immediate angioplasty compared with the administration of a thrombolytic agent followed by conservative treatment for myocardial infarction. N Engl J Med 1993;328:685-691.

31. Every NR, Parsons LS, Mark Hlatky BS, et al. for the Myocardial Infarction Triage and Intervention Investigators. A comparison of thrombolytic therapy with primary coronary angioplasty for acute myocardial infarction. N Engl J Med 1996;335:1253-1317.

32. Weiss AT, Fine DG, Applebaum D, et al. Prehospital coronary thrombolysis: A new strategy in acute myocardial infarction. Chest 1987;92:124-128.

33. Koren G, Weiss AT, Hasin Y, et al. Prevention of myocardial damage in acute myocardial ischemia by early treatment with intravenous streptokinase. N Engl J Med 1985;313:1384-1389.

34. Weaver WD, Eisenberg MS, Martin JS, et al. Myocardial infarction triage and intervention project-Phase I: Patient characteristics and feasibility of prehospital initiation of thrombolytic therapy. J Am Coll Cardiol 1990;15:925-931.

35. Grijseels EWM, Deckers JW, Hoes AW, et al. Prehospital triage of patients with suspected myocardial infarction: Evaluation of previously developed algorithms and new proposals. Eur Heart J 1995;16:325-332.

36. Kereiakes DJ, Weaver WD, Anderson JL, et al. Time delays in the diagnosis and treatment of acute myocardial infarction: A tale of eight cities. Am Heart J 1990;120:773-780.

37. Ho MT, Eisenberg MS, Litwin PE, et al. Delay between onset of chest pain and seeking medical care: The effect of pub-

lic education. Ann Emerg Med 1989;18: 727-731.

38. Rogers WJ, Bowlby LJ, Chandra NC, et al. Treatment of myocardial infarction in the United States (1990 to 1993): Observations from the National Registry of myocardial infarction. Circulation 1994;90:2103-2114.

39. Appelbaum D, Weiss AT, Koren G, et al. Feasibility of prehospital fibrinolytic therapy of acute myocardial infarction by emergency medical services. J Am Emerg Med 1986;4:207-210.

40. Koren G, Luria MH, Weiss AT, et al. Early treatment of acute myocardial infarction with intravenous streptokinase. Arch Intern Med 1987;147:237-240.

41. Grijseels EWM, Bouten MJM, Lenderink T, et al. Prehospital thrombolytic therapy with either alteplase or streptokinase: Practical applications, complications and long-term results in 529 patients. Eur Heart J 1995;16: 1833-1838.

42. Rawles J, on Behalf of the GREAT Group. Halving of mortality at 1 year by domiciliary thrombolysis in the Grampian Region Early Anistreplase Trial (GREAT). J Am Coll Cardiol 1994; 23:1-5.

43. More R, Moore K, Quinn E, et al. Delay times in the administration of thrombolytic therapy: The Brighton experience. Int J Cardiol 1995;49:S39-S46.

44. Coccolini S, Berti G, Bosi S, et al. Prehospital thrombolysis in rural emergency room and subsequent transport to a coronary care unit: Ravenna myocardial infarction (RAMI) trial. Intern J Cardiol 1995;49:S47-S58.

45. Ottesen MM, Kober L, Jorgensen S, et al. on behalf of the TRACE Study Group. Determinants of delay between symptoms and hospital admission in 5978 patients with acute myocardial infarction. Eur Heart J 1996;17:429-437.

46. National Heart, Lung and Blood Institute: Patient/bystander recognition and action: Rapid identification and treatment of acute myocardial infarction. National Heart Attack Alert Program (NHAAP). Bethesda, Md: National Institutes of Heaith: 1993; NIH Publication No. 93-3303.

47. Rozenman Y, Gotsman MS. Selected Topics in the Clinical Sciences: The earliest diagnosis of acute myocardial infarction. Ann Rev Med 1994;44:31-44.

48. Simoons ML, Arnold AE. Tailored thrombolytic therapy. Circulation 1993; 88:2556-2564.

49. Chesebro JH, Knatterud G, Roberts R, et al. Thrombolysis in myocardial infarction (TIMI) Trial, Phase I: A comparison between intravenous tissue plasminogen activator and intravenous streptokinase: Clinical findings through hospital discharge. Circulation 1987;76:142-154.

50. Collen D, Van de Werf F. Coronary thrombolysis with recombinant staphylokinase in patients with evolving myocardial infarction. Circulation 1993; 87:1850-1853.

51. Weaver WD. Results of the RAPID 1 and RAPID 2 thrombolytic trials in acute myocardial infarction. Eur Heart J 1995;17:14-20.

52. Cannon CP, McCabe CH, Gibson M, et al. and the TIMI 10A Investigators. TNK-tissue plasminogen activator in acute myocardial infarction: Results of the Thrombolysis in Myocardial Infarction (TIMI) 1OA Dose-Ranging Trial. Circulation 1997;95:351-356.

53. The International Study Group. In-hospital mortality and clinical course of 20,891 patients with suspected acute myocardial infarction randomized between alteplase and streptokinase with or without heparin. Lancet 1990;336: 71-75.

54. Hsia J, Hamilton WP, Kleiman N, et al. A comparison between heparin and low-dose aspirin as adjunctive therapy with tissue plasminogen activator for acute myocardial infarction. Heparin-Aspirin Reperfusion Trial (HART) Investigators. N Engl J Med 1990;323: 1433-1437.

55. The EPIC Investigators. Prevention of ischemic complications in high-risk angioplasty by a chimeric monoclonal antibody c7E3 Fab fragment directed against the platelet glycoprotein IIb/IIIa receptor. N Engl J Med 1994; 330: 956-961.

56. Tcheng JE. Glycoprotein IIb/IIIa receptor inhibitors: Putting the EPIC, IMPACT II, RESTORE, and EPILOG Trials into perspective. Am J Cardiol 1996;78:35-40.

57. Antman EM. Hirudin in acute myocardial infarction: Safety report from the Thrombolysis and Thrombin Inhibition in Myocardial Infarction (TIMI) 9A Trial. Circulation 1994;90:1624-1630.

58. Fibrinolytic Therapy Trialist's (FTT)

Collaborative Group: Indications for fibrinolytic therapy in suspected acute myocardial infarction: Collaborative overview of early mortality and major morbidity results from all randomized trials of more then 10000 patients. Lancet 1994;343:311-322.

59. De Bono DP, Simoons ML, Tijssen J, et al. for the European Cooperative Study Group. Effect of early intravenous heparin on coronary patency, infarct size and bleeding complications after alteplase thrombolysis: Results of a randomized double blind European Cooperative Study Group trial. Br Heart J 1992;67:122-128.

60. Berger PB, Ruocco NA, Ryan TJ, et al. Incidence and significance of ventricular tachycardia and fibrillation in the absence of hypotension or heart failure in acute myocardial infarction treated with recombinant tissue-type plasminogen activator: Results from the Thrombolysis in Myocardial Infarction (TIMI) Phase II Trial. J Am Coll Cardiol 1993;22:1773-1779.

61. Welber S, Gotsman MS, Sapoznikov D, et al. Left ventricular function after prompt thrombolysis in acute myocardial infarction. In: Sideman S, Beyar R. eds. Simulation and Control of the Cardiac System, Volume II. Boca Raton: CRC Press, Inc., 1985, pp. 43-60.

62. Serruys PW, Arnold AER, Brower RW, et al. Acute coronary reocclusion after thrombolysis with recombinant human tissue-type plasminogen activator: Pevention by a maintenance infusion. Circulation 1986;73:347-351.

63. Zahger D, Gotsman MS. Effect of reperfusion therapy for acute myocardial infarction, ventricular function and heart failure. Heart Failure Reviews 1996;1: 97-104.

64. Zahger D, Gotsman MS. Thrombolysis in the era of the randomized trials. Curr Opinion Cardiol 1995;10:372-380.

65. Gotsman MS, Rozenman Y, Admon D, et al. Changing paradigms in thrombolysis in acute myocardial infarction. Int J Cardiol 1997;59:227-242.

66. Uebis R. How to estimate reocclusion risk? In: Effert S, von Essen R, Hugenholtz PG, Uebis R, Verstraete M. Facts and Hopes in Thrombolysis in Acute Myocardial Infarction, (International Symposium Aachen) Steinkopff Verlag Darmstadt. New York: Springer-Verlag, New York, 1985.

67. Weaver WD. Results of the RAPID I and RAPID 2 thrombolytic trials in acute myocardial infarction. Eur Heart J 1996;17:14-20.

68. Meijer A, Verheugt FWA, van Eenige MJ, et al. Left ventricular function at 3 months after successful thrombolysis: Impact of reocclusion without reinfarction on ejection fraction, regional function, and remodelling. Circulation 1994;90:1706-1714.

69. Von Essen R, Schmidt W, Uebis R, et al. Myocardial infarction and thrombolysis: Electrocardiographic short-term and long-term results using precordial mapping. Br Heart J 1985;54:6-10.

70. Krukoff MW, Croll MA, Pope JE, et al. Continuously updated ST-segment recovery analysis for myocardial infarct artery patency assessment and its correlation with multiple simultaneous early angiographic observations. Am J Cardiol 1993;72:145-151.

71. Kruckoff MW, Croll MA, Pope JE, et al. Continuous 12-lead ST segment recovery analysis: A non-invasive method for real time detection of failed myocardial reperfusion. Circulation 1993;88:437-446.

72. White HD, Cross DB, Elliott JM, et al. Long-term prognostic importance of patency of the infarct-related coronary artery after thrombolytic therapy for acute myocardial infarction. Circulation 1994;89:61-67.

73. Marber MS, Brown DL, Kloner RA. The open artery hypothesis: To open, or not to open, that is the question. Eur Heart J 1996.17:505-509.

74. TIMI Study Group: Comparison of invasive and conservative strategies after treatment with intravenous tissue plasminogen activator in acute myocardial infarction. Results of the Thrombolysis in Myocardial Infarction (TIMI) Phase II Trial. N Engl J Med 1989;320:618-627.

75. Ryan TJ, Anderson JL, Antman EM, et al. and the Task Force Members. ACC/AHA guidelines for the management of patients with acute myocardial infarction: A report of the American College of Cardiology/American Heart Association Task Force on practice guidelines (Committee on Management of Acute Myocardial Infarction). J Am Coll Cardiol 1996;28:1328-1428.

76. Behar S, Abinader E, Caspi A, et al. Frequency of use of thrombolytic ther-

apy in acute myocardial infarction in Israel. Am J Cardiol 1991;58:1291-1294.

77. Lincoff AM, Topol EJ. Illusion of reperfusion. Circulation 1993;88:1361-1374.

78. Randomized trial of cholesterol lowering in 4444 patients with coronary heart disease: The Scandinavian Simvastatin Survival Study (4S). Lancet 1994;344:1383-1389.

Chapter 13

Left Ventricular Function Following Thrombolytic Therapy for Myocardial Infarction

John K. French M.B., FRACP, Ph.D., Thomas A. Hyde, M.B., B.S., BSc, MRCP, and Harvey D. White, M.B., DSc, FRACP, FACC, FESC

From the Cardiology Department, Green Lane Hospital, Auckland, New Zealand

The introduction of thrombolytic therapy to treat eligible patients with acute infarction has markedly reduced deaths from left ventricular (LV) failure. Following reperfusion therapy for acute myocardial infarction (MI), LV function remains the single most significant prognostic factor. Three trials have shown that LV function and survival improved in concert, following randomization to receive thrombolytic therapy. The Global Utilization of Strategies to Open Occluded Coronary Arteries study (GUSTO-I) showed that end-systolic volume at 90 minutes (or 180 minutes) after starting thrombolytic therapy correlates with early thrombolysis in myocardial infarction (TIMI) flow grades as well as survival. *(J Interven Cardiol 1998;11:9-18)*

Introduction

Most patients presenting in the few hours after symptom onset with acute myocardial infarction (MI) have occlusive intracoronary thrombi.[1] Among patients with infarction, those presenting within 12 hours of symptom onset with ST elevation or bundle branch block should be considered thrombolytic-eligible,[2] as they have a mortality benefit following randomization to receive thrombolytic agents.[3] The mechanism of this beneficial therapeutic effect is the early restoration of normal infarct related artery flow, which is associated with preservation of left ventricular (LV) function.[4,5] This article reviews the evidence that relates treatment benefit of thrombolytic therapy to ventricular function.

Ventricular Function after Thrombolytic Therapy

Preservation of LV function occurs after acute MI following randomization to receive streptokinase,[6-10] rt-PA (recombinant tissue plasminogen activator),[11-14] or anistreplase[15,16] (Table 1).

In three trials randomization to receive thrombolytic therapy has also been shown

Table 1. Effect of Administration of Intravenous Thrombolytic Agents on Left Ventricular Function

Study	Number of Patients	% of Eligible Patients	First Infarction	Time to Treatment	Dose	Time of Evaluation	Method	Ejection Fraction	P	Difference (95% Confidence Interval)
Intravenous streptokinase versus placebo										
Schreiber et al.[62]	38	82%	No	< 5 hours	1 MU	Predischarge	Contrast	Streptokinase 47% Control 42%	NS	5% (NA)
ISAM[6]	1741	49%	No	< 6 hours	1.5 MU	1 month	Contrast	Streptokinase 57% Placebo 54%	< 0.005	2.9% (2.8 – 3)
White et al.[9]	172	90%	Yes	< 4 hours	1.5 MU	21 days	Contrast	Streptokinase 59% Placebo 53%	< 0.005	6% (2.8 – 9.3)
Intravenous streptokinase versus control										
Bassand et al.[7]	107	90%	Yes	< 5 hours	1.5 MU	21 days	RVG	Streptokinase 45% Control 44%	NS	1% (– 2.1 – 4.1)
Durand et al.[8]	64	70%	Yes	< 3 hours	1.5 MU	5 weeks	Contrast	Streptokinase 57% Control 49%	< 0.02	8% (1.4 – 15.8)
Kennedy et al.[10]	368	46%	No	< 6 hours	1.5 MU	14 days	RVG	Streptokinase 54% Control 51%	NS	3% (– 0.1 – 6.1)
Anistreplase versus heparin										
Meinertz et al.[15]	313	82%	No	< 4 hours	30 U	2–3 weeks	Contrast	Anistreplase 53% Heparin 54%	NS	1% (– 3.9 – 5.9)
APSAC[16]	231	90%	Yes	< 6 hours	30 U	2–7 days	Contrast	Anistreplase 53% Heparin 47%	0.002	6% (5.9 – 6)
						2–3 weeks	Contrast	Anistreplase 43% Heparin 39%	NS	4% (– 4.6 – 2.6)
rt-PA versus placebo										
Guerci et al.[11]	138	85%	No	< 4 hours	80–100 mg	10 days	RVG	rt-PA 53% Placebo 46%	< 0.02	7% (– 0.1 – 12.1)
National Heart Foundation of Australia[12]	144	72%	No	< 4 hours	100 mg	7 days	Contrast	rt-PA 58% Placebo 52%	0.05	6% (– 0.1 – 12.1)
		72%	Yes					rt-PA 59% Placebo 53%	0.05	6% (– 0.1 – 12.5)
European Cooperative Study[18]	721	79%	No	< 5 hours	rt-PA 100 mg	10–22 days	Contrast	rt-PA 51% Placebo 49%	< 0.05	2% (0.3 – 3.7)
O'Rourke et al.[63]	145	81%	No	< 2.5 hours	100 mg	21 days	Contrast	rt-PA 61% Placebo 54%	< 0.005	7% (2.2 – 11.8)
		88%	No				RVG	rt-PA 52% Placebo 48%	0.08	4% (– 0.6 – 8.6)
Armstrong et al.[14]	115	90%	No	< 4 hours	Duteplase*	4 hours	RVG	rt-PA 49% Placebo 45%	0.02	4% (0.6 – 7.8)
						9 days	RVG	rt-PA 54% Placebo 48%		6% (5.3 – 6.8)
Intravenous rt-PA + heparin versus rt-PA										
TAMI-3[64]	134	NA	No	< 6 hours	rt-PA 90 mg	7 days	Contrast	rt-PT + heparin 49% rt-PA 50%	NS	– 1% (– 4.6 – 2.6)

NA = not available; NS = not significant; rt-PA = recombinant tissue plasminogen activator; RVG = radionuclide ventriculography.

* Weight adjusted 0.4 MU/kg for 1 hour, 0.08–0.14 MU/kg for 1 hour, and 0.03 MU/kg for 4–8 hours.

Table 2. Relationship Between TIMI Flow at 90 Minute and Left Ventricular Function in GUSTO-I

	TIMI 0–2	TIMI 3	P
EF (%)	57	61	< 0.001
ESV (mL)	30	27	< 0.05
Infarct zone wall motion (SD of chords)	− 2.2	− 1.8	< 0.01

ESV = End-systolic volume; EF = ejection fraction; GUSTO = Global Utilization of Strategies to Open Occluded Coronary Arteries; TIMI = thrombolysis in myocardial infarction.

to improve both LV function and survival.[9,17,18] The Interuniversity Study was designed to achieve as high infarct related artery patency rate as possible with the best treatments available in the early 1980s.[19] Randomization of patients to control compared intracoronary streptokinase and/or intravenous streptokinase and/or angioplasty was associated with a 6% reduction in ejection fraction (EF) and an 8% increase in 1-year mortality.[17,19] In our study of 172 patients with first infarctions randomized to receive intravenous streptokinase, EF was 6% higher compared with that in patients randomized to receive placebo, and survival improved (12.5% vs 2.9%, P = 0.02).[9] In the European Cooperative Study Group trial of 721 patients, randomization to receive rt-PA was associated with 2.2% higher EFs and reduced mortality from 5.7% to 2.8% compared to placebo.[18] Finally, the recent RAPID I and II studies[20]-Reteplase Angiographic Phase II International Dose Finding Study and Reteplase Versus Alteplase Patency Investigation During Acute MI Study-which examined TIMI flow 90 minutes after thrombolysis with either r-PA (recombinant plasminogen activator) or accelerated rt-PA, showed that patients with preserved ventricular function had improved survival.

While independently these trials are too small to draw definitive conclusions about mortality benefit, together they show that LV function and survival improve in concert. The significant correlation between LV function and survival (P < 0.01), was confirmed in GUSTO-I (Global Utilization of Strategies to Open Occluded Coronary Arteries) of patients comparing four different thrombolytic regimens, which evaluated LV function angiographically (Table 2).

Timing of Assessment of Left Ventricular Function

Following the onset of occlusion of a coronary artery there is decreased regional systolic contraction in the area of myocardium supplied by the occluded artery. Usually, compensating hyperkinesis of the contralateral wall occurs as a result of increased circulating catecholamines. Thus, global LVEF may be relatively unchanged in the initial days after onset of infarction. Over the next few days the hyperkinesis of the noninfarct zones attenuates, and the EF may then decrease. Assessment of "net" LV impairment at this stage may be overestimated due to myocardial stunning.[21] Over subsequent days and weeks improvement in LV function is variable,[22,23] and reliable assessment of the "net" effect of acute infarction on LV function should be deferred. However, a limitation of this approach is that some patients with poor LV function may die before measurement of LV function can be performed.

End-systolic Volume

Although resting global EF is a very powerful prognostic factor, end-systolic volume has been shown to be an even more important prognostic factor.[24] The effects of thrombolytic therapy on end-systolic volume are summarized in Table 3. The additional prognostic value to EF becomes evident when the EF is reduced to < 50%. Thrombolytic therapy results in smaller end-systolic volumes and affects the healing phase of infarction.[9]

Interestingly, GUSTO-I has reported recently that the relationship between end-systolic volume index and thrombolysis in MI (TIMI)-3 flow 90-180 minutes following the initiation of thrombolytic therapy was shown to be inverse curvilinear (P = 0.006, Fig. 1).[25] Furthermore, an end-systolic volume ≥ 40 mL/m^2 at 90-180 minutes is inde-

pendently predictive of 30-day (odds ratio 3:4 [2-5.8]) and 1-year mortality (odds ratio 3:8 [(1.7-8.3]).

The limitation of LV dilatation following infarction by ACE (angiotensin-converting enzyme) inhibitor therapy has been established,[26-29] and these observations provided the rationale for large clinical trials[30-33] that showed a mortality reduction in patients randomized to receive ACE inhibitor therapy. In a preliminary report[34] we have shown that randomization to ACE inhibition with captopril 2 hours after starting streptokinase has a greater effect on limiting infarct-zone dilatation at 3 weeks, especially when infarct-artery blood flow is abnormal.

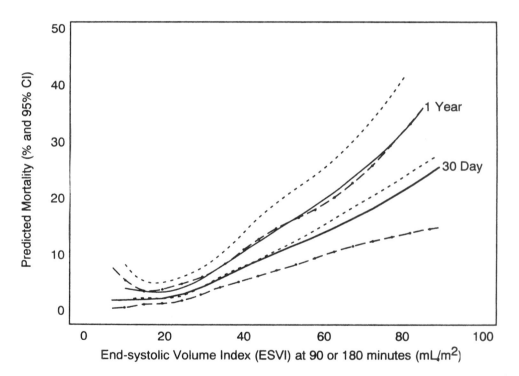

Figure 1. A model of the relationship between ESVI and 30-day and 1-year mortality; 4 df were used for each spline model. This is comparable in terms of df to a predictor variable that is broken into five categories; however, the cubic spline provides a smooth curve describing the possibly nonlinear relationship. For the purpose of these plots, no adjustment was made for covariates. Adjusted odds ratios are described elsewhere in tabular form. The underlying general model for 30-day mortality is logistic regression, whereas Cox regression is used to assess 1-year mortality. Dashed lines indicate 95% CI for 1-year mortality; dotted dashed lines, 95% CI for 30-day mortality. (From Migrino et al. End-systolic volume index at 90 to 180 minutes into reperfusion therapy for acute MI is a strong predictor of early and late mortality. Circulation 1997;96:116-121. Copyright 1997 American Heart Association, reproduced with permission.) CI = confidence interval; df = degrees of freedom; ESVI = end-systolic volume index.

Table 3. Effect of Intravenous Thrombolytic Therapy on End-Systolic Volume

Study	Number of Patients	% of Eligible Patients	First Myocardial Infarction	Time to Treatment	Dose	Time of Evaluation	Method	End-Systolic Volume*	P	Difference (95% Confidence Interval)
Intravenous streptokinase versus placebo										
White et al.[9]	182	85%	Yes	< 4 hours	1.5 MU	21 days	Contrast	Streptokinase 55 mL Placebo 73 mL	< 0.05	− 18 mL (− 36.3 − − 3)
rt-PA versus placebo										
European Cooperative Study Van de Werf et al.[18]	721	78%	No	< 5 hours	rt-PA 100 mg over 3 hours	10–22 days	Contrast	rt-PA 60 mL Placebo 66 mL	NS	− 6 mL (− 10.6 − 1)
Intravenous streptokinase versus rt-PA										
White et al.[65]	270	89%	Yes	< 4 hours	Streptokinae 1.5 MU rt-PA 100 mg over 3 hours	21 days	Contrast	Streptokinase 61 mL rt-PA 66 mL	NS	− 5 mL (− 12.7 − 2.7)
Anistreplase versus rt-PA										
Anderson et al.[66]	325	82%	No	< 4 hours	Anistreplase 30 U rt-PA 100 mg over 3 hours	10 days	RVG	Anistreplase 82 mL rt-PA 74 mL	0.02	− 8 mL (− 7.5 − − 8.7)
						1 month	RVG	Anistreplase 86 mL rt-PA 77 mL	0.06	− 9 mL (− 7.6 − − 9.2)
Intravenous streptokinase versus rt-PA versus streptokinase + rt-PA										
GUSTO-I[4]	733	75%	No	< 6 hours	Streptokinase 1.5 MU + subcutaneous heparin	5–7 days	Contrast	31 mL	NS	
					Streptokinase 1.5 MU + intravenous heparin			29 mL	NS	− 2 mL (− 5 − 1)†
					rt-PA 100 mg over 90 minutes			28 mL	NS	− 3 mL (− 5.7 − 0.3)†
					Streptokinase 1.5 MU, rt-PA 1 mg/kg over 1 hour			30 mL	NS	− 1 mL (− 4.1 − 2.1)†

NS = not significant, rt-PA = recombinant tissue plasminogen activator, RVG = radionuclide ventriculography.

* Defined as the left ventricular volume at end-systole (Whitlock & Bass).[67]

† Versus streptokinase + subcutaneous heparin.

The Healing and Early Afterload Reducing Therapy study,[35] which commenced ACE inhibitor therapy within 24 hours of anterior infarction, showed that early "full" dose ramipril showed the greatest improvement in EFs between days 1 and 14 compared with early "low dose" or "delayed" ramipril.

Regional Wall Motion Assessment

Function in the noninfarct region is important, and the ability of the noninfarct zone to compensate for hypokinesis of the infarct zone may be critical for patient survival.[23] As there are variable changes in the function of the noninfarct zone and its capacity to become hyperkinetic, assessment of global EF may not accurately reflect the size of the infarct or infarct zone contractility.[36] Regional wall motion assessment is therefore able to give additional information to global assessment alone. In the GUSTO Trial, even as early as 90 minutes after the onset of infarction, the wall motion of the infarct zone was better in patients treated with an accelerated rt-PA regimen than in patients treated with streptokinase.[5]

The RAPID I and II studies both showed that the increased 90-minute TIMI-3 flow achieved by double bolus r-PA (10 mg), compared with accelerated rt-PA (63% vs 49% and 60% vs 45%, respectively; both $P < 0.05$), was associated with better regional wall motion mean (chord score) in the infarct zone on the predischarge ventriculogram.[37,38]

Relation of Patency of the Infarct Related Artery to LV Function and Survival

Preservation of ventricular function, as measured by the EF, occurs following successful reperfusion of the ischemic myocardium compared with unsuccessful reperfusion.[23] Patients treated earlier have greater preservation of LV function,[17,39,40] and sustained patency of the infarct related artery is closely related to preservation of LV function.[23] In the GUSTO Trial, TIMI-3 flow at 90 minutes was already associated with less infarct zone wall motion impairment.[4]

There have been no trials to show that the infarct related artery TIMI flow grade is superior to LV function, assessed after the first day, in predicting survival. In 1994, we reported long-term follow-up of 312 patients with first MI treated within 4 hours with thrombolytic therapy that ventricular function and infarct artery patency 4 weeks after infarction are independent prognostic factors.[41] The flow of the infarct related artery was assessed by the TIMI scoring system and by a scoring system relating coronary stenoses and flow to the amount of myocardium supplied. On univariate and multivariate analysis, ventricular function (EF, $P = 0.006$ and 0.02, or end-systolic volume index, $P = 0.01$ and 0.06) was the most important prognostic factor. Patency of the infarct related artery measured as TIMI-3 flow was marginally significant on univariate analysis ($P = 0.08$) but not on multivariate analysis ($P = 0.2$). Patency was an independent prognostic factor on univariate and multivariate analysis when measured as an occlusion score (amount of myocardium supplied by an occluded artery, $P = 0.01$ and < 0.05). When the EF was $\geq 50\%$, only occluded arteries supplying $> 25\%$ of the LV adversely affected prognosis. If the EF was $< 50\%$, occluded arteries supplying $< 25\%$ of myocardium also adversely affected prognosis.

The Interuniversity Study showed that at 5-year follow-up EF was the most important prognostic factor, although TIMI-3 flow at 3 weeks in the infarct related artery on the hospital discharge angiogram was also important.[42] Also, we have shown that patients with TIMI-3 flow in the infarct related artery at 3 weeks have enhanced 5-year, but not 10-year, survival, irrespective of randomization to receive streptokinase or placebo.[43] The Western Washington Intracoronary Streptokinase Trial showed improved 12-month mortality following administration of intracoronary streptokinase.[44] One-year survival was related to whether the infarct artery had complete reperfusion. In this trial, there was no improvement in LV function because of the late intervention, up to 12 hours after the onset of infarction. However, when the EF was analyzed on day 3 (when significant myocardial stunning was present), EF was the most important prognostic factor, and patency was not a prognostic factor.

The Thrombolysis and Angioplasty in Myocardial Infarction Trials have also shown EF to be the most important predictor of hospital survival on multivariate analysis.[45] On 18-month follow-up, EF continued to be the most important factor, although it is possible that patency of the infarct related artery has not been shown to be prognostically important because of the high rate of patency achieved in these trials.[46] The Western Washington Intravenous rt-PA Trial also showed that LV function was the most important prognostic factor at 1-year follow-up, and patency of the infarct related artery at the time of hospital discharge did not appear to give prognostic information.[47]

Possible mechanisms of benefit of a patent infarct related artery include reduction of ventricular remodeling and ventricular dilatation,[48] reduction of ventricular arrhythmias,[49] and provision of collaterals to a later infarct in another coronary artery, the most frequent cause of late reinfarction.

Cardiogenic Shock and Mortality

After the introduction of coronary care units, there was a dramatic decrease in the number of patients dying from ventricular fibrillation. Following the adoption of thrombolytic therapy, the impairment of LV function in survivors has been dramatically reduced,[9,19,50] and the incidence of cardiogenic shock may have been reduced.[9,19] In the Interuniversity Study comparing three different strategies to open infarct arteries with control, the incidence of cardiogenic shock was reduced from 9.1% to 4.8%.[19] In our trial with streptokinase, the percentage of patients dying from cardiogenic shock was reduced from 8% to 2%, and the percentage of patients with EFs < 40% was reduced from 15.1% to 3.8%, P < 0.01[9] (Fig. 2). The number of patients dying from ventricular fibrillation has remained about the same as before the thrombolytic era,[51] but there has been an increase in cardiac rupture on day 1.[51,52] The number of patients dying from stroke has increased slightly.[3]

The long-term mortality reduction following thrombolytic therapy has been as equally impressive as the early reduction in mortality,[46,53-55] although the survival curves may not be diverging.[45,56] The lack of continuing divergence of survival curves may be because more patients with low EFs survive following thrombolytic therapy. Also the incidence of reocclusion of infarct related arteries is 24%-30% during the first year,[57,58] which is often clinically silent, and relates to infarct artery flow.[59]

Trial Sizing for Different End Points

In randomized trials of thrombolytic therapy with mortality as the primary end point, several thousand patients are required for sufficient statistical power to detect small differences between treatments. If the 35-day mortality in the 1990s for patients aged < 65 years who are thrombolytic-eligible is approximately 5%,[4,60] for a new treatment to reduce mortality by 15% to 4.2% at least 21,490 patients would be required for an α of 0.05 and a β of 80%. If, however, the mortality is 10.5%, as it was for all patients in the third International Study of Infarct Survival (ISIS) without age restrictions, then 10,726 patients are required to have the same power to show a 15% reduction. Mortality trials therefore require large numbers of patients or a high proportion of high risk patients.

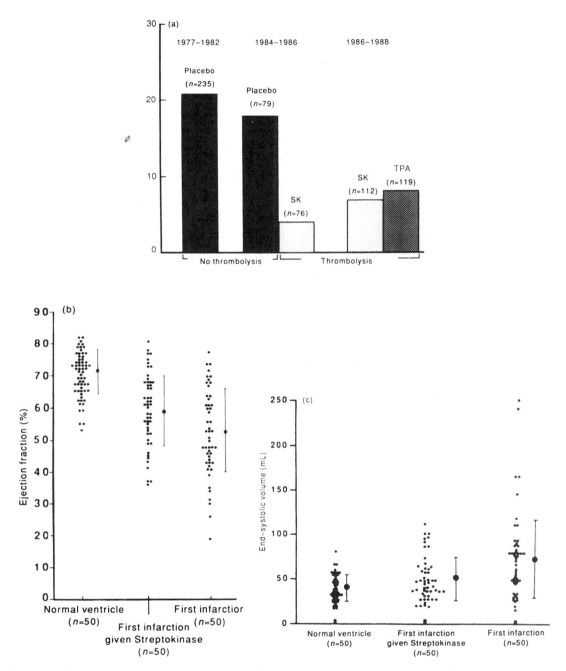

Figure 2. Ventricular function approximately 1 month after MI: the effect of thrombolysis. (A) The percentage of patients with EFs < 40% at cardiac catheterization after MI (Norris et al. 1984, White et al. 1987a, White et al. 1989). (B) Effect of streptokinase on EF after MI. C) Effect of streptokinase on end-systolic volume after MI. (From French and White. LV function following thrombolytic therapy for MI. Clin Exp Pharmacol Physiol 1995;22:173-179, reproduced with permission.) EF = ejection fraction; LV = left ventricular; MI = myocardial infarction.

As LV function is measured as a continuous variable rather than as a discrete variable, an improvement in EF from 50% to 55% requires only 100 patients, and from 50% to 53%, only 300 patients. A LV function trial of 200-300 patients can therefore have the same statistical power as a mortality trial of 10,000-20,000 patients.

For patency trials the numbers of patients required are much larger. For example, if the patency achieved with a particular treatment is 70%, then to show an improvement to 76% would require 1,784 patients, and an improvement in patency to 80%, 626 patients. For reocclusion, if the rate is 10%, to show a decrease to 8% would require 6,626 patients, and to 5%, 948 patients.

Intracranial hemorrhage is the most devastating adverse event of thrombolytic therapy, and it is critical that the safety of a new thrombolytic regimen is accurately assessed. As the incidence of intracranial hemorrhage in thrombolytic trials is low, large numbers of patients are required to show a difference in incidence with various treatments. If the rate is 1.5%, to show a 33% reduction to 1% requires 16,290 patients. However, the absolute differences in intracranial hemorrhage rates between various thrombolytic and adjuvant treatment regimens may be $< 0.5\%$,[61] necessitating greater numbers to demonstrate clinically important differences.

Conclusion

In thrombolytic trials the three most important assessments of overall patient benefit are survival, LV function, and freedom from disabling stroke.[61] Infarct related artery TIMI-3 flow has also been shown to be of independent prognostic benefit at 5 years.[41-43] Clinical trials should have the statistical power for each of these assessments to enable firm conclusions to be drawn. LV function remains the most important potentially modifiable prognostic factor. As new thrombolytic and antithrombotic regimens are developed, assessment of LV function will remain an important end point of clinical trials.

References

1. DeWood MA, Spores J, Notske R, et al. Prevalence of total coronary occlusion during the early hours of transmural myocardial infarction. N Engl J Med 1980;303:897-902.
2. French JK, Williams BF, Hart HH, et al. Prospective evaluation of eligibility for thrombolytic therapy in acute myocardial infarction. Br Med J 1996;312: 1637-1641.
3. Fibrinolytic Therapy Trialists' (FTT) Collaborative Group. Indications for fibrinolytic therapy in suspected acute myocardial infarction: Collaborative overview of early mortality and major morbidity results from all randomised trials of more than 1000 patients. Lancet 1994;343:311-322.
4. The GUSTO Investigators. An international randomized trial comparing four thrombolytic strategies for acute myocardial infarction. N Engl J Med 1993; 329:673-682.
5. The GUSTO Angiographic Investigators. The effects of tissue plasminogen activator, streptokinase, or both on coronary-artery patency, ventricular function, and survival after acute myocardial infarction [published erratum appears in N Engl J Med 1994;330: 516]. N Engl J Med 1993;329:1615-1622.
6. The ISAM Study Group. A prospective trial of intravenous streptokinase in acute myocardial infarction (ISAM): Mortality, morbidity, and infarct size at 21 days. N Engl J Med 1986; 314:1465-1471.
7. Bassand JP, Faivre R, Becque O, et al. Effects of early high-dose streptokinase intravenously on left ventricular function in acute myocardial infarction. Am J Cardiol 1987;60:435-439.
8. Durand P, Asseman P, Pruvost P, et al. Effectiveness of intravenous streptokinase on infarct size and left ventricular function in acute myocardial infarction: Prospective and randomized study. Clin Cardiol 1987;10:383-392.
9. White HD, Norris RM, Brown MA, et al. Effect of intravenous streptokinase on left ventricular function and early sur-

vival after acute myocardial infarction. N Engl J Med 1987;317:850-855.

10. Kennedy JW, Martin GV, Davis KB, et al. The Western Washington intravenous streptokinase in acute myocardial infarction randomized trial [published erratum appears in Circulation 1988;77:1037]. Circulation 1988;77:345-352.

11. Guerci AD, Gerstenblith G, Brinker JA, et al. A randomized trial of intravenous tissue plasminogen activator for acute myocardial infarction with subsequent randomization to elective coronary angioplasty. N Engl J Med 1987;317:1613-1618.

12. National Heart Foundation of Australia coronary thrombolysis group. Coronary thrombolysis and myocardial salvage by tissue plasminogen activator given up to 4 hours after onset of myocardial infarction. Lancet 1988;I:203-208.

13. O'Rourke M, Baron D, Keogh A, et al. Limitation of myocardial infarction by early infusion of recombinant tissue-type plasminogen activator. Circulation 1988;77:1311-1315.

14. Armstrong PW, Baigrie RS, Daly PA, et al. Tissue plasminogen activator: Toronto (TPAT) placebo-controlled randomized trial in acute myocardial infarction. J Am Coll Cardiol 1989;13:1469-1476.

15. Meinertz T, Kasper W, Schumacher M, et al. The German multicenter trial of anisoylated plasminogen streptokinase activator complex versus heparin for acute myocardial infarction. Am J Cardiol 1988;62:347-351.

16. Bassand JP, Machecourt J, Cassagnes J, et al. Multicenter trial of intravenous anisoylated plasminogen streptokinase activator complex (APSAC) in acute myocardial infarction: Effects on infarct size and left ventricular function. J Am Coll Cardiol 1989;13:988-997.

17. Serruys PW, Simoons ML, Suryapranata H, et al. Preservation of global and regional left ventricular function after early thrombolysis in acute myocardial infarction. J Am Coll Cardiol 1986;7:729-742.

18. Van de Werf F, Arnold AER, for the European Cooperative Study Group for Recombinant Tissue Type Plasminogen Activator. Intravenous tissue plasminogen activator and size of infarct, left ventricular function, and survival in acute myocardial infarction. Br Med J 1988;297:1374-1379.

19. Simoons ML, Serruys PW, van den Brand M, et al. Improved survival after early thrombolysis in acute myocardial infarction: A randomised trial by the Interuniversity Cardiology Institute in the Netherlands. Lancet 1985;II:578-582.

20. Smalling RW, Bode C, Weaver WD, et al. Favorable impact of early patency and a third generation thrombolytic agent on left ventricular function and survival in acute myocardial infarction: A meta analysis of the RAPID I and RAPID II trials. Circulation. In press.

21. Braunwald E, Kloner RA. The stunned myocardium: Prolonged, postischemic ventricular dysfunction. Circulation 1982;66:1146-1149.

22. Ellis SG, Henschke CI, Sandor T, et al. Time course of functional and biochemical recovery of myocardium salvaged by reperfusion. J Am Coll Cardiol 1983;1:1047-1055.

23. Sheehan FH, Doerr R, Schmidt WG. Early recovery of left ventricular function after thrombolytic therapy for acute myocardial infarction: An important determinant of survival. J Am Coll Cardiol 1988;12:289-300.

24. White HD, Norris RM, Brown MA, et al. Left ventricular end-systolic volume as the major determinant of survival after recovery from myocardial infarction. Circulation 1987;76:44-51.

25. Migrino RQ, Young JB, Ellis SG, et al. End-systolic volume index at 90 to 180 minutes into reperfusion therapy for acute myocardial infarction is a strong predictor of early and late mortality. Circulation 1997;96:116-121.

26. Pfeffer JM, Pfeffer MA, Braunwald E. Influence of chronic captopril therapy on the infarcted left ventricle of the rat. Circ Res 1985;57:84-95.

27. Pfeffer MA, Pfeffer JM, Steinberg C, et al. Survival after an experimental myocardial infarction: Beneficial effects of long-term therapy with captopril. Circulation 1985;72:406-412.

28. Pfeffer MA, Lamas GA, Vaughan DE, et al. Effect of captopril on progressive ventricular dilatation after anterior myocardial infarction. N Engl J Med 1988;319:80-86.

29. Sharpe N, Murphy J, Smith H, et al. Treatment of patients with symptomless left ventricular dysfunction after myocardial infarction. Lancet 1988;I:255-259.

30. ISIS-4 (Fourth International Study of

Infarct Survival) Collaborative Group. ISIS-4: A randomised factorial trial assessing early oral captopril, oral mononitrate, and intravenous magnesium sulphate in 58,050 patients with suspected acute myocardial infarction. Lancet 1995;345:669-685.

31. Gruppo Italiano per lo Studio della Sopravvivenza nell'Infarto Miocardico. GISSI-3: Effects of lisinopril and transdermal glyceryl trinitrate singly and together on 6-week mortality and ventricular function after acute myocardial infarction. Lancet 1994;343:1115-1122.

32. Chinese Cardiac Study Collaborative Group. Oral captopril versus placebo among 13,634 patients with suspected acute myocardial infarction: Interim report from the Chinese Cardiac Study (CCS-1). Lancet 1995;345:686-687.

33. Swedberg K, Held P, Kjekshus J, et al. Effects of the early administration of enalapril on mortality in patients with acute myocardial infarction: Results of the Cooperative New Scandinavian Enalapril Survival Study II (CONSENSUS II). N Engl J Med 1992;327:678-684.

34. French JK, Amos DJ, Cross DB, et al. Captopril within 6 hours of streptokinase in patients with reduced TIMI flow improves ventricular function in the area at risk. (abstract) Circulation 1996;94(Suppl I):I-189.

35. Pfeffer MA, Greaves SC, Arnold JMO, et al. Early versus delayed angiotensin-converting enzyme inhibition therapy in acute myocardial infarction: The Healing and Early Afterload Reducing Therapy Trial. Circulation 1997;95:2643-2651.

36. Sheehan FH. Determinants of improved left ventricular function after thrombolytic therapy in acute myocardial infarction. J Am Coll Cardiol 1987;9:937-944.

37. Smalling RW, Bode C, Kalbfleisch J, et al. More rapid, complete, and stable coronary thrombolysis with bolus administration of reteplase compared with alteplase infusion in acute myocardial infarction. Circulation 1995;91:2725-2732.

38. Bode C, Smalling RW, Berg G, et al. Randomized comparison of coronary thrombolysis achieved with double-bolus reteplase (recombinant plasminogen activator) and front-loaded, accelerated alteplase (recombinant tissue

plasminogen activator) in patients with acute myocardial infarction. Circulation 1996;94:891-898.

39. Schwarz F, Schuler G, Katus H, et al. Intracoronary thrombolysis in acute myocardial infarction: Duration of ischemia as a major determinant of late results after recanalization. Am J Cardiol 1982;50:933-937.

40. Mathey DG, Sheehan FH, Schofer J, et al. Time from onset of symptoms to thrombolytic therapy: A major determinant of myocardial salvage in patients with acute transmural infarction. J Am Coll Cardiol 1985;6:518-525.

41. White HD, Cross DB, Elliott JM, et al. Long-term prognostic importance of patency of the infarct-related coronary artery after thrombolytic therapy for acute myocardial infarction. Circulation 1994;89:61-67.

42. Lenderink T, Simoons ML, van Es GA, et al. Benefit of thrombolytic therapy is sustained throughout five years and is related to TIMI perfusion grade 3 but not grade 2 flow at discharge. The European Cooperative Study Group. Circulation 1995;92:1110-1116.

43. French JK, Amos D, Webber B, et al. TIMI 3 flow at 3 weeks following myocardial infarction determines long-term mortality in patients randomized to streptokinase or placebo. (abstract) J Am Coll Cardiol 1997;29(Suppl A):71A.

44. Kennedy JW, Ritchie JL, Davis KB, et al. The Western Washington Randomized Trial of Intracoronary Streptokinase in Acute Myocardial Infarction: A 12-month follow-up report. N Engl J Med 1985;312:1073-1078.

45. Topol EJ, Califf RM, George BS, et al. Insights derived from the thrombolysis and angioplasty in myocardial infarction (TAMI) trials. J Am Coll Cardiol 1988;12:24A-31A.

46. Muller DW, Topol EJ, George BS, et al. Long term follow-up in the thrombolysis and angioplasty in myocardial infarction (TAMI) trials: Comparison with trials of thrombolysis alone (abstract). Circulation 1989:80 Suppl II:520.

47. Flygenring BP, Althouse RG, Sheehan FH, et al. Does vessel patency at the time of hospital discharge following thrombolytic therapy predict survival? (abstract) J Am Coll Cardiol 1990;15:202A.

48. Hochman JS, Choo H. Limitation of

myocardial infarct expansion by reperfusion independent of myocardial salvage. Circulation 1987;75:299-306.

49. Sager PT, Perlmutter RA, Rosenfeld LE, et al. Electrophysiologic effects of thrombolytic therapy in patients with a transmural anterior myocardial infarction complicated by left ventricular aneurysm formation. J Am Coll Cardiol 1988;12:19-24.

50. White HD. Relation of thrombolysis during acute myocardial infarction to left ventricular function and mortality. Am J Cardiol 1990;66:92-95.

51. ISIS-2 (Second International Study of Infarct Survival) Collaborative Group. Randomised trial of intravenous streptokinase, oral aspirin, both, or neither among 17,187 cases of suspected acute myocardial infarction: ISIS-2. Lancet 1988;II:349-360.

52. Gruppo Italiano per lo Studio della Streptochinasi nell'Infarto Miocardico (GISSI). Effectiveness of intravenous thrombolytic treatment in acute myocardial infarction. Lancet 1986;I:397-402.

53. Gruppo Italiano per lo Studio della Streptochi-nasi nell'Infarto Miocardico (GISSI). Long-term effects of intravenous thrombolysis in acute myocardial infarction: Final report of the GISSI Study. Lancet 1987;II:871-874.

54. AIMS Trial Study Group. Long-term effects of intravenous anistreplase in acute myocardial infarction: Final report of the AIMS Study. Lancet 1990; 335:427-431.

55. Wilcox RG, von der Lippe G, Olsson CG, et al. Effects of alteplase in acute myocardial infarction: 6-month results from the ASSET Study. Lancet 1990; 335: 1175-1178.

56. Baigent C, Collins R, for the ISIS collaborative group. ISIS-2: 4-year mortality follow-up of 17,187 patients after fibrinolytic and antiplatelet therapy in suspected acute myocardial infarction. (abstract) Circulation 1993;88: I-291.

57. White HD, French JK, Hamer AW, et al. Frequent reocclusion of patent infarct-related arteries between 4 weeks and 1 year: Effects of antiplatelet therapy. J Am Coll Cardiol 1995;25:218-223.

58. Meijer A, Verheugt FWA, Werter CJPJ, et al. Aspirin versus coumadin in the prevention of reocclusion and recurrent ischemia after successful thrombolysis: A prospective placebo-controlled

angiographic study: Results of the APRICOT Study. Circulation 1993;87: 1524-1530.

59. French JK, Ellis CJ, Webber BJ, et al. Abnormal coronary flow in infarct arteries 1 year after myocardial infarction is predicted at 4 weeks by corrected TIMI frame count and stenosis severity. Am J Cardiol. In press.

60. ISIS-3 (Third International Study of Infarct Survival) Collaborative Group. ISIS-3: A randomised comparison of streptokinase vs tissue plasminogen activator vs anistreplase and of aspirin plus heparin vs aspirin alone among 41,299 cases of suspected acute myocardial infarction. Lancet 1992;339: 753-770.

61. Topol EJ, Califf RM, Van de Werf F, et al. Perspectives on large-scale cardiovascular clinical trials for the new millenium. Circulation 1997;95:1072-1082.

62. Schreiber TL, Miller DH, Silvasi DA, et al. Randomized double-blind trial of intravenous streptokinase for acute myocardial infarction. Am J Cardiol 1986; 58:47-52.

63. O'Rourke M, Keogh A, Kelly R, et al. Improved LV ejection fraction at 21 days following coronary occlusion treated by early intravenous rt-PA infusion (abstract). Aust N Z J Med 1988;18:351.

64. Topol EJ, George BS, Kereiakes DJ, et al. A randomized controlled trial of intravenous tissue plasminogen activator and early intravenous heparin in acute myocardial infarction. Circulation 1989;79:281-286.

65. White HD, Rivers JT, Maslowski AH, et al. Effect of intravenous streptokinase as compared with that of tissue plasminogen activator after first myocardial after first myocardial infarction. N Engl J Med 1989;320:817-821.

66. Anderson JL, Becker LC, Sorensen SG, et al. Anistreplase versus alteplase in acute myocardial infarction: Comparative effects on left ventricular function, morbidity and 1-day coronary artery patency. J Am Coll Cardial 1992;20:753-766.

67. Whitlock RML, Bass NM. Left ventricular volume estimation by single-plane right anterior oblique cine angiocardiography. Proceedings of the Biological Engineering Society 20th Anniversary International Conference; London; 1980.

Chapter 14

New Thrombolytic Agents

Allan M. Ross, M.D.

From the Cardiovascular Research Institute, George Washington University, Washington, D.C.

Introduction

The decade of the 1990s has witnessed an intense rebirth of enthusiasm for the development of new thrombolytic agents. This activity can be directly traced to an understanding that higher total rates of successful restoration of normal velocity infarct artery coronary flow or achieving such flow faster is the key to promoting an improved postinfarction clinical outcome. The acceptance of this principle relates to the large Global Utilization of Streptokinase and tPA for Occluded Arteries (GUSTO-1) trial,[1,2] which demonstrated the link between early complete flow restoration and improved survival when more effective regimens (at promoting rapid clot lysis) were compared with less effective ones. Prior to the GUSTO trial interest in designing and developing new agents had been effectively inhibited by the failure of initial comparative drug trials (notably the Gruppo Italiano per lo Studio della Sopravvivenza nell'Infarto Miocardico [GISSI]-2 and the Third International Study of Infarct Survival [ISIS-3] studies)[3,4] to show important clinical outcome differences based on treatment assignment. In retrospect, those neutral results can likely be ascribed to a combination of research protocol design issues including the drugs and dosing plans of the drugs selected for testing, the timing of therapy, patient selection issues, and adjunctive therapy choices.

While there is now little residual debate over the desirability to design faster and more effective pharmacological reperfusion regimens, it is not widely appreciated how very substantial must be the augmentation of patency rates and/or how much faster acting must therapies be to effect further measurable clinical advantages. Hence a review of new thrombolytic drugs logically begins with a discussion of the quantitative patency-survival relationship.

In the GUSTO-1 trial, identification of restored fully normal infarct related vessel flow (thrombolysis in myocardial infarction [TIMI] grade 3) within 90 minutes of the start of therapy was associated with a 30-day mortality rate of approximately 4%. In contrast, the finding of a persistently closed artery at that time point correlated to a mortality rate of about 9%. It should be appreciated that successful reperfusion does not equate to survival for all patients any more than does failure to reperfuse result in extraordinarily high fatality rates. These values form the basis of the aforementioned need for very substantial patency augmentation to produce further recognizable clinical benefits. Simple algebra would lead to an expectation that one would need to open about 20 arteries per 100 infarct patients to lessen mortality by 1 per 100 patients (or 20 additional arteries with a new regimen to show superiority compared with an existing treatment).[5] In actuality, of course, the relationship is more complex and is altered by many factors, including time to treatment, infarct location, patient age, reocclusion rate, etc.; but the broad relationship of 20 or so extra open arteries for one extra survivor appears to hold up reasonably well. In the GUSTO-1 study the accelerated tPA treatment group produced 23 more open (TIMI grade 3) arteries per 100 patients than the streptokinase-treated patients. This corresponded to an absolute reduction in 30-day mortality, from 7.3%–6.3%.

Although it might be assumed that measurement of the reperfusion efficacy of new treatments is a straightforward, reproducible, and highly reliable exercise, in actuality there are many pitfalls in the estimate of success rates produced by a new treatment, particularly since they are often based on rather small patient experiences. For example, the 95% confidence intervals (CIs) around a point estimate of 60% patency derived from a 150 patient sample is approximately ± 8%. Furthermore, patency is not simply a function of the treatment administered but is significantly influenced by the following: patient body weight (higher weight, lower patency),[6] smoking status (smokers are more likely to reperfuse),[7] time to treatment,[8] adjunctive drugs administered,[9] etc. The variability in patency with the same treatment regimen but in different clinical trials can be appreciated by inspecting Figure 1.

While there is a substantial improvement in outcome when treatment rapidly produces grade 3 patency (normal flow), reopening to only sluggish flow (TIMI grade 2) is not associated with equivalent benefits. The difference between these two grades of patency is qualitative, however, and categorical assignment at the time of analysis is somewhat imprecise. There is a gray zone, and even experienced angiographers may not agree on the flow grade in up to 15% of films. All of these baseline variable and interpretive issues add to the requirement that very large patency differences, demonstrated in large trials, are required before reaching conclusions on a new treatment's benefit profile.

Regarding the development of new regimens to accomplish the related goal of faster patency restoration, complexities similar to those regarding production and proof of higher total patency are encoun-

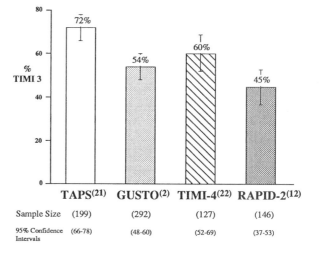

Figure 1. The accelerated tPA regimen: 90 minutes patency in four trials.

	TAPS[21]	GUSTO[2]	TIMI-4[22]	RAPID-2[12]
Sample Size	(199)	(292)	(127)	(146)
95% Confidence Intervals	(66-78)	(48-60)	(52-69)	(37-53)

tered. To improve outcome by accomplishing faster reperfusion, a considerable savings in time to artery reopening must occur. Furthermore, it is more difficult to define the magnitude of additional mortality benefit accomplished by reducing minutes to lysis. This is so because in most trials with a wide range of pain onset to treatment times, there is little information on actual time to reperfusion. Recorded time to treatment clearly does not equate to time of reopening, and in most studies we can only estimate both the incidence of reperfusion success and the timing of its occurrence, since angiograms have been infrequently performed in mortality trials. Nonetheless, Cannon et al.,[10] in a review of the importance of the time factor in reperfusion, have calculated that in relating time to treatment with survival, each hour saved in a group of infarct patients reduces the absolute mortality by 1%. This estimate obviously reflects a blend of reperfusion grades and times and hence is only an approximation of the actual relationship. One could theoretically bypass these issues and problems by evaluating all new and experimental thrombolytic regimens by performing large (20,000 or so) comparative mortality trials, but that is impractical if not impossible. Hence, our initial opinions regarding new treatments (and the important decision to pursue or abandon them) tend to be made on the basis of preliminary patency and speed data plus early observations on safety (usually major bleeding).

What Features Are Sought in New Fibrinolytics, and What Are the Sources of the New Agents?

The quest for faster, more effective activators has focused on increasing their resistance to inactivation by natural antagonists (e.g., plasminogen activator inhibitor 1 [PAI-1]), increasing their fibrin selectivity, and inducing alterations in active halflife following infusion or, increasingly, after bolus administration.

Table 1.
The New Thrombolytics

a) Derived from wild-type tPA
   rPA (reteplase)
   TNK-tPA
   nPA (lanoteplase)
b) Derived from other sources
   staphylokinase
   dsPA

The principal source of new lytics (Table 1) has been the result of purposeful modifications of "wild type" or human tPA. These drugs have been created either by affecting selective deletions of specific domains of the tPA molecule or by specific substitution of a few of its amino acids known or suspected to influence the properties of interest.

The other important source of lytics under evaluation has been isolation and then duplication by recombinant techniques of substances elicited by bacteria, insects, and animals, and which are known to be plasminogen activators.

Reteplase (rPA) is the sole agent in Figure 2 to have secured FDA approval for clinical use. It is a deletion mutant of tPA that exhibits several differences compared to its parent compound. Compared with the wild type, it is modestly less fibrin selective and has a modestly prolonged half-life of about half an hour. This latter property permits bolus dosing, but two injections of 10 mega units 30 minutes apart are recommended. This fixed dose without weight adjustment is used for all patients. Several small to moderate size patency trials have been reported.[11,12] In the Rapid 1 and 2 trials comprising under 300 patients, the 90-minute posttreatment TIMI grade 3 patency rate was 61% with a 95% CI between 52% and 68%. In the 6,000-patient Inject Trial[13] the 30-day rPA mortality rate was 9.0% compared with 9.5% for patients randomized to 1.5 million units of streptokinase (SK, P = ns). This study was prespecified as an equivalence trial with equivalence prespecifed as 95% CIs excluding the likelihood of rPA producing an absolute increase in deaths of 1% compared with SK. The CI did not overlap that prespecified boundary. Bleeding with the two agents was rather high, 15% in both treatment groups. The most recent GUSTO-3 trial[14] tested the hypothesis that rPA would produce a significant mortality reduction when tested in a randomized comparison against human type tPA. It did not, with a 30-day fatality rate among 10,000 rPA patients of 7.2% versus 7.0% among 5,000 tPA patients (a 2:1 randomization scheme). While not designed as an equivalence trial, the study investigators nonetheless pointed out that the 95% CI included the possibility that the mortality effect of rPA included its being 1.1% worse than rtPA in absolute terms. In GUSTO-3 both the overall mortality and stroke rates were higher than expected.

The TNK mutant of tPA alters the molecule by amino acid substitutions to increase (compared to native tPA) fibrin selectivity 10 fold and PAI-1 resistance 80 fold and produces an 8 fold prolongation in the half-life. This latter feature permits single bolus dosing. TNK has been tested across a wide range of doses with 30 and 40 mg having been selected for further clinical evaluation. In the initial patency studies,[15] boluses of 30–50 mg all produced patency rates of 57%–64% at 90 minutes. Encouragingly, such rates of opening had already been achieved in patients who had their first endpoint angiogram 60 minutes after the bolus suggested that the goal of altering the tPA molecule to increase its speed of action may be achievable. Larger patency and clinical endpoint studies with this agent are nearing completion.

Another tPA mutant (of the deletion variety) similarly designed to increase the speed of patency achievement is nPA (lanoteplase). In the InTime angiographic trial[16] this activator's use was associated with a 51% TIMI-3 rate 60 minutes after a single bolus. Clinical results following the administration of nPA are currently being investigated in the large InTime-2 study.

Staphylococcal products, like those from the Streptococcus, are known to activate plasminogen. Filtration and other physical and chemical purification techniques have been inadequate to produce a sufficiently pure product for clinical use. With the advent of recombinant methods, however, staphylokinase can now be produced in a clinically usable form. Patency trials of this agent in patients[17] have shown the highest 90-minute TIMI-3 patency rates seen with any activator tested to date. These results are ascribed to near absolute fibrin selectivity for the products obtained when staphylokinase interacts with plasma proteins. There is, however, some concern about residual antigenicity, and the development of this novel agent has been slow.

Finally, for several years there has been some interest in another extremely effective fibrinolytic agent: "bat" PA (more appropriately called dsPA). The vampire bat (desmodus rotundus, hence ds) secretes in its saliva the most potent activator yet identified. In a very small number of myocardial infarction patients it has been remarkably successful in promoting coronary clot lysis. Whether a usable pharmaceutical, sufficiently free of associated bleeding complications, can be developed from this source remains to be shown.

From this brief description of agents under development it might be concluded that the apparent improvements over wild type tPA (with the possible exception of the last agents mentioned) are in fact rather modest and possibly insufficient to be reflected in clear-cut clinical gains. With the spectrum of recently developed lytics providing overall patency of about 80%, with 60% of patients demonstrating TIMI-3 flow at 90 minutes, there is clearly room for a significant advance in the efficiency of fibrinolytics (Fig. 2). Whether it will be pharmacologically achieved is not yet established.

Such observations have stimulated a parallel line of investigation in which faster and more complete reperfusion is sought by combinations of lytic drugs with potent newer antithrombin and antiplatelet drugs.

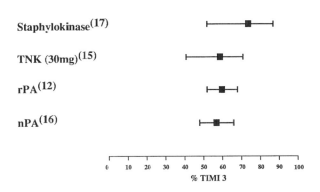

Figure 2. Some recently reported 90-minute TIMI-3 flow rates (with 95% confidence intervals) using new thrombolytic regimens.

Generally, both unfractionated heparin and aspirin are part of the infarct therapeutic package. While initially utilized to prevent postreperfusion reocclusion, it is now appreciated that the newer drugs in these classes—direct thrombin inhibitors, low molecular weight heparin, platelet glycoprotein receptor antagonists, etc.—actually contribute to faster reduction in net thrombus mass. Early clinical studies utilizing hirulog,[18] hirudin[19] and integrilin[20] have been at least in part encouraging, although very effective doses of Hirudin with lytics has produced excess bleeding, and yet other combinations are under investigation.

In the space of a very few years we have gone from infrequent use of prototype fibrinolytics with older adjunctive antithrombotics to the development of an extensive array of specifically designed second and third generation drugs intended to augment the gains already achieved. To what degree that goal will be accomplished, how soon, and with which new agents remains to be seen.

References

1. The GUSTO Investigators . An international randomized trial comparing four thrombolytic strategies for acute myocardial infarction. N Engl J Med 1993: 329:673-682.

2. The GUSTO Angiographic Investigators. The effects of tissue plasminogen activator, streptokinase, or both on coronary artery patency, ventricular function, and survival after acute myocardial infarction. N Engl J Med 1993: 329:1615-1622.

3. Gruppo Italiano per lo Studio della Sopravvivenza nell'lnfarto Miocardico. GISSI-2: A factorial randomised trial of alteplase versus streptokinase and heparin versus no heparin among 12,490 patients with acute myocardial infarction. Lancet 1990:336:65-71.

4. ISIS-3 (Third International Study of Infarct Survival) Collaborative Group. ISIS-3: A randomised comparison of streptokinase vs tissue plasminogen activator vs anistreplase and of aspirin plus heparin vs aspirin alone among 41,299 cases of suspected acute myocardial infarction. Lancet 1993:339: 753-770.

5. Simes RJ, Topol EJ, Holmes DR, et al. for the GUSTO-1 Investigators. Link between the angiographic substudy and mortality outcomes in a large randomized trial of myocardial reperfusion. Circulation 1995;91.7:1923-1928.

6. Lundergan CF, Reiner JS, McCarthy WF, et al. Clinical predictors of early infarct related artery patency following thrombolytic therapy: Importance of body weight, smoking history, infarct related artery, and choice of thrombolytic regimen: the GUSTO-1 experience. J Am Coll Cardiol 1997; in press.

7. Barbash GL, Reiner J, White H, et al. for the GUSTO-1 Investigators. Evaluation of paradoxic beneficial effects of smoking in patients receiving thrombolytic therapy for acute myocardial infarction: Mechanism of "Smoker's

Paradox" from the GUSTO-1 Trail, with angiographic insights. J Am Coll Cardiol 1995;26:1222-1229.

8. Chesebro JH, Knatterud G, Roberts R, et al. Thrombolysis in Myocardial Infarction (TIMI) trial, phase 1: A comparison between intravenous tissue plasminogen activator and intravenous streptokinase: Clinical findings through hospital discharge. Circulation 1987;76:142-154.

9. Hsia J, Hamilton WP, Kleiman N, et al. A comparison between heparin and low-dose aspin as adjunctive therapy with Tissue Plasminogen Activator for Acute Myocardial Infarction. N Engl J Med 1990;323:1433-1437.

10. Cannon CP, Antman EM, Walls R, et al. Time as an adjunctive agent to thrombolytic therapy. J Thromb Thrombolysis 1994;1:27-34.

11. Bode C, Smalling RW, Berg G, et al. Randomized comparison of coronary thrombolysis achieved with double-bolus reteplase (recombinant plasminogen activator) and front-loaded, accelerated alteplase (recombinant tissue plasminogen activator) in patients with acute myocardial infarction. Circulation 1996;94:891-898.

12. Smalling RW, Bode C, Kalbfleisch J, et al. More rapid, complete and stable coronary thrombolysis with bolus administration of reteplase compared with alteplase infusion in acute myocardial infarction. Circulation 1995; 91:2725-2732.

13. Hampton JR, Schroder R, Wilcox RG, et al. Randomised, double-blind comparison of reteplase double-bolus administration with streptokinase in acute myocardial infarction (INJECT): Trial to investigate equivalence. Lancet 1995;346:329-336.

14. The GUSTO III Investigators. A comparison of reteplase with alteplase for acute myocardial infarction. New Engl J Med 1997;337:1118-1123.

15. Cannon CP, McCabe CH, Gibson CM, et al. TNK-Tissue plasminogen activator in acute myocardial infarction: Results of the thrombolysis in myocardial infarction (TIMI) 10a dose-ranging trail. Circulation 1997;95:351-356.

16. Chew P. Presented at the 1996 AHA National Meeting. Personal communication.

17. Vandersheren S, Barrios L, Kerdsinchai P, et al. A randomized trial of recombinant staphylokinase versus alteplase for coronary artery patency in acute myocardial infarction. Circulation 1995;92:2044-2049.

18. Maraganore JM, Adelman BA. Hirulog: A direct thrombin inhibitor for management of acute coronary syndromes. Coron Artery Dis 1996;7:438-448.

19. Antman EM. Hirudin in acute myocardial infarction. Thrombolysis and thrombin inhibition in myocardial infarction (TIMI) 9B trial. Circulation 1996;94:911-921.

20. Ohman EM, Kleiman NS, Gacioch G, et al. Combined accelerated tissue-plasminogen activator and platelet glycoprotein IIb/IIIa integrin receptor blockade with Integrilin in acute myocardial infarction. Results of a randomized, placebo-controlled, dose-ranging trial. IMPACT-AMI Investigators. Circulation 1997;95:846-854.

21. Neuhaus KL, Von Essen R, Tebbe U, et al. Improved thrombolysis in acute myocardial infarction with front-loaded administration of alteplase: Results of the rt-PA-APSAC patency study (TAPS). J Am Coll Cardiol 1992;19: 885-891.

22. Cannon CP, McCabe CH, Diver DJ, et al. Comparison of front-loaded recombinant tissue-type plasminogen activator, anistreplase and combination thrombolytic therapy for acute myocardial infarction: Results of the Thrombolysis in Myocardial Infarction (TIMI) 4 trial. J Am Coll Cardiol 1994; 24:1602-1610.

Chapter 15

New Thrombolytics, Adjunctive Therapies, and Mechanical Interventions for Acute Ischemic Syndromes: A Current Perspective

George P. Hanna, M.D. and Richard W. Smalling, M.D., Ph.D.

From the Department of Internal Medicine, Division of Cardiology, The University of Texas Medical School and The Hermann Heart Center, Hermann Hospital, Houston, Texas

Significant advances occurred in the management of acute coronary syndromes over the past two decades that have resulted in > 25% reduction in mortality from myocardial infarction (MI).[1] The incorporation of early thrombolysis and promptly recanalizing the occluded coronary artery receive the major credit along with improvements in intensive coronary care units (CCUs), chest pain centers, and activation of advanced emergency medical services (EMS) for prehospital treatment and resuscitation. However, acute MI (AMI) and its complications remain the leading causes of death and disability in the western world. In the past few years, aggressive interventions such as angioplasty, stents, and intra-aortic balloon pumping (IABP) for managing acute coronary syndromes have received significant attention. However, controversy regarding their usefulness in this setting remains. In this review article, we will address some of the pros and cons of such interventions, as well as potential roles of newer thrombolytics and adjunctive therapies. (J Interven Cardiol 1998; 11:415–426)

Pathophysiology of Acute Coronary Syndromes

In 1980, DeWood et al. demonstrated thrombus formation by angiography in the majority of patients in the first 4 hours of AMI.[2] Since then, our understanding of the pathophysiology underlying acute coronary syndromes evolved rapidly in an attempt to devise strategies through which therapeutic interventions could be implemented to reduce the high mortality rates associated with this syndrome. As a result, we now know that AMI is a consequence of series of events: plaque rupture and fissuring in the atherosclerotic coronary artery, platelet aggregation, and thrombus formation play critical roles. As the plaque ruptures, it exposes several elements that are potent thrombogenic stimuli, including fibrillar collagen type 1. Endothelial cell dysfunction in the region of the plaque may result in vasoconstriction of the involved coronary segment, thus worsening coronary luminal diameter. Platelet aggregation ensues, and with activation of the coagulation system, a thrombus is generated, producing a marked decrease in blood flow to the corresponding myocardium, which is then in jeopardy of irreversible necrosis. Reimer et al. demonstrated, in the canine model, that myocardial necrosis proceeds from the subendocardium to the epicardium in a wavefront pattern, and minimal myocardium remains to be salvaged after 3 hours of coronary occlusion.[3,4] Theroux et al. demonstrated that reperfusion salvaged myocardial function, and this implied infarct salvage as well.[5] Subsequently, Rentrop et al.[6] demonstrated the feasibility of coronary thrombolysis in humans, and more effective treatment regimens evolved.

Why the Emphasis Now?

Early reperfusion is beneficial in many respects. Based on the premise that in-hospital mortality correlates directly with the degree of left ventricular dysfunction, reducing infarct size with early reperfusion should result in a decline in mortality rates.[7–9] In addition, prompt recanalization has been shown to reduce the incidence of malignant arrhythmias,[10] promote myocardial healing,[11] limit infarct expansion and ventricular aneurysm formation during remodelling,[12] and result in a higher grade of angiographic coronary flow and sustained patency of the infarct related artery.[13–15] Early coronary artery recanalization with restoration of TIMI 3 flow is presently the current goal of therapy of patients who present with AMI.

A number of large clinical trials in the U.S.A. and Europe demonstrated the beneficial effect of thrombolytic agents both in the short- and intermediate-terms[13,16,17] in reducing mortality. Thrombolytic therapy with intravenous tPA results in infarct-related artery patency (TIMI 2 or 3 flow) in 70%–80% of patients presenting with AMI within 90 minutes of intravenous administration, which is higher than that observed with streptokinase or anistreplase.[13,18] Even

with the accelerated form of tPA, however, the GUSTO angiographic investigators observed TIMI 3 flow in only 54% of patent arteries (Table 1). Mortality reduction was observed mainly in those with TIMI 3 flow, while the clinical outcome of patients with TIMI 2 flow were comparable to those without evidence of reperfusion. This suggests that thrombolysis alone, even with second-generation agents, is less than optimal in achieving adequate coronary flow demonstrable on early angiography in a large number of patients with acute MI.

Third-Generation Thrombolytics

r-PA.

r-PA (recombinant plasminogen activator: Reteplase) is a deletion mutant of the second kringle and protease domains of tPA molecule and has recently been approved by the Food and Drug Administration (FDA) for clinical use. The molecule is deglycosylated, as it is produced in *E. Coli* since bacterial expression lacks posttranslational modification. Reteplase has several advantages over tPA: the fibrin binding capacity of this molecule is five times lower and its half-life ninefold higher and possesses better clot penetration than t-PA.[19] In addition, r-PA can be administered as a double bolus dosing of 10 U 30 minutes apart with high incidence of TIMI 3 flow, allowing ease of administration and potential use for prehospital treatment of acute MI.[20] The RAPID II and the larger inject trials further determined the clinical efficacy, safety, and low mortality associated with r-PA.[21,22] However, GUSTO III, a large multicenter international trial of r-PA versus t-PA, failed to demonstrate an advantage of r-PA in the absence of rescue or early percutaneous transluminal coronary angioplasty (PTCA), presumably due to reclosure of the infarct-related artery in the first 24 hours after drug administration.[23]

Table 1. Properties of the Main Thrombolytic Agents in Acute Myocardial Infarction

	rt-PA	SK	APSAK	UK	scu-PA**	r-PA	TNK-tPA*	N-PA*
Peak effect	45 min	20 min to 2 hr	45 min	20 min–2 hr	60 min	—	—	—
Duration of effect	6 hr to 2 d	6 to 24 hr	6 hr to 2 d	6–24 hr	3–4 hr	—	—	—
Dose	100 mg	1.5 million IU	30 IU	3 million IU	80 mg	20 million U	1.5 mg/kg	50 KU/kg
Coronary patency rate at 90 minutes(%)	70–75	50–70	55–75	50–70	70–75	70–80	77	74%**
Coronary reperfusion rate at 90 minutes(%)	60–70	35–60	45–65	40–60	—	78	80–95	—
Drug ½ life (min)	2 to 6	23	70–90	14	6 to 10	10	(A) 9, (B) 31	(A) 10, (B) 30–55
TIMI 3	49	40–50	40	35–45	—	63–71	57–64	43**

* Experimental drugs.

** At 60 minutes

Adapted from Smalling and Hanna, *AJC* cont'd. educ series 1997.

TNK-PA. TNK-PA is a multiple point mutation variant of wild-type t-PA, which has an increased half-life but has intense fibrin binding and specificity. Although its plasma half-life would suggest it should be given as a double bolus, due to its intense fibrin binding, its biological half-life is longer, allowing it to be given as a single bolus. The TIMI 10a and ASSENT I dose ranging trials suggest that the 60- and 90-minute TIMI 3 flow with TNK-tPA are comparable to front loaded tPA with acceptable bleeding risk.[24,25] Consistent with the theory advanced by Kohnert and colleagues that intense fibrin binding may be deleterious to early clot lysis,[26,27] TNK-tPA failed to improve the incidence of TIMI-3 flow early but did allow single bolus administration. A large mortality trial evaluating TNK-PA is presently under way (ASSENT II).

Lanoteplase. Lanoteplase is a deletion and point mutation mutant tPA, which has a longer half life (30–40 minutes) and has less fibrin affinity and more lytic activity than wild-type tPA. With these pharmacological characteristics, it can be administered as a single bolus. In the InTIME I dose ranging trial at the highest dose, it achieved better 60-minute and 90-minute TIMI 3 patency than front loaded t-PA without an increase in bleeding complications.[28] A large mortality trial with this agent (lnTIME 2) has recently begun.

The Role of Angioplasty in Acute Myocardial Infarction

The primary advantages of direct coronary angioplasty over thrombolysis are the avoidance of the risk of hemorrhagic stroke, as well as achieving higher recanalization rates of 85% to 95% and possibly a decreased recurrent ischemic event rate.[29,30]

To determine the time required to achieve reperfusion with tPA versus primary angioplasty, 56 patients were randomized to thrombolysis and 48 patients to PTCA[31] in one study. Reperfusion rates from the TIMI 1 trial were used for comparison. The mean time for randomization to thromblysis was 20 minutes versus 45 minutes for PTCA. At 50, 80, and 110 minutes after randomization, the reperfusion rates for direct PTCA were 12%, 54%, and 83%. These rates are similar to previously reported reperfusion rates for tPA, and higher than for streptokinase. Therefore, primary PTCA can be performed rapidly and can result in reperfusion rates comparable to thrombolytics.

De Boer et al.[32] randomized 301 patients with AMI to receive streptokinase or undergo primary PTCA (ZWOLLE trial). The in-hospital mortality rate was 7% and 2% for the streptokinase and PTCA groups, respectively (Fig. 1). Reinfarction was observed in 10% in the thrombolytic group versus 1% in the angioplasty group. Combined death and AMI were observed in 15% versus 3% in the streptokinase and PTCA groups, respectively. Left ventricular ejection fraction (LVEF) was 44% and 50% in the thrombolytic and PTCA groups, respectively. This study suggests that PTCA may be superior to thrombolytics with regard to the above parameters.

In two prospective randomized trials, primary angioplasty was compared to t-PA (PAMl-l and GUSTO-llB). In the PAMI trial,[33] PTCA was superior to tPA in reducing in-hospital mortality (2.6% vs 6.5%; P = 0.039) (Fig. 1). The reduction in in-hospital death or reinfarction with angioplasty versus tPA was particularly marked in patients ≥ 65 years of age (8.6% vs 20%; P = 0.048). Primary management with PTCA was the most powerful multivariate correlate of freedom from recurrent ischemic events (10.3% vs 28%; P = 0.0001). These benefits of PTCA over tPA were maintained at 6-month follow-up (8.2% vs 17%; P = 0.02), and at 2-year follow-up a trend toward lower mortality or reinfarction was observed (14.4% vs 21%; P = 0.07). In GUSTO-llb,[34] an angioplasty substudy,

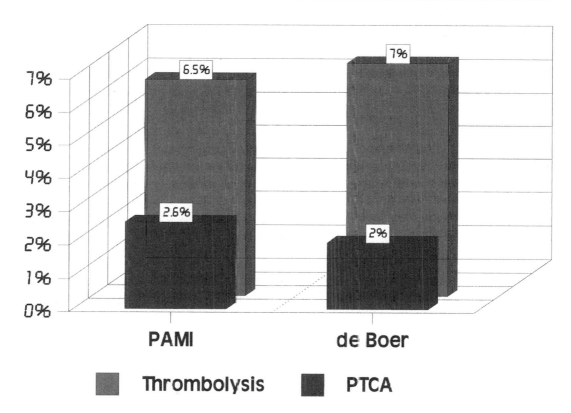

Figure 1. Bar graph representing percent in-hospital mortality post-PTCA versus thrombolysis for both PAMI I and ZWOLLE study by de Boer et al. See text for details.

1138 patients from 57 hospitals were randomized within 12 hours of an AMI to receive primary angioplasty or accelerated recombinant tPA therapy. The primary study end-point was composite outcome of death, nonfatal reinfarction, and nonfatal disabling stroke at 30 days. The incidence of the primary end-point in the PTCA and tPA groups was 9.6% and 13.7%, respectively ($P = 0.033$). Death occurred in 5.7% and 7.0% ($P = 0.037$), reinfarction in 4.5% versus 6.5%, and disabling stroke in 0.2% and 0.9% ($P = 0.11$) in the PTCA and tPA groups, respectively. At 6 months, there was no significant difference in the incidence of composite end-point. Therefore, GUSTO-IIb showed PTCA to be superior to tPA early, but this advantage was lost over 6 months. Once again, when a broad spectrum of acute intervention centers are in-

cluded in the analysis, the final results are less favorable than were previously seen in smaller studies.

Primary Angioplasty in Myocardial Infarction (PAMI) II was designed to determine whether coronary angiography performed acutely in the setting of AMI is helpful in stratifying patients into high- and low-risk groups on the one hand, and to address the issue of post-PTCA intra-aortic balloon pump in AMI on the other. Of the 1,100 patients enrolled, 89% of patients and 96.4% of occluded vessels underwent percutaneous angioplasty. Six percent of patients were treated medically, and 5% were referred for coronary artery bypass graft (CABG) due to life-threatening anatomy. Overall mortality was a low 2.9%. Patients stratified as high- and low-risk groups had a 5.5% and 0.3% mortality rate, respectively.

Multivariate analysis was utilized to determine clinical and catheterization variables predictive of poor prognosis; age > 70, Killip class > 1, TIMI < 2, LVEF < 45%, and three-vessel disease were predictive of higher mortality. In fact, patients with low EF, three-vessel disease, and TIMI 0–1 were associated with 3.8 times the risk of death.

In the setting of cardiogenic shock, Eckman et al.'s meta analysis suggested a superior role for angioplasty with an in-hospital mortality of 35% to 53% with direct angioplasty versus 63% to 77% for thrombolytic therapy and 69% to 81% for conservative therapy.[35]

Every et al.,[36] however, compared in-hospital and long-term mortality, as well as the use of resources among 1,050 patients in a primary angioplasty group and 2,095 patients in a thrombolytic therapy group. Patients were selected from the Myocardial Infarction Triage and Intervention (MITI) project registry cohort of 12,331 consecutive patients admitted with AMI to 19 Seattle hospitals. To avoid potential selection bias, the author performed several subgroup analyses that included patients eligible for thrombolysis, high-risk patients, and patients in the primary angioplasty group who were treated at hospitals with high volumes of angioplasty. No significant difference in mortality was observed (5.5% in the angioplasty vs 5.6% in the t-Pa group; P = 0.93). Also, no difference in mortality in high-risk patients between the two groups was observed. Moreover, the rates of procedures and costs were lower in the thrombolysis-treated patients versus PTCA at hospital discharge and at 3-year follow-up (30% fewer coronary angiograms, 15% fewer angioplasties, and 13% lower costs after 3 years in terms of follow-up). Therefore, in a community setting, there was no observed benefit in terms of reducing mortality or the use of resources with primary angioplasty rather than thrombolytic therapy in a large cohort of patients with AMI. However, this study was a retrospective nonrandomized study with a large number of centers participating. The possibility that results from low-volume interventional centers biased the results adversely is real.

Acute Angioplasty Immediately after Thrombolysis for Acute Myocardial Infarction

Since the underlying pathophysiology of acute coronary syndromes involves a combination of atheroma and thrombus, many have attempted a multifaceted approach for their therapeutic schemes: a combination of thrombolysis and percutaneous angioplasty. Three randomized trials were designed to determine the outcome of AMI patients receiving both tPA and angioplasty. The Thrombolysis and Angioplasty in Myocardial Infarction Study-1 (TAMI-I),[37] where 386 patients received 150 mg tPA, and those successfully reperfused were randomized to undergo acute or delayed PTCA at 7 days. The European Co-operative Study Group[38] enrolled 367 patients who received 100 mg tPA, and those eligible were randomized to have immediate or no PTCA. TIMI-IIA[39] study enrolled 389 patients who received 100 to 150 mg tPA and then randomized to immediate or delayed PTCA at 18 to 24 hours. No benefit in mortality reduction was observed in any of the three studies (Fig. 2). In fact, the mortality rate, bleeding complications, and referral for emergency bypass tended to be higher in the immediate angioplasty groups. No improvement in predischarge LVEF was observed. These studies, however, did not address the role of angioplasty in patients who had unsuccessful thrombolysis or thrombolysis with other thrombolytic agents. The high rate of early reclosure in these patients may be eliminated by acute stenting and newer thrombolytics using today's techniques.

Rescue PTCA

Compared to patients with normal flow after thrombolysis, patients with TIMI-2 flow or less may have worse LV

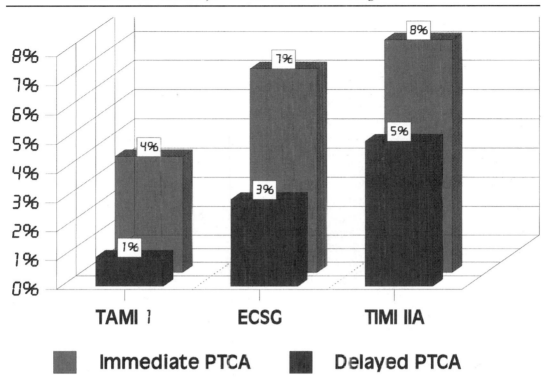

Figure 2. Bar graph representing percent mortality for immediate versus delayed PTCA for TAMI I, European Co-operative Study Group, and TIMI IIA studies. See text for details.

function and higher mortality. Rescue PTCA is often performed in this group of patients to re-establish normal flow, salvage myocardium, and improve LV performance. Early reports of rescue PTCA show acute patency of 70% to 100% of occluded coronary arteries after failed thrombolysis. Reocclusion rates, however, are high at 18%, and in-hospital mortality around 10%. Failed rescue PTCA is associated with a 28% to 39% mortality.[40,41] In the multicenter international RESCUE trial (Randomised Evaluation of Salvage angioplasty with Combined Utilisation of Endpoints),[42] rescue PTCA patients had better left ventricular function, less congestive heart failure, and lower mortality at 1-month and 1-year than medically treated patients. Therefore, the prognosis of patients receiving rescue PTCA is similar to that of successful thrombolysis. However, patients requiring rescue PTCA are at in-

creased risk for reocclusion compared to patients treated with primary PTCA or successful thrombolysis, and early mortality seems to be high if rescue PTCA is unsuccessful.

Adjunctive Therapies

Antiplatelet therapy with c7E3 in conjunction with primary or rescue PTCA in the setting of AMI has been shown to reduce the incidence of ischemic events and clinical restenosis, as was evident in the EPIC and EPILOG trials.[43,44] In the EPIC trial, the primary composite points comprised death, reinfarction, bypass surgery, or repeat intervention. Outcomes were assessed at 30 days and 6 months. The composite end-points were reduced by 83% (26% placebo vs 4.5% c7E3 bolus and infusion; P = 0.06). No reinfarctions or repeat urgent interventions occurred in the c7E3 groups at 30 days, although there was a trend toward more deaths in c7E3-treated patients. There was increased bleeding with c7E3 (24% vs 13%; P = 0.28). At 6 months, ischemic events were reduced from 47.8% with placebo to 4.5%o with c7E3 bolus and infusion (P = 0.002). Data from the EPILOG trial also showed markedly reduced risk of ischemic complications in patients undergoing PTCA without increasing the risk of hemorrhage. At 30 days, the composite event rate (death, MI, and urgent revascularization) was 11.7% in the group assigned to placebo with standard dose heparin and 5.5% in the group assigned to GP IIb/IIIa (P < 0.001), and 5.4% in the group assigned to GP IIb/IIIa with standard low dose heparin (P < 0.001). Therewas no significant increase in risk of major bleeding complications. In addition, preliminary data from the European CAPTURE[45] trial demonstrated a reduction in 30-day combined end-points of death, MI, or urgent reinterventions for unstable angina patients treated with ReoPro for 18–24 hours prior to PTCA; this effect was mainly due to CPK level reduction (4.4% vs 9.4% for ReoPro and placebo, respectively). The RAPPORT[46] trial enrolled 483 patients with AMI to receive ReoPro or placebo prior to PTCA. The in-hospital mortality for the whole group was 1.2%, and the total 30-day mortality was 2.7%. There was no intracranial hemmorrhage. Major bleeding occurred in 6%, and 13% had bail-out stenting. These data provided evidence of benefit of GP IIb/IIIa receptor blockade during PTCA in AMI. Oral forms of Gp IIb/IIIa receptor inhibitors are presently being investigated in conjunction with PTCA and stent deployment.

The Role of Stents

Although beneficial in AMI, percutaneous transluminal angioplasty has many limitations; there is an increased incidence of recurrent ischemia, reinfarction rate of 3% to 6% of cases, and reocclusion of the infarct related artery in 5% to 10% of cases. More importantly still is the high rate of restenosis at 6 months from 25% to 50% of cases. The use of ReoPro has been shown to reduce the restenosis rate; however, the cost and risk of vascular complications limit its routine use. Some centers are presently addressing the role of coronary stenting as an option to achieve the beneficial effects of PTCA, but with a reduced rate of associated untoward events. The multicenter PAMI Stent Pilot Study is presently under way, and some of the early data were presented recently by Dr. Cindy Grines at an Interventional Symposium; preliminary results are promising.[47] Analysis of 275 cines of patients undergoing coronary intervention within 12 hours of symptom onset of AMI in the PAMI Stent Pilot Study was presented at the 70th Scientific Session of the American Heart Association (AHA). It was observed that dissections were present in 6.5%, spasm in 0.5%, distal embolization in 1.5%, and no reflow in 0.5%. Stent placement was feasible in 75% of patients with AMI, associated with a very low (12%) residual stenosis, and resulted in TIMI 3 flow in 95% of cases.[48] At the same AHA meeting, Patrick Serruys presented a pilot study data, a preamble to a large randomized trial of 900 patients with AMI presently under way, regarding the feasibility and safety of heparin-coated stents in AMI in 101 patients. No patient received adjunctive lytic therapy, and only three patients received IIb/IIIa receptor inhibitors. Minimal luminal diameter (MLD) post procedure was 2.5 mm with an average residual diameter of stenosis (DS) of 17%. At 6 months, MLD was 1.95 mm with an average DS of 32%.[49] Restenosis at 6 months was 15.3%. Suryapranata et al.[50] conducted a randomized comparison study of primary stenting (S) with primary angioplasty (B) in AMI. A total of 204 patients were randomized. The clinical end-points at 30 days were death, stroke, recurrent MI, and subsequent reintervention. Subacute occlusion occurred in 5% of patients allocated to B, and one patient allocated to S. Three patients in B and one patient in S died. Reinfarction was observed in four patients in B and one patient allocated to S. Target vessel revascularization was necessary in 10 patients after B, and in 2 patients after S (P = 0.0331). The cardiac event-free survival rate of 97% in the S group was significantly higher than the 87% observed in the B group (P = 0.02). This study showed that primary stenting in acute MI can be performed safely, effectively, and can result in reduced composite end-points at 30 days compared to angioplasty.[50] In the FRESCO trial (Florence Randomised Elective Stenting in Acute Coronary Occlusion),[51] a prospective randomized trial, enrolled 150 patients with AMI. Stenting was feasible in all patients. The cumulative 6-month major adverse events (death, re-MI, and reintervention mortality) were significantly lower in the stented group versus the primary angioplasty group (3 vs 15; P = 0.001). The above data demonstrate that stenting of the infarct related artery is not only highly feasible, but is also associated with better clinical outcome than conventional coronary angioplasty.

Intra-aortic Balloon Pump in Acute Myocardial Infarction

High-risk patients presenting with hypotension, tachycardia, or pulmonary edema, usually in association with extensive anterior MI, prior MI, and frequently diabetes, have an expected mortality of 80%. Placement of an intra-aortic balloon pump preintervention will improve overall hemodynamic status during cardiac catheterization, accelerate thrombolysis, potentially limit additional injury to jeopardized myocardium during reperfusion, and enhance coronary patency following angioplasty.[52–54] With adequate blood volume and systemic vascular resistance, a properly timed balloon inflation augments diastolic blood pressure, improving coronary perfusion, while balloon deflation effectively unloads the left ventricle, improving cardiac output and reducing myocardial oxygen demand.[55]

In PAMI-II, high-risk patients were randomized to IABP or no IABP after angioplasty. Unfortunately, patients with cardiogenic shock were excluded. Despite the fact that IABP placement proved to be safe overall with regard to vascular complications, infection, and need for transfusions, there was a slight increase of transient ischemic attacks and strokes. Moreover, IABP placement post-PTCA did not impact the primary end-point of cumulative death, reinfarction, or congestive heart failure.[56] In addition, IABP did not improve left ventricular function determined at predischarge catheterization and at 6 weeks. However, a lower rate of recurrent ischemia was observed. Unfortunately, this study used left ventricular (LV) assist post-reperfusion, while experimental data have suggested that LV assist is most helpful when implemented prior to reperfusion.[57]

Ohman et al.[58] randomized 182 patients post-PTCA within 24 hours of AMI to receive IABP for 48 hours, excluding patients in cardiogenic shock. Cardiac catheterization was performed at a median of 5 days after randomization in 89% in the IABP group and 90% in the control group. Both groups had similar rates of bleeding complications, blood transfusions, and vascular repair or thrombectomy. Patients randomized to IABP had significantly lower rates of reocclusion of the infarct related artery (8% vs 21%; P < 0.03). In addition, there were significantly lower event rates in terms of composite clinical end-points (death, stroke, reinfarction, need for emergency revascularization, or recurrent ischemia: 13% vs 24%; P < 0.04). Once again, however, the maximum potential benefit was not achieved since the IABP was placed after reperfusion.

Angioplasty for Unstable Angina

Unstable angina is characterized by acute coronary ischemia with a high predilection for progression to AMI, if not managed promptly. However, USA is an umbrella syndrome that can be further classified into subgroups with varying prognosis. Patients with rest ischemia and those with post-infarction angina have high mortality and complication rates that may warrant acute intervention both medically and invasively.

In the 1985–1986 NHLBI PTCA registry report,[59] a 5-year follow-up of 857 patients from 15 clinical centers with unstable angina who underwent PTCA, a higher crude mortality rate was observed in patients with post-infarction angina and "acute coronary insufficiency" group (P < 0.05) than for other subsets. There were similar rates of restenosis for all subsets of USA. Complicated failures such as dissections, CABG surgery, or death were also similar in all groups. Therefore, since in-hospital incidence of post-MI in these patients ranges from 18% to 57%,[60–63] and since reported success rates of PTCA in this setting range from 76% to 91% with low complication rates,[64] aggressive interventions are indicated to pacify the unstable active plaque to prevent infarct extension, salvage myocardium, and preserve ventricular function.

The TAUSA trial was conducted to evaluate the adjunctive use of thrombolytics with PTCA for treating rest ischemia.[65] This trial randomized 469 patients undergoing PTCA for rest pain (with or without recent [< 1 month] infarct) to receive intracoronary urokinase (UK) or placebo. Acute closure was higher in the UK arm versus placebo (10.2% vs 4.3%; P < 0.02). Adverse in-hospital events (ischemia, infarction, or emergency CABG) were also increased with UK versus placebo (12.9% vs 6.3%, respectively; P < 0.02). These data suggest that at last some thrombolytics do not mix well with PTCA alone. However, their role in stenting has not been tested.

Future Directions

So what is optimal therapy for AMI? Is it primary intervention or thrombolysis? This article underscores the fact that primary intervention is at least equivalent to thrombolysis and in experienced centers may in fact edge thrombolysis. It is important to note, however, that neither therapy is perfect when instituted alone, and implementation of a series of therapies may be warranted.

Since time to patency of the infarct-related artery is important, interest in prehospital thrombolysis has been rekindled. The feasibility and safety of prehospital thrombolysis have been documented in many studies. The European Myocardial Infarction Project[66] enrolled 5,469 patients in 16 countries in a double-blind, placebo-controlled study using anistreplase and documented 16% reduction in cardiac death and 13% reduction in overall 30-day mortality (P = 0.049 and 0.08, respectively) in favor of the prehospital group. Grijseels et al.[67] conducted a retrospective analysis of 529 patients who received prehospital alteplase or streptokinase demonstrating the feasibility, safety, significant time gain, and excellent long-term prognosis in these patients. The GREAT study[68] was conducted to determine the time saved by administration of thrombolytic therapy at home rather than in the hospital and to assess whether earlier thrombolysis resulted in decreased mortality from AMI. It was a randomized, double-blind parallel-group clinical trial of 311 patients with suspected AMI seen by their general practitioners within 4 hours of symptom onset. These patients were given intravenous anistreplase (30 U) either at home or later, after arrival in the hospital. Anistreplase was given at home or in the hospital at median times of 101 and 240 minutes, respectively, after symptom onset. The median time saved by domiciliary thrombolysis was 130 minutes. By the end of 1 year after trial entry, 17 (10.4%) of 163 patients given anistreplase at home died compared with 32 (21.6%) of 148 in those allotted anistreplase in the hospital (relative reduction 52%, 95% confidence interval 14% to 89%; P = 0.007). In this trial, the time saved by domiciliary thrombolysis by primary care physicians was > 2 hours. It is

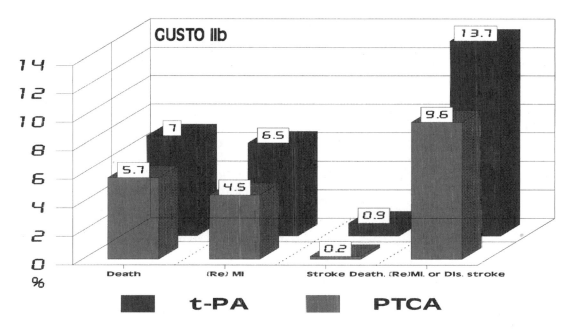

Figure 3. Bar graph showing end-points of Gusto IIb direct angioplasty substudy. See text for details.

likely that a similar time saving would be achieved if prehospital thrombolysis were to become an established practice. Prehospital thrombolysis resulted in a halving of the mortality rate from AMI.

In the USA, the IPTARS study, a placebo-controlled multicenter trial to assess prehospital thrombolysis with r-Pa followed by urgent angiography and stenting is presently being planned. However, as mentioned earlier, it is less likely that thrombolysis alone, even when administered to AMI patients en route to the hospital, will be adequate therapy to achieve TIMI 3 flow and maintain long-term coronary patency in the majority of these patients. An analysis of GUSTO III patients with early angiography demonstrated high TIMI 3 flow at 90 minutes, but also revealed a trend toward higher reocclusion rates beyond 24 hours in patients receiving r-Pa. In addition, a study by Van Belle et al. using coronary angioscopy revealed persistent coronary thrombus on ulcerated plaques in the infarct-related artery in the majority of patients evaluated by angiography up to 30

days after thrombolysis for AMI.[69]

Therefore, based on available data, it appears that optimal therapy for AMI will likely be a series of therapies. Prehospital thrombolysis with second or third generation lytics, perhaps in a reduced dose to reduce the risk of intracranial bleeding that can be administered by experienced EMS personnel, should be instituted early prior to patient arrival to the emergency room (ER). On arrival to the ER, the patient should be taken to the cardiac catheterization laboratory and should undergo stenting of the infarct-related artery to passivate the active plaque and ensure long-term patency. Intravenous agents that block GP IIb/IIIa may be beneficial acutely as well, but oral IIb/IIIa blockers may need to be administered for at least another month to reduce the risk of rethrombosis.

Conclusion

Achieving prompt reperfusion in patients presenting with acute coronary occlusion and maintaining TIMI 3 flow is the main goal of modern therapy for MI. Thrombolytic therapy results in angiographic coronary artery patency of 70% to 80%. However, TIMI 3 flow is observed in 50% to 60% of cases only. Primary angioplasty/stenting is an attractive alternative to thrombolysis due to high coronary patency and TIMI 3 flow rates, and improved clinical outcome in terms of reinfarction and mortality, as well as reduced risk of intracranial bleeding in experienced centers. The use of stents in these syndromes combined with aspirin and ticlopidine (and possibly GP IIb/IIIa inhibitors) is particularly attractive and may lead to much better late outcomes. Left ventricular assist devices may be especialiy useful in patients who present late in their course with borderline hemodynamics. However, in order to achieve the most benefit from LV assistance, it should be instituted prior to restoring coronary perfusion.

References

1. American Heart Association: Heart Facts. Dallas, TX, American Heart Association National Center, 1987.
2. DeWood MA, Spores J, Notchke R, et al. Prevalence of total coronary occlusion during the early hours of transmural myocardial infarction. N Engl J Med 1980;303:897-902.
3. Reimer KA, Jennings RB. The "wave front phenomenon" of myocardial ischemic cell death. II. Transmural progression of necrosis within the framework of ischemic bed size, (myocardium at risk) and collateral flow. Lab Invest 1979;40:633-644.
4. Reimer KA, Lowe JE, Rasmussen MM, et al. The "wavefront phenomenon" of ischemic cell death. I. Myocardial size vs duration of coronary occlusion in dogs. Circulation 1977;56:786-793.
5. Theroux P, Ross J Jr, Kemper WS, et al. Coronary arterial reperfusion. III. Early and late effects on regional myocardial function and dimensions in conscious dogs. Am J Cardiol 1976;38:599-606.
6. Rentrop KP, Feit F, Blanke H, et al. Effects of intracoronary streptokinase and intracoronary nitroglycerin infusion on coronary angiographic patterns and mortality in patients with acute myocardial infarction. N Engl J Med 1984;311:1457-1463.
7. Feld S, Li G, Amirian J, et al. Enhanced thrombolysis, reduced coronary reocclusion and limitation of infarct size with liposomal prostaglandin E_1 in a canine thrombolysis model. JACC 1994;24:1382-1390.
8. Kelly MJ, Thompson PL, Quinlan MF. Prognostic significance of left ventricular ejection fraction after acute myocardial infarction: A bedside radionuclide study. Br Heart J 1985;53:16-24.
9. Shah PK, Pichler M, Berman DS, et al. Left ventricular ejection fraction determined by radionuclide ventriculography in early stages of first transmural myocardial infarction: Relation to short term prognosis. Am J Cardiol 1980;45:542-546.
10. Saeger P, Perlmuher R, Rosenfeld L, et al. Thrombolysis decreases sudden death and arrhythmogenic potential after anterior myocardial infarction with aneurysm formation. Circulation 1987;76(Suppl.):IV-261.
11. Hochman JS, Choo H. Limitation of myocardial infarct expansion by reperfusion independent of myocardial salvage. Circulation 1987;75:299-306.
12. Topol EJ, Califf RM, Vandormeal M, et al. A randomized trial of late reperfusion therapy for acute myocardial infarction. Circulation 1992;85:2090-2099.
13. The GUSTO Angiographic Investigators. The effects of tissue plasminogen activator, streptokinase, or both on coronary artery patency, ventricular function, and survival after acute myocardial infarction. N Engl J Med 1993;329:1615-1622.
14. Anderson JL, Karagounis LA, Becker LC, et al. TIMI perfusion grade 3 but not 2 results in improved outcome after thrombolysis for myocardial infarction. Ventriculographic, enzymatic, and electrocardiographic evidence from the TEAM-3 study. Circulation 1993;87:1829-1839.
15. Belenkie I, Thompson CR, Manyari DE,

et al. Importance of effective, early and sustained reperfusion during acute myocardial infarction. Am J Cardiol 1989; 63:912-916.

16. Gruppo Italiano per lo Studio della Streptochinasi nell'Infarto Miocardico (GISSI). Effectiveness of intravenous thrombolytic treatment in acute myocardial infarction. Lancet 1986;I:397-401.

17. ISIS-2 (Second International Study of Infarct Survival) Collaborative Group: Randomised trial of intravenous streptokinase, oral aspirin, both, or neither among 17,187 cases of suspected acute myocardial infarction: ISIS-2. Lancet 1988;II:349-360.

18. Neuhaus KL, von Essen, Tebbe U. et al. Improved thrombolysis in acute myocardial infarction with front loaded administration of alteplase: Results of the r-tPA-APSAC patency study (TAPS). JACC 1992;19:885-891.

19. Califf RM. Thrombolytic therapy. New standards of care. Part 1. The science of plasminogen activators. Continuing education series.

20. Smalling RW, Bode C, Kalbfleisch J, et al. More rapid, complete and stable coronary thrombolysis with bolus administration of reteplase compared with alteplase infusion in acute myocardial infarction. Circulation 1995;91:2725-2732.

21. Smalling RW, Bode C, Kalbfleisch J, et al. Improvement of global and regional LV-function by the bolus administration of recombinant plasminogen activator (r-PA) in acute myocardial infarction: A comparison with standard dose alteplase. (abstract) Circulation 1994; 90(Suppl. I):1-562.

22. International Joint Efficacy Comparison of Thrombolytics. Randomised, double blind comparison of reteplase double bolus administration with streptokinase in acute myocardial infarction (INJECT): Trial to investigate equivalence. Lancet 1995;346:320-336.

23. GU5TO 3. A comparison of reteplase with alteplase for acute myocardial infarction. N Engl J Med 1997;337:1118-1123.

24. Cannon CP, McCabe CH, Gibson CM, et al. TNK-tissue plasminogen activator in acute myocardial infarction. Results on the Thrombolysis in Myocardial Infarction (TIMI) 10A dose ranging trial. Circulation 1997;21:95:351-356.

25. Preliminary data of ASSENT I were presented at the 70th scientific session of the American Heart Association, November 1997.

26. Kohnert U, Rudolph R, Verheijen JH, et al. Biochemical properties of the Kringle 2 and protease domains are maintained in the refolded t-PA deletion variant BM 06.022. Protein Eng 1992;5.93-100.

27. Hu CK, Kohnert Ü, Sturzebecher J, et al. Complexation of the tissue plasminogen activator protease with benzamidine-inhibitors: Interference by the Kringle 2 module. Biochemistry 1996; 35:3270-3276.

28. Liao WC, Beierle FA, Stoufer BC, et al. Single bolus regimen of lanoteplase (nPA) in acute myocardial infarction: Pharmakokinetic evaluation from in-TIME 1 study. Circulation 1997;96:I-260.

29. Rothbaum DA, Linnemeier TJ, Landin RJ, et al. Emergency percutaneous coronary angioplasty in acute myocardial infarction: A three year experience. JACC 1987;10:264-272.

30. Stack RS, O'Conner CM, Mark KDB, et al. Coronary perfusion during acute myocardial infarction with a combined therapy of coronary angioplasty and high dose intravenous streptokinase. Circulation 1988;77:151-161.

31. Berger PB, Bell MR, Holmes DR Jr, et al. Time to reperfusion with direct coronary angioplasty and thrombolytic therapy in acute myocardial infarction. Am J Cardiol 1994;73:231-236.

32. de Boer JM, Noorntje JCA, Ottervanger JP, et al. Immediate coronary angioplasty versus intravenous streptokinase in acute myocardial infarction: Left ventricular ejection fraction, hospital mortality and reinfarction. JACC 1994;23:1004-1008.

33. O'Neill WW, Brodie BR, Ivanhoe R, et al. Primary coronary angioplasty for acute myocardial infarction (the Primary Angioplasty registry). Am J Cardiol 1994;73:627-634.

34. Ellis S. Gusto IIB angioplasty substudy. A clinical trial comparing primary coronary angioplasty with tissue plasminogen activator for acute myocardial infarction. N Engl J Med 1997;336:1621-1628.

35. Eckman MH, Wong JB, Salem DN, et al. Direct angioplasty for acute myocardial infarction; A review of outcomes in

clinical subsets. Ann Intern Med 1992; 117:667-676.

36. Every NR, Parsons LS, Hlatky M, et al. A comparison of thrombolytic therapy with primary coronary angioplasty for acute myocardial infarction. Myocardial Infarction Triage and Intervention Investigators. N Engl J Med 1996;335: 1253-1260.

37. Topol EJ, Califf RM, George BS, et al. A randomised trial of immediate versus elective angioplasty after intravenous tissue plasminogen activator in acute myocardial infarction. N Engl J Med 1987;317:581-588.

38. Simoons ML, Betriu A, Col J, et al. Thrombolysis with tissue plasminogen activator in acute myocardial infarction: No additional benefit from immediate percutaneous coronary angioplasty. Lancet 1988;1:197-202.

39. The TIMI Research Group. Immediate versus delayed catheterization and angioplasty following thrombolytic therapy for acute myocardial infarction. JAMA 1988;260:2849-2858.

40. Gibson CM, Cannon CP, Piana RN, et al. Rescue PTCA in the TIMI 4 trial. JACC 1994;1A-484A:225A.

41. Wnęk A, Krupa H, Gasior M, et al. Results of rescue angioplasty after unsuccessful intracoronary streptokinase therapy in patients with acute myocardial infarction. Eur Heart J 1995; 16(Suppl.):125.

42. Ellis SG, Ribeiro da Silva E, Heyndrickx G, et al. Randomised comparison of rescue angioplasty with conservative management of patients with early failure of thrombolysis for acute anterior myocardial infarction. Circulation 1994;90:2280-2284.

43. Lefkovits J, Ivanhoe RJ, Califf RM, et al. Effects of platelet glycoprotein IIb/IIIa receptor blockade by a chimeric monoclonal antibody (Abciximab) on acute and six-month outcomes after percutaneous transluminal angioplasty for acute myocardial infarction. Am J Cardiol 1996;77:1045-1050.

44. The EPILOG Investigators. Platelet glycoprotein IIb/IIIa receptor blockade and low-dose heparin during percutaneous coronary revascularization. N Engl J Med 1997;336:1689-1696.

45. Simoons M. The CAPTURE study, as presented at the 45th Annual Session of The American College of Cardiology in Orlando, Fla, USA, March 1996.

46. Brener SJ, Barr LA, Burchenal J, et al. A randomised, placebo controlled trial of Abciximab with primary angioplasty for acute MI. The RAPPORT trial. Circulation 1997;96(Suppl.):I-473.

47. Grines CL. Aggressive intervention for myocardial infarction: Angioplasty, stents, and intra-aortic balloon pumping. Am J Cardiol 1996;78(Suppl. 3A): 29-34.

48. Abizaid AS, Stone GW, Rothbaum DA, et al. Quantitative angiographic outcomes for stenting in acute myocardial infarction: Core lab analysis from the PAMI stent pilot study. Circulation 1997;96(Suppl.): I-327.

49. Serruys PW, Garcia-Fernandez E, Kiemeney F, et al. Stenting in acute MI: A pilot study as preamble to a randomised trial comparing balloon angioplasty and stenting. Circulation 1997; 96(Suppl.):I-326.

50. Suryapranata H, Hoorntje JC, de Boer MJ, et al. Randomised comparison of primary stenting with primary balloon angioplasty in acute myocardial infarction. Circulation 1997;96(Suppl.):I-327.

51. Antoniucci D, Santoro GM, Bolognese L, et al. A prospective randomised trial of elective stenting in acute myocardial infarction-Preliminary results of the FRESCO study. (Florence Randomised Elective Stenting in Acute Coronary Occlusion). Circulation 1997; 96(Suppl.):I-327.

52. Ohman EM, Califf RM, George BS, et al. The use of intraaortic balloon pumping as an adjunct to reperfusion therapy in acute myocardial infarction. Am Heart J 1991;121:895-901.

53. Smalling RW, Cassidy DB, Barrett R, et al. Improved regional myocardial blood flow, left ventricular unloading, and infarct salvage using an axial-flow, transvalvular, left ventriciular assist device. A comparison with intra-aortic balloon counterpulsation and reperfusion alone in a canine infarction model. Circulation 1992;85:1152-1159.

54. Smalling RW. The use of mechanical assist devices in the management of cardiogenic shock secondary to acute myocardial infarction. Tex Heart Inst J 1991;18:275-281.

55. Feld S, Kjellgren O, Smalling RW. Aggressive interventional treatment of acute myocardial infarction; Lessons from the animal laboratory applied to the catheterization suite. Cardiology 1995;86:365-373.

56. Grines CL, Brodie BR, Griffin JJ, et al. Prophylactic intraaortic balloon pumping for acute myocardial infarction does not improve left ventricular function. JACC 1996;27(Suppl. A):167.

57. Allen BS, Okamoto F, Buckberg GD, et al. Studies of controlled reperfusion after ischemia. XIII. Reperfusion conditions: Critical importance of total ventricular decompression during regional reperfusion. J Thorac Cardiovasc Surg 1986;92:605-612.

58. Ohman ME, George BS, White CJ, et al. Use of aortic counterpulsation to improve sustained coronary artery patency during acute myocardial infarction. Circulation 1994;90:792-799.

59. Bentivoglio LG, Detre K, Yeh W, et al. Outcome of percutaneous transluminal coronary angioplasty in subsets of unstable angina pectoris: A report of the National Heart, Lung, and Blood Institute Percutaneous Transluminal Coronary Angioplasty Registry. JACC 1994;24:1195-1206.

60. Stenson RE, Flamm MD, Zaret BL, et al. Transient ST segment elevation with post myocardial infarction angina: Prognostic significance. Am Heart J 1975;89:449-454.

61. Fraker TD, Wagner GS, Rosati RA. Extention of myocardial infarction: Incidence and prognosis. Circulation 1979;60:1126-1129.

62. Schuster EH, Bulkley BH. Early postinfarction angina: Ischemia at a distance and ischemia in the infarct zone. N Engl J Med 1981;305:110-115.

63. Gibson RS, Beller GA, Gheorghiade M, et al. The prevelance and clinical significance of myocardial ischemia 2 weeks after uncomplicated non Q wave infarction: A prospective natural history study. Circulation 1986;73:1186-1189.

64. de Feyter PJ, Serruys PW, vd Brand M, et al. Percutaneous transluminal coronary angioplasty for unstable angina. Am J Cardiol 1991;68:125B-135B.

65. Ambrose JA, Almeida OD, Sharma SK, et al. Adjunctive thrombolytic therapy during angioplasty for ischemic rest angina. Results of the TAUSA Trial. Circulation 1994;90:69-77.

66. Boissel JP. The European Myocardial Infarction Project: An assessment of pre-hospital thrombolysis. Int J Cardiol 1995;49(Suppl.):S29-S37.

67. Grijseels EW, Bouten MJ, Lenderink T, et al. Pre-hospital thrombolytic therapy with either alteplase or streptokinase. Practical applications, complications, and long term results in 529 patients. Eur Heart J 1995;16:1833-1838.

68. Rawles J. Halving of mortality at 1 year by domiciliary thrombolysis in the Grampian Region Early Anistreplase Trial (GREAT). JACC 1994;23:1-5.

69. Van Belle E, Lablanche JM, Bauters C, et al. Coronary angioscopic findings in the infarct-related vessel within 1 month of acute myocardial infarction. Natural history and the effect of thrombolysis. Circulation 1998;97:26-33.

Chapter 16

The Primary Angioplasty in Myocardial Infarction Studies: An Overview

Cindy L. Grines, M.D., FACC*, Gregg W. Stone, M.D., FACC,[†] and William W. O'Neill, M.D., FACC*

From the *Division of Cardiology, William Beaumont Hospital, Royal Oak, Michigan; and the [†]Division of Cardiology, El Camino Hospital, Mountain View, California

Introduction

The purpose of the Primary Angioplasty in Myocardial Infarction (PAMI) study group is to conduct high quality scientific research with a specific focus on mechanical reperfusion strategies in acute myocardial infarction (MI). Our research ideas and hypotheses originate from joint collaboration of practicing physicians, and not the medical device or pharmaceutical industries. Specific objectives have included determination of the best methods of achieving high rates of normal coronary flow and low rates of reocclusion, determining the safest and most cost-effective reperfusion strategy, and how to effectively deliver acute MI treatments to patients regardless of their geographical location.

PAMI-1

Observational trials had demonstrated that primary percutaneous transluminal coronary angioplasty (PTCA) was associated with early patency rates exceeding 90%, and low rates of intracranial bleeding, recurrent ischemia and death.[1] However, randomized trials of primary PTCA compared to thrombolytic therapy were necessary to determine which reperfusion strategy was superior. The PAMI-1 study involved 12 clinical centers that enrolled 395 patients within 12 hours of the onset of MI.[2] Patients were treated with intravenous heparin and aspirin, then randomly assigned to undergo PTCA as the primary reperfusion strategy (without previous thrombolytic therapy) or to receive intravenous tissue plasminogen activator (tPA) followed up by conservative care (Fig. 1). Among the patients randomly assigned to PTCA, all patients underwent catheterization, and in 90%, anatomy was appropriate for angioplasty. The PTCA success rate was 97%, and no patient required emergency coronary artery bypass surgery. In-hospital mortality rates in the PTCA and tPA groups were 2.6% and 6.5%, respectively (P = 0.06). In patients classified as "not low risk" (age > 70 years, anterior MI or admission heart rate > 100 beats per minute), mortality rates in PTCA and tPA groups

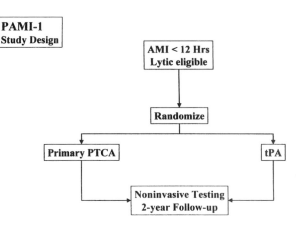

Figure 1. PAMI-1 study design algorithm.

* Primary Endpoint: Combined death or recurrent MI

were 2.0% and 10.4%, respectively (P = 0.01). As demonstrated in Figure 2, the primary end point of in-hospital reinfarction or death occurred in 5.1% of patients treated with PTCA and 12% of patients treated with tPA (P = 0.02). Intracranial bleeding occurred less frequently among patients who received PTCA (0% vs 2.0%, P = 0.05). Recurrent ischemia (including reinfarction) occurred in 10.3% of patients treated with PTCA compared to 28% of patients treated with tPA (P < 0.001). Therefore, primary PTCA reduced the combined occurrence of nonfatal reinfarction or death and was associated with a lower rate of intracranial bleeding, recurrent ischemia, and a shorter length of hospital stay compared to tPA therapy.

To determine long-term event rates, PAMI-1 patients were reevaluated at 1 month, 6 months, 1 year and 2 years.[3] At 2 years' follow-up, patients randomized to primary PTCA had reduced rates of recurrent ischemia (36.4% vs 48% for tPA patients, P = 0.026) and reintervention (27.2% vs 46.5%, P < 0.0001). The combined primary end point of death or reinfarction was significantly reduced in PTCA-treated patients (14.9% vs 23% for tPA patients, P = 0.034). Therefore, the initial benefit of primary angioplasty appeared to be maintained over a 2-year follow-up with improved infarct-free survival and reduced reintervention rate.

Primary PTCA has been criticized on the theoretical basis that it may be more expensive than thrombolysis. To determine the relative cost-effectiveness of the two treatment strategies, we obtained detailed in-hospital charge data from all patients randomized in the PAMI-1 trial who were recruited within the United States.[4] Patients

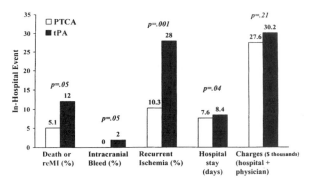

Figure 2. PAMI-1 events during the index hospital admission.

treated with primary PTCA in the United States had lower in-hospital rates of death (2.3% vs 7.2%, P = 0.03), reinfarction (2.8% vs 7.2%, P = 0.06), death or reinfarction (5.1% vs 13.3%, P = 0.008), and recurrent ischemia (11.3% vs 28.7%, P = 0.0001). Despite the initial cost of cardiac catheterization in all patients with invasive strategy, the total mean hospital charges were $3,436 lower per patient treated with PTCA compared to tPA (P = 0.04), primarily due to the reduction in adverse in-hospital outcomes. However, professional fees were higher after primary PTCA, and thus total charges, although favoring PTCA, were not significantly different ($27,653 ± $13,709 vs $30,227 ± $18,903, P = 0.21). At a mean follow-up time of 2.1 ± 7 years, no major differences in postdischarge events or functional class were present between PTCA- and tPA-treated patients, suggesting similar late resource consumption. Thus, given the greater clinical benefit with similar cost, primary PTCA appears to be more cost-effective than intravenous thrombolysis. Moreover, the potential to acutely risk stratify patients and discharge low risk patients early has subsequently made the relative cost even more favorable for primary PTCA (See PAMI-2 trial, below).

We found that development of recurrent ischemia adversely affected patient outcome and increased morbidity, mortality, and resource utilization.[5] To determine the predictors of recurrent ischemia during the index hospitalization, sixteen clinical variables were examined in a multiple logistic regression analysis. Treatment with PTCA rather than tPA was the strongest predictor of freedom from recurrent ischemia (P < 0.0001). The only other significant predictor was an admission Killip class of ≥ 2, (P = 0.026). Although the incidence of recurrent ischemia after angioplasty and tPA was similar within the first two days of admission (9.2% vs 14.5%, P = 0.11), after the second hospital day recurrent ischemia occurred in only 1.1% of patients who received primary PTCA compared to 13.5% of patients treated with tPA (P < 0.0001).

Given the fact that recurrent ischemia was uncommon after the second hospital stay in patients treated with primary PTCA, we speculated that early discharge on day 3 could be feasible in selected patients treated with primary PTCA. This hypothesis was to be tested in the PAMI-2 trial.

PAMI-1

Subgroup Analyses. In some hospitals, primary PTCA may not be uniformly applied to all patients. Therefore, we performed several subgroup analyses to determine which patients benefit the most from primary PTCA.

Anterior MI patients are known to have a higher mortality risk than those with inferior MI, and thus may have a greater benefit from PTCA.[6] Among the 138 patients with anterior MI in the PAMI-1 trial, in-hospital mortality was significantly reduced by treatment with PTCA compared to tPA (1.4% vs 11.9%, P = 0.01). The benefit of primary PTCA was confirmed by multivariate analysis and interaction testing. Although the in-hospital mortality in patients with inferior MI was similar between PTCA and tPA treated groups, even low risk, inferior MI patients who were treated with primary PTCA experienced a reduced rate of recurrent ischemia (9.7% vs 27.8%, P = 0.0002), fewer unscheduled catheterization and revascularization procedures, and a shorter hospital stay (7.0 vs 8.6 days, P = 0.01).

Women have an increased risk of intracranial bleeding and early and late morbidity and mortality following treatment for MI compared to men. The 107 women enrolled in the PAMI-1 trial were found to be older and to have a higher prevalence of diabetes, hypertension, and congestive heart failure presented later after symptom onset compared with the 288 men.[7] Although the in-hospital mortality was 3.3-fold higher than men (9.3% vs 2.8%, P = 0.0005), after adjustment for comorbidities, only advanced age independently correlated with mortality. Among patients treated with tPA, mortality was significantly higher in women than in men, as was the rate of intracranial hemorrhage (5.3% vs 0.7%, P = 0.037). In contrast, women and men had similar in-hospital mortality after primary PTCA (4.0% vs 2.1%, P = 0.46), and no intracranial bleeding occurred in PTCA-treated patients. By multiple logistic regression analysis of 15 clinical variables, a younger age and treatment with PTCA rather than tPA were independently predictive of in-hospital survival in women. Thus, primary PTCA may be ideally suited to women with acute MI, with reduced rates of death and intracranial bleeding.

Thrombolytic ineligibility results in up to 75% of MI patients being excluded from reperfusion therapy. Current recommendations have suggested expanding the eligibility criteria for thrombolytic therapy to allow more patients to benefit from reperfusion. However, these recommendations may also increase the complication rate of thrombolytic therapy. In the PAMI-1 trial, all patients were thrombolytic eligible based on expanded criteria; however, 151 patients would have had contraindications for thrombolytic therapy based on former restrictive criteria (age > than 70 years, symptom duration > 4 hours, or prior bypass surgery).[8] In-hospital mortality was higher in patients with former thrombolytic contraindications, compared to thrombolytic-eligible patients (8.6% vs 2.0%, P =

0.002). When patients with former thrombolytic contraindications were treated with primary PTCA compared to tPA, in-hospital mortality (2.9% vs 13.2%, P = 0.025) and 6-month mortality rates (2.9% vs 15.7%, P = 0.009) were significantly reduced. By logistic regression analysis, treatment with PTCA rather than tPA was the strongest predictor of survival in these patients. Thrombolytic-eligible patients treated with tPA and PTCA had similar in-hospital mortality (1.7% vs 2.4%, P = NS). Therefore, patients with conditions formerly contraindicating thrombolytic therapy constitute a high risk group with significant morbidity and mortality after thrombolysis. Our data suggest that these patients may benefit from preferential management with primary PTCA without antecedent thrombolysis. Figure 3 summarizes late outcome emphasizing the durability of these effects.

Paradoxically, smokers who present with an acute MI have been reported to have a favorable prognosis compared to nonsmokers. Given the hypercoagulable state and less atherosclerotic burden, smokers may have a more thrombotic lesion with the potential for better response to thrombolytic therapy. To evaluate this issue, we stratified patients who were current smokers and those who had never smoked.[9] In smokers, the treatment strategy did not significantly affect in-hospital outcomes. However, nonsmokers appeared to have more benefit from PTCA, with a lower frequency of death and nonfatal MI (7% vs 18%, P = 0.05), in-

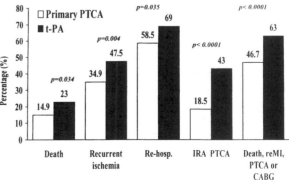

Figure 3. PAMI-1 long-term follow-up. The initial benefit of primary PTCA over tPA is sustained over 2 years, with improved infarct free survival and a reduced rate of reintervention. PTCA 5 percutaneous transluminal coronary angiography; tPA 5 tissue plasminogen activator.

hospital ischemia (11% vs 33%, P = 0.004), or the combined event (13% vs 40%, P = 0.001), compared to tPA. This observation may reflect the ability of angioplasty to achieve a high reperfusion rate, even in nonsmokers who have a predominantly atherosclerotic occlusion that may not respond favorably to thrombolysis.

TX:In the PAMI-1 study, we proved that primary PTCA was superior to thrombolysis. We then moved on to investigate methods of reducing cost and improving prognosis using primary PTCA as the reperfusion strategy. Few data existed regarding the need for intensive care unit admission, noninvasive testing, and the appropriate length of stay after reperfusion of MI patients at low clinical risk. Conversely, high-risk MI patients have a poor prognosis despite reperfusion therapy. Since the majority of deaths occur within the first 48 hours, risk stratification and therapeutic interventions ideally should occur acutely. The PAMI-2 study prospectively evaluated the hypotheses that emergency catheterization could acutely risk stratify MI patients, that early discharge on day 3 is safe and cost-effective in low risk patients treated with PTCA, and that intraaortic balloon pump (IABP) counterpulsation could improve clinical outcomes and reduce reocclusion in high risk patients.[10-13]

Thirty-four clinical sites from five countries recruited 1,100 MI patients into the PAMI-2 study (Fig. 4), making PAMI-2 the largest multicenter primary PTCA experi-ence to date. Patients who presented within the first 12 hours of symptom duration underwent emergency catheterization, with PTCA when appropriate. Patients were then stratified into low risk (age ≤ 70, ejection fraction [EF] > 45%, 1-2 vessel disease, successful PTCA of a native coronary artery, and the absence of persistent arrhythmias after reperfusion) or high risk groups. Low risk patients were randomized to accelerated care (admission to a nonintensive care unit, 48 hours full-dose heparin followed by 12 hours half-dose heparin, no noninvasive testing, and discharge on day 3) or traditional care. High risk patients were randomized to IABP for 36 to 48 hours versus no balloon pump, with predischarge catheterization performed to determine infarct vessel patency and ventricular function.

Among the 1,100 patients enrolled, primary PTCA was performed in 89% (with an angiographic success rate of 96.1%), primary bypass surgery in 5%, and medical therapy alone in 6%. Based on the PAMI-2 definition of risk, we identified high and low risk groups (5.5% and 0.3% mortality, P = 0.0001). To determine whether the catheterization was necessary to acutely risk stratify, the prognostic importance of clinical and catherization variables was analyzed. Reinfarction was predicted only by catherization variables (EF < 45%, P < 0.001 or suboptimal PTCA, P = 0.009). The multivariable predictors of the combined end point (death, heart failure, reinfarction, stroke), were age > 70 years, lytic ineligible, heart

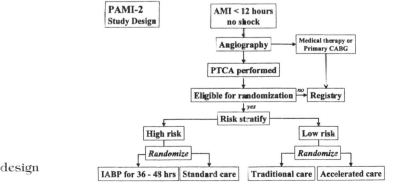

Figure 4. PAMI-2 study design algorithm.

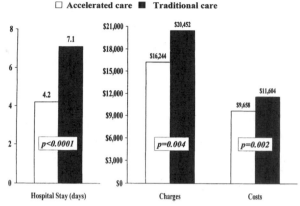

☐ Accelerated care ■ Traditional care

Figure 5. PAMI-2 low risk strata. Low risk patients randomized to accelerated care (omission of intensive care unit and noninvasive testing with discharge on day 3) were discharged on average 3 days earlier with resultant cost savings.

rate > 100, Killip class > 1, acute EF < 45% and final thrombolysis in myocardial infarction (TIMI) flow 0-1. Even after accounting for the "best" clinical predictors, catherization variables identified patients who were 2.8 times more likely to have an event. Thus, the acute catherization provides prognostic information (beyond what can be determined clinically), and the ability to triage MI patients to the appropriate therapies, resulting in a low overall mortality.[12]

In PAMI-2, 908 patients were randomized (471 patients in the low risk strata, 437 patients in the high risk strata). One hundred ninety-two patients were not randomized, but followed in the registry. Low risk patients randomized to accelerated care had similar in-hospital outcomes (death

0.4% vs 0.4%, reinfarction 0.4% vs 0.4%) but were discharged 3 days earlier (4.2 vs 7.1 days, P < 0.0001) with reduced hospital costs of $2,000 (P = 0.002), compared to the traditional care group (Fig. 5). At 6 months, accelerated and traditional care groups had similar rates of death (0.8% vs 0.4%, P = 0.38), unstable ischemia, reinfarction, stroke, heart failure, or the combined occurrence (15.6% vs 17.5%, P = 0.58). Within the low risk group, we identified a cohort of 150 patients who were "ultra low risk" (age < 60 years, single vessel disease, residual stenosis < 30% with TIMI-3 flow, and no thrombus or dissection after primary PTCA).[14] The hospital course in these patients was so benign (Table 1), that they were potentially eligible for discharge at 48

Table 1

Comparison of Pami-2 Ultra Low Risk Patients to the Remaining Low Risk Group

End Point	ULR* (N = 150)	Other Low Risk (N = 309)	P
Death	0.0%	0.65%	0.32
Reinfarction	0.67%	3.88%	0.05
Reocclusion	0.67%	4.21%	0.03
CVA/TIA	0	1.09%	0.11
CHF	0.67%	3.88%	0.05
Combined	1.33%	8.74%	0.002

* ULR = Ultra Low Risk.
Age ≤ 60, single vessel disease, residual stenosis < 30% with TIMI-3 flow and no thrombus or dissection after primary PTCA.

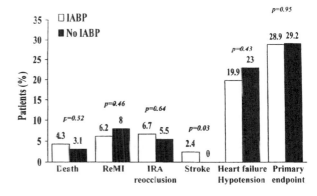

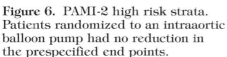

Figure 6. PAMI-2 high risk strata. Patients randomized to an intraaortic balloon pump had no reduction in the prespecified end points.

hours. Based on these data in low risk patients, in the absence of clinical contraindications, early discharge without noninvasive testing appears to be safe and cost-effective.

Among patients stratified as high risk, prophylactic placement of an IABP following the angioplasty procedure proved to be of little benefit with regard to clinical events of death, reinfarction, reocclusion, congestive heart failure, or the primary combined end point (Figure 6).[10,11] In addition, there was a slight increase in strokes in patients randomized to IABP. This may have been due to preexisting conditions in some patients; nonetheless, it was disturbing. EF improvement over 1 week was similar in IABP and non-IABP groups (2.6% vs 2.2%). Moreover, there were no differences in infarct zone function at 1 week, or resting and exercise EF measured at 1 month. Balloon pumping did, however, reduce the incidence of recurrent ischemia requiring repeat catheterization. However, this was not a primary end point of the trial, and since ischemia was readily treated, "hard" events remained similar for the two groups. Based on these data, we reserve IABP use for patients with hemodynamic compromise or ongoing ischemia.

PAMI-2

Subgroup Analyses. To help answer clinically relevant questions, we also performed several analyses in the PAMI-2 database. It has been suggested that primary PTCA for acute MI is applicable only for a small number of experienced, high volume PTCA centers. We determined the impact of operator and institutional volume on procedural outcome and hospital course in PAMI-2.[15] Centers were divided based on overall yearly volume (low ≤ 500, medium 501-1,000, high > 1,000); operators were similarly divided (low ≤ 75, medium 76-200, high > 200). Angioplasty success, emergency bypass for failed PTCA, reinfarction, and mortality rates did not differ between any groups. This demonstrates that among sites motivated enough to participate in the trial and willing to perform primary PTCA "the PAMI way," high success and low complication rates can be achieved, irrespective of operator or institutional volume.

Primary PTCA is limited by logistical difficulties and time delays in mobilizing on-call teams during off hours. Subsequently, many hospital have adopted the approach of performing primary PTCA during the day and giving thrombolytics in the evening. In PAMI-2, 470 patients were randomized during evening and weekends (off-shift), and 434 patients were treated during usual business hours.[16] No differences in age, gender, or risk stratification were apparent between on- and off-shift patients. As expected, the time from emergency room (ER) arrival to angiography was delayed during the off-shift (130 vs 95 min, P = 0.00001). However, PTCA success

(98% vs 98%) and catherization lab complications i.e., arrhythmias, hypotension, etc., were similar between on- and off-shifts. Furthermore, the combined end point of death, reinfarction, stroke, or heart failure occurred with similar frequencies (15.7% vs 12.6%, P = 0.18) in on- and off-shift treated patients. Although use of primary PTCA during off hours is associated with greater delay, these data suggest that the delay in mobilizing the catherization lab and the potential for operator fatigue do not affect PTCA success, complications, or clinical outcome.

For primary PTCA to be widely applied, patients must be transferred to hospitals with catherization lab facilities, necessitating inherent delays in reperfusion. To study the effect of delayed presentation on mortality after PTCA, we examined the PAMI-2 database.[17] Outcomes stratified by the time from chest pain onset to ER arrival appear in Table 2. By multivariate analysis, the strongest correlates of survival were age and restoration of TIMI-3 flow; mortality was 2.0% with TIMI-3 flow versus 12.7% with TIMI 0-2 flow (P < 0.001). In contrast, there was no difference in the mean time from chest pain to ER time in survivors versus nonsurvivors (146 ± 144 vs 157 ± 151 mins, P = 0.66). Unlike thrombolysis, patients who present late achieve high patency rates and have excellent survival when managed by primary PTCA. The low mortality rate after primary PTCA is primarily dependent on the high rate of TIMI-3 flow achieved rather than the rapidity of treatment. These data suggest that the time

delay inherent in transferring patients to tertiary centers for primary PTCA may not be prohibitive, and that randomized trials are warranted.

Studies of acute PTCA of infarct vessels after successful thrombolysis have shown no benefit and a trend toward increased complications. This lack of benefit may have been due to dilation of insignificant (60%) stenoses, increased platelet aggregation due to thrombolytics, or the fact that these studies did not pretreat patients with aspirin, used low doses of heparin, did not monitor activated clotting times (ACTs), and utilized nonionic contrast (which has more clotting potential than ionic agents). In PAMI-2, angioplasty was performed avoiding these potential sources of complications. Infarct vessels were dilated if they had < TIMI-2 flow or patent with > 70% stenosis, at operator discretion. Vessels were patent on the first angiogram in 219 patients (20%), and we performed an analysis to determine the outcome.[18] PTCA was performed on 154 (70%) with a 95% success rate; 1 (0.6%) required emergency bypass for PTCA failure. Of the 200 patients with > 70% stenosis of patent infarct-related arteries (IRAs), there was no significant difference between groups with or without PTCA in recurrent ischemic events (19.5% vs 15.2%), reinfarction (2.6% vs 4.3%), repeat catherization ± PTCA (5.8% vs 2.2%), coronary artery bypass graft (CABG) for recurrent ischemia or failed PTCA (3.2% vs 4.4%), or in-hospital death (3.9 vs 6.5%). Therefore, primary PTCA of patent IRAs was performed safely, with

Table 2.

Chest Pain—ER

Hours	0–1	1–2	2–3	3–6	6–12	P value
N	288	336	191	189	95	—
Age (mean 6 SD)	59 ± 12	60 ± 12	61 ± 12	62 ± 12	61 ± 11	0.06
TIMI-3 flow restored	93%	95%	91%	93%	88%	0.31
Death in-hospital	2.8%	1.8%	3.7%	3.7%	3.2%	0.66

ER = emergency room.

success and complication rates similar to elective PTCA. Although subsequent in-hospital ischemic events were not increased by withholding PTCA of patent vessels, there may have been selection bias to perform PTCA in vessels perceived to be at high risk of reocclusion.

Patients with acute MI and prior CABG have suboptimal outcomes after thrombolytic therapy. We therefore examined the combined randomized PAMI-1 and PAMI-2 trials, in which primary PTCA was performed in 1,103 patients.[19] Compared to patients without prior CABG (N = 1,061), patients with prior CABG (N = 42) were older (64 ± 10 years vs 59 ± 12 years, P = 0.02) and more likely to have prior MI (60% vs 15%, P < 0.0001) and three vessel disease (60% vs 15%, P < 0.0001). The infarct vessel in patients with prior CABG was a bypass graft in 19 patients (45%), a native coronary artery in 22 patients (53%) and unidentified in 1 patient (2%). TIMI-3 flow (84% vs 91%) and death/reinfarction (5% vs 4%) rates were similar in patients with prior CABG when the infarct vessel was a bypass graft versus a native coronary artery. Despite the increased frequency of comorbid risk factors, in-hospital outcomes were similar between patients with and without prior CABG: death (2.4% vs 2.1%), reinfarction (2.4% vs 4.7%), recurrent ischemia (17% vs 11%, P = 0.24) stroke (0 vs 0.8%) and hospital stay (6.8 vs 7.8 days). Due to the small sample size, strong conclusions cannot be drawn. However, these data suggest that primary PTCA may be a good reperfusion strategy for patients with prior CABG.

It has been suggested that new devices or potent pharmacological agents may reduce abrupt closure and recurrent ischemia when PTCA is performed on unstable plaques. However, due to the cost and bleeding associated with those technologies, their use should be targeted at patients most likely to experience an adverse event. To investigate this issue we reviewed the 982 PAMI-2 patients who underwent primary PTCA.[20] Infarct vessel patency was achieved in 97.4% and TIMI-3 flow in 92.8%. Among patients with unsuccessful PTCA, 42% were attributed to abrupt closure, 25.6% to inability to cross, and 32.6% for other reasons. Suboptimal angiographic results (operator assessment) include post-PTCA dissection in 20.3%, thrombus in 18%, and residual stenosis > 30% in 14.4%. Important ischemic events defined as reinfarction, or urgent recatheterization, repeat PTCA, or CABG occured in 116 patients (11.8%). In multivariate analysis, ischemia occurred more frequently in patients with EF < 45% (17.3% vs 10.0%, P = 0.004), stenosis > 30% (19.9% vs 10.5%, P = 0.001), or dissection (18.7% vs 9.7%, P = 0.001). Post-PTCA thrombus was not predictive, and a trend for more ischemia occurred when thrombus was treated with lytics (18.8% vs 9.0%, P = 0.08). These data show that although primary PTCA can be performed with high clinical and angiographic success, ischemia remains a problem. Patients with poor EF, post-PTCA dissection, or stenosis > 30% may benefit from new mechanical or pharmacological approaches.

Local PAMI

Limitations of reperfusion by primary PTCA include recurrent ischemia in 10%-15% of cases, restenosis in 40%, and late infarct vessel reocclusion in 10%-15%. Coronary angioplasty causes immediate endothelial denudation and deep medial injury resulting in ex-posure of collagen, elastin, and smooth muscle cells to circulating blood. Within minutes of intimal and medial disruption, platelet deposit occurs. This interaction of platelets and thrombin with the surface of injured blood vessels are major factors in coronary artery thrombosis and reocclusion after PTCA procedures. Although antithrombin or antiplatelet agents may reduce ischemia, systemic administration requires high doses and is limited by the cost and bleeding potential.

An alternative approach is to administer a small dose of heparin locally at the site of the lesion. Heparin infused locally into the vessel wall adheres to and permeates the

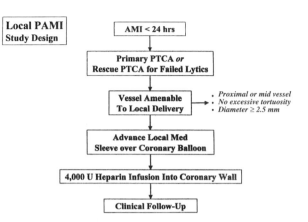

Figure 7. Local PAMI algorithm.

intima of arteries, resulting in a high concentration locally that persists for several hours to days. A variety of different delivery devices used to infuse local heparin have consistently demonstrated reduced platelet deposition, and local heparin infusions in animals have been demonstrated to reduce intimal hyperplasia. An additional benefit of local heparin delivery is the potential to reduce the dose and duration of systemic heparin, which may minimize bleeding complications.

We examined the safety of local heparin delivery in 120 acute MI patients treated with primary PTCA. Angioplasty was performed using standard techniques, after which heparin (4,000 U) was delivered via the LocalMed InfusaSleeve drug delivery catheter (Local Med, Inc., Palo Alto, CA, USA) into the coronary wall (Fig. 7). Reduction in TIMI flow due to progression of dissection, was noted in two patients following heparin infusion. Final procedural success (TIMI flow $\geq$ 2, residual stenosis < 50%) occurred in 99% of patients, and stents were placed at the operator's discretion in 24% of cases. Serious complications prior to hospital discharge were reported in 7.5% of patients (deaths 1.7%, abrupt closure 1.7%, infarct artery revascularization 3.3%, reinfarction 0.8). In the final phase no additional heparin was given postprocedure in low risk patients; no complications were noted. At 6 months the infarct vessel revascularization rate was 7.5%. Therefore, local delivery of heparin in the setting of primary PTCA for acute MI was feasible and safe, was associated with low rates of reocclusion and target vessel revascularization at 6 months, and may eliminate the need for systemic heparin.

PAMI Stent Pilot Study

In the PAMI-2 study, we demonstrated that residual stenosis > 30% or coronary dissection was associated with an increased risk of recurrent ischemia and reocclusion.[20] Since coronary stenting can lower the residual stenosis and seal dissection planes created by PTCA, primary stenting may further improve short- and long-term outcomes after mechanical reperfusion. The PAMI stent pilot study (Fig. 8) determined the safety and feasibility of using the commercially available Palmaz-Schatz (Johnson & Johnson Interventional Systems, Warren, NJ, USA) stent in 312 patients who were treated with primary PTCA.[21,22] Following PTCA, stenting was attempted in all eligible lesions (vessel size $\geq$ 3 mm diameter, ability to cover lesion with 2 stents, and the absence of major side branch jeopardy, excessive proximal tortuosity, calcification, or no reflow). Stented patients were treated with aspirin, ticlopidine, and a 60-hour heparin regimen (48 hours full dose, 12 hours half dose). Stenting was attempted in

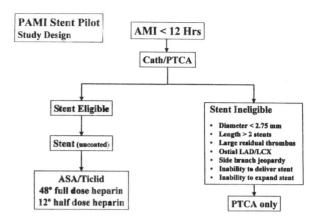

Figure 8. PAMI Stent Pilot algorithm.

77% of cases and was successful in 98% of attempts, and TIMI-3 flow was restored in 96% of stented patients. Stented patients experienced low rates of in-hospital death (0.8%), reinfarction (1.7%), recurrent ischemia (3.8%), and predischarge target vessel revascularization (1.3%). At 30-day follow-up, no additional deaths or reinfarctions occurred among stented patients. Comparing the outcomes of the entire 312-patient population (both stented patients and those ineligible for stenting) to patients treated with primary PTCA in the PAMI-2 trial, the strategy of stenting all eligible lesions was associated with lower rates of death (0.6% vs 2.7%, P = 0.03), recurrent ischemia (3.5% vs 11.5%, P = 0.001), and repeat PTCA of the infarct vessel (2.9% vs 6.0%, P = 0.06). Therefore, primary stenting appears to compare favorably to primary PTCA with regard to reduction of early and late ischemic events. To further elucidate this issue, well-designed prospective randomized trials were necessary.

Stent PAMI

The development of a heparin-coated stent combines the mechanical benefits of the stent (ability to enlarge the lumen and seal dissection planes) with the pharmacological advantage of a drug (to reduce thrombosis). In an in vitro model of pulsatile blood flow, platelet deposition was reduced by 95% with the heparin-coated Palmaz-Schatz stent compared to the non-coated stent. In animals that were pretreated with aspirin and intravenous heparin, by 4-12 weeks the heparin-coated stent resulted in 0% thrombosis compared to 37% in stents that were not heparin-coated (P < 0.01). The heparin-coated stent was placed electively in 200 patients in the Benestent II Pilot study with no subacute thrombosis and an angiographic restenosis rate of only 13%. In the Benestent II trial, which randomized patients to PTCA versus heparin-coated stenting, subacute thrombosis (0.2%) and restenosis rates (16%) were lower than those observed in other stent trials.

We speculated that since the heparin-coated stent reduces platelet deposition and reocclusion, it may be ideally suited for implantation into the thrombotic milieu of acute MI. Moreover, the heparin coating may obviate the need for intravenous heparin infusion post-MI. To determine the feasibility and safety, we performed a pilot study in which 101 MI patients received the Palmaz-Schatz heparin-coated stent as the primary reperfusion strategy.[23] If the stent result was optimal (≤ 10% residual stenosis with the absence of dissection, thrombus, or no reflow) no further heparin was given. Stent implantation was successful in 97% of cases; subacute thrombosis did not occur, and angiographic restenosis at 6 months was only 17%.

Based on the favorable pilot study results, we proceeded with a randomized trial.

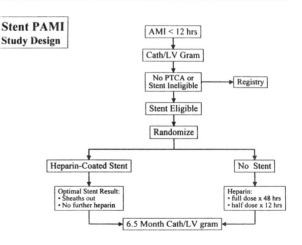

Figure 9. Heparin-Coated Stent PAMI Study algorithm.

The Stent PAMI trial incorporated 64 international sites that randomized 901 patients to receive primary PTCA alone versus primary stenting with the heparin-coated device (Fig. 9). Recruitment was completed in November 1997, but the results are not yet available. The primary end point of the study is the 6-month composite incidence of death, nonfatal reinfarction, disabling stroke, or ischemia-driven target vessel revascularization. Six-month angiographic follow-up will allow determination of reocclusion, restenosis, and left ventricular functional recovery in primary PTCA and primary stent arms. Our hypothesis is that the heparin-coated stent will reduce recurrent ischemia, reocclusion, and restenosis and early bleeding complications compared to primary PTCA.

Controlled Abciximab and Device Investigation to Lower Late Angioplasty Complications

Platelet activation and aggregation likely contributes to vessel thrombosis and reocclusion after primary PTCA in acute MI. At clinically useful doses, abciximab results in blockade of the IIb/IIIa receptors on the platelet, reducing platelet aggregation to < 20% of baseline levels. In the Evaluation of 7E3 for the Prevention of Ischemic Complications (EPIC) and Evaluation of PTCA to Improve Long-term Outcome by C7E3 Glycoprotein IIb/IIIa Receptor Blockade (EPILOG) trials, abiximab was superior to placebo at reducing urgent revascularization and creatine kinase (CK) leaks after elective PTCA. The ReoPro in AMI Primary PTCA Organization and Randomized Trial (RAPPORT) which enrolled 483 acute MI patients treated with primary PTCA, demonstrated no difference in death, reinfarction, or the combined study end point of death, reinfarction, or revascularization at 6 months. Although there was a reduced rate of urgent target vessel revascularization favoring abciximab over placebo, a significant increase in bleeding occurred. Whether abciximab is superior to placebo if PTCA is performed the PAMI way (ticlopidine and aspirin in emergency room, ionic contrast, ACT > 350 seconds, stent for suboptimal result)[24] is unknown; however, if the plaque is stabilized enough to allow early discharge, abciximab may be of great advantage.

The Controlled Abciximab and Device Investigation to Lower Late Angioplasty Complications (CADILLAC, Fig. 10) is an ongoing multicenter international trial that will randomize 2,000 patients to the flexible,

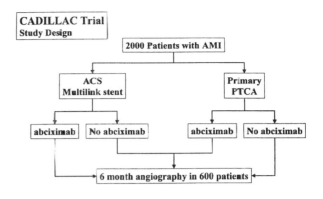

Figure 10. CADILLAC Study algorithm.

nonarticulated ACS MultiLink stent (Santa Clara, CA, USA) with or without abciximab, versus primary PTCA with or without abciximab. The hypotheses of this trial are that primary stenting will result in a greater minimal luminal diameter, reduced rates of recurrent ischemia, target vessel revascularization, and the 6-month incidence of angiographic restenosis and infarct vessel reocclusion compared to patients undergoing primary PTCA. Secondly, compared to stenting or PTCA with a traditional heparin regimen, the use of abciximab may obviate the need for postprocedural heparin, thereby allowing a 2-3 day discharge strategy to be safe and cost-effective. The CADILLAC trial started in November 1997, and results should be available in 1999.

Air PAMI

Advanced age, anterior infarction, admission tachycardia, hypotension, and higher Killip classes have been associated with increased mortality with MI, despite administration of thrombolytic therapy.[25] Randomized trials have demonstrated that primary PTCA is superior to thrombolytics with regard to greater TIMI-3 flow rates and reduced frequency of recurrent ischemia, reinfarction, stroke, and death.[26] For these reasons, primary PTCA is considered the treatment of choice when an acute MI patient is admitted to a PTCA facility.[27]

However, the majority of hospitals in the United States do not have PTCA facilities. Therefore, when patients present to a hospital where PTCA is not readily available, a thrombolytic agent is usually administered. Alternatively, transfer of high risk patients for primary PTCA may occur, but there is some concern that delay in reperfusion may adversely affect outcome. A third practice that exists in some hospitals that have catheterization laboratories but no elective PTCA or cardiac surgery is to perform primary PTCA on site (by experienced interventionalists who routinely perform elective PTCA at tertiary centers).

Whether the best treatment is on-site thrombolysis, on-site primary PTCA, or transfer to a tertiary care center for primary PTCA is unknown. To address these issues, the Air PAMI study was designed (Fig. 11). Patients with acute MI who are thrombolytic eligible and meet at least one high risk criteria (age > 70 years, heart rate > 100, blood pressure < 100, Killip Class 2 or 3, or electorcardiogram demonstrating anterior MI or left bundle branch block) are enrolled. If the participating institution does not perform PTCA, patients are randomized to either immediate intravenous thrombolysis or emergent transfer for cardiac catheterization and intervention. If the patient presents to a participating hospital that is able to perform emergency PTCA (but does not perform elective PTCA and

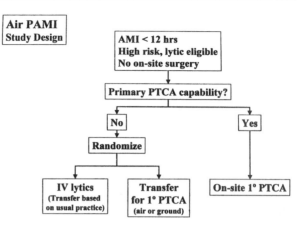

Figure 11. Air PAMI Study algorithm.

does not have surgery on site [SOS]) the patient is not transferred, but is treated with primary PTCA at that institution. The Air PAMI study is an ongoing multicenter international trial, the results of which should be available in 1998.

Therefore, the PAMI study group has made major advances in determining the best mechanical reperfusion strategies for acute MI patients. Future directions will include continued efforts at expanding the applicability of primary PTCA and investigating the role of new devices and pharmacological adjuncts.

Acknowledgment: The authors wish to thank Monica Kusak for manuscript preparation.

PAMI-1 Investigators.

C. Grines, William Beaumont Hospital, Royal Oak, Michigan; K. Browne, Lakeland Regional Medical Center, Lakeland, Florida; J. Marco, Clinique Pasteur, Toulouse, France; D. Rothbaum, St. Vincent Hospital, Indianapolis, Indiana; G. Stone, El Camino Hospital, Mountain View, California; G. Hartzler, Mid-America Heart Institute, Kansas City, Missouri; J. O'Keefe and C. Dreiling, St. Mary of the Plains, Lubbock, Texas; P. Overlie and M. Quijada, Allegheny General Hospital, Pittsburgh, Pennsylvania; B. Donohue, Allegheny General Hospital, Pittsburgh, Pennsylvania; N. Chelliah, United Hospital, Grand Forks, North Dakota; C. Cates, The Heart Institute of St. Joseph Hospital, Atlanta, Georgia; R. Ivanhoe, Florida Hospital South, Orlando, Florida; J. Freeman, Central Heart Clinic, Wausau, Wisconsin.

PAMI-2 Investigators.

C. Grines, William Beaumont Hospital, Royal Oak, Michigan; B. Brodie, Moses H. Cone Hospital, Greensboro, North Carolina; J. Griffin, Virginia Beach General Hospital, Virginia Beach, Virginia; B. Donohue, Allegheny General Hospital, Pittsburgh, Pennsylvania; C. Costantini, Hospital Santa Case De Misericordia, Curitiba, Brazil; C. Balestrini, Instituto Modelo de Cardiologia, Cordoba, Argentina; G. Stone, El Camino Hospital, Mountain View, California; T. Wharton, Jr., Exeter and Portsmouth Regional Hospitals, Exeter, New Hampshire; P. Esente, St. Joseph's Hospital, Syracuse, New York; M. Spain, St. Francis Hospital, Tulsa, Oklahoma; J. Moses, Lenox Hill Hospital, New York, New York; M. Nobuyoshi, Kokura Memorial Hospital, Kitakyushu, Japan; M. Ayers, Fort Sanders Regional Medical Center, Knoxville, Tennessee; T. Shimshak, Mid-America Heart Institute,

Kansas City, Missouri; N. Chelliah, United Hospital, Grand Forks, North Dakota; J. Delcan and E. Garcia, Hospital General, Madrid, Spain; K. Browne, Lakeland Regional Medical Center, Lakeland, Florida; P. Overlie, Methodist Hospital of Lubbock, Lubbock, Texas; W. Stan Wilson, St. Patrick Hospital, Missoula, Montana; D. Westerhausen, Jr., St. Joseph Medical Center/Elkhart General Hospital, South Bend, Indiana; M. Sodums, Guthrie Healthcare System, Sayre, Pennsylvania; B. Evans, Providence Hospital, Portland, Oregon; R. Ivanhoe, Florida Hospital South, Orlando, Florida; C. Cates, The Heart Institute of St. Joseph Hospital, Atlanta, Georgia; A. Kahn, Eastern Carolina University School of Medicine, Greenville, North Carolina; N. Kander, Riverside Hospital, Columbus, Ohio; S. Katz, North Shore University Hospital, Manhasset, New York; J. Schneider, Wake Medical Center, Raleigh, North Carolina; J. Dervan, S.U.N.Y. at Stony Brook, Stony Brook, New York; T. Schreiber, St. John Hospital, Detroit, Michigan; M.J. Samaha, Baptist Memorial Hospital, Memphis, Tennessee; D. Rothbaum, St. Vincent Hospital, Indianapolis, Indiana; J. Hines, Hinsdale Hospital, Hinsdale, Illinois; B. Lew, The Heart Center of Fort Wayne, Fort Wayne, Indiana.

Local PAMI Investigators.

P. Esente, St. Joseph's Hospital and Health Center, Syracuse, New York: J. Martin, Bryn Mawr Hospital, Bryn Mawr, Pennsylvania; K. Ford, Western Baptist Hospital, Paducah, Kentucky; M. Ayers, Fort Sanders Regional Medical Center, Knoxville, Tennessee; D. Lasorda, Allegheny General Hospital, Pittsburgh, Pennsylvania; E. Kosinski, St. Vincents Medical Center, Bridgeport, Connecticut; C. Grines, William Beaumont Hospital, Royal Oak, Michigan; N. Gaither, Winchester Hospital, Winchester, Virginia; DS Gantt, Scott and White Clinic, Temple, Texas.

PAMI Stent Pilot Investigators.

G. Stone, F. St. Goar, El Camino Hospital, Mountain View, California; C. Grines, William Beaumont Hospital, Royal Oak, Michigan; M. Claude-Morice, Clinique du Bois de Verrieres, France; J. Griffin, Virginia Beach General Hospital, Virginia Beach, Virginia; B. Brodie, Moses Cone Memorial Hospital, Greensboro, North Carolina; P. Overlie, Methodist Hospital of Lubbock, Lubbock, Texas; T. Linnemeier, Indiana Heart Institute, Indianapolis, Indiana; T. Shimshak, Mid-America Heart Institute, Kansas City, Missouri; C. Costantini, Hospital Santa Case De Misericordia, Curitiba, Brazil; J. Moses, Lenox Hill Hospital, New York, New York.

Stent PAMI Investigators.

G. Stone, El Camino & Stanford University Medical Center, Mountain View, California; D. Cox, Presbyterian Hospital, Charlotte, North Carolina; E.G. Fernandez, Hospital Universitario Gregorio Maranon, Madrid, Spain; C.L. Grines, William Beaumont Hospital, Royal Oak, Michigan; S. Katz, North Shore University Hospital, Manhasset, New York; B.R. Brodie, LeBauer Health Care, PA, Greensboro, North Carolina; J.E. De Sousa, Instituto Dante Pazzanese de Cardiologia, Sao Paulo, Brazil; A. Giambartolomei, St. Joseph's Hospital, Syracuse, New York; B.C. Donohue, Allegheny General Hospital, Pittsburgh, Pennsylvania; J. Griffin, Virginia Beach General Hospital, Virginia Beach, Virginia; P. Casale, Lancaster Heart Foundation, Lancaster, Pennsylvania; M. Vandormael, Clinique Generale Saint Jean, Brussels, Belgium; P. Materne, Hospital de la Citadelle, Liege, Belgium; T. Lefevre, Institut Cardiovasculaire Paris Sud, Massy, France; G. J. Karrillon, Institut Cardiovasculaire Paris Sud, Quincy-Sous-Senart, France; J.A. Werner, Overlake Hospital Medical Center, Bellevue, Washington; J. Martin, Bryn Mawr

Hospital, Bryn Mawr, Pennsylvania; T. J. Linnemeier, Indiana Heart Institute, Indianapolis, Indiana; P. Overlie, Methodist Heart Center, Lubbock, Texas; K. Niazi, King Faisal Specialist Hospital, Riyadh, Saudi Arabia; W. Van der Giessen, Thoraxcentrum AZR Dijkzigt, Rotterdam, the Netherlands; M. Novuyoshi, Kokura Memorial Hospital, Kitakyushu, Japan; J. Marco, Clinique Pasteur, Toulouse, France; S.H. West, Lakeview Hospital, Bountiful, Utah; J. Belardi, Instituto Cardiovascular de Cardiologia, Buenos Aires, Argentina; I. Penn, Vancouver Hospital and Health Science Center, Vancouver, BK (Canada); P. Probst, Universitatsklinik fur Innere Medizin, Vienna, Austria; T. Feldman, University of Chicago, Chicago, Illinois; P. Kraft, Henry Ford Hospital, Detroit, Michigan; C. Conti, Instituto de Cardiologia, Buenos Aires, Argentina; A. Bartorelli, University of Milano, Milano, Italy; B. Glatt, Centre Cardiologique de Nord, Saint Denis, France; C. Cates, The Atlanta Cardiology Group, Atlanta, Georgia; L. Grinfeld, Hospital Italiano de Buenos Aires, Buenos Aires, Argentina; J. Goy, Centre Hospitalier Universitaire Vaudois, Lausanne, Switzerland; F. Fernandez-Aviles, Hospital Universitario de Valladolid, Valladolid, Spain; N. Kander, Riverside Hospital, Columbus, Ohio; J. Burke, Temple Cardiology, Philadelphia, Pennsylvania; R. Heuser, Columbia Medical Center, Phoenix, Arizona; D. Williams, Rhode Island Hospital, Providence, Rhode Island; J.M. Lasala, Barnes Hospital, St. Louis, Missouri; M.B. Leon, Washington Hospital Center, Washington, DC

Air PAMI Investigators.

C. Balestrini, Instituto Modelo De Cardiologia, Cordoba, Argentina; D.

Westerhausen, St. Joseph Medical Center, South Bend, Indiana; T. Hanlon, St. Charles Medical Center, Bend, Oregon; M. Niemelä, Oulu University Hospital, Oulu, Finland; T. Logemann, Wausau Hospital, Wausau, Wisconsin; C. Grines, William Beaumont Hospital, Royal Oak, Michigan; C. Vozzi, Sanatorio Los Arroyos, Argentina; N. Bhalla, New York University Medical Center/Brooklyn Hospital Center, New York, New York; C. Allen, Allegheny General Hospital, Pittsburgh, Pennsylvania; N. Howard Kander, Riverside Methodist Hospital, Columbus, Ohio; A. Riba, Oakwood Hospital and Medical Center, Dearborn, Michigan; C. Conti, Instituto De Cardiologia, Buenos Aires, Argentina.

No SOS Investigators.

J. Johnston, Hilton Head Hospital, Hilton Head Island, South Carolina; M. Turco, Doylestown Hospital, Doylestown, Pennsylvania; J. Souther, Blount Memorial Hospital, Maryville, Tennessee; T. Wharton, Exeter/Portsmouth Hospital, Exeter, New Hampshire; D. Lew, Leesburg Regional Medical Center, Leesburg, Florida; W. Bilnoski, Auburn Regional Medical Center, Auburn, Washington; S. Singhi, Piedmont Medical Center, Rock Hill, South Carolina; A. Atay, Mercy Medical Center, Cedar Rapids, Iowa; V. Reyes, Tuality Community Hospital, Hillsboro, Oregon; S. Defehr, Jane Phillips Medical Center, Bartlesville, Oklahoma; C. Sholes, Columbia North Side Hospital, Johnson City, Tennessee; J. Elliott, Christ Church Hospital, Christ Church, New Zealand; A. Shaikh, St. Joseph Community Hospital, Mishawaka, Indiana; Y. Moosa, St. Lukes, Sioux City, Iowa; D. Hansen, Highline Community Hospital, Seattle, Washington.

References

1. O'Neill WW, Brodie BR, Ivanhoe R, et al. Primary coronary angioplasty for acute myocardial infarction (the Primary Angioplasty Registry). Am J Cardiol 1994;73:627-634.
2. Grines CL, Browne KF, Marco J, et al. A comparison of immediate angioplasty with thrombolytic therapy for acute myocardial infarction. N Engl J Med 1993;328:673-679.
3. Nunn C, O'Neill W, Rothbaum D, et al. Primary angioplasty for myocardial infarction improves long-term survival: PAMI-1 follow-up. J Am Coll Cardiol 1996;27(Suppl A):153A.
4. Stone GW, Grines CL, Rothbaum D, et al. Analysis of the relative costs and effectiveness of primary angioplasty compared to tissue plasminogen activator: The Primary Angioplasty in Myocardial Infarction trial. J Am Coll Cardiol 1997;29:901-907.
5. Stone GW, Grines CL, Browne KF, et al. Implications of recurrent ischemia after reperfusion therapy in acute myocardial infarction: A comparison of thrombolytic therapy and primary angioplasty. J Am Coll Cardiol 1995; 26:66-72.
6. Stone GW, Grines CL, Browne KF, et al. Influence of acute myocardial infarction location on in-hospital and late outcome after primary percutaneous transluminal coronary angioplasty versus tissue plasminogen activator therapy. Am J Cardiol 1996; 78:19-25.
7. Stone GW, Grines CL, Browne KF, et al. Comparison of in-hospital outcome in men versus women treated by either thrombolytic therapy or primary coronary angioplasty for acute myocardial infarction. Am J Cardiol 1995; 75:987-992.
8. Stone GW, Grines CL, Browne KF, et al. Primary angioplasty in myocardial infarction (PAMI) investigators. Outcome of different reperfusion strategies in patients with former contraindications to thrombolytic therapy: A comparison of primary angioplasty and tissue plasminogen activator. Cathet Cardiovasc Diagn 1996;39:333-339.
9. Bowers TR, Terrien EF, O'Neill WW, et al., for the PAMI investigators. Effect of reperfusion modality on outcome in nonsmokers and smokers with acute myocardial infarction (A primary angioplasty in myocardial infarction [PAMI] substudy). Am J Cardiol 1996; 78:511-515.
10. Grines CL. Aggressive intervention for myocardial infarction: Angioplasty, stents, and intra-aortic balloon pumping. Am J Cardiol 1996;78(Suppl 3A):29-34.
11. Stone GW, Marsalese D, Brodie BR, et al. A prospective, randomized evaluation of prophylactic intraaortic balloon counterpulsation in high risk patients with acute myocardial infarction treated with primary angioplasty. J Am Coll Cardiol 1997;29:1459-1467.
12. Grines C, Marsalese D, Brodie B, et al. Acute catherization provides the best method of risk stratifying MI patients. Circulation 1995;92(Suppl I):I-531.
13. Grines CL, Marsalese D, Brodie B, et al., for the PAMI-II Investigators. Safety and cost effectiveness of early discharge after primary angioplasty in low risk patients with acute myocardial infarction. J Am Coll Cardiol 1998; in press.
14. Schreiber T, Marsalese D, Griffin J, et al. Identification of ultra low-risk patients following primary angioplasty for acute myocardial infarction. J Am Coll Cardiol 1996;27(Suppl A):83A.
15. Hollingsworth V, Marsalese D, Brodie B, et al. Should primary PTCA be performed around the clock? Circulation 1995;92(Suppl I):I-663.
16. Stone GW, Brodie B, Griffin J, et al. Should the risk of delaying reperfusion prohibit inter-hospital transfer to perform primary PTCA in acute myocardial infarction? Circulation 1996; 94(Suppl I):I-331.
17. O'Neill WW, Griffin JJ, Stone G, et al. Operator and institutional volume do not affect the procedural outcome of primary angioplasty therapy. J Am Coll Cardiol 1996;27(Suppl A):13A.
18. Wharton TP, Marsalese D, Brodie B, et al. How often do infarct-related arteries show early perfusion without prior thrombolytic therapy, and should these vessels be dilated acutely? Results from PAMI-2. Circulation 1995;92(Suppl I):I-530.
19. Stone GW, Brodie B, Griffin J, et al. Primary angioplasty in patients with

prior bypass surgery. Circulation 1996;94(Suppl I):I-243.

20. Grines C, Brodie B, Griffin J, et al. Which primary PTCA patients may benefit from new technologies? Circulation 1995;92(Suppl I):I-146.

21. Stone GW, Brodie BR, Morice MC, et al, for the PAMI Stent Pilot Trial Investigators. Primary stenting in acute myocardial infarction: Design and interim results of the PAMI stent pilot trial. J Invasive Cardiol 1997;9(Suppl B):24B-30B.

22. Stone GW, Brodie BR, Griffin JJ, et al. Prospective, multi-center study of the safety and feasibility of primary stenting in acute myocardial infarction: In-hospital and 30-day results of the PAMI stent pilot trial. J Am Coll Cardiol 1998;31:23-30.

23. Grines CL, Morice MC, Mattos L, et al. A prospective multicenter trial using the JJIS heparin-coated stent for primary reperfusion of acute myocardial infarction. J Am Coll Cardiol 1997;29(Suppl A):389A.

24. Grines CL, Stone GW, O'Neill WW. Establishing a program and performance of primary PTCA-The PAMI way. J Invasive Cardiol 1997;9(Suppl B):44B-52B.

25. Grines CL. Transfer of high-risk myocardial infarction patients for primary PTCA. J Invasive Cardiol 1997;9(Suppl B):13B-19B.

26. Weaver WD, Simes RJ, Betriu A, et al. Comparison of primary coronary angioplasty and intravenous thrombolytic therapy for acute myocardial infarction: A quantitative review. JAMA 1997;278:2093-2098.

27. Grines CL. Primary Angioplasty-The strategy of choice. New Engl J Med 1996:335:1313-1317.

Chapter 17

The Restoration of Coronary Blood Flow in Acute Myocardial Infarction

Gerald C. Timmis, M.D., and Steven B.H. Timmis, M.D.

From the Division of Cardiology, William Beaumont Hospital, Royal Oak, Michigan

When an acute coronary syndrome degenerates into a myocardial infarction the centerpiece of therapy is the normalization of myocardial blood flow to the extent that it can be achieved in the shortest interval possible after the onset of symptoms. A variety of strategies including mechanical intervention have been used to achieve this goal. but the benchmark therapy to which all other therapeutic alternatives must be compared involves the use of thrombolytic agents. However, given the availability of catheter laboratories and interventional expertise, mechanical reperfusion appears to be at least as good and probably better than thrombolytic therapy. Because of the universal access to thrombolytic therapy, certain clinical issues must be underscored. More important than pursuing the ideal thrombolytic agent is the administration of thrombolytic therapy at the earliest possible juncture after the onset of symptoms heralding myocardial infarction. Adjunctive therapy includes aspirin and intravenous heparin. Altering platelet activity by glycoprotein IIb/IIIa receptor blockers holds enormous promise for thrombolytic therapy and PTCA, but as yet enjoys limited availability on a global scale.(J Interven Cardiol 1998; 11[Suppl.]:S9–S17)

Early Trials

When an acute coronary syndrome degenerates into a myocardial infarction, the centerpiece of therapy is the normalization of myocardial blood flow to the extent that this can be achieved in the shortest interval possible after the onset of symptoms. A variety of strategies including mechanical intervention have been used to achieve this goal, but the benchmark therapy to which all other therapeutic alternatives must be compared involves the use of thrombolytic agents. Numerous trials using various species of thrombolysis in more than 100,000 patients worldwide have documented improved survival and myocardial salvage. At the forefront of these trials are the second International Study of Infarct Survival (ISIS) experience,[1] the first Gruppo Italiano per lo Studio della Streptochinasi nell'Infarto Miocardico (GISSI) Trial,[2] the APSAC Intervention Mortality Study,[3] the Thrombolysis in Myocardial Infarction (TIMI) Trials,[4] and most recently the first Global Utilization of Streptokinase and tPA for Occluded Arteries (GUSTO) experience.[5] Only the earliest of these trials sought to measure the efficacy of thrombolysis in comparison to no such treatment using a randomized double-blind placebo-controlled model.[6] These early studies documented a survival advantage of > 20% in the recipients of thrombolytic therapy compared to those in whom no specific attempt to reestablish myocardial blood flow was attempted. Subsequent trials attempted to identify the ideal thrombolytic agent with variable results. ISIS-3 and GISSI-2 failed to show a clear superiority among the three lytic agents most frequently used, streptokinase (SK), tissue plasminogen activator (tPA), and anistreplase (APSAC).[7,8] By using a weight-adjusted front-loaded administration of tPA, the GUSTO Trialists teased out an approximate 1% net survival advantage of weight-adjusted front-loaded tPA compared with SK, APSAC, or the combination of SK and tPA.[5]

As we pursued identification of the ideal agent, several lessons emerged, the most important of which was that regardless of the agent used, the earliest possible administration of *any* thrombolytic choice probably salvaged more muscle and saved more lives. The Fibrinolytic Therapy Trialists' (FTT) group estimated that every hour of delay from symptom onset to the initiation of fibrinolysis resulted in a loss of benefit amounting to 1.6 lives per thousand in the first 24 hours after infarction.[6] Others have shown this relationship to be less linear with an even greater loss of survival advantage within the first several hours of symptoms.[9] A number of trials have explored the administration of therapy before hospital admission in the frontier, the transporting ambulance, or immediately on arrival in the emergency care center.[10–16] On combining seven such trials in which patients were randomized to receive prehospital or early in-hospital thrombolytic therapy, a 17% reduction in early mortality was shown with prehospital treatment (21 lives saved per thousand patients treated; P = 0.02). The later administration of thrombolytic therapy, especially beyond 6 hours, has been debated extensively.[1,17,18] There is a general

consensus that significant benefit is realized if thrombolytic therapy is used within 12 hours after the onset of symptoms. Other trials have shown that this may be true beyond this point.[1] A singularly provocative revelation on subgroup analysis of a study exploring late thrombolytic reperfusion was that patients with ST segment depression, while showing no survival advantage when administered thrombolytic therapy in the first 6 hours may do so with later administration of this therapy.[18,19] This is in contrast to earlier trials showing no thrombolytic advantage when ST depression exists.[1,20,21] The final clinical significance of this phenomenon remains unexplained and is not totally logical when juxtaposed to established pathophysiologic concepts. In considering the ideal lytic agent in the context of time to treatment, it should be understood that agents of lesser lytic potency such as SK administered *very early* after the onset of symptoms may achieve the same late patency rates as with accelerated weight-adjusted tPA when administered more than 4 hours after symptom onset. Moreover, the higher reocclusion risk following tPA compared with SK, APSAC, or urokinase further supports the importance of time to treatment over the selection of the "ideal lytic agent.[22] Studies have shown that the survival advantage measured in the first month or two following myocardial infarction is sustained for years, especially with the reestablishment of TIMI-3 coronary blood flow.[23,24]

Eligibility

Another compelling lesson has arisen from the changing definition of eligibility for thrombolytic therapy. Numerous papers have suggested that eligibility averages 20%.[25] This is particularly true in the Western world. Eligibility in these studies was based on a limited time window of approximately 4 hours from symptom onset, men and non-menstruating women < 76 years of age, ischemic chest pain lasting at least 30 minutes, and at least 1-mm ST segment elevation in two contiguous leads. In reality, menstruation and atraumatic cardiopulmonary resuscitation probably do not contraindicate thrombolytic therapy.[26,27] The issue of time has already been discussed. Patients excluded on the basis of the criteria described previously have a mortality rate five times greater than those randomized to thrombolysis in accordance with these inaugural eligibility criteria (19% vs 3.8%).[25] In a recent study, more than 50% of patients from four different institutions in New Zealand were deemed eligible for reperfusion therapy on the basis of electrocardiographic (ECG) criteria including, ST segment elevation or new left bundle branch block who presented within 12 hours of symptom onset.[28] Presumably age did not contravene eligibility in this study (age has been a particularly vexing issue in determining eligibility for thrombolytic therapy). Patients 75 years of age and older are far less likely to receive thrombolytic therapy than younger patients. While a variety of reasons such as less typical clinical presentation, nondiagnostic ECGs, higher incidence of comorbidities, and greater risk of stroke may explain this, the benefit of thrombolytic therapy in this older group has been clearly established. This was shown to be the case as early as ISIS-2 and has been reconfirmed in the GUSTO-1 Trial where no upper age limit was imposed.[1,5] One reason why age looms as a particularly ominous consideration is that death rates are twice as high for those patients > 70 years of age. Nevertheless, the clinical benefit, notwithstanding the greater mortality and increased risk of disabling stroke, is in favor of treating patients without consideration of age as an absolute issue.[29] For patients in GUSTO-1 > 85 years of age the safest regimen appeared to be SK plus subcutaneous heparin in contrast to the reported superiority of tPA in other subgroups of this study.

New Thrombolytic Agents and Strategies

The clinical significance of these foregoing issues must be reassessed as we continue to explore new thrombolytic agents in the pursuit of earlier and more complete myocardial reperfusion. There are a variety of reasons why thrombolytic reperfusion may fail, including nonthrombotic reocclusion, coronary hypoperfusion leading to reduced thrombolytic efficacy, and a "dead-end" phenomenon where the infarct related arterial vessel may preclude lytic access to the thrombus; thus incomplete obstruction is associated with a much higher rate of reperfusion than with total obstruction (78% with TIMI grade 1 flow vs 48% with initial TIMI grade 0 flow).[30] Moreover, the clot becomes more resistant to thrombolysis as it ages with greater cross-linking of fibrinogen. A platelet-rich composition also may resist fibrinolysis. Accordingly, new lytic agents have been developed to circumvent these problems.[31] These new fibrinolytic agents have been designed to improve on some of the shortcomings of SK, tPA, and urokinase, such as susceptibility to inactivation by natural antagonists, including plasminogen activator inhibitor 1 (PAI-1), a relatively nonselective complexing antagonist with fibrin and an excessively short half-life. By increasing resistance to inactivation, improving fibrin selectivity, and lengthening half-life, administration of thrombolytic agents would be facilitated significantly even allowing bolus administration. Most of the new agents have been derived from modifying the wild type tPA molecule by domain deletions or amino acids substitutions and include reteplase (rPA), TNK-tPA, and lanoteplase (nPA). Other new agents such as staphylokinase and dSPA are obtained from the *Staphylococcus* bacterium and the vampire bat saliva (*desmodus rotundus*), respectively. Moreover, recent trials such as TIMI 14 and GUSTO IV pilot (SPEED Trial) have been designed to explore the potential of platelet inhibition combined with thrombolytic therapy and will be discussed shortly.[32,33]

The major "new" thrombolytic agents under study include rPA, a modified wild type tPA known as TNK-tPA, lanoteplase, staphylokinase, and saruplase. With the exception of reteplase and saruplase all have only investigational status. Of these new agents, rPA has been the most thoroughly investigated. Reteplase is a nonglycosylated deletion mutant of wild type tPA; it consists of the kringle-2 and protease domains of the latter but lacks the kringle-1, finger and growth factor domains of tPA. This modification imparts a longer half-life and greater thrombolytic potency than tPA but with less high affinity fibrin binding. In a phase II trial, 606 patients with acute myocardial infarction were randomized to one of four treatment arms, three of which involved rPA dose escalation (15-MU single bolus, 10-MU bolus followed by 5 MU 30 minutes later or 10-MU bolus followed by an additional 10 MU 30 minutes later). The fourth arm was randomized to tPA (100 mg IV over 3 hours) administered in a conventional fashion.[34] The RAPID Trial was intended to test the hypothesis that bolus administration of one or more of rPA doses would result in more rapid, complete, and sustained coronary perfusion compared with a standard dose of tPA. Using global ejection fraction and regional wall motion as a surrogate end point, both were found to improve significantly at discharge in the 10 + 10 MU rPA group (53 ± 1.3% vs 49 ± 1.3%, P = 0.034; −2.19 ± 0.10 vs −2.61 ± 0.13 SD per cord, P = 0.02, respectively). The results with the other two rPA arms were similar to the tPA arm, all of which were inferior to those of the 10 + 10 MU rPA group. Ninety-minute patency rates were significantly greater with the 10 + 10 MU regimen than tPA (85.2% vs 77.2%) as was TIMI grade 3 flow (62.7% vs 49%, P < 0.01). The same was true at discharge with an overall patency of 95.1% versus 87.8% for tPA, P < 0.05 and for TIMI grade 3 flow, 87.8% with rPA versus 70.7% for tPA, P < 0.01.[34] The INJECT Trial randomized 6,010 patients from 208 centers in 9 countries with ECG criteria consistent with acute myocardial infarction to receive in a double-blind fashion SK 1.5 MU intravenously over 60 minutes or two 10 MU boluses of reteplase given 30 minutes apart; all pa-

tients received intravenous heparin for at least 24 hours.[35] At 35 days there were 270 deaths in the rPA group (9%) and 285 deaths in the SK group (9.5%, P = NS). Bleeding events were similar in the two treatment groups as was recurrent myocardial infarction, but there were significantly fewer cases of atrial fibrillation, cardiogenic shock, heart failure, and hypotension in the rPA group. In the RAPID II Trial, 324 patients with acute myocardial infarction were randomized to receive 10 + 10 MU double bolus rPA or front-loaded tPA.[36] This phase II study used the primary end point of 90-minute patency as was the case in RAPID I; background therapy of heparin and aspirin was used. The patency of the infarct related coronary artery (TIMI grade 2 or 3) and complete patency (TIMI grade 3) at 90 minutes after the initiation of thrombolysis were significantly higher in the rPA arm (TIMI grade 2 or 3: 83.4% vs 73.3% for front-loaded tPA, P = 0.03; TIMI grade 3: 60 % vs 45%, P = 0.01). Superiority of rPA was evident at 60 minutes as well (TIMI grade 2 or 3: 82% vs 66%, P = 0.01; TIMI grade 3: 51% vs 37%, P < 0.03). The rPA arm required fewer postlysis coronary interventions (14% vs 27%, P < 0.01); moreover, 35-day mortality also was less for the rPA arm (4% vs 8.4%, P = NS). There was no significant difference in bleeding in the two arms or in hemorrhagic stroke (12.4% vs 9.7% and 1.2% vs 1.9%, respectively). On the basis of these data at least an equivalent performance of rPA versus tPA was anticipated in the Global Use of Strategies To Open Occluded Coronary Arteries Trial III (GUSTO III).[37] A total of 15,059 myocardial infarction patients from 807 hospitals in 20 countries presenting within 6 hours of symptom onset with ST segment elevation or bundle branch block were randomly assigned in a 2 to 1 ratio to receive rPA in two bolus doses of 10 MU each 30 minutes apart or an accelerated infusion of tPA up to 100 mg over a period of 90 minutes. It was hypothesized that mortality would be less with rPA. In fact, the mortality at 30 days was 7.47% for the rPA arm and 7.24% for the tPA arm (odds ratio, 1.03; 95% CI, 0.91–1.18). For absolute difference in mortality, the confidence interval ranged from −1.1% to 0.66%; stroke was distributed equally (1.4% and 1.79% with rPA and tPA, respectively). The combined end point of death or nonfatal disabling stroke was also the same (7.89% and 7.91% for rPA and tPA, respectively). Accordingly, rPA did not provide any additional survival advantage in the treatment of acute myocardial infarction. Notwithstanding the ensuing debate as to whether rPA was truly equivalent to tPA, it is anticipated that the ease and abbreviated time period of administration of rPA will facilitate the successful clinical introduction of this drug, which has been approved by the United States Food and Drug Administration as standard therapy.

Lanoteplase, a novel plasminogen-activator (nPA) is a third generation derivative of tPA in which the finger and endothelial growth factor-like domains have been deleted and Asn-36 has been mutated to Gln-36. There are no glycosidic side chains. These changes prolong in vivo half-life of nPA without affecting its lytic efficacy at therapeutic concentrations.[38] The deletion mutant nPA was administered to 590 patients in escalating doses (five randomization arms) from a 15 to 120 KU/kg bolus in the InTIME-1 Trial.[39] The highest dose achieved overall patency of 83% at 90 minutes, 57% of whom displayed TIMI grade 3 flow compared with 46.4% in patients treated with tPA. This agent is under study in InTIME-2, a phase III investigation using mortality as a primary end point in a large number of patients; it will be completed in 1999.

By modifying wild type tPA somewhat less aggressively, TNK-tPA has been genetically modified as follows: a threonine (T) has been replaced by asparagine adding a glycosylation site to position 103 of the tPA molecule; an asparagine (N) in turn has been replaced by glutamine resulting in removal of glycosylation site from position 117; and a tetra-alanine (A) has been substituted for lysine (K) histidine and arginine at

sites 296 to 299. The change of the glycosylation sites in kringle-1 (T and N replacements) decreases the clearance rate of TNK-tPA, while the tetra-alanine substitution confers enhanced fibrin specificity and resistance to PAI-1 inhibition.[40] Animal studies have shown more complete recanalization of occluded arteries and less platelet activation. In a dose-ranging pilot trial, 113 patients were enrolled in 18 hospitals (TIMI 10A).[41] Because of its prolonged half-life of 17 ± 7 minutes, TNK-tPA was administered as a single bolus. TIMI grade 3 flow at 90 minutes was achieved in 57% to 64% of patients at the 30- to 50-mg dose level; major hemorrhage occurred in 7 patients (6.2%), but was localized to the vascular access site in 6 patients. TIMI-10B was a large phase II efficacy trial in which a single 40-mg bolus of TNK-tPA produced a 63% TIMI grade 3 flow rate at 90 minutes, which was identical to that observed in the tPA randomization arm.[42] The best angiographic results were obtained with dose rate-adjusting (0.5 mg/kg). In a larger safety trial 3,325 patients were randomized in ASSENT-1 to escalating doses of TNK-tPA; the 40-mg dose was deemed to be relatively safe based on a 0.76% intracranial hemorrhage rate, which was considered acceptable because almost 15% of the patients were > 75 years old.[43] More than 16,000 additional patients will be studied in ASSENT-2, a phase III mortality trial comparing weight-adjusted TNK-tPA to tPA in a double-blind manner. This study will be concluded in 1999.

The fourth new agent to be discussed in this article is staphylokinase, a derivitive of *Staphylococcus aureus*, which has the advantage of fibrin selectivity. This agent has been under study for decades, but because of its immunogenicity has not gained widespread clinical applicability. However, recent efforts to reduce immunoreactivity have been successful, enabling > 200 patients to be studied in two different trials comparing staphylokinase to tPA.[44,45] In the STAR Trial 100 patients presented within 6 hours of an acute myocardial infarction. Recombinant staphylokinase (STAR) was administered to

48 patients (10 to 20 mg over 30 minutes) and the remainder received accelerated weight-adjusted tPA over 90 minutes.[46] TIMI grade 3 flow at 90 minutes was achieved in 62% of STAR patients versus 58% of tPA patients. However, with a 20-mg dose TIMI grade 3 flow was achieved in 74%! A more recent study of 102 patients found that two 15-mg doses of STAR administered as a bolus 30 minutes apart achieved TIMI grade 3 flow in 68% of patients compared to 57% for the tPA arm (P = NS).[47] Double-bolus STAR was significantly more fibrin-specific than with tPA (residual fibrinogen at 90 minutes; 105 ± 4.1% and 68 ± 7.5%, respectively, P < 0.0001). While allergic reactions were not seen, neutralizing antibodies developed in 73% of patients at two weeks. Intraarterial instillation of STAR has been used successfully in peripheral arterial occlusion as well.[48]

Saruplase (prourokinase, SCUPA) is a naturally occurring glycoprotein that is converted by plasmin into urokinase. It has been reproduced in mass by recombinant engineering, and it has been shown that in comparison to streptokinase there is less fibrinogen breakdown. Reperfusion rates have been shown to be similar to those of tPA. In a recent equivalence trial (COMPASS; 3,089 patients), patients in the saruplase arm (20-mg bolus, 60-mg infusion over 60 minutes) displayed a lower all-cause mortality at 30 days (5.7%) than those in the streptokinase arm (6.7%; odds ratio 0.84, P < 0.01 for equivalence). There were more hemorrhagic strokes in the saruplase group (0.9% vs 0.3%); otherwise the rate of bleeding was similar.[49]

There are several less completely studied thrombolytic agents. One example is E6010, a novel modified tPA with a single amino acid substitution, cysteine 84, having been replaced by serine in the epidermal growth factor domain, resulting in a prolongation of half-life from 4 minutes (wild type tPA) to > 23 minutes.[50] Accordingly, it can be administered as a bolus and has shown to achieve a higher rate of reperfu-

sion (TIMI grade 2 or 3) at 60 minutes (79% compared to 65% with native tPA, P = 0.032). Another extremely effective fibrinolytic agent, a plasminogen activator obtained from the vampire bat (batPA) has been shown to be very effective in a small number of patients with myocardial infarctions achieving high rates of reperfusion.[31] The risk of bleeding has yet to be established. If this can be controlled, batPA may be an extremely important contribution.

Adjunctive Strategies

A number of studies have explored the effects of antiplatelet and antithrombin agents on the efficacy of thrombolysis. Antithrombin therapy generally has been ineffective with the exception of the Hirulog Early Reperfusion/Occlusion (HERO) Trial, which showed that patients with acute myocardial infarction presenting within 3 hours who were treated with SK and high dose hirulog achieved a 73% TIMI grade 3 flow rate at 90 minutes![51] However, there appears to be greater promise with the use of antiplatelet strategies as suggested by the TIMI-14 Trial in which 681 patients presenting with ischemic pain and ST segment elevation in two adjacent leads were enrolled.[32] Patients were administered accelerated tPA in a standard dose (100 mg, group 1), ascending doses of tPA (35–65 mg, group 2), ascending doses of SK (.5–1.5 MU, group 3), or no lytic therapy (group 4). Standard dose heparin was administered to group 1 and ascending doses of abciximab, a GPIIb/IIIa inhibitor, to groups 2, 3, and 4 in doses ranging from 0.25 to 0.3 mg/kg 3 minutes before thrombolytic therapy. The primary end point, TIMI grade 3 flow at 90 minutes, was achieved in 58% in group 1, 53% to 79% in group 2, 42% to 80% in group 3, and in 32% in group 4. A combination of 1.5 MU of SK plus abciximab resulted in a 15% intracranial bleed rate and was therefore abandoned. Abciximab with reduced tPA appears to be promising at this juncture. In the GUSTO IV pilot trial (SPEED; 170 patients), rPA in single doses ranging from 5 to 10 units was administered with abciximab and compared with abciximab alone. TIMI grade 3 flow rates at 90 minutes of up to 52% were achieved (abciximab plus 10 units rPA). This may be compared to a TIMI grade 3 flow rate of 45% for tPA in 12 meta-analyzed studies.[33]

Adjunctive Angioplasty

Depending on agent and adjunctive therapy, thrombolytic failure ranges from 15% to 25%. Accordingly, strategies have been explored to resolve this using mechanical adjuncts such as balloon angioplasty (PTCA). The Thrombolysis and Angioplasty in Myocardial Infarction-1 (TAMI-1) Trial,[52] TIMI-2 Trial,[53] the fifth European Co-operative Study Group (ECSG-5) Trial, [54] and the Should We Intervene Following Thrombolysis (SWIFT) Trial[55] have attested to the relative inefficacy of adjunctive PTCA on the heels of thrombolytic therapy. Similarly, our investigation of Streptokinase and Angioplasty in Myocardial Infarction (SAMI) Trial has shown that the administration of intravenous SK prior to angioplasty in a placebo-controlled investigation of 122 patients with evolving myocardial infarction failed to improve arterial patency rates, enhance ventricular function, or affect restenosis rates of PTCA.[56] Against this background of uncertainty as to the place of adjunctive angioplasty in the context of thrombolysis, this issue was revisited in the Plasminogen Activator and Angioplasty Compatibility Trial (PACT). This randomized placebo-controlled study of 606 patients with acute myocardial infarction within 6 hours of symptom onset was designed to compare primary angioplasty to fibrin selective short-acting thrombolytic therapy followed by truly immediate angioplasty if necessary in a design similar to that of the SAMI Trial.[56,57] Against a therapeutic background of aspirin and heparin, patients were randomized to a 50-mg bolus

of tPA or placebo and then were taken to the catheterization laboratory for angiography. Immediate angioplasty was performed in those with TIMI grade 0 to 2 flow rates. A second bolus of the study drug or placebo was given to those with TIMI grade 3 flow. Patients displaying TIMI grade 3 flow on arrival to the cath lab had an ejection fraction (EF) of 62% at hospital discharge compared to an EF of 58% if TIMI grade 3 flow was achieved only after angioplasty and 55% if TIMI grade 3 flow was never achieved. Urgent revascularization was more likely (P = 0.07) in patients not receiving pre-PTCA lytic therapy. Patients achieving TIMI grade 3 flow with thrombolytic therapy alone did so at 51 minutes compared to the longer interval of 93 minutes when PTCA was required. This study shows that the technical efficacy of PTCA is not diminished by prior administration of thrombolytic therapy.

Primary Angioplasty

Although not as universally applicable as thrombolysis, at least on a global scale, primary angioplasty for myocardial infarction has become an increasingly important means of establishing high grade myocardial reperfusion. In the mid-1980s, we randomly assigned 56 patients presenting within 12 hours of symptoms heralding myocardial infarction to intracoronary streptokinase or primary PTCA.[58] Coronary recanalization was achieved in 83% of patients treated with PTCA and in 85% of those receiving intracoronary SK. Contrast ventriculography confirmed a higher EF at discharge and better wall motion in the PTCA group (increase of 8% ± 7% vs 1% ± 6%, P < 0.001 and +1.32 ± 1.32 SD vs +0.59 ± 0.79 SD, P < 0.05, respectively). This was the first study to suggest the therapeutic superiority of primary PTCA for acute myocardial infarction. We revisited this issue on a larger scale in the early 1990s having randomized 395 patients within 12 hours of myocardial infarction symptom onset to immediate PTCA (195 patients) or intravenous tPA (200 patients).[59] In-hospital mortality rates for the two groups were 2.6% and 6.5%, respectively (P = 0.06). In-hospital reinfarction or death rates were 5.1% and 12.0%, respectively (P = 0.02). Intracranial bleeding occurred in 2% of the tPA group. Ventricular function was similar in the two groups at 6 weeks. At 6 months, death and reinfarction occurred in 8.5% and 16.8%, respectively (P = 0.02). This investigation followed on the heels of a smaller study of 107 patients with single-vessel coronary artery disease primarily in the *absence* of myocardial infarction.[60] Patients were randomized to PTCA or best medical management (nitrates, calcium channel blockers, beta-adrenergic blockers, aspirin, and/or dipyridamole). This trial (ACME) showed that in patients with single-vessel coronary artery disease, PTCA yields earlier and more complete relief of angina than medical therapy and is associated with a better subsequent performance of exercise testing. Two other studies in the context of acute myocardial infarction were reported at about the same time. Gibbons and colleagues[61] at the Mayo Clinic randomized a small group of patients to PTCA (47) or tPA (56).Using tomographic imaging (Technetium-99m sestamibi) as the primary end point, they found that myocardial salvage was slightly less with tPA (27% ± 21% of the left ventricular mass for tPA versus 31% ± 21% for PTCA). This was interpreted as showing no biologically meaningful difference in salvage between the two strategies. However, Zijlstra's group studied 301 patients with acute myocardial infarction, randomizing 149 to intravenous SK and 152 to PTCA. Mortality rates were 7% versus 2%, respectively (P = 0.024). Reinfarction rates similarly favored PTCA (10% vs 1%, P < 0.001). The benefit of PTCA over thrombolytic therapy also was observed in a group of 95 patients characterized as being at low risk.[62–64]

The Myocardial Infarction Triage and Intervention (MITI) group[65] reviewed 1,050 PTCA patients and 2,095 patients treated with thrombolytic therapy all of whom were selected from a registry of 12,331 consecutive patients admitted with acute myocardial infarction to 19 Seattle hospitals (1988 to 1994). Efforts were made to avoid bias by selecting only patients eligible for thrombolysis, high risk patients, and patients in the PTCA group who were treated only in institutions with high PTCA volumes. They concluded that in a community setting there was no benefit in terms of mortality or the use of resources using a strategy of primary PTCA compared with thrombolytic therapy. The GUSTO IIb angiographic substudy analyzed 1,138 patients from 57 hospitals presenting within 12 hours of acute myocardial infarction randomized to PTCA (565) or tPA (573).[66] The primary end point was a composite of death, reinfarction, or nonfatal disabling stroke at 30 days. The end point incidence was 9.6% for PTCA versus 13.7% for tPA (odds ratio, 0.67; 95% CI, 0.47–0.97; P = 0.033). There was, however, no significant difference in any of the three components of the composite end point. Moreover, at six months the composite end point narrowed to 14.1% and 16.1% for PTCA and tPA, respectively (P = NS). Accordingly, this study was interpreted as showing that the advantage of primary angioplasty over thrombolytic was small to moderate and limited to the short term.

Weaver and colleagues[67] attempted to put this issue into perspective by analyzing 10 randomized trials from 1985 through 1996 involving 2,606 patients who were assigned to PTCA or thrombolytic therapy (4 trials using SK, 3 using standard dose tPA, and 3 using accelerated tPA administered over 90 minutes as opposed to 3–4 hours in the previous three studies). Thirty-day mortality was 4.4% for 1,290 patients treated with PTCA compared with 6.5% for 1,316 patients treated with thrombolytic therapy (34% reduction; odds ratio, 0.66; 95% CI, 0.46–0.94; P = 0.02). Results were similar among various thrombolytic regimens. There was an additional significant reduction in total stroke and hemmoraghic stroke favoring PTCA (0.7% vs 2.0%, P = 0.007 and 0.1% vs 1.0%, P < 0.001, respectively). They concluded that angioplasty appears to be superior to thrombolytic therapy for acute myocardial infarction with the proviso that PTCA success rates are as good in other institutions as those achieved in the trials reviewed. In a critique of this analysis several points were emphasized.[68] First, in trials other than GUSTO IIb the composite clinical outcome of death, reinfarction, and stroke was not defined in advance (posthoc analysis). Moreover, the benefit of PTCA was attenuated substantially at 6 months, suggesting that the foregoing meta-analysis is more of an observational nature than a prospective well-designed study. Additionally, assuming a 30-day mortality rate of 7% in the thrombolytic group, a much larger number of patients (12,700) would be needed to arrive at reasonably sound conclusions (based on a two-tailed alpha level of 0.05 with a power of 0.90). Finally, the risk of hemorrhagic stroke from the meta-analysis in question (1.1%) is higher than the 0.3% in patients receiving thrombolysis in previous trials.[6]

Conclusion

Notwithstanding the plethora of studies extolling the virtues of pharmacological and mechanical reperfusion strategies, a few truths are worthy of emphasis. Based on worldwide availability of facilities, logistics, and therapeutic opportunity, the benchmark reperfusion strategy remains thrombolytic therapy. However, given the availability of catheter laboratories, interventional expertise, and the ability to manage the short-term economic burdens of mechanical reperfusion, this therapy appears to be at least as good as and probably better than thrombolytic therapy. This is certainly the case in some institutions. Because of the universal access to thrombolytic therapy, certain clinical issues must be underscored. More important than pursuing the ideal thrombolytic agent is the need to administer thrombolytic therapy at the earliest possible juncture after the onset of symptoms heralding myocardial infarction. It is important to use those agents that the practitioner knows best. The earliest administration of *any* agent is better than the delayed administration of the *best* agent. The reperfusion rate 4 to 5 hours after the very early administration of SK, for example, approaches the 90-minute reperfusion rates achieved only after a delay of several hours observed with the best available thrombolytic agents that appear to be limited by a "reperfusion ceiling." Adjunctive therapy has been mentioned sparsely in this article; the most important universally available example of which is aspirin. Intravenous heparin also has been used universally (if not universally agreed upon) until now as an essential adjunct to thrombolytic therapy. Altering platelet activity by glycoprotein IIb/IIIa receptor blockers holds enormous promise for thrombolytic therapy and PTCA, but enjoys limited availability on a global scale. Nevertheless, it is reasonable to expect that the greatest gains, at least in the area of pharmacological reperfusion, may be obtained from therapy other than the thrombolytic agent.

References

1. ISIS-2 (Second International Study of Infarct Survival) Collaborative Group. Randomised trial of intravenous streptokinase, oral aspirin, both, or neither among 17,187 cases of suspected acute myocardial infarction: ISIS-2. Lancet 1988;II:349-360.

2. GISSI (Gruppo Italiano per lo Studio della Streptochinasi nell'Infarto miocardico). Effectiveness of intravenous thrombolytic treatment in acute myocardial infarction. Lancet 1986;I:397-401.

3. AIMS (APSAC Intervention Mortality Study) Trial Study Group. Effects of intravenous APSAC on mortality after acute myocardial infarction: Preliminary report of a placebo-controlled clinical trial. Lancet 1988;I:545-549.

4. Cannon CP, Braunwald E, McCabe CH, et al. The Thrombolysis In Myocardial Infarction (TIMI) Trials: The first decade. J Interven Cardiol 1995;8:117-135.

5. Califf RM, White HD, Van de Werf F, et al. One-year results from the Global Utilization of Streptokinase and TPA for Occluded Coronary Arteries (GUSTO-I) Investigators. Circulation 1996;94:1233-1238.

6. Fibrinolytic Therapy Trialists' (FTT) Collaborative Group. Indication for fibrinolytic therapy in suspected acute myocardial infarction: Collaborative overview of early mortality and major morbidity results from all randomised trials of more than 1000 patients. Lancet 1994;343:311-322.

7. ISIS-3 (Third International Study of Infarct Survival) Collaborative Group. ISIS-3: A randomised trail of streptokinase vs tissue plasminogen activator vs anistreplase and of aspirin plus heparin vs aspirin alone among 41, 299 cases of suspected acute myocardial infarction. Lancet 1992;339:753-770.

8. Gruppo Italiano per lo Studio della Streptochinasi nell'Infarto Miocardico (GISSI). Effectiveness of intravenous thrombolytic treatment in acute myocardial infarction. Lancet 1986;I:397-401.

9. Boersma E, Maas ACP, Deckers JW, et al. Early thrombolytic treatment in acute myocardial infarction: Reappraisal of the golden hour. Lancet 1996;348:771-775.

10. McNeill AJ, Cunningham SR, Flannery DJ, et al. A double blind placebo controlled study of early and late administration of recombinant tissue plasminogen activator in acute myocardial infarction. Br Heart J 1989;61:316-321.

11. Schofer J, Büttner J, Geng G, et al. Prehospital thrombolysis in acute myocardial infarction. Am J Cardiol 1990;66:1429-1433.

12. Barbash GI, Roth A, Hod H, et al. Improved survival but not left ventricular function with early and prehospital treatment with tissue plasminogen activator in acute myocardial infarction. Am J Cardiol 1990;66:261-266.

13. McAleer B, Ruane B, Burke E, et al. Prehospital thrombolysis in a rural community: Short-and long-term survival. Cardiovasc Drugs Ther 1992;6: 369-372.

14. The GREAT Group. Feasibility, safety, and efficacy of domiciliary thrombolysis by general practitioners: Grampian Region Early Anistreplase Trial. Br Med J 1992;305:548-553.

15. The European Myocardial Infarction Project Group. Prehospital thrombolytic therapy in patients with suspected acute myocardial infarction. N Engl J Med 1993;329:383-389.

16. Weaver WD, Cerqueira M, Hallstrom AP, et al. Prehospital-initiated vs hospital-initiated thrombolytic therapy. JAMA 1993;270:1211-1216.

17. EMERAS (Estudio Multicéntrico Estreptoquinasa Repúblicas de América del Sur) Collaborative Group. Randomised trial of late thrombolysis in patients with suspected acute myocardial infarction. Lancet 1993;342: 767-772.

18. LATE Study Group. Late Assessment of Thrombolytic Efficacy (LATE) study with alteplase 6-24 hours after onset of acute myocardial infarction. Lancet 1993;342:759-766.

19. Langer A, Goodman SG, Topol EJ, et al. Late assessment of thrombolytic efficacy (LATE) study: Prognosis in patient with non-Q wave myocardial infarction. JACC 1996;27:1327-1332.

20. DeWood MA, Stifter WF, Simpson CS, et al. Coronary arteriographic findings soon after non-Q wave myocardial infarction. N Engl J Med 1986;315:417-423.

21. The TIMI IIIA Investigators. Early effects of tissue-type plasminogen activator added to conventional therapy on the culprit lesion in patients presenting with ischemic cardiac pain at rest: Results of the Thrombolysis in Myocardial Ischemia (TIMI IIIA) trial. Circulation 1993;87:38-52.

22. Granger CB, Califf RM, Topol EJ. Thrombolytic therapy for acute myocardial infarction. A review. Drugs 1992; 44:293-325.

23. Lenderink T, Simoon ML, Van Es G-A, et al. Benefit of thrombolytic therapy is unstained throughout five years and is related to TIMI perfusion grade 3 but not grade 2 flow at discharge. Circulation 1995;92:1110-1116.

24. Ross AM, Coyne KS, Moreyra E, et al.

Extended mortality benefit of early postinfarction reperfusion. Circulation 1998;97:1549-1556.

25. Cragg DR, Friedman HZ, Bonema JD, et al. Outcome of patients excluded from thrombolytic therapy. Ann Intern Med 1991;115:173-177.

26. Karnash SL, Granger CB, White HD, et al. Treating menstruating women with thrombolytic therapy: Insights from the Global Utilization of Streptokinase and Tissue Plasminogen Activator for Occluded Coronary Arteries (GUSTO-1) Trial. JACC 1995;26:1651-1656.

27. Neches RB, Goldfarb AM. Thrombolytic therapy after cardiopulmonary resuscitation in acute myocardial infarction. Am J Cardiol 1993;71:258.

28. French JK, Williams BF, Hart HH, et al. Prospective evaluation of eligibility for thrombolytic therapy in acute myocardial infarction. Br Med J 1996;312: 1637-1641.

29. White HD, Barbash GI, Califf RM, et al. Age and outcome with contemporary thrombolytic therapy. Results from the GUSTO-I Trial. Circulation 1996;94: 1826-1833.

30. Anderson JL. Why does thrombolysis fail? Breaking through the reperfusion ceiling. Am J Cardiol 1997;80:1588-1590.

31. Ross AM. New thrombolytic agents. J Interven Cardiol 1997;10:395-399.

32. Antman EM. TIMI 14: Abciximab plus thrombolytic therapy. Presented at the George Washington University 13th International Workshop: Thrombolysis and Interventional Therapy in Acute Myocardial Infarction. Orlando, FL, November 1997.

33. Ohman EM. GUSTO-IV pilot. Presented at the Myocardial Reperfusion XI: Concepts and Controversies (Cleveland Clinic Foundation). Atlanta, GA, March 1998.

34. Smalling RW, Bode C, Kalbfleisch J, et al. More rapid, complete, and stable coronary thrombolysis with bolus administration of reteplase compared with alteplase infusion in acute myocardial infarction. Circulation 1995;91: 2725-2732.

35. International Joint Efficacy Comparison of Thrombolytics. Randomised, double-blind comparison of reteplase double-bolus administration with streptokinase in acute myocardial infarction (INJECT): Trial to investigate equivalence. Lancet 1995;346:329-336.

36. Bode C, Smalling RW, Berg G, et al. Randomized comparison of coronary thrombolysis achieved with double-bolus reteplase (recombinant plasminogen activator) and front-loaded, accelerated alteplase (recombinant tissue plasminogen activator) in patients with acute myocardial infarction. Circulation 1996;94:891-898.

37. The Global Use of Strategies to Open Occluded Coronary Arteries (GUSTO III) Investigators. A comparison of reteplase with alteplase for acute myocardial infarction. N Engl J Med 1997; 337:1118-1123.

38. Larsen GR, Timony GA, Horgan PG, et al. Protein engineering of novel plasminogen activators with increased thrombolytic potency in rabbits relative to activase. J Biol Chem 1991;266: 8156-8161.

39. Chew P. Presented at the 1996 AHA National Meeting. Personal communication.

40. Benedict CR, Refino CJ, Keyt BA, et al. New variant of human tissue plasminogen activator (TPA) with enhanced efficacy and lower incidence of bleeding compared with recombinant human TPA. Circulation 1995;92:3032-3040.

41. Cannon CP, McCabe CH, Gibson M, et al. TNK-tissue plasminogen activator in acute myocardial infarction. Results of the Thrombolysis in Myocardial Infarction (TIMI) 10A Dose-Ranging trial. Circulation 1997;95:351-356.

42. Cannon CP, McCabe CH. TNK-tissue plasminogen activator compared with front-loaded tissue plasminogen activator in acute myocardial infarction: Primary results of the TIMI 10B trial. (abstract) Circulation 1997;96(Suppl I): I-206.

43. White HD, Van de Werf FJJ. Thrombolysis for acute myocardial infarction. Circulation 1998;97:1632-1646.

44. Collen D, De Cock F, Demarsin E, et al. Recombinant staphylokinase variants with altered immunoreactivity. III: Species variability of antibody binding patterns. Circulation 1997;95:455-462.

45. Collen D, Stockx L, Lacroix H, et al. Recombinant staphylokinase variants with altered immunoreactivity. IV: Identification of variants with reduced antibody induction but intact potency. Circulation 1997;95:463-472.

46. Vanderschueren S, Barrios L, Kerdsinchai P, et al. A randomized trial of recombinant staphylokinase versus

alteplase for coronary artery patency in acute myocardial infarction. Circulation 1995;92:2044-2049.

47. Vanderschueren S, Dens J, Kerdsinchai P, et al. Randomized coronary patency trial of double-bolus recombinant staphylokinase versus front-loaded alteplase in acute myocardial infarction. Am Heart J 1997;134:213-219.

48. Vanderschueren S, Stockx L, Wilms G, et al. Thrombolytic therapy of peripheral arterial occlusion with recombinant staphylokinase. Circulation 1995; 92:2050-2057.

49. Tebbe U, Michels R, Adgey J, et al. Randomized, double-blind study comparing saruplase with streptokinase therapy in acute myocardial infarction: The COMPASS Equivalence Trial. JACC 1998;31:487-493.

50. Kawai C, Yui Y, Hosoda S, et al. A prospective, randomized, double-blind multicenter trial of a single bolus injection of the novel modified t-PA E6010 in the treatment of acute myocardial infarction: Comparison with native t-PA. JACC 1997;29:1477-1453.

51. White HD, Aylward PE, Frey MJ, et al. Randomized, double-blind comparison of hirulog versus heparin in patients receiving streptokinase and aspirin for acute myocardial infarction (HERO). Circulation 1997;96:2155-2161.

52. Topol EJ, Califf RM, George BS, et al. A randomized trail of immediate versus delayed elective angioplasty after intravenous tissue plasminogen activator in acute myocardial infarction. N Engl J Med 1987;317:581-588.

53. TIMI Study Group. Comparison of invasive and conservative strategies after treatment with intravenous tissue plasminogen activator in acute myocardial infarction: Results of the Thrombolysis in Myocardial Infarction (TIMI) Phase II Trial. N Engl J Med 1989;320:618-627.

54. Arnold AER, Serruys PW, Rutsch W, et al. For the European Cooperative Study Group for rtPA. Reasons for no additional benefit of angioplasty immediately after recombinant tissue plasminogen activator for acute myocardial infarction: A regional wall motion analysis. JACC 1991;17:11-21.

55. SWIFT Trial Study Group. SWIFT trial of delayed elective intervention versus conservative treatment after thrombolytic therapy for acute myocardial infarction. Br Med J 1991;302:555-560.

56. O'Neill WW, Weintraub R, Grines CL, et al. A prospective, placebo-controlled, randomized trial of intravenous streptokinase and angioplasty versus lone angioplasty therapy of acute myocardial infarction. Circulation 1992;86:1710-1717.

57. Ross AM. The Plasminogen Activator-Angioplasty Compatibility Trial (PACT). Presented at the George Washington University 13th International Workshop: Thrombolysis and Interventional Therapy in Acute Myocardial Infarction. Orlando, FL, November 1997.

58. O'Neill W, Timmis GC, Bourdillon PD, et al. A prospective randomized clinical trial of intracoronary streptokinase versus coronary angioplasty for acute myocardial infarction. N Engl J Med 1986; 314:812-818.

59. Grines CL, Browne KF, Marco J, et al. A comparison of immediate angioplasty with thrombolytic therapy for acute myocardial infarction. N Engl J Med 1993; 328:673-679.

60. Parisi AF, Folland ED, Hartigan P. A comparison of angioplasty with medical therapy in the treatment of single-vessel coronary artery disease. N Engl J Med 1992;326:10-16.

61. Gibbons RJ, Holmes DR, Reeder GS, et al. Immediate angioplasty compared with the administration of a thrombolytic agent followed by conservative treatment for myocardial infarction. N Engl J Med 1993;328:685-691.

62. Zijlstra F, De Boer MJ, Hoorntje JCA, et al. A comparison of immediate coronary angioplasty with intravenous streptokinase in acute myocardial infarction. N Engl J Med 1993;328:680-684.

63. Zijlstra F, Beukema WP, van't Hof AWJ, et al. Randomized comparison of primary coronary angioplasty with thrombolytic therapy in low risk patients with acute myocardial infarction. JACC 1997;29:908-912.

64. De Boer MJ, Hoorntje JCA, Ottervanger JP, et al. Immediate coronary angioplasty versus intravenous streptokinase in acute myocardial infarction: Left ventricular ejection fraction, hospital mortality and reinfarction. JACC 1994;23: 1004-1008.

65. Every NR, Parsons LS, Hlatky M, et al. A comparison of thrombolytic therapy

with primary coronary angioplasty for acute myocardial infarction. N Engl J Med 1996;335:1253-1260.

66. The Global Use of Strategies to Open Occluded Coronary Arteries in Acute Coronary Syndromes (GUSTO IIb) Angioplasty Substudy Investigators. A clinical trial comparing primary coronary angioplasty with tissue plasminogen activator for acute myocardial infarction. N Engl J Med 1997;336:1621-1628.

67. Weaver WD, Simes J, Betriu A, et al. Comparison of primary coronary angioplasty and intravenous thrombolytic therapy for acute myocardial infarction. A quantitative review. JAMA 1997;278:2093-2098.

68. Yusuf S. Primary angioplasty compared with thrombolytic therapy for acute myocardial infarction. (Editorial). JAMA 1997;278:2110-2111.